American Hospital Association Hospital Statistics

1991-92 Edition

Data compiled from the
American Hospital Association
1990 Annual Survey of Hospitals

AHA American Hospital Association
840 North Lake Shore Drive
Chicago, Illinois 60611-2431

AHA members $50.00
Nonmembers $125.00
AHA product no. H01-082091
Telephone orders 1-800-AHA-2626

ISSN 0090-6662
ISBN 0-87258-606-5

840 North Lake Shore Drive
Chicago, Illinois 60611-2431

Printed in the U.S.A.

Contents

Contents continued on following page.

Acknowledgements

The *American Hospital Association Hospital Statistics* is published annually by the American Hospital Association, Richard J. Davidson, President.

Division of Data Services

Deborah L. Frett, General Manager
Alisa A. Kurakazu, Secretary

Randall L. Heiser, Manager of Client Services
Limmie Batchelor, Secretary
Margie Berry, Service Assistant
Lachelle Curry, Service Analyst
Marcia R. Foley, Senior Service Consultant
George J. Krueger, III, Service Consultant
Brenda Maass, Senior Service Consultant
Colin K. McKenzie, Senior Service Consultant
Mary Scanlon, Service Representative
Sharon A. Zinkula, Technical Writer

Karen M. McGannon, Product Manager
Jo Ann Adad, Secretary
Mary T. Krzywicki, Production Specialist
Sandra Sloan, Assistant Product Manager
Jeanette Spears, Data Verifier
Michelle R. Tribue, Production Clerk
Julie A. Utroska, Assistant Product Manager

Jane M. B. Olson, Product Manager
Cheryl Allen, Administrative Assistant
Cynthia Jackson, Secretary
Diane Costa Rote, Production Specialist
Pamela L. Sutton, Data Verifier
Christine M. Wack, Assistant Product Manager

Health System Information and Evaluation

Joseph R. Martin, Senior Director

Health Data Base Services

Robert Bergmann, Associate Director
Lloyd R. Wackerling, Project Manager
Robert L. Davis, Programmer/Analyst II
Ollie Williams, Project Specialist

Hospital Data Center

Peter D. Kralovec, Director

Annual Survey Department

Elaine R. Singh, Manager
Michael J. Jankowiak, Project Director
Steve Reczynski, Project Director
Gary Vacha, Senior Programmer
Clisby Jackson, Research Assistant
Angeline Choate, Data Analyst
Allen Griffin, Data Analyst
Dorian McCraney, Data Analyst
Terrie A. Micelli, Data Analyst
Stephanie Moore, Data Analyst
Donna M. Moran, Data Analyst
Doris D. Valdez, Data Analyst
Dinah Woods, Data Analyst

Division of Marketing Services

Henrie Moise, Manager, Marketing and Promotions
Wendy Zimberoff, Graphic Designer

Division of Strategic Planning & Marketing

Deborah Reczynski, Senior Staff Specialist

Printing Services Group

Ron Stamp, Director
Vito Benigno, Manager
Gary Rothmund, Production Planner

Typesetting provided by:

Graphic Image Corporation
300 West Grand Avenue
Chicago, IL 60610

Printing provided by:

IPC Publishing Services
501 Colonial Drive
St. Joseph, MI 49085

FOR FURTHER INFORMATION

For questions and general information please contact Client Services, Division of Data Services at 800/621-8096.

The data published here should be used with the following advisements: The data are based on replies to an annual survey that seeks a variety of information, not all of which is published in this book. The information gathered by the survey includes specific services, but not all of each hospital's services. Therefore, the data do not reflect an exhaustive list of all services offered by all hospitals. For information on the availability of additional data, please contact the American Hospital Association's Data Services Division, 800/621-8096.

The American Hospital Association does not assume responsibility for the accuracy of information voluntarily reported by the individual institutions surveyed. The purpose of this publication is to provide basic data reflecting the delivery of health care in the United States and associated areas, and is not to serve as an official and all-inclusive list of services offered by individual hospitals.

How To Use *AHA Hospital Statistics*

Introduction

This introduction is designed to help you use and interpret the wealth of data included in *AHA Hospital Statistics*. The aggregate data published are an ideal resource for comparative and trending analyses. However, the economic climate, demographic characteristics, personnel issues, and local health care financing and payment policies differ by region, state, and city across the country. *Differences in these factors must be taken into account when using the data.* In addition, the profile of hospitals across comparison groups vary. For example, states will differ in terms of the number and percentage of hospitals by size, ownership, services provided, teaching hospital status, types of patients treated and so forth. *Differences in these variables must also be taken into consideration when doing a comparative analysis.*

This section includes highlights of the 1991-92 edition and a description of each table. Following are the Definitions of Terms and Technical Notes.

Hospital Trends

Hospital Trends provides both narrative and visual highlights of key issues and trends facing hospitals. It covers a range of subjects including financial, utilization, hospital facilities and services, medical technologies, and personnel. Hospital Trends begins on page xxxiii.

Tables

AHA Hospital Statistics is composed of 25 statistical tables based on data from the American Hospital Association 1990 Annual Survey of Hospitals. Tables begin on page 1.

Data for each table are predominantly based on all AHA-registered hospitals in the United States and U.S.-associated areas and AHA-registered community hospitals in the United States.

An institution may be **registered by the AHA** as a hospital if it is accredited as a hospital by the Joint Commission on Accreditation of Healthcare Organizations or is certified as a provider of acute services under Title 18 of the Social Security Act and has provided the AHA with documents verifying the accreditation or certification.

Community hospitals are nonfederal short-term general and other special hospitals, excluding hospital units of institutions, whose facilities and services are available to the public.

The statistical tables present a profile of financial, utilization, personnel, and hospital facilities and services of U.S. hospitals.

Financial data refers to expenses such as payroll, employee benefits, and total expenses.

Utilization data refers to hospital usage patterns, such as the number of beds, admissions, average daily census, and occupancy percent.

Personnel data refers to full-time equivalent (FTE) personnel and trainees, such as the number of physicians and dentists, registered nurses, and other salaried personnel.

Hospital facilities and services data refers to the number of facilities, services, and inpatient service areas provided in hospitals, such as acquired immune-deficiency syndrome (AIDS), cardiac, geriatric services, and more.

Data are organized by geographical areas, bed-size categories, type of organizational control, type of service provided, and length of stay.

Geographical areas include the 9 U.S. census regions, metropolitan statistical areas (MSAs), U.S. states and U.S. associated areas, and the 100 largest U.S. cities.

Bed-size categories include: 6-24 beds, 25-49 beds, 50-99 beds, 100-199 beds, 200-299 beds, 300-399 beds, 400-499 beds, and 500 or more beds.

Control refers to who owns and operates a hospital. Types of controls include government, nonfederal; nongovernment, not-for-profit; investor-owned (for-profit); and government, federal.

Service refers to the type of primary care provided to the majority of admissions. Types of services include general medical and surgical; psychiatric; tuberculosis and other respiratory diseases; and other specialty services.

Length of stay refers to short-term or long-term hospitals. Short-term hospitals are those where the average length of stay is less than 30 days. Long-term hospitals are those where the average length of stay is 30 days or more.

For more definitions, please refer to Definitions of Terms beginning on page xxiii.

For information regarding the data collection process of the AHA Annual Survey of Hospitals, please refer to Technical Notes beginning on page xxxi.

New Features

This edition features 30 new hospital facilities and services in Table 12A and Table 12B. Some of these include:

AIDS services including general inpatient care for AIDS/ARC, AIDS/ARC unit, and specialized outpatient program for AIDS/ARC.

Geriatric services including comprehensive geriatric assessment, geratic acute care unit, adult day care program, senior membership, Alzheimer's diagnostic/assessment services, emergency response (geriatric), respite care, and geriatric clinic.

Cardiac services including angioplasty, cardiac catheterization laboratory, cardiac rehabilitation program, non-invasive cardiac assessment services, and open-heart surgery.

For a comprehensive listing of the hospital facilities and services included, please refer to page 206.

What's in the Tables

Table 1 — Trends in Utilization, Personnel, and Finances for Selected Years from 1946 through 1990

Table 1 classifies hospitals by *control* and *service.* Control refers to who owns and operates a hospital. Service refers to the type of primary care provided to the majority of patients.

Types of controls include:

* Government, nonfederal
* Nongovernment, not-for-profit
* Investor-owned (for-profit)
* Government, federal

Types on services include:

* General medical and surgical
* Psychiatric
* Tuberculosis and other respiratory diseases
* Other specialty services

Table 1 contains utilization, personnel and financial data for all U.S. AHA-registered hospitals for selected years from 1946 through 1990.

Utilization data includes the following:

* Number of hospitals
* Number of beds
* Number of admissions
* Average daily census
* Adjusted average daily census
* Occupancy percent
* Average length of stay in days
* Number of outpatient visits
* Newborns (bassinets, births)

Personnel data includes the total number of FTE personnel and FTE personnel per 100 adjusted census.

Financial data covers hospital expenses. The major categories are labor and total.

Labor includes:

* Payroll
* Employee benefits
* Adjusted labor expenses per inpatient day

Total includes:

* Total expenses
* Adjusted total expenses per admission
* Adjusted total expenses per inpatient day

Table 2A Utilization, Personnel, and Finances in Short-Term Hospitals

Table 2A describes *short-term hospitals* those where the average length of stay is less than 30 days, classified as follows:

* General
* Psychiatric
* TB and other respiratory diseases
* All other

These classifications are then further divided by bed-size category and control.

Table 2A contains utilization, personnel, and financial data for short-term hospitals.

Utilization data includes the following:

* Number of hospitals
* Number of beds
* Number of admissions
* Occupancy percent
* Average daily census
* Adjusted average daily census
* Average length of stay in days
* Number of surgical operations
* Number of outpatient visits
* Newborns (bassinets, births)

Personnel data includes total number of FTE personnel.

Financial data includes the following:

* Payroll (labor)
* Employee benefits (labor)
* Total expenses (labor)
* Total expenses (labor and nonlabor)

Table 2B Utilization, Personnel, and Finances in Long-Term Hospitals

Table 2B has the same structure as Table 2A, but is based on *long-term hospitals.* Long-term hospitals are those where the average length of stay is 30 days or more. Please refer to Table 2A for a more detailed explanation.

Table 3 Utilization, Personnel Per Census, and Finances Per Inpatient Day

Table 3 divides hospitals by:

* Total United States by bed-size category
* Federal by service
* Nonfederal by service, control, and bed-size category

Table 3 contains utilization, personnel, and financial data for all U.S. AHA-registered hospitals.

Utilization data includes the following:

* Number of hospitals
* Number of beds
* Number of admissions
* Occupancy percent
* Average daily census
* Adjusted average daily census
* Average length of stay in days
* Surgical operations
* Newborns (bassinets, births, and days)
* Outpatient visits (emergency, other, total)

Personnel data show how many employees a certain type of hospital has for every 100 patients, with separate figures provided for:

* FTE personnel
* Registered nurses only
* Licensed practical nurses

Financial data covers hospital expenses. The three expense categories are labor, other, and total. Labor includes:

* Payroll
* Employee benefits
* Total (includes adjusted total *labor* expenses per admission and per inpatient day.)

Total Expenses includes:

* Adjusted total expenses per admission
* Adjusted total expenses per inpatient day

Table 4A Utilization of Hospital Units and Nursing-Home-Type Units Operated by Hospitals

Table 4A divides hospitals by:

* Total United States by bed-size category
* Federal by service
* Nonfederal by service, control, and bed-size category

Table 4A contains utilization data on hospital units and nursing-home-type units for all U.S. AHA-registered hospitals.

A nursing-home-type unit is a separate hospital-managed unit offering primarily only the following types of service to the majority of its patients:

* Skilled nursing
* Intermediate care
* Personal care
* Sheltered/residential care

The three major categories are total facilities, hospital units and nursing-home-type units.

Subcategories include:

* Number of facilities
* Number of beds
* Number of admissions
* Number of inpatient days

Table 4B Utilization of Hospital Units and Nursing-Home-Type Units Operated by Community Hospitals, by State

Table 4B divides community hospitals by:

* Total United States by bed-size category
* U.S. Census Division by state within that division

Table 4B contains utilization data on hospital units and nursing-home-type units for AHA-registered community hospitals.

The three major categories are total facilities, hospital units and nursing-home-type.

Subcategories include:

* Number of facilities
* Number of beds
* Number of admissions
* Number of inpatient days

Table 4C Personnel and Finances in Hospital Units and Nursing-Home-Type Units Operated by Hospitals

Table 4C divides hospitals by:

* Total United States by bed-size category
* Federal by service
* Nonfederal by services, control, and bed-size category

Table 4C contains personnel and financial data on hospital units and nursing-home-type units for U.S. AHA-registered hospitals.

The three major categories are total facilities, hospital units and nursing-home-type units.

Subcategories include:

* Number of facilities
* Number of FTEs
* Payroll expenses
* Total expenses

Table 4D Personnel and Finances in Hospital Units and Nursing-Home-Type Units Operated by Community Hospitals, by State

Table 4D divides community hospitals by:

* Total United States, by bed-size category
* U.S. Census Division by state, within division

Table 4D contains personnel and financial data on hospital units and nursing-home-type units for U.S. AHA-registered community hospitals.

The three major categories are total facilities, hospital units and nursing-home-type units.

Subcategories include:

* Number of facilities
* Number of FTEs
* Payroll expenses
* Total expenses

Table 5A Utilization, Personnel, and Finances in U.S. AHA-Registered Hospitals

Table 5A divides hospitals by:

* Total United States by bed-size category
* Federal by service
* Nonfederal by services, control and bed-size category

Table 5A contains utilization, personnel, and financial data for all U.S. AHA-registered hospitals.

Utilization data includes the following:

* Number of hospitals
* Number of beds
* Number of admissions
* Number of inpatient days
* Adjusted patient days
* Occupancy percent
* Average daily census
* Adjusted average daily census
* Average length of stay in days
* Surgical operations
* Outpatient visits (emergency, other, total)
* Newborns (bassinets, births)

Personnel data divides hospital employees by two categories: full-time equivalent personnel, and full-time equivalent trainees. The term "full-time equivalent" indicates that the data listed for these categories take into account both full and part-time employees. Categories for full-time equivalent personnel include the following:

* Physicians and dentists
* Registered nurses
* Licensed practical nurses
* Other salaried personnel
* Total personnel

Trainees are divided into the following categories:

* Medical and dental residents
* Other trainees
* Total trainees

Expenses are divided into labor and total labor categories as follows:

* Payroll
* Employee benefits
* Total (in thousands of dollars and as a percentage of overall expenses)

For community hospitals, the total expense categories also include statistics for adjusted total expenses per admission and per inpatient day.

Table 5B Utilization, Personnel, and Finances in Census Divisions

Table 5B divides hospitals by U.S. census division within:

* Bed-size category
* Service
* Federal by service
* Nonfederal by service, control, and bed-size category

The U.S. census divisions are:

* U.S. Census Division 1 - New England
* U.S. Census Division 2 - Middle Atlantic
* U.S. Census Division 3 - South Atlantic
* U.S. Census Division 4 - East North Central
* U.S. Census Division 5 - East South Central
* U.S. Census Division 6 - West North Central
* U.S. Census Division 7 - West South Central
* U.S. Census Division 8 - Mountain
* U.S. Census Division 9 - Pacific

Table 5B contains utilization, personnel, and financial data for all U.S. AHA-registered hospitals. Please refer to the description of the utilization, personnel, and financial data items included in Table 5A.

Table 5C Utilization, Personnel, and Finances in States

Table 5C divides hospitals by state within:

* Bed-size category
* Service
* Federal by service
* Nonfederal by service, control, and bed-size category

Table 5C contains utilization, personnel, and financial data for all U.S. AHA-registered hospitals. Please refer to the description of the utilization, personnel, and financial data items included in Table 5A.

Table
5D
Utilization, Personnel, and Finances in U.S. Associated Areas

Table 5D divides hospitals by the U.S. associated areas (except Puerto Rico) within:

* Bed-size category
* Service
* Federal by service
* Nonfederal by service, control and bed-size category

The U.S. associated areas included are:

* American Samoa
* Guam
* Marshall Islands
* Virgin Islands

Table 5D contains utilization, personnel, and financial data for all AHA-registered hospitals in those U.S.-associated areas. Please refer to the description of the utilization, personnel, and financial data items included in Table 5A.

Table
5E
Utilization, Personnel, and Finances in Puerto Rico

Table 5E divides hospitals in Puerto Rico by:

* Bed-size category
* Service
* Federal by service
* Nonfederal by service, control, and bed-size category

Table 5E contains utilization, personnel, and financial data for all AHA-registered hospitals in Puerto Rico. Please refer to the description of the utilization, personnel, and financial data items included in Table 5A.

Table
6
Utilization, Personnel, and Finances in Community Hospitals, by Metropolitan Statistical Area

Table 6 divides community hospitals by:

* U.S. census divisions
* State
* Metropolitan statistical areas (MSAs)

A metropolitan statistical area (MSA) is defined as a city or urbanized area of at least 50,000 population, with a total metropolitan area of at least 100,000. For a more detailed definition, please refer to page 147.

Table 6 contains utilization, personnel, and financial data for all U.S. AHA-registered community hospitals. Please refer to the description of the utilization, personnel, and financial data items included in Table 5A.

Table 7
Utilization, Personnel, and Finances in Community Hospitals, for the 100 Largest Central Cities

Table 7 divides hospitals by the 100 largest U.S. central cities based on the 1980 U.S. census data.

Table 7 contains utilization, personnel, and financial data for all AHA-registered community hospitals. Please refer to the description of the utilization, personnel, and financial data items included in Table 5A.

Table 8
Utilization, Personnel, and Finances in Community Hospitals Affiliated with Medical Schools

Table 8 divides hospitals by the total United States *and* for each U.S. census division. Each is further divided as follows:

* Nongovernment
* State and local government

Each of these subcategories is then further divided by the following bed-size categories:

* less than 300 beds
* 300-399
* 400-499
* 500 or more

Table 8 contains utilization, personnel, and financial data for all AHA-registered community hospitals. Please refer to the description of the utilization, personnel, and financial data items included in Table 5A.

Table 9
Utilization, Personnel Per Census, and Finances Per Inpatient Day in Accredited Hospitals

Table 9 presents data only for hospitals accredited by the Joint Commission on Accreditation of Healthcare Organizations (JCAHO). These accredited hospitals are divided by:

* Total United States by bed-size category
* Federal by service
* Nonfederal by service, control, and bed-size category

Table 9 contains utilization, personnel, and financial data for all AHA-registered hospitals who are accredited by JCAHO. Please refer to the description of the utilization, personnel, and financial data items included in Table 3.

Table 10A AHA Membership, Approval, and Affiliation Status in the United States

Table 10A divides hospitals by:

* Total United States by bed-size category
* Federal by service
* Nonfederal by service, control, and bed-size category

Table 10A contains AHA membership, approval, and affiliation status information as of January 1991. Categories for AHA member hospitals include the number of hospitals, beds, and admissions.

Approval and affiliation status categories are as follows:

* Accreditation (A-1)
* Cancer program (A-2)
* Residency (A-3)
* Medical School Affiliation (A-5)
* Professional nursing school (A-6)
* Council of teaching hospitals (A-8)
* Blue Cross participation (A-9)
* Medicare certification (A-10)

Table 10B AHA Membership, Approval, and Affiliation Status in States

Table 10B divides hospitals by state and U.S.-associated area.

Table 10B contains AHA membership, approval, and affiliation status information. Please refer to the description of this information in Table 10A.

Table 11 Revenue in Community Hospitals

Table 11 divides hospitals by:

* Total United States by bed-size category
* U.S. Census Division by state within division

Table 11 is two tables in one. The first part presents revenue data for all U.S. AHA-registered community hospitals. The second part presents revenue data for all AHA-registered nongovernment not-for-profit hospitals only, a subcategory of community hospitals.

Gross patient revenue data includes percent of total for inpatient gross revenue and percent of total for outpatient gross revenue.

There are also breakdowns for net patient revenue (gross patient revenue less deductions for contractual adjustments, bad debts, charity, and so forth), and net total revenue, which consists of net patient revenue plus all other revenue (contributions, endowment revenue, government grants, and all other payments not made on behalf of individual patients).

Consistent with recent developments in hospital financial reporting practices which recognize the limitations of gross patient revenue as a meaningful financial indicator, this edition of *AHA Hospital Statistics* now only presents percentages of gross inpatient and outpatient revenue to total gross patient revenue. Net patient revenue which reflects the actual dollars received for patient care and net total revenue which reflects the actual dollars received from both patient and nonpatient revenue sources continue to be presented because of their general utility.

Table

12A

Facilities and Services in the United States

Table 12A divides hospitals by:

* Total United States by bed-size category
* Federal by service
* Nonfederal by service, control and bed-size category

This table provides two kinds of data for each of the 70 facilities and services. It first lists how many hospitals within each classification report providing a particular facility or service. It then provides this same number as a percentage of the total number of hospitals reporting.

For a comprehensive listing of all of the facilities and services, please turn to page 206.

Table

12B

Facilities and Services in U.S. Census Divisions and States

Table 12B divides hospitals by:

* Total United States
* U.S. Census Division by state within division

This table provides two kinds of data for each of the 70 facilities and services. It first lists how many hospitals within each classification report providing a particular facility or service. It then provides this same number as a percentage of the total number of hospitals reporting.

For a comprehensive listing of all of the facilities and services, please turn to page 206.

Table

13A

Hospitals, Units, and Beds, by Inpatient Service Area in the United States

Table 13A divides hospitals by:

* Total United States by bed-size category
* Federal by service
* Nonfederal by service, control, and bed-size category

This table provides data for the number of hospitals and number of beds for inpatient service areas. They are the following:

* General medical and surgical
  (divided into adult and pediatric subcategories)
* Obstetrics
* Burn care
* Neonatal intermediate care
* Intensive care
  (divided into neonatal, pediatric, cardiac, and mixed or other intensive care subcategories)
* Long-term care unit
  (divided into skilled nursing and other subcategories)
* Psychiatric
* Mental retardation
* Alcoholism/chemical dependency
* Rehabilitation
* Other

For definitions, please refer to Definitions of Terms beginning on page xxiii.

Table
13B Hospitals, Units, and Beds, by Inpatient Service Area in U.S. Census Divisions and States

Table 13B divides hospitals by:

* Total United States
* U.S. Census Divisions by state within division

This table provides data for the number of hospitals and number of beds for inpatient service areas. They are the following:

* General medical and surgical
  (divided into adult and pediatric subcategories)
* Obstetrics
* Burn care
* Neonatal intermediate care
* Intensive care
  (divided into neonatal, pediatric, cardiac, and mixed or other intensive care subcategories)
* Long-term care unit
  (divided into skilled nursing and other subcategories)
* Psychiatric
* Mental retardation
* Alcoholism/chemical dependency
* Rehabilitation
* Other

For definitions, please refer to Definitions of Terms beginning on page xxiii.

Table
14 Utilization, Personnel, and Finances in U.S. AHA-Nonregistered Hospitals

Table 14 has the same structure as Table 5A, but is based on AHA-nonregistered hospitals. Please refer to Table 5A for a more detailed explanation.

DATA COMPARABILITY

Questions may arise about the comparability of data from different tables, that is, if the same hospitals are represented when two or more tables are being used. The most reliable method of determining whether identical groups of hospitals are being dealt with is to compare the number of hospitals. In most tables, the number of hospitals is given in the first column. If the numbers and characteristics of the hospitals are identical, then the data are comparable.

Please note: The economic climate, demographic characteristics, personnel issues, and health care financing and payment policies differ by region, state, and city across the country. *Differences in these factors must be taken into account when using the data.* In addition, the profile of hospitals across comparison groups vary. For example, states will differ in terms of the number and percentage of hospitals by size, ownership, services provided, teaching hospital status, types of patients treated and so forth. *Differences in these variables must also be taken into consideration when doing a comparative analysis.*

CHARACTERISTICS OF TABLES

The chart entitled "Contents of Tables" on page xx presents a capsule guide to the statistical tables. The first two left-hand columns indicate the table number and give a general description of the data contained in the table. The next three columns indicate whether estimates for nonreporting hospitals have been included, whether the data are for AHA-registered hospitals only, and whether data for community hospitals are included. The remaining columns fall into three broad categories. For each table, these columns indicate the hospital characteristics that the table features, the types of data it presents, and the geographic breakdowns it provides.

The chart directs users to the tables that include the desired information. For example, a user may be interested in financial data for psychiatric hospitals in Indiana. The chart indicates that state data are to be found in tables 4B, 4D, 5C, 6, 10B, 11, 12B and 13B. However, tables 6 and 11 contain data for community hospitals only and, therefore, do not contain data for psychiatric hospitals. Tables 4B, 10B, 12B, and 13B do not present financial data. However, the chart indicates that table 5C presents financial data classified by state and by the type of service the hospital provides. Thus, table 5C is the proper one to consult for financial data on psychiatric hospitals in Indiana.

CONTENTS OF TABLES

Table		Description	Estimated Data for Nonreporters	Data for AHA-Registered Hospitals Only	Community Hospital Data	Control	Service	Detailed Service	Short-term vs. Long-term data	Bed Size	Utilization	Finances	Personnel	Approvals	Facilities and Services	AHA Membership	Total U.S.	U.S. Census Division	State	MSA	City	U.S. Associated Areas
			Hospital Characteristics							Data Characteristics							Geographic Characteristics					
1		Historical trends	●	●	●	●	●				●	●	●				●					
2	A	Short-term hospitals	●	●		●	●		●	●	●	●	●				●					
	B	Long-term hospitals	●	●		●	●		●	●	●	●	●				●					
3		Federal by service/nonfederal by service and control	●	●	●	●	●			●	●	●	●				●					
4	A	Hospital utilization	●	●	●	●	●		●	●	●	●					●					
	B	Community hospital utilization (Total facility, hospital units, and NHT[d] unit data)	●	●	b				●	●	●						●	●	●			
	C	Hospital personnel and finances (Total facility, hospital units, and NHT[d] unit data)	●	●	●	●	●		●	●		●	●				●					
	D	Community hospital personnel and finances (Total facility, hospital units, and NHT[d] unit data)	●	●	b				●	●		●	●				●	●	●			
5	A	U.S. AHA-registered hospitals (Detailed service and community hospital data)	●	●	●	●	●	●		●	●	●	●				●					
	B	U.S. census division (Detailed service and community hospital data)	●	●	●	●	●	●		●	●	●	●					●				
	C	State (Detailed service and community hospital data)	●	●	●	●	●	●		●	●	●	●						●			
	D	U.S. associated areas (Detailed service and community hospital data)	●	●	●	●	●	●		●	●	●	●									●
	E	Puerto Rico (Detailed service and community hospital data)	●	●	●	●	●	●		●	●	●	●									c
6		Metro-nonmetro (community hospitals)	●	●	b				b		●	●	●				●	●	●	●		
7		Largest U.S. central cities (community hospitals)	●	●	b				b		●	●	●								●	
8		Medical school affiliation (community hospitals)	●	●	b	●			b	●	●	●	●				●	●				
9		Accredited hospitals	●	●	●	●	●			●	●	●	●				●					
10	A	Membership and approvals by control, service, and size		●	●	●	●			●				●		●	●					
	B	Membership and approvals by state		●										●		●	●		●			●
11		Revenue (community hospitals)	●	●	b				b	●		●					●	●	●			
12	A	Facilities and services by control, service, and size		●	●	●	●			●					●		●					
	B	Facilities and services by state		●											●		●	●	●			
13	A	Hospitals, units, and beds, by inpatient service area		●	●	●	●			●						●	●					
	B	Hospitals, units, and beds, by inpatient service area		●												●	●	●	●			
14		Nonregistered U.S. hospitals	●	a	●	●	●	●		●	●	●	●		●							

[a]Table contains data for nonregistered hospitals only.
[b]Table contains data for community hospitals only.
[c]Table contains data for Puerto Rico hospitals only.
[d]NHT = nursing-home-type.

TABLE 5C (Continued)/INDIANA

CLASSIFICATION	HOSPITALS	BEDS
INDIANA	**135**	**26,501**
6-24 beds	2	37
25-49	16	635
50-99	39	2,701
100-199	33	4,327
200-299	15	3,885
300-399	9	3,241
400-499	10	4,416
500 or more	11	7,259
Psychiatric	17	3,834
Hospitals	17	3,834
Institutions for mentally retarded	0	0
General	114	22,244
Hospitals	113	22,227
Hospital units of institutions	1	17
TB and other respiratory diseases	0	0
Obstetrics and gynecology	1	144
Eye, ear, nose, and throat	0	0
Rehabilitation	1	60
Orthopedic	0	0
Chronic disease	1	159
All other	1	60
Federal	4	1,205
Psychiatric	1	580
General and other special	3	625
Nonfederal	131	25,296
Psychiatric	16	3,254
Hospitals	16	3,254
Institutions for mentally retarded	0	0
TB and other respiratory diseases	0	0
Long-term general and other special	1	159
Short-term general and other special	114	21,883
Hospital units of institutions	1	17
Community Hospitals*	113	21,866
6-24 beds	0	0
25-49	14	552
50-99	32	2,155
100-199	29	3,707
200-299	15	3,885
300-399	8	2,851
400-499	6	2,577
500 or more	9	6,139
Nongovernment not-for-profit	56	14,944
Investor-owned (for-profit)	7	960
State and local government	50	5,962

*For information on community hospitals that excludes nursing-home-type data, refer to Hospital Units columns in tables 4A through 4D.

TABLE FORMATS

Table 5 was selected to illustrate how to read the tables because it is the most useful for general purposes. It includes detailed community hospital data for the total United States (5A), for each U.S. census division (5B), and for each state (5C). To the left, column 1 of table 5C for Indiana is reproduced. Note that the data have been broken down into three subsections: bed size, service, and Federal vs. Nonfederal. Nonfederal hospitals are also divided by service, and within community hospitals there is a further subdivision by bed size. The number of hospitals in each subsection adds up to the total number for the state of Indiana, and each subsection thus represents a complete set of data for Indiana hospitals. Note that an indentation within a subsection represents the subtotal of the line preceding the indentation. For example, in the second subsection, the line *Psychiatric* is further broken down into psychiatric hospitals proper and institutions for the mentally retarded. In the third subsection, *Community hospitals* is broken down by bed size and by control.

ISSUES OF *AHA GUIDE AND AHA HOSPITAL STATISTICS*

From 1946 through 1971, data from the AHA Annual Survey of Hospitals were published as part two of the August 1 issue of *Hospitals, J.A.H.A.* The data represented the annual period ending September 30 of the preceding year. Thus, the August 1, 1971, *Guide Issue* contained 1970 data, in both aggregate and directory format. Beginning in 1972, the *American Hospital Association Guide to the Health Care Field* and *AHA Hospital Statistics* were issued as separate publications; the *AHA Guide* contained individual hospital data in directory format, and *AHA Hospital Statistics* contained aggregate data. As in the past, the 1972 edition of the *AHA Guide* contained 1971 data. However, its companion publication was titled *AHA Hospital Statistics, 1971.* The companion publication of the 1973 *AHA Guide* was called *AHA Hospital Statistics, 1972.* To clarify the relationship between the *AHA Guide* and *AHA Statistics,* the companion edition of the 1974 *AHA Guide* was titled *AHA Hospital Statistics, 1974 Edition: 1973 Data from the American Hospital Association Annual Survey.* Succeeding editions of *AHA Hospital Statistics* have carried a similar subtitle. To clarify the time period during which each edition of *AHA Hospital Statistics* is most current, beginning with the 1989-90 edition the year is given as bridging two years, e.g., *AHA Hospital Statistics,* 1991-92 edition. The following chart assists users in referencing the two publications.

Issues of *AHA Guide* and *AHA Hospital Statistics*

Data for the year	Title of *AHA Guide*	Title of *AHA Hospital Statistics*
1946 through 1970		*AHA Guide* and *AHA Hospital Statistics* issued jointly as an issue of *Hospitals*
1971	1972 *AHA Guide*	*AHA Hospital Statistics, 1971*
1972	1973 *AHA Guide*	*AHA Hospital Statistics, 1972*
1973	1974 *AHA Guide*	*AHA Hospital Statistics, 1974 edition;* 1973 data
1974	1975 *AHA Guide*	*AHA Hospital Statistics, 1975 edition;* 1974 data
1975	1976 *AHA Guide*	*AHA Hospital Statistics, 1976 edition;* 1975 data
1976	1977 *AHA Guide*	*AHA Hospital Statistics, 1977 edition;* 1976 data
1977	1978 *AHA Guide*	*AHA Hospital Statistics, 1978 edition;* 1977 data
1978	1979 *AHA Guide*	*AHA Hospital Statistics, 1979 edition;* 1978 data
1979	1980 *AHA Guide*	*AHA Hospital Statistics, 1980 edition;* 1979 data
1980	1981 *AHA Guide*	*AHA Hospital Statistics, 1981 edition;* 1980 data
1981	1982 *AHA Guide*	*AHA Hospital Statistics, 1982 edition;* 1981 data
1982	1983 *AHA Guide*	*AHA Hospital Statistics, 1983 edition;* 1982 data
1983	1984 *AHA Guide*	*AHA Hospital Statistics, 1984 edition;* 1983 data
1984	1985 *AHA Guide*	*AHA Hospital Statistics, 1985 edition;* 1984 data
1985	1986 *AHA Guide*	*AHA Hospital Statistics, 1986 edition;* 1985 data
1986	1987 *AHA Guide*	*AHA Hospital Statistics, 1987 edition;* 1986 data
1987	1988 *AHA Guide*	*AHA Hospital Statistics, 1988 edition;* 1987 data
1988	1989 *AHA Guide*	*AHA Hospital Statistics, 1989-90 edition;* 1988 data
1989	1990 *AHA Guide*	*AHA Hospital Statistics, 1990-91 edition;* 1989 data
1990	1991 *AHA Guide*	*AHA Hospital Statistics, 1991-92 edition;* 1990 data

Definitions of Terms

CLASSIFICATION OF HOSPITALS

Community hospitals: All nonfederal short-term general and other special hospitals, excluding hospital units of institutions, whose facilities and services are available to the public.

Note: As defined later (under nursing-home-type unit), a hospital may include a nursing-home-type unit and still be classified as short-term, provided that the majority of its patients are admitted to units where the average length of stay is less than 30 days. Therefore, statistics for community hospitals often include some data about such nursing-home-type units.*

Note: Before 1972, hospital units of institutions, such as prison and college infirmaries, were included in the category of community hospitals. Including these units made this category equivalent to the short-term general and other special hospitals category. Although hospital units are few in number (approximately 50) and small in size, this change in definition should be taken into consideration when community hospital data from 1972 and after are compared with data from earlier years.

Noncommunity hospitals: Includes federal hospitals, long-term hospitals, hospital units of institutions, psychiatric hospitals, hospitals for tuberculosis and other respiratory diseases, chronic disease hospitals, institutions for the mentally retarded, and alcoholism and chemical-dependency hospitals.

*An example is furnished by Montana, where 55.55 percent of all hospitals classified as community hospitals include nursing-home-type units. Expense, revenue, utilization, and personnel data for these hospitals include data about their nursing-home-type units. Thus, total admissions to Montana community hospitals in 1990 were 105,405; total inpatient days, 1,035,165; total expenses, $552,973,000; and total payroll expenses, $249,505,100. If nursing-home-type unit data were excluded, these same items would be 104,077; 594,834; $522,578,000; and $232,679,000, respectively.

Control: The types of organization responsible for establishing policy concerning the overall operation of hospitals. The four major categories are government, nonfederal; nongovernment, not-for-profit; investor-owned (for-profit); and government, federal.

Nursing-home-type unit/facility: A unit or facility owned and operated by the hospital, offering primarily only the following types of service to the majority of all admissions: (a) Skilled nursing: the provision of medical and nursing care services, therapy, and social services under the supervision of a licensed registered nurse on a 24-hour basis. (b) Intermediate care: the provision, on a regular basis, of health-related care and services to individuals who do not require the degree of care or treatment that a skilled nursing unit is designed to provide. (c) Residential care: elderly housing the provision of residential services for those who do not need nursing or medical services but may need some assistance in activities of daily living. Services may include sheltered care facilities for the developmentally disabled or long term psychiatric patients, as well as elderly housing.

Short-term and long-term: Hospitals are classified either short-term or long-term according to the average length of stay. A short-term hospital is one in which the average length of stay is less than 30 days. A long-term hospital is one in which the average length of stay is 30 days or more.

Service: The type of service provided to the majority of admissions. There are four general hospital service categories: general medical and surgical; psychiatric, including care for the mentally retarded and treatment of alcoholism and other chemical dependencies; tuberculosis and other respiratory diseases; and all other specialty services, such as obstetrics and gynecology, rehabilitation, orthopedics, chronic disease, and eye, ear, nose, and throat.

Bed Size: *Number of beds* set up and staffed for use in the hospital. Most of the tables in *AHA Hospital Statistics* contain breakdowns by the following bed size categories: 6 to 24 beds, 25 to 49, 50 to 99, 100 to 199, 200 to 299, 300 to 399, 400 to 499, and 500 or more.

UTILIZATION, FINANCES, PERSONNEL

Adjusted average daily census: Average number of patients (inpatients plus an equivalent figure for outpatients) receiving care each day during the reporting period, which is usually 12 months. Derived by dividing the number of inpatient day equivalents (also called *adjusted inpatient days*) by the number of days in the reporting period.

Adjusted expenses per admission: Average expense to the hospital in providing care for one hospital inpatient stay. Adjusted expenses is derived by removing expenses incurred for the provision of outpatient care from total expenses. (See formula 2 under *adjusted expenses per inpatient day*, below). This number, representing the expenses incurred for inpatient care only, is divided by total admissions to derive the average expense per hospital stay.

Adjusted expenses per inpatient day (formerly called **expenses per adjusted patient day**): Expenses incurred for inpatient care only, and derived by dividing total expenses by inpatient day equivalents (adjusted inpatient days). This computation can be further expanded as shown in formula 1, below:

The term *expenses per adjusted patient day* was at times misinterpreted to mean the average expenses of two services: a high-priced inpatient service and a low-priced outpatient service. Formula 2 shows that this is not the case. Dividing total expenses by the composite figure, which represents inpatient days plus outpatient visits converted into equivalent inpatient days (formula 1) is *exactly equal* to the removal from total expenses of that part incurred for outpatient care and then the division of the residual by inpatient days (formula 2).

Formula 1:

$$\frac{\text{total expenses}}{\text{inpatient days} + \text{outpatient visits}\left(\dfrac{\dfrac{\text{outpatient revenue}}{\text{per outpatient visit}}}{\dfrac{\text{inpatient revenue}}{\text{per inpatient day}}}\right)}$$

which is equivalent to

Formula 2:

$$\frac{\text{total expenses}\left(\dfrac{\text{inpatient revenue}}{\text{total patient revenue}}\right)}{\text{inpatient days}}$$

Adjusted inpatient days: See *Inpatient day equivalents.*

Admissions: Number of patients, excluding newborns, accepted for inpatient service during the reporting period.

Approvals: Eight types of approvals, as reported by various approving bodies, are listed on page 195.

Average daily census: Average number of inpatients, excluding newborns, receiving care each day during the reporting period.

Average length of stay (also **average stay**): Average stay of inpatients during the reporting period. Derived by dividing the number of inpatient days by the number of admissions.

Bassinets: Number of newborn infant bassinets set up and staffed for use at the end of the reporting period. Bassinets are not included in the bed total and do not include isolettes or neonatal intensive care units, which are included under beds.

Beds: Average number of beds, cribs, and pediatric bassinets regularly maintained (set up and staffed for use) for inpatients during the reporting period; also referred to as *statistical beds.* Derived by adding the total number of beds available each day during the hospital's reporting period and dividing this figure by the total number of days in the reporting period.

Births: Total number of infants born in the hospital during the reporting period. Births do not include infants transferred from other institutions and are excluded from admission and discharge figures.

Census divisions: Division of the 50 states and the District of Columbia into nine geographical regions as defined by the U.S. Department of Commerce, Bureau of the Census. These are listed and illustrated on page 19.

Employee benefits: The component of nonpayroll expenses, which includes hospital expenditures for employees' Social Security, group insurance, and retirement benefits. A component of *labor expenses.* (See *Expenses.*)

Expenses: Includes all expenses for the reporting period. *Payroll expenses* includes all salaries and wages, except those paid to medical and dental residents and interns and other trainees, that is, medical technology trainees, x-ray therapy trainees, administrative residents, and so forth. All professional fees and those salary expenditures excluded from payroll are defined as nonpayroll expenses and are included in total expenses. *Labor-related expenses* is defined as payroll expenses plus employee benefits. *Non-labor-related expenses* is all other nonpayroll expenses. In accordance with the revised AICPA Audit Guide, within the Annual Survey of Hospitals, 'bad debt' has been reclassified from a "deduction in revenue" to an expense. However, for historical consistency purposes, the expense total that appears throughout *AHA Hospital Statistics, does not include 'bad debt' as an expense item.*

Note: Financial data may not add due to rounding.

Facilities and services: A selection of 70 facilities and services is listed in tables 12A and 12B; they are defined on pages xxvi-xxx.

FTE: Full-time equivalent personnel. (See *Personnel.*)

Inpatient days: Number of adult and pediatric days of care, excluding newborn days of care, rendered during the entire reporting period.

Inpatient day equivalents (also called **adjusted inpatient days**): An aggregate figure reflecting the number of days of inpatient care, plus an estimate of the volume of outpatient services, expressed in units equivalent to an inpatient day in terms of level of effort. Derived by multiplying the number of outpatient visits by the ratio of outpatient revenue per outpatient visit to inpatient revenue per inpatient day, and adding the product (which represents the number of patient days attributable to outpatient services) to the number of inpatient days.

Metropolitan statistical area (MSA): Revised classification of a geographic area based on population information collected from the 1980 U.S. census, including definitions through June 1989. The U.S. Office of Management and Budget defines an MSA as a "city or urbanized area of at least 50,000 population, with a total metropolitan area of at least 100,000." A more detailed definition is presented on page 147, and maps of MSAs begin on page 149.

Occupancy: Ratio of average daily census to the average number of beds, that is, statistical beds, maintained during the reporting period.

Note: The number of statistical beds may differ from the actual bed count at the close of the reporting period.

Outpatient visits: Visits by patients who are not lodged in the hospital while receiving medical, dental, or other services. Each appearance by an outpatient to each unit of the hospital counts as one outpatient visit. A visit consists of one or more *occasions of service.* (Each test, examination, treatment, or procedure rendered to an outpatient counts as one occasion of service.)

Because at one time some hospitals reported occasions of service rather than visits, hospitals were asked to report them both from 1977 to 1981. This procedure made it possible to verify outpatient visit data and to separate these data from occasions of service data. Since 1978, outpatient visits, the most convenient measure of outpatient utilization, has been divided into two categories, emergency and other. The other category combines the previous categories of clinic and other (referred). In 1982 both categories of outpatient visits, emergency and other, were further divided into three subcategories, professional contact visits, outpatient therapy and treatment visits, and ancillary service visits. Hospitals were not asked to report separate occasions of service data in 1982. In 1983, the occasions of service category was again used as a visit verification measure.

Personnel: Number of persons on the hospital payroll as of September 30, 1990. Personnel are recorded in *AHA Hospital Statistics* as full-time equivalents (FTEs), which are calculated by adding the number of full-time personnel to one-half the number of part-time personnel, excluding medical and dental residents and interns and other trainees. *Per 100 adjusted census* indicates the ratio of personnel to adjusted average daily census, each on a 100-census basis.

Revenue: *Gross patient revenue* (inpatient and outpatient) consists of revenue from services rendered to patients, including payments received from or on behalf of individual patients. *Net patient revenue* consists of gross patient revenue less deductions for contractual adjustments, bad debts, charity, and so forth. *Net total revenue* consists of net patient revenue plus all other revenue, including contributions, endowment revenue, government grants, and all other payments not made on behalf of individual patients.

Surgical operations: Those surgical operations, whether major or minor, performed in the operating room(s). A surgical operation can involve one or more surgical procedures, but is still considered only one surgical operation.

FACILITIES AND SERVICES

Adult day care program: Program providing supervision, medical and psychological care, and social activities for older adults who live at home or in another family setting, but cannot be alone or prefer to be with others during the day. May include intake assessment, health monitoring, occupational therapy, personal care, noon meal, and transportation services.

AIDS/ARC unit: Special unit or team designated and equipped specifically for diagnosis, treatment, continuing care planning, and counseling services for AIDS/ARC patients and their families.

Alcohol/drug abuse or dependency outpatient services: Organized hospital services that provide medical care and/or rehabilitative treatment services to outpatients for whom the primary diagnosis is alcoholism or other chemical dependency.

Alzheimer's diagnostic/assessment services: Specially organized program to diagnose and evaluate people suspected of having Alzheimer's disease. Includes the assessment of medical, social and behavioral conditions and development of a treatment plan addressing family preferences and financial options as well as medical concerns.

Angioplasty: The reconstruction or restructuring of a blood vessel by operative means or by nonsurgical techniques such as balloon dilation or laser.

Arthritis treatment center: Specifically equipped and staffed center for the diagnosis and treatment of arthritis and other joint disorders.

Birthing room/LDRP room: A hospital-managed combination labor and delivery unit with a homelike setting for parents who have completed specified childbirth courses and wish to participate jointly in the birth of their child.

Blood bank: A medical facility with the responsibility for each of the following: blood procurement, drawing, processing, and distribution.

Cardiac catheterization laboratory: Facility for special diagnostic procedures necessary for the care of patients with cardiac conditions. Available procedures must include, but need not be limited to, introduction of a catheter into the interior of the heart by way of a vein or artery or by direct needle puncture.

Cardiac rehabilitation program: Restorative services whereby a patient is reconditioned from a state of cardiac injury or high risk, to resume daily activities of living at an optimum level. Programs often include counseling, education and exercise. Patient instruction in self monitoring of their cardiac condition, stress management and dietary counseling are often components of these programs. Cardiac rehab services are used after open heart surgery, angioplasty, acute myocardial infarction (heart attack), and for patients identified as being at high risk for adverse cardiovascular events.

Chronic obstructive pulmonary disease services: Services provided for the treatment of disorders such as asthma, chronic bronchitis, and emphysema which are marked by persistent obstruction of bronchial air flow.

Community health promotion: Similar to patient education, but for individuals in the community, not within a place of employment or as a patient.

Comprehensive geriatric assessment: Diagnostic and evaluation services that determine elderly patients' short-term and long-term needs for health care and related services. Includes the assessment of medical conditions, functional activities, mental and emotional conditions and incorporates these into a treatment plan incorporating family and financial concerns as well as medical needs.

CT scanner: Computerized tomographic scanner for head and/or whole body scans.

Diagnostic radioisotope facility: The use of radioactive isotopes (radiopharmaceuticals) as tracers or indicators to detect an abnormal condition or disease.

Emergency department: Organized hospital facility for the provision of unscheduled outpatient services to patients whose conditions are considered to require immediate care. Must be staffed 24 hours a day.

Emergency department social work services: Social work services provided to emergency department patients by social workers dedicated to the emergency department or on call.

Emergency response (geriatric): A program for disabled and/or homebound elderly individuals whereby subscribers have an emergency response unit attached to their telephone, linking them to the hospital emergency department, and can automatically call for help by pressing a button.

Extracorporeal shock wave lithotripter (ESWL): A medical device used for treating stones in the kidney or ureter. The device disintegrates kidney stones noninvasively through the transmission of acoustic shock waves directed at the stones.

Fitness center: Provides exercise, testing or evaluation programs and fitness activities to the community and hospital employees.

General inpatient care for AIDS/ARC: Inpatient diagnosis and treatment for AIDS/ARC patients, but dedicated unit is not available.

Genetic counseling/screening services: A service equipped with adequate laboratory facilities and directed by a qualified physician to advise parents and prospective parents on potential problems in cases of genetic defects. Service provides antenatal diagnosis including aminocentesis, chorionic villi sampling, fetal blood sampling, and MRI imaging. Service shall have appropriate ultrasound evaluation capacity.

Geriatric acute care unit: Provides acute care to elderly patients in a special unit in the hospital. Care is provided by a multi-disciplinary team trained in geriatrics. Unit may also offer architectural modifications to accommodate the needs of older adults.

Geriatric clinics: Special medical or surgical clinics providing services targeted to older adults such as arthritis, primary geriatric and podiatric clinics.

Health sciences library: A facility that maintains an organized collection of printed and/or other library materials, has a staff trained to provide and interpret such materials as required to meet informational or educational needs, and keeps an established schedule in which services of the staff are available to clientele.

Hemodialysis: Provision of equipment and personnel for the treatment of renal insufficiency on an inpatient or outpatient basis.

Histopathology laboratory: A laboratory in which tissue specimens are examined by a qualified pathologist.

Home health services: An organized program administered by the hospital that provides medical, nursing, other treatment, and social services to patients in their places of residence.

Hospice: A program providing palliative care, chiefly medical relief of pain and supportive services, addressing the emotional, social, financial, and legal needs of terminally ill patients and their families. Care can be provided in a variety of settings, both inpatient and at home.

Hospital auxiliary: A volunteer community organization formed to assist the institution in carrying out its purpose and to serve as a link between the institution and the community.

Magnetic resonance imaging (MRI): The use of a uniform magnetic field and radio frequencies to study tissue and structure of the body. This procedure enables the visualization of biochemical activity of the cell *in vivo* without the use of ionizing radiation, radioisotopic substances, or high-frequency sound.

Megavoltage radiation therapy: The use of specialized equipment in the supervoltage and megavoltage (above one million volts) ranges for deep therapy treatment of cancer. This would include cobalt units, linear accelerators with or without electron beam therapy capability, betatrons, and Van de Graff machines.

Non-invasive cardiac assessment services: Includes cardiac studies, tests and evaluations not conducted in the cardiac Catheterization laboratory or operating room. Services include at a minimum: echocardiography and exercise stress testing (stress EKG); and may additionally include cardiac nuclear medicine studies.

Occupational health services: Includes services designed to protect the safety of employees from hazards in the work environment.

Occupational therapy services: Facilities for the provision of occupational therapy services prescribed by physicians and administered by or under the direction of a qualified occupational therapist.

Open-heart surgery facilities: Heart surgery where the chest has been opened and the blood recirculated and oxygenated with the proper equipment and the necessary staff to perform the surgery.

Organ/tissue transplant: Service offering specially trained and equipped staff qualified to perform the surgical removal of viable human tissue or organs from either a living donor or a deceased person immediately after death, and the surgical grafting of the tissue or organ into a suitably evaluated and prepared patient.

Organized outpatient services: Health care services offered by appointment on an ambulatory basis. Services may include outpatient surgery; examination, diagnosis and treatment of a variety of medical conditions on a nonemergency basis; and laboratory and other diagnostic testing as ordered by staff or outside physician referral.

Organized social work services: Services that are properly directed and sufficiently staffed by qualified individuals who provide assistance and counseling to patients and their families in dealing with social, emotional, and environmental problems associated with illness or disability, often in the context of financial or discharge planning coordination.

Orthopedic surgery: Surgical treatment of the skeletal system, its articulations, and associated structures.

Outpatient social work services: Social work services provided in ambulatory care areas.

Outpatient surgery services: Scheduled surgical services provided to patients who do not remain in the hospital overnight. The surgery may be performed in operating suites also used for inpatient surgery, specially designated surgical suites for ambulatory surgery, or procedure rooms within an ambulatory care facility.

Patient education: Written goals and objectives for the patient and/or family related to therapeutic regimens, medical procedures and self care.

Patient representative services: Organized hospital services providing personnel through whom patients and staff can seek solutions to institutional problems affecting the delivery of high-quality care and services.

Physical therapy services: Services and use of facilities prescribed by physicians and administered by or under the direction of a qualified physical therapist.

Psychiatric child/adolescent services: Provides care to emotionally disturbed children and adolescents, including those admitted for diagnosis and those admitted for treatment.

Psychiatric consultation and/or liaison services: Provides organized psychiatric consultation/liaison services to nonpsychiatric staff and/or departments on psychological aspects of medical care that may be generic or specific to individual patients.

Psychiatric educational services: Provides psychiatric educational services to community agencies and workers such as schools, police, courts, public health nurses, welfare agencies, clergy, and so forth. The purpose is to expand the mental health knowledge and competence of personnel not working in the mental health field and to promote good mental health through improved understanding, attitudes, and behavioral patterns.

Psychiatric emergency services: Hospital facilities for the provision of unscheduled outpatient care to psychiatric patients whose conditions are considered to require immediate care. Staff must be available 24 hours a day.

Psychiatric geriatric services: Provides care to emotionally disturbed elderly patients, including those admitted for diagnosis and those admitted for treatment.

Psychiatric outpatient services: Hospital services for the diagnosis and treatment of psychiatric outpatients.

Psychiatric partial hospitalization program: Organized hospital facilities and services for day care and/or night care of psychiatric patients who do not require inpatient care 24 hours a day.

Radioactive implants: The use of radioactive material (radium, cobalt-60, cesium-137, or iridium-192 implants) for the treatment of malignancies.

Recreational therapy: Facilities for the provision of recreational therapy services prescribed by physicians and administered by or under the direction of a qualified recreational therapist.

Rehabilitation outpatient services: Provision of coordinated multidisciplinary physical restorative services to ambulatory patients under the direction of a physician knowledgeable and experienced in rehabilitative medicine.

Reproductive health services: Organized clinic offering family planning information and services, child-spacing assistance, and fertility testing.

Respiratory therapy services: The equipment and staff necessary for the administration of oxygen and certain potent drugs through inhalation or positive pressure.

Respite care: Facilities and services that provide for short-term placement of individuals to help meet family emergencies, planned absences (such as vacations or hospitalization), or to allow the family caregivers to shop or do errands.

Senior membership program: A senior enrollment program which offers older adults service benefits such as information, claims assistance, education and senior wellness programs, and discounts for other hospital services. May or may not charge an application fee.

Single photon emission computerized tomography (SPECT): A nuclear medicine imaging technology which combines existing technology of gamma camera imaging with computed tomographic imaging technology to provide a more precise and clear image.

Specialized outpatient program for AIDS/ARC: Special outpatient program providing diagnostic, treatment, continuing care planning, and counseling services for AIDS/ARC patients and their families.

Speech therapy services: Service providing evaluation and treatment to inpatients or outpatients with speech and language disorders.

Sports medicine clinic/services: Provision of diagnostic screening and assessment, clinical and rehabilitation services for the prevention and treatment of sports related injuries.

Therapeutic radioisotope facility: The use of radioactive isotopes (radiopharmaceuticals) for the treatment of malignancies.

Trauma center (certified): State certified facility that provides emergency and specialized intensive care to critically ill and injured patients.

Ultrasound: The use of acoustic waves above the range of 20,000 cycles per second to visualize internal body structures for diagnostic purposes.

Volunteer services department: An organized hospital department responsible for coordinating the services of volunteers working within the institution.

Women's Center: An area set aside for coordinated education and treatment services specifically for and promoted to women as provided by this special unit. Services may or may not include obstetrics, but include a range of services other than OB.

Worksite health promotion: Similar to patient education, but for employees of a company implemented by the hospital and sponsored by their employer.

X-ray radiation therapy: The treatment of disease by roentgen rays or other radiant energy, with the exception of radium, cobalt, or radioisotopes.

INPATIENT SERVICE AREAS

Alcohol/drug abuse or dependency: Provides diagnosis and therapeutic services to patients with alcoholism or other drug dependencies. Includes care for inpatient/residential treatment for patients whose course of treatment involves more intensive care than provided in an outpatient setting or where patient requires supervised withdrawal. Beds must be set up and staffed in a unit(s) specifically designated for this service.

Burn care: Provides care to severely burned patients. Severely burned patients are those with any of the following: 1) second-degree burns of more than 25% total body surface area for adults or 20% total body surface area for children; 2) third-degree burns of more than 10% total body surface area; 3) any severe burns of the hands, face, eyes, ears, or feet; or 4) all inhalation injuries, electrical burns, complicated burn injuries involving fractures and other major traumas, and all other poor risk factors. Beds must be set up and staffed in a unit(s) specifically designated for this service.

General medical and surgical: Provides acute care to patients in medical and surgical units on the basis of physicians' orders and approved nursing care plans. Beds must be set up and staffed in a unit specifically designated for this service.

Intensive care (cardiac care only): Provides patient care of a more specialized nature than the usual medical and surgical care, on the basis of physicians' orders and approved nursing care plans. The unit is staffed with specially trained nursing personnel and contains monitoring and specialized support or treatment equipment for patients who, because of heart seizure, open-heart surgery, or other life-threatening conditions, require intensified, comprehensive observation and care. May include myocardial infarction, pulmonary care, and heart transplant units. Beds must be set up and staffed in a unit(s) specifically designated for this service.

Intensive care (mixed or other): Provides patient care of a more intensive nature than the usual medical and surgical care, on the basis of physicians' orders and approved nursing care plans. These units are staffed with specially trained nursing personnel and contain monitoring and specialized support equipment for patients who, because of shock, trauma, or other life-threatening conditions, require intensified, comprehensive observation and care. Includes mixed intensive care units. Beds must be set up and staffed in a unit(s) specifically designated for this service.

Intensive care (neonatal): A unit that must be separate from the newborn nursery providing intensive care to all sick infants including those with the very lowest birth weights (less than 1500 grams). NICU has potential for providing mechanical ventilation, neonatal surgery and special care for the sickest infants born in the hospital or transferred from another institution. A full-time neonatologist serves as director of the NICU. Beds must be set up and staffed in a unit(s) specifically designated for this service.

Intensive care (pediatric): Provides care to pediatric patients that is of a more intensive nature than that usually provided to pediatric patients. The unit is staffed with specially trained personnel and contains monitoring and specialized support equipment for treatment of patients who, because of shock, trauma, or other life-threatening conditions, require intensified, comprehensive observation and care. Beds must be set up and staffed in a unit specifically designated for this service.

Long-term care (skilled nursing): Provides physicians' services and continuous professional nursing supervision to patients who are not in an acute phase of illness and who currently require primarily convalescent rehabilitative and/or restorative services. May include extended care units. Can include, but not restricted to, Medicare/Medicaid-certified skilled nursing care. Beds must be set up and staffed in unit(s) specifically designated for this service.

Long-term care (other): Provides care and services to persons who do not require the degree of care or treatment that a skilled nursing unit is designed to provide. May include intermediate, residential, or other long-term care. Beds must be set up and staffed in unit(s) specifically designated for this service.

Mental retardation: Provides, on a regular basis, health-related care and services to patients with developmental impairment who do not require the degree of care or treatment that a skilled nursing unit is designed to provide. Beds must be set up and staffed in a unit specifically designated for this service.

Neonatal intermediate care: A unit that must be separate from the normal newborn nursery and that provides intermediate and/or recovery care and some specialized services, including immediate resuscitation, intravenous therapy, and capacity for prolonged oxygen therapy and monitoring. Beds must be set up and staffed in a unit(s) specifically designated for this service.

Obstetric care: Levels should be designated: (1) unit provides services for uncomplicated maternity and newborn cases; (2) unit provides services for uncomplicated cases, the majority of complicated problems, and special neonatal services; and (3) unit provides services for all serious illnesses and abnormalities and is supervised by a full time maternal/fetal specialist. Beds must be set up and staffed in a unit(s) specifically designated for this service.

Pediatric: Provides acute care to pediatric patients on the basis of physicians' orders and approved nursing care plans. Beds must be set up and staffed in a unit specifically designated for this service.

Psychiatric care: Provides care to emotionally disturbed patients, including patients admitted for diagnosis and for treatment of psychiatric problems, on the basis of physicians' orders and approved nursing care plans. May also include the provision of medical care, nursing services, and supervision to the chronically mentally ill, mentally disordered, or other mentally incompetent persons. Beds must be set up and staffed in unit(s) specifically designated for this service.

Rehabilitation: Provides coordinated multidisciplinary physical restorative services to inpatients under the direction of a physician knowledgeable and experienced in rehabilitative medicine. Beds must be set up and staffed in a unit specifically designated for this service.

Technical Notes

The 1991-92 edition of *The American Hospital Association Hospital Statistics* is the statistical complement to the 1991 edition of the *American Hospital Association Guide to the Health Care Field,* which contains selected data about individual hospitals. Both publications use data from the 1990 AHA Annual Survey of Hospitals, conducted by the Hospital Data Center of the American Hospital Association.* This survey was mailed to all hospitals, both AHA-registered and nonregistered, in the United States and its associated areas: American Samoa, Guam, the Marshall Islands, Puerto Rico, and the Virgin Islands. U.S. government hospitals located outside the United States were not included. Of the hospitals included, 6,261 responded—a response rate of 91.1 percent.

The 1990 AHA Annual Survey of Hospitals was mailed to 6,710 AHA-registered hospitals. Of these, 6,648 were located in the 50 states and the District of Columbia, and 62 were located in U.S. associated areas. Of these, 6,104 or 91.8 percent responded from the U.S., and 42 or 67.7 percent responded from the U.S. associated areas. Overall, 6,146

Text Table A

AHA-Registered Hospitals Responding to the 1990 AHA Annual Survey of Hospitals, by Bed Size

Hospital bed-size category	Percent
6-24 beds	84.1
25-49	88.9
50-99	88.5
100-199	91.9
200-299	96.7
300-399	96.5
400-499	95.3
500 or more	96.4

Text Table B

AHA-Registered Hospitals Responding to the 1990 AHA Annual Survey of Hospitals, by U.S. Census Division

U.S. Census division	Percent
New England	92.4
Middle Atlantic	93.8
South Atlantic	91.7
East North Central	95.7
East South Central	92.5
West North Central	95.7
West South Central	91.4
Mountain	91.0
Pacific	81.5

Text Table C

Reporting Periods of Responding AHA-Registered Hospitals

Last month of reporting period	Percent of hospitals
Dec. 1989	3.0
Jan. 1990	0.0
Feb. 1990	0.2
Mar. 1990	1.9
Apr. 1990	1.4
May 1990	2.1
June 1990	28.2
July 1990	0.5
Aug. 1990	5.4
Sept. 1990	38.1
Oct. 1990	0.9
Nov. 1990	0.7
Dec. 1990	17.5

*Data gathered by the 1990 AHA Annual Survey of Hospitals but not presented in the aggregate format of the *AHA Hospital Statistics* are available from the computer files of the Hospital Data Center, Information Systems and Services, American Hospital Association. However, revenue data for individual hospitals are confidential and are not released.

AHA-registered hospitals reported data, a response of 91.59 percent.

The percentages of response were generally related to hospital size. For example, 84.1 percent of hospitals with fewer than 25 beds responded, but more than 96.4 percent of hospitals with 500 or more beds responded (see text table A).

Percentages of response were also related to type of hospital control (management). Nongovernment not-for-profit hospitals had a response rate of 95.6 percent, followed by 91.7 percent for state and local government hospitals, 89.2 percent for federal hospitals, and 80.4 percent for investor-owned hospitals.

Among nonregistered U.S. hospitals, 114 of 160, or 71.3 percent responded.

Regionally, hospitals in the East North Central and West North Central states responded at a 95.7 percent rate, the highest among the U.S. census divisions (see text table B). The lowest response rate, 81.5 percent, was among Pacific hospitals.

Hospitals were requested to report data for a full year, preferably ending September 30, 1990. Approximately 38.1 percent of the responding AHA-registered hospitals used this reporting period; 28.2 percent used the year ending June 30, 1990; and the remaining hospitals used various reporting periods (see text table C).

The statistical tables, beginning on page 2, present data reported or estimated for a 12-month period, except for data on personnel and facilities, which represent situations as they existed at the end of the reporting period. The tables are based on data from all 1990 AHA Annual Survey questionnaires that had been received and processed by June 1, 1991.

The data for tables 1 through 13B include the 6,648 AHA-registered hospitals in the United States and the District of Columbia. Tables 5D, 5E, and 10B, however, include data on the 62 AHA-registered hospitals in U.S. associated areas. Table 14 presents data on U.S. nonregistered hospitals. Data on community hospitals only are presented in tables 4B, 4D, 6, 7, 8, and 11. Data on reporting hospitals only are tabulated in tables 12A, 12B, 13A, and 13B. Data on accredited hospitals only are given in table 9. The information on approvals and affiliations reported in tables 10A and 10B is based on the AHA's current membership file, which includes information supplied by national approving organizations. In tables 2A and 2B, bed-size categories are listed only if one or more hospitals fit into that particular group. In table 8, the five smallest bed-size categories are all combined into one group, entitled "less than 300 beds." In all the other statistical tables, whenever bed-size categories are listed, all eight categories are given whether or not there are hospitals in each of the categories.

The AHA-registered hospitals included in the *AHA Guide* are not necessarily identical with those included in the *AHA Hospital Statistics*. The institutions listed in the 1991 edition of the *AHA Guide* include all of those institutions registered as of April 1991. The tables in the *AHA Hospital Statistics,* present data for both AHA-registered hospitals (tables 1 through 13B) and nonregistered hospitals (table 14) that were in operation during the 12-month reporting period ending September 30, 1990. Thus, hospitals not included in the *AHA Guide,* for example, those that closed between October 1990 and April 1991 and nonregistered hospitals, would be included in the *AHA Hospital Statistics.* Hospitals registered between October 1990 and April 1991, however, would be included in the *AHA Guide,* but would not necessarily be included in AHA-registered hospital data in the *AHA Hospital Statistics.* Data on those hospitals dropped from AHA registration because of mergers or consolidation with another hospital are reported in combined form and are not counted individually.

Both AHA-registered and nonregistered osteopathic hospitals are included in the *AHA Guide.* Data for AHA-registered osteopathic hospitals are included in tables 1 through 13B of the *AHA Hospital Statistics,* and data for nonregistered osteopathic hospitals are included in table 14. As of May 1991, 7 osteopathic hospitals were not registered by the American Hospital Association.

Estimates were made of data for nonreporting hospitals and for reporting hospitals that submitted incomplete AHA Annual Survey questionnaires. Estimates were not made for beds, bassinets, and facilities. Data for beds and bassinets of nonreporting hospitals were based on the most recent information available from those hospitals. Facilities and services and inpatient service area data include only reporting hospitals and, therefore, do not include estimates (see statistical tables 12 and 13).

Estimates for missing revenue, expenses, admissions, inpatient days, outpatient visits, and full-time equivalent personnel were based on data reported the previous year, if available. If the previous year's data were not available, the estimates were based on data furnished by reporting hospitals that are similar in size, control, major service provided, length of stay, and geographic and demographic characteristics to the hospitals that did not report this information.

Hospital Trends

U.S. Registered Hospitals

Since 1946, the American Hospital Association (AHA) has conducted a national inventory of hospitals through its Annual Survey of Hospitals. With the cooperation of participating hospitals and allied hospital associations, the AHA collects data on facilities, services, utilization, personnel, and finances in the nation's hospitals. This survey provides the basis for the following analysis of the key trends impacting hospitals in the United States today (see text table 1).

Setting the Environment

A variety of forces, including economic trends, demographic characteristics, and payer efforts to hold down health care costs affected the performance of hospitals in 1990.[1]

Economics

The economic factors that faced the nation's hospitals changed dramatically in 1990. Throughout the year, the housing and automobile industries slumped badly, unemployment rose, consumer spending was down and corporate profits declined. Before the year was over, sharp declines in consumer and business confidence along with higher oil prices arising from Iraq's invasion of Kuwait in August 1990, had driven the U.S. economy into a recession.

Recessionary problems in the economy threatened hospitals' financial stability. The recession sharpened employer's needs to cut costs. Public and private payers stepped up efforts to reduce health care outlays. Lower payments to hospitals and increased financial pressures were the outcomes. In 1990, community hospitals were able to maintain a total net margin of 3.8 percent. The 1990 figure represents a slight increase from the 3.4 percent margin reported in 1989. Although the total net margin was positive at the aggregate national level, 1,500 hospitals reported negative total margins. In addition, patient revenues did not cover total expenses and the net patient revenue margin for all community hospitals was −4.2 percent.

In addition, the recession increased the numbers of unemployed and uninsured individuals which increased hospitals' Medicaid and uncompensated care burdens. Higher oil and energy prices added to hospitals' non-labor expenses, which rose at a rate of 11.8 percent in 1990. Finally as

Text Table 1 **Selected Measures in U.S. Registered Hospitals, 1980 and 1989-90**

	Year			Percent Change*	
Measure	1980	1989	1990	1980-90	1989-90
Hospitals	6,965	6,720	6,649	− 4.5%	−1.1%
Beds (000s)	1,365	1,226	1,213	−11.1%	−1.0%
Average number of beds per hospital	196	182	182	− 6.9%	0.1%
Admissions (000s)	38,892	33,742	33,774	−13.2%	0.1%
Average daily census (000s)	1,060	853	844	−20.4%	−1.0%
Average length of stay, days	10.0	9.2	9.1	− 8.5%	−1.1%
Inpatient days (000s)	387,557	311,079	307,871	−20.6%	−1.0%
Occupancy, percent	77.7	69.6	69.5	−10.5%	0.0%
Surgical operations (000s)	19,530	22,512	23,091	18.2%	2.6%
Bassinets (000s)[a]	80	71	71	−11.7%	−1.3%
Births (000s)[a]	3,500	3,920	4,047	15.6%	3.2%
Outpatient visits (000s)[b]	262,951	352,248	368,184	40.0%	4.5%

[a] Based only on hospitals reporting newborn data.
[b] Based only on hospitals reporting outpatient visits.
*Percent changes are based on actual figures, not rounded.

capital markets tightened in response to the failing economy, hospitals found it increasingly difficult to access capital for needed improvements.

Pressures to control costs also intensified for hospitals in 1990. Public and private payers implemented numerous measures to reduce their outlays for health care services; providers worked to improve productivity and efficiency through such efforts as changes in staffing and reductions in bed capacity. Hospitals also faced inadequate Medicaid reimbursements, proposals for further reductions in Medicare payments, and demands for more favorable pricing arrangements from private payers. Managed care plans accounted for a growing proportion of hospital revenues as both public and private payers continue to explore managed care options as one means of controlling health care costs.

The focus of efforts to control health care spending has increasingly shifted from inpatient care to outpatient and physician services. In 1990, whereas admissions increased slightly by 0.1 percent, outpatient visits increased by 4.5 percent compared to a 4.8 percent increase reported in 1989. Since 1980, admissions have declined by 13.1 percent despite a 10 percent increase in the U.S. population. During this same period, outpatient visits have increased by 40 percent. The federal government is in the process of implementing reforms in Medicare payments and is attempting to develop a prospective pricing system for outpatient services.

Demographics

The U.S. Census Bureau reports that between 1980 and 1990 the U.S. population increased by approximately 10 percent, to 249 million. However, all states did not share equally in this growth. Generally, states in the southern and western parts of the country gained population at a faster rate than did those in the Northeast and Midwest. In general, the South and the West also fared better economically in 1990 than did those in the Northeast and Midwest. During this period, the rural population declined by 1.4 percent.

In 1990, according to the U.S. Census Bureau, 33.6 million Americans were poor.[2] The 1990 poverty rate of 13.5 percent was higher than the rate of 12.8 for 1989. Continued recessionary conditions are likely to push poverty rates even higher. Of special concern is the fact that 20 percent of all U.S. children live in poverty. Many of the poor lack adequate health insurance coverage to seek necessary care. The U.S. Census Bureau reports that 34.4 million Americans—up from 31 million in 1987—lacked health coverage of any kind in 1990. In addition, it is estimated that as many as 1 out of 4 Americans will lose their health insurance for at least some period of time in the next two years thereby further increasing the number of uninsured. Growth in the numbers of the poor and uninsured further increased hospitals' uncompensated care burdens in 1990.

Many of the uninsured are among the "working poor" who cannot obtain employer-sponsored coverage but are also ineligible for Medicaid. Nearly 50 percent of the uninsured are ineligible for Medicaid. It is widely acknowledged that the Medicaid program is not doing an adequate job of providing health coverage for the poor. Medicaid now covers only 40 percent of those living in poverty, down from 65 percent in the 1970s. Moreover, Medicaid dollars increasingly are going toward coverage of long-term care for the aged, blind, and disabled rather than toward primary care for poor children and their parents. Also, where Medicaid does pay for services, in many states, the payment does not cover the costs incurred. For example, in 1989, it was estimated that on average Medicaid paid only 78.8 percent of costs, down from 90.5 percent paid in 1980. This underpayment resulted in a national shortfall of 4.1 billion for which the hospitals were responsible, thereby further increasing their uncompensated care burdens. Given the rising numbers of poor and uninsured, and inadequacies of the Medicaid program, the hospitals will feel heightened financial pressure.

In 1990, elderly people comprised 12.6 percent of the U.S. population and numbered approximately 31 million. The proportion of elderly persons will continue to rise well into the 21st century. For this segment of the population, Medicare is the primary source of health care coverage. Medicare currently accounts for 40.4 percent of community hospital patient revenues somewhat up from 39.9 percent in 1989.

With respect to Medicare, hospitals will continue to be squeezed financially under the prospective pricing system (PPS) as budget considerations drive government payment policies. For example, the Omnibus Reconciliation Act of 1990 called for nearly $17 billion in cuts in Medicare payments to hospitals over a five year period. Cuts in reimbursement for capital, outpatient care and medical education coupled with increases in DRG prices that fell below market basket inflation rates have resulted in inadequate Medicare payments to hospitals in recent years. It is estimated that more than 60 percent of hospitals lost money on Medicare patients in 1990. Although the elderly will continue to comprise a significant percentage of hospital admissions, Medicare payments will in many cases not cover costs, further straining hospitals' financial position.

Private Health Insurance

The health insurance industry underwent significant change in the 1980s as a result of employer and insurer attempts to control ever-escalating health care costs. By 1989, 82 percent of Americans with employer-sponsored health care coverage were enrolled in managed care plans including HMOs, PPOs, and managed fee-for-service plans. In the 1990s, managed care will become even more important as a payer for hospital services. Typically, managed care includes utilization review, pre-admission screening, and case management and attempts to ensure that only medically necessary services are provided and that the services are provided in the most appropriate setting. Managed care incentives, in addition to various technological advancements, have contributed to the significant growth in outpatient services in recent years. As managed care arrangements grow, hospitals will face more requests for deeper discounts or other favorable pricing arrangements.

Regulatory Pressures

In addition to the increased financial pressures that hospitals will feel from all payers, additional issues must be faced in the 1990s.

Hospitals will continue to face increased scrutiny of virtually all of their activities as a result of legislative and regulatory actions. Government bodies are questioning tax exemptions for non-profit hospitals. Ethics in Patient Referral legislation and anti-kickback regulations will subject hospital-physician joint business ventures to increased government review, and hospitals considering mergers may well be challenged on anti-trust grounds. Federal and state regulatory activities relating to environmental issues such as

Text Table 2 **Selected Measures in Community Hospitals, 1980 and 1989-90**

	Year			Percent Change*	
Measure	**1980**	**1989**	**1990**	**1980-90**	**1989-90**
Hospitals	5,830	5,455	5,384	− 7.7%	−1.3%
Beds (000s)	988	933	927	− 6.2%	−0.6%
Average number of beds per hospital	170	171	172	1.6%	0.7%
Admissions (000s)	36,143	31,116	31,181	−13.7%	0.2%
Average daily census (000s)	747	618	619	−17.1%	0.2%
Average length of stay, days	7.6	7.2	7.2	− 4.1%	0.0%
Inpatient days (000s)	273,085	225,437	225,972	−17.3%	0.2%
Occupancy, percent	75.6	66.2	66.8	−11.6%	0.9%
Surgical operations (000s)	18,768	21,340	21,915	16.8%	2.7%
Bassinets (000s)[a]	78	69	68	−11.8%	−1.4%
Births (000s)[a]	3,408	3,831	3,958	16.1%	3.3%
Outpatient visits (000s)[b]	202,310	285,712	301,329	48.9%	5.5%

[a] Based only on hospitals reporting newborn data.
[b] Based only on hospitals reporting outpatient visits.
*Percent changes are based on actual figures, not rounded.

infection control and waste management are likely to result in higher costs. The need to develop systems designed to measure and review "quality of care" will intensify in response to demands from both payers and consumers.

Conclusion

Recognizing the importance of their community service missions, hospitals in the 1990s will become increasingly responsive to community needs. They will continue to diversify and provide more outpatient, long-term, and preventive care services. Hospitals will also play a greater role in the delivery of primary care services. Hospitals must be sensitive to the needs of their communities and be in a position to change as the communities' needs change.

In the previous section, environmental factors that impacted on the nation's hospitals were described. In the next section, specific hospital performance trends in 1990 will be analyzed for community hospitals (see text table 2).

Community Hospital Distribution Trends

Community hospitals include institutions that are nonfederal, short-term, general and other special hospitals whose facilities are open to the public. Not included in the community hospital category are hospital units of institutions, long-term hospitals, psychiatric hospitals, and alcoholism and chemical dependency facilities. Over the past 10 years, the total number of U.S. community hospitals has been declining, especially since 1985. Reductions in the number of hospitals occur as hospitals close, merge, or are acquired by other facilities. In 1990, 50 community hospitals closed down from the 65 reported closures in 1989. Since 1980, 558 community hospitals have closed, ceasing to provide inpatient acute care services.[3] In the same period, many hospitals merged with or were acquired by other hospitals, resulting in fewer hospitals after these transactions were concluded. Each year, reductions in the number of hospitals are offset in part by new hospital openings as well as facility reopenings. In 1990, although 43 hospitals opened, only 6 of the new hospitals were identified as being community hospitals.

Urban versus Rural

In 1990, there were fewer rural hospitals and fewer small hospitals than in 1980 (see text table 3). The number of rural community hospitals decreased 14.4 percent in 10 years. By comparison, the number of urban hospitals remained relatively steady, 1.0 percent decrease from 1980 to 1990 (see figure 1).

Bed size

Since 1980, the number of community hospitals fell by 7.7 percent or by 446 hospitals. During this ten year period, the number of hospitals in all bed-size categories declined with the exception of the 200-299 bed-size category which increased

Figure 1 **Distribution of Community Hospitals by Urban versus Rural, 1980-90**

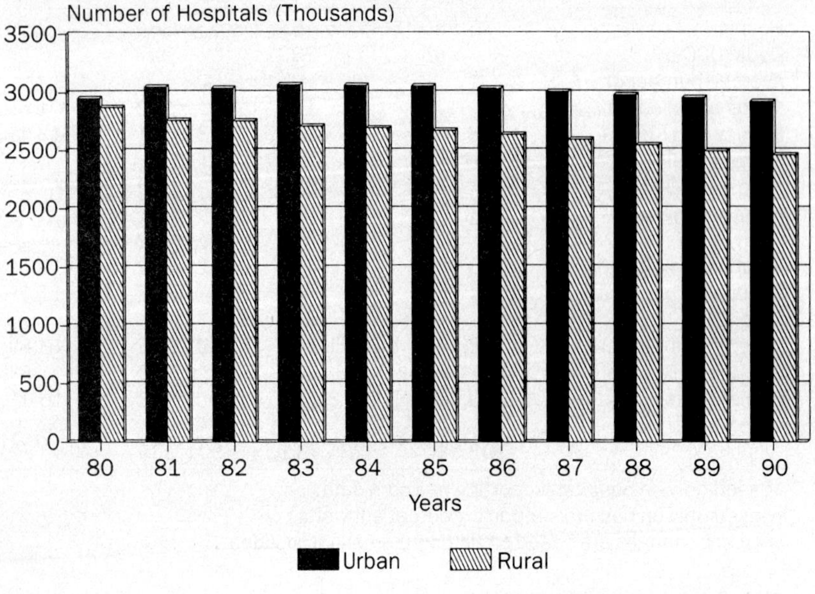

Text Table 3 **Distribution of Community Hospitals, 1980 and 1989-90**

	Number of Hospitals			Percent Change	
	1980	**1989**	**1990**	**1980-90**	**1989-90**
Total community hospitals	5,830	5,455	5,384	− 7.7%	− 1.3%
Urban community hospitals	2,955	2,958	2,924	− 1.0%	− 1.1%
6-24 Beds	46	36	34	−26.1%	− 5.6%
25-49	211	182	174	−17.5%	− 4.4%
50-99	456	448	439	− 3.7%	− 2.0%
100-199	756	801	785	3.8%	− 2.0%
200-299	553	625	619	11.9%	− 1.0%
300-399	371	369	375	1.1%	1.6%
400-499	251	208	218	−13.1%	4.8%
500 or more	311	289	280	−10.0%	− 3.1%
Rural community hospitals	2,875	2,497	2,460	−14.4%	− 1.5%
6-24 Beds	213	203	192	− 9.9%	− 5.4%
25-49	818	767	761	− 7.0%	− 0.8%
50-99	1,006	840	824	−18.1%	− 1.9%
100-199	614	530	521	−15.1%	− 1.7%
200-299	162	117	120	−25.9%	2.6%
300-399	41	32	33	−19.5%	3.1%
400-499	15	3	4	−73.3%	33.3%
500 or more	6	5	5	−16.7%	0.0%

Figure 2 **Distribution of Community Hospitals by U.S. Census Region**

1990 **Percent Change 1980-90**

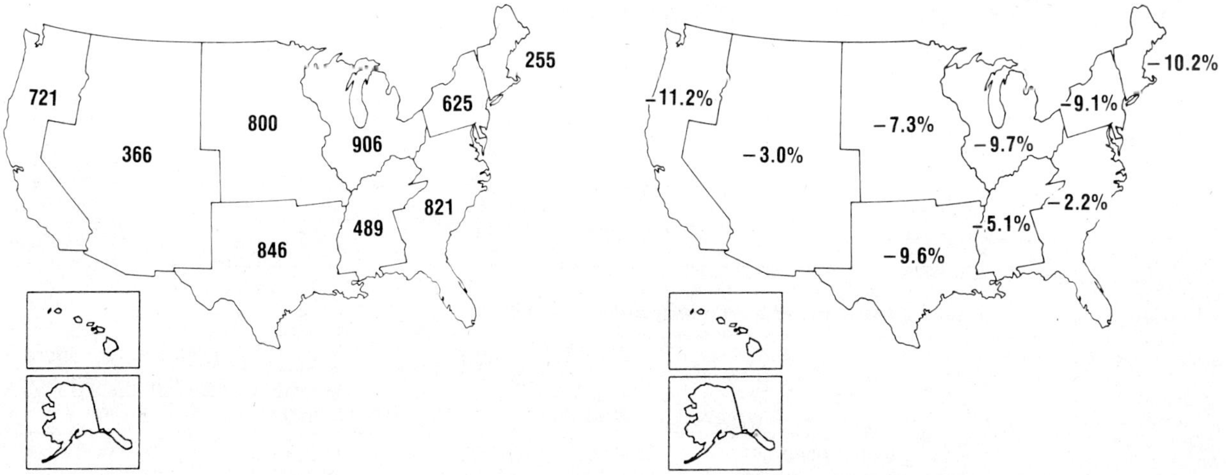

by 3.4 percent. The largest declines, which were ten percent or more, were recorded for hospitals in the 6-24, 50-99, 400-499, and 500 or more bed-size categories. The smallest declines, which were less than 5 percent, were recorded for hospitals in the 100-199 and 300-399 bed-size categories.

U.S. Census Regions

Regional data show a disproportionate reduction in the number of hospitals available in some areas. In the Pacific and New England regions, the number of community hospitals has dropped over 10 percent in the past 10 years. The East North Central, West South Central, and the Middle Atlantic regions lost between 9 and 10 percent of their hospitals. The other regions lost between 2.2 and 7.3 percent with no region registering an increase in the number of hospitals over the time period (see figure 2).

Beds

A decline in the number of hospital beds set up and staffed for use has accompanied the decline in hospitals. This is in response to the reduction in average length of hospital stays and total inpatient days. The number of beds in U.S. community hospitals peaked in 1983, slightly over one million. Significant reductions in the number of beds started in 1986. In 1986 and 1987, 23,000 and 20,000 beds were removed from service respectively. In 1988 and 1989, the absolute reduction in the number of beds slowed somewhat. In 1988 and 1989 approximately 11,000 and 14,000 beds were removed from service. In 1990, the national bed complement was reduced by approximately 6,000 beds which represented the smallest absolute reduction in beds since 1984. Over time, the majority of reductions occurred in rural hospitals and 1990 was no exception. By bed size, hospitals with 50-99 beds and those in the 400-499 bed-size category removed a larger share of their beds from service (see text table 4).

Financial Trends

Expenses

Hospital financial trends have been affected by the changes in hospital reimbursement policies, medical practice patterns, and medical technology. Between 1983 and 1986 hospital expense growth averaged eight percent annually. In the past three years, however, expenses have begun to rise more rapidly.

Community hospital expenses rose 10.6 percent in 1988, 9.6 percent in 1989, and 10.2 percent in 1990. Urban

Text Table 4 **Distribution of Community Hospital Beds, 1980 and 1990**

	1980		1990		Percent Change in No. of Beds
	Number of Beds	Percent of Total Beds	Number of Beds	Percent of Total Beds	
Total community hospitals	988,387	100.0%	927,360	100.0%	– 6.2%
Urban community hospitals	738,561	74.7%	721,141	77.8%	– 2.4%
Rural community hospitals	249,826	25.3%	206,219	22.2%	–17.5%
Bed-size category					
6-24 Beds	4,932	0.5%	4,427	0.5%	–10.2%
25-49	37,478	3.8%	35,420	3.8%	– 5.5%
50-99	105,278	10.7%	90,394	9.7%	–14.1%
100-199	192,892	19.5%	183,867	19.8%	– 4.7%
200-299	172,390	17.4%	179,670	19.4%	4.2%
300-399	139,434	14.1%	138,938	15.0%	– 0.4%
400-499	117,724	11.9%	98,833	10.7%	–16.0%
500 or more	218,259	22.1%	195,811	21.1%	–10.3%

Text Table 5 **Total Expenditures of Community Hospitals, 1989-90**

	Total Expenditures (Millions)[a]		Percent Change	Average Expenditure per Hospital (Millions)
	1989	1990		1990
Total community hospitals	$184,898	$203,693	10.2%	$ 38
Urban community hospitals	161,228	177,480	10.1%	61
Rural community hospitals	23,669	26,213	10.7%	11
Bed-size category				
6-24 Beds	456	473	3.7%	2
25-49	3,766	4,012	6.5%	4
50-99	11,638	12,590	8.2%	10
100-199	30,801	33,282	8.1%	25
200-299	35,435	38,698	9.2%	52
300-399	29,842	33,137	11.0%	81
400-499	21,277	25,297	18.9%	114
500 or more	51,683	56,205	8.7%	197

[a]Figures have been rounded to the nearest million; therefore, entries in vertical columns will not necessarily add to the totals given.

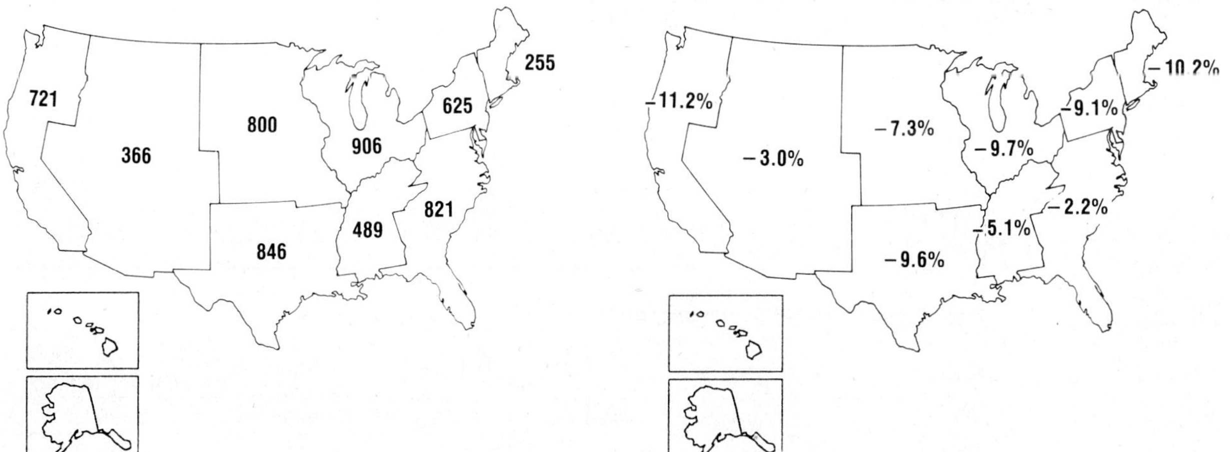

hospital expenses grew at a 10.1 percent rate in 1990, while rural hospital expenses rose 10.7 percent (see text table 5).

In 1990, payroll and benefits were almost 54.4 percent of total expenses. Thus, wages, salaries, and employee benefits represent more than half of the aggregate community hospital expenses. Another third of hospital expenses are for medical supplies, pharmaceuticals, utilities, food, housekeeping supplies, and administrative costs. The remainder of hospital expenses are capital costs, (interest and depreciation on a hospital's facilities and equipment) and fees paid for contracted professional and administrative services (see figure 3).

Revenue

Growth in total community hospital revenues is parallel to the trend in total expense growth. Since 1983, growth in revenues was reduced to an average annual rate of about eight percent. Total revenues in 1990 increased 10.7 percent, somewhat faster than the 9.6 percent growth reported in 1989. Net patient revenues, the revenue hospitals actually receive from the care they provide to patients, rose 10.5 percent in 1990, compared with 9.8 percent in 1989.

Payer Sources

Gross patient revenue reflects the amount hospitals would have received if all patients paid at full "retail" charges.[4] Gross patient revenues are not used to evaluate hospitals' financial position, but can indicate the level of services rendered and provide revenue source information. In 1990, Medicare represented approximately 40 percent of the total community hospital gross patient revenue while Medicaid represented 11.4 percent. Third-party payers accounted for 32.2 percent, and patients who pay for hospital services themselves or from other government and nongovernment sources accounted for 8.8 percent (see figure 4).

Figure 3 **Community Hospital Expenditures, 1990**

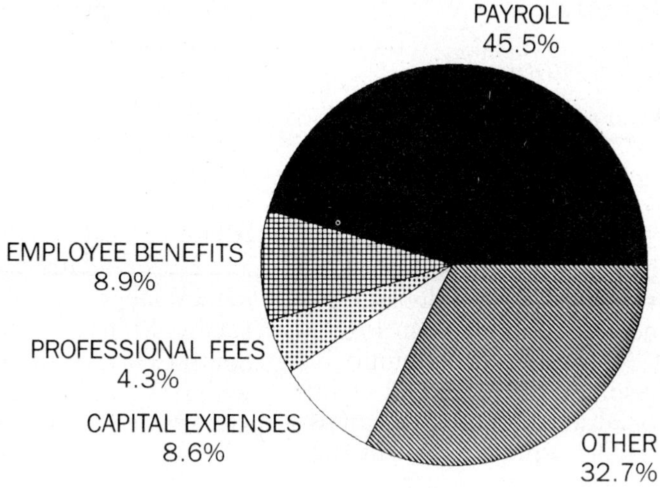

Figure 4 **Community Hospital Gross Patient Revenue by Payer Source, 1990**

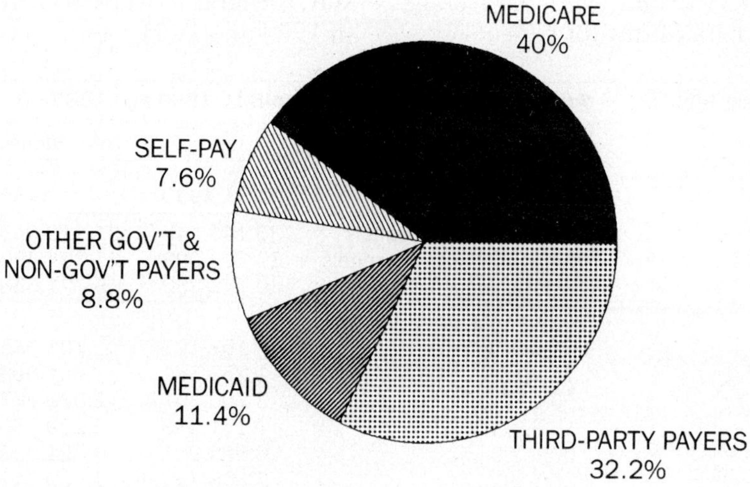

Utilization Trends

Trends in the utilization of hospital services have been varied. Declines in inpatient use and simultaneous growth in outpatient care depict what is perhaps the most significant change in health care delivery in the past 10 years.

Changes in Inpatient Activity

Admissions

Total admissions have decreased 13.7 percent from 1980 to 1990. In 1990, admissions in registered community hospitals totalled 31.1 million, a slight 0.2 percent increase from 1989 (see text table 6). Admissions increased slightly from 1989 to 1990 for urban community hospitals and decreased slightly for rural community hospitals. Urban hospitals experienced a 0.4 percent increase in admissions compared to last year's 0.7 percent drop. Rural hospitals continued to feel more pressure as admissions were off 0.5 percent in 1990 and 2.7 percent in 1989 (see figure 5).

Average Length of Stay

In 1989 and 1990, the average length of stay for patients admitted to U.S. community hospitals was 7.2 days. In 1980, the length of stay was 7.6 days. Since 1984, where the length of stay was 7.3 days, the average length of stay has stabilized declining by only one tenth of a day. The decline in length of stay from the early 1980s coincides with the beginning of Medicare prospective pricing and likely reflects hospitals' response to the payment system's incentives, encouraging cost efficient treatment methods.

Length of stay, however, varies, considerably across regions. Hospitals in the Middle Atlantic, West North Central, and New England had the highest length of stay. The Pacific, Mountain, and West South Central had the lowest with stays under the national average of 7.2 days.

Inpatient Days

Inpatient days slightly increased by 0.2 percent in 1990. As stated previously, the change in inpatient days in the past 10 years has been dramatic. The decline began in 1981, but as with admissions and length of stay, the largest drops occurred in 1984 and 1985 after PPS was initiated. Since 1980, inpatient days have fallen a total of 15 percent after peaking at 278 million in 1981 (see figure 6).

Hospital occupancy rates have also declined, both in urban and rural hospitals. The aggregate occupancy rate for community hospitals was 66.8 percent in 1990, down from 75.6 percent in 1980.

Occupancy tends to rise with hospital size, ranging from 32.3 percent in 1990 among hospitals with 6 to 24 beds to 77.3 percent among those with 500 or more beds.

Changes In Outpatient Activity

While hospital reimbursement policies and medical technologies have contributed to the decrease in inpatient use, they have conversely affected outpatient visits. In 1990 community hospitals reported 301 million outpatient visits, up 5.5 percent from 1989. Outpatient visits increased at a relatively slow rate until 1986, at which time it rose roughly 6 percent in both 1986 and 1987, and nearly 10 percent in 1988.

Contributing to the rapid

Text Table 6 **Admissions in Community Hospitals, 1980 and 1989-90**

	Total Admissions			Percent Change	
	1980	1989	1990	1980-90	1989-90
Total community hospitals	36,143,445	31,116,048	31,181,046	−13.7%	0.2%
Urban community hospitals	27,102,093	25,394,492	25,490,254	− 5.9%	0.4%
Rural community hospitals	9,041,352	5,721,556	5,690,792	−37.1%	−0.5%
Bed-size category					
6-24 Beds	158,797	101,085	95,487	−40.0%	−5.5%
25-49	1,253,581	881,695	869,830	−30.6%	−1.3%
50-99	3,700,367	2,536,377	2,474,497	−33.1%	−2.4%
100-199	7,161,988	5,939,666	5,832,890	−18.6%	−1.8%
200-299	6,595,911	6,321,333	6,333,181	−40.0%	0.2%
300-399	5,358,161	4,999,912	5,091,049	− 5.0%	1.8%
400-499	4,401,325	3,386,017	3,643,952	−17.2%	7.6%
500 or more	7,513,315	6,949,963	6,840,160	− 9.0%	−1.6%

growth in outpatient visits is the increase in outpatient surgical procedures, both in urban and rural settings. In 1984, just over one quarter of all surgeries performed in community hospitals were done on an outpatient basis. By 1990, that proportion had risen to nearly half. Almost all U.S. community hospitals, regardless of size or location, provided some type of ambulatory surgical service to their patients. As the number of non-invasive surgical methods increases, so will the growth in ambulatory surgery (see text table 7).

Figure 5 **Admissions in Community Hospitals, 1980-90**

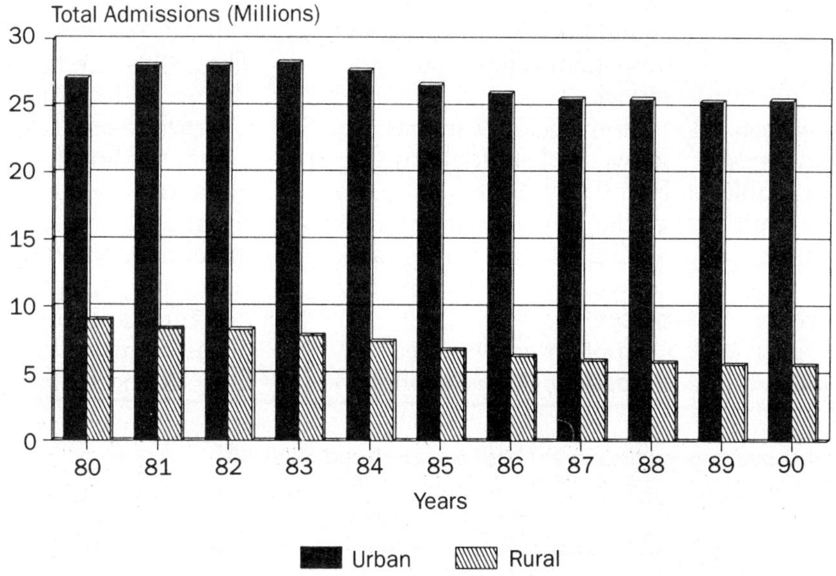

Figure 6 **Community Hospital Inpatient Days versus Outpatient Visits, 1980-90**

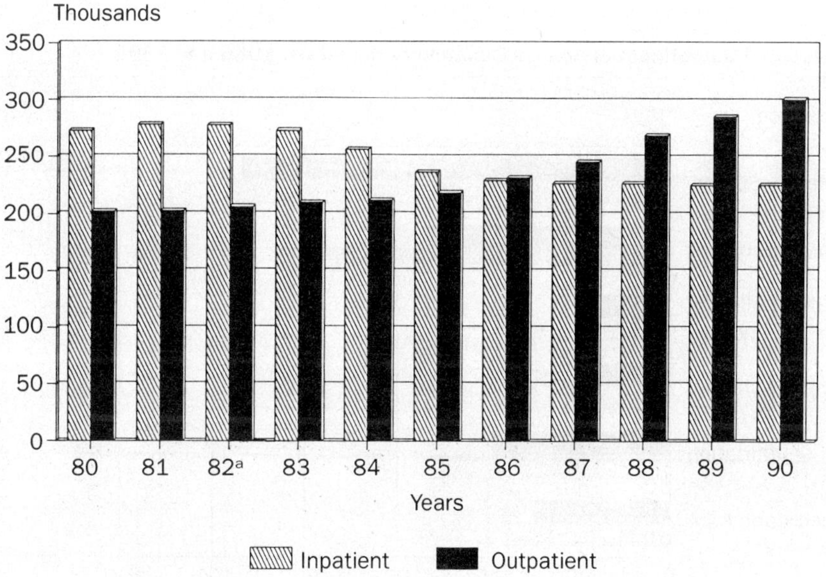

[a]Outpatient visit data for 1982 has been estimated using statistical techniques in order to compensate for a change in the reporting method for outpatient visits in 1982.

Trends In Health Care Services

Because of the shift towards more outpatient treatment as well as technological innovations, hospitals are also able to offer more types of procedures and treatments to their patients.

Outpatient Services

As established, there has been a surge in the number and types of outpatient services available. In 1985, more than half of all community hospitals offered outpatient departments to their communities. Just five years later, more than three-quarters of all community hospitals have an outpatient department (see figure 7).

Outpatient rehabilitation had also experienced significant growth. In 1985, the number of hospitals reporting outpatient rehabilitation services was 2,086. In 1990, that figure increased to 2,606. As a result , half (51.5 percent) of all community hospitals provide outpatient rehabilitation services.

Home health care has also showed substantial growth. Home health services are now available in almost 36 percent of all community hospitals compared to approximately 30 percent in 1985.

Another growth area in outpatient care is alcohol and chemical dependency treatment. In 1990, nearly one-fifth of community hospitals provide treatment for alcohol and drug abuse problems in their communities on an outpatient basis.

Emergency and Trauma Services

The 1980s also marked a change in the nature of emergency services offered. The number of hospitals equipped to handle emergency medical situations has been steadily increasing. Nearly all community hospitals (93.5 percent) have emergency departments staffed 24 hours a day (see text table 8).

Text Table 7 **Surgical Operations in Community Hospitals, 1980 and 1989-90**

	Number of Surgeries			Percent Change	Percent Change
	1980	1989	1990	1980-90	1989-90
Total surgical operations	18,767,666	21,340,280	21,914,868	16.8%	2.7%
Inpatient	15,714,062	10,989,409	10,844,916	– 31.0%	–1.3%
Outpatient	3,053,604	10,350,871	11,069,952	262.5%	6.9%

Figure 7 **Trends in Selected Outpatient Services in Community Hospitals, 1985 and 1990**

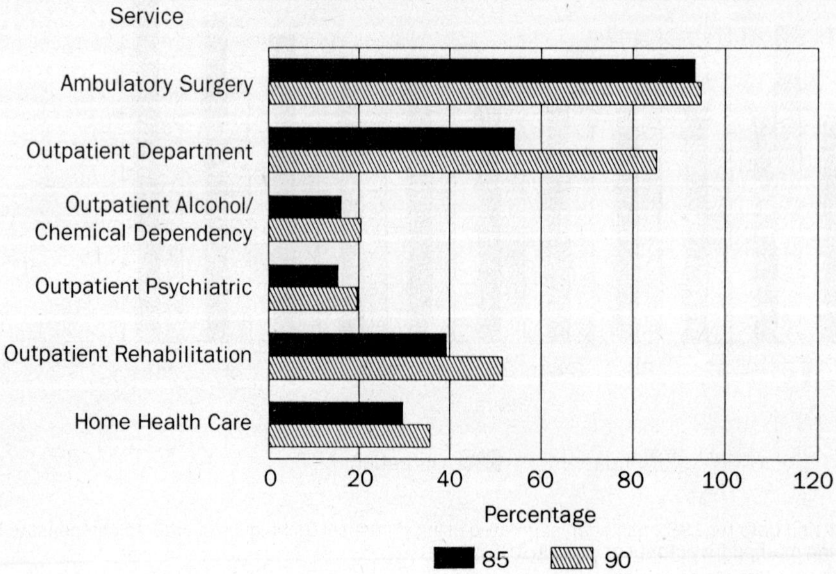

Text Table 8 **Trends in Selected Services of Community Hospitals, 1985 and 1989-90 (Number/Percentage of Reporting Hospitals with Selected Services)**

	1985		1989		1990	
	No. of Hospitals	Percent	No. of Hospitals	Percent	No. of Hospitals	Percent
Ambulatory surgery	4,961	93.4%	4,886	95.2%	4,788	94.7%
Birthing rooms	2,698	50.8%	3,351	65.3%	3,292	65.1%
Blood bank	3,910	73.6%	3,589	69.9%	3,493	69.1%
Emergency department	5,057	95.2%	4,846	94.4%	4,728	93.5%
Outpatient alcoholism/ chemical dependency	853	16.1%	1,037	20.2%	1,035	20.5%
Physical therapy	4,842	91.1%	4,338	84.5%	4,271	84.5%
Trauma care	1,097	20.6%	629	12.3%	651	12.9%
Volunteer services	3,765	70.9%	3,427	66.8%	3,427	67.8%
Outpatient rehabilitation	2,086	39.3%	2,501	48.7%	2,606	51.5%
Outpatient department	2,873	54.1%	4,153	80.9%	4,309	85.2%
Home health care	1,580	29.7%	1,784	34.7%	1,801	35.6%
Hospice	687	12.9%	804	15.7%	817	16.2%
Number of hospitals reporting	5,313		5,134		5,056	

Figure 8 **Long-Term Care Units in Community Hospitals, 1980-90**

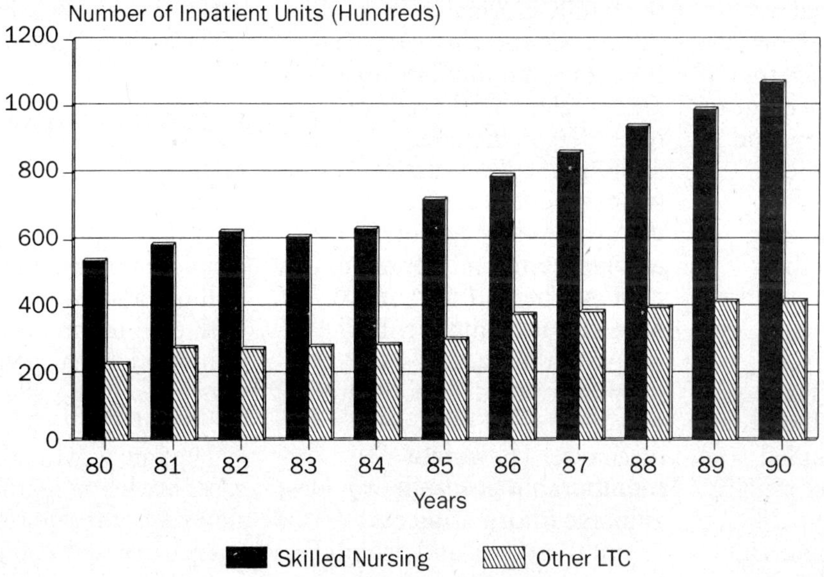

Trauma is one of the leading causes of death in the United States. The number of hospitals with trauma centers providing specialized intensive care to critically injured patients has increased slightly with 22 more state-certified trauma centers than 1989, stopping the downward trend that started in 1985. However, there are currently 446 fewer state-certified trauma centers operating than in 1985, representing a significant decrease over that time span[5]. This is in response to the high cost of operating trauma centers. Trauma care demands highly qualified medical personnel, state-of-the-art communications, and a strong emergency response team. Unfortunately, this specialized network is expensive. Annual operating costs can exceed $5 million.

Long-Term Care Services

Responding to the growth in the over 65 population and the number of children and disabled adults requiring long-term, nonacute care, hospitals have expanded their long-term care services. Ensuring sufficient and affordable long-term care services has been a prominent issue in Capitol Hill and will continue to be one of

Text Table 9 **Trends in Selected Geriatric Services of Community Hospitals, 1989-90 (Number/Percentage of Reporting Hospitals with Selected Services)**

	1989		1990	
	No. of Hospitals	Percent	No. of Hospitals	Percent
Adult day care program	332	6.5%	321	6.4%
Alzheimer's diagnostic/assessment services	373	7.3%	395	7.8%
Comprehensive geriatric assessment	928	18.1%	918	18.2%
Emergency response system	1,629	31.7%	1,776	35.1%
Geriatric acute care unit	526	10.2%	507	10.0%
Geriatric clinics	292	5.7%	320	6.3%
Respite care	800	15.6%	840	16.6%
Senior membership program	1,007	19.6%	1,142	22.6%
Geriatric services	2,937	57.2%	3,071	60.7%
Number of hospitals reporting	5,134		5,056	

the major health care challenges of the 1990s. Congress has considered a wide range of long-term care proposals, ranging from consumer, private, long-term care insurance to extending Medicare coverage to include home health care and nursing home care services.

A growing number of hospitals have separate long-term care units within the hospital providing physician services and continuous professional nursing supervision to patients not requiring acute care.. Today hospitals have more skilled nursing units and other long-term care units than in 1980. The number of skilled nursing units and other long-term care units have each increased by over 80 percent in the past 10 years (see figure 8).

Geriatric Services

Hospitals have developed a spectrum of services and programs to meet the needs of older adults in their communities. Eight such services are surveyed, each with a different focus.

Of the services listed, **adult day care** and **respite care** programs focus on supporting the family caregivers of an older person. Outpatient services that focus on examining the medical and psycho-social needs of the older person include **Alzheimer's diagnostic/ assessment services, comprehensive geriatric assessment,** and **geriatric clinics**. The **geriatric acute care unit** is an inpatient program that targets select hospitalized older people who may be at risk of delayed discharge. The **senior membership program** provides valuable information on hospital services and usually offers social activities and health/wellness programs to an older person. The **emergency response system** monitors the older person in his/her home, helping to link that individual to the hospital in case of an accident.

The number of hospitals offering these geriatric services has remained relatively stable. A few, like emergency response system and senior membership programs have shown a modest rise between 1989 and 1990. These two programs are also the most frequently reported geriatric services among the eight surveyed (see text table 9).

AIDS-Related Services

Nationwide, the number of persons diagnosed with AIDS exceeds 150,000 and it is estimated that as many as 1.5 million persons may be infected with the human immunodeficiency virus (HIV), many of which will develop full-blown AIDS.

The rate at which new AIDS cases are being reported has slowed. Total reported AIDS cases increased 220 percent from 1985 to 1987 compared to 135 percent from 1987 to 1989. AIDS is, however, present in every state. AIDS is also on the rise in smaller urban and rural areas.

Although homosexual and bisexual males account for more than half of the AIDS cases, the disease, at this time, is spreading most rapidly among women, children, and IV drug users and their sexual partners. Hospitals are playing a key role in the continuum of care for persons with AIDS or other symptoms of HIV infection, sometimes referred to as AIDS related complex (ARC).

When the first cases of AIDS were diagnosed in the late 1970s the disease was treated primarily on an inpatient basis. Although inpatient care is typically required during the first and last stages of the disease, more care in the interim is provided on an outpatient basis now. Health care needs are also being addressed through other community sources; home health care, hospice, and other services to AIDS and ARC patients. Through discharge planning and case management programs, hospitals can coordinate these outpatient services for their patients. With improvements in drug therapy, fewer days of hospitalization and more outpatient care, the cost of treating an AIDS patient has been reduced. Even with these reductions in costs, additional funding must become available to ease the burden on hospitals treating large numbers of AIDS patients.

Since 1988, the AHA Annual Survey of Hospitals has collected information on the specific types of hospital-based services available for AIDS and ARC patients. In 1990, 67.5 percent of hospitals provided general inpatient care for AIDS and ARC patients up from 64 percent in 1989. Also, in 1990, 5.7 percent of hospitals offered specialized outpatient programs for AIDS and ARC patients. Hospital-based services for AIDS patients are likely to continue to change as the promise of new drugs such as AZT and Pentamidine continue to advance the treatment of AIDS and required routine administration of intravenous medications or specialized physical or respiratory therapies continues (see text table 10).

In treating AIDS patients, hospitals are undertaking intensive efforts to educate their staffs on the risks of AIDS transmission and on minimizing those risks.

Evolving Medical Technologies

Technological advances have also contributed to the number of services available today. One of the most significant changes in medical technology is the growth in outpatient applications. Many new procedures and techniques are now available in settings outside the hospital. Less invasive procedures made possible by advances in radiology and surgery have made diagnosis and treatment of disease less traumatic for patients and have allowed more care to be provided in outpatient settings. It is likely that the 1990s will see an increase in cancer care being treated on an outpatient basis. The growing need for around-the-clock, ambulatory cancer care will reinforce the trend toward the establishment of outpatient cancer centers supported by home health services, including home infusion therapy. In addition, many nonhospital centers have been opened offering access to diagnostic and therapeutic units have also increased accessibility to cardiac catheterization, MRI, mammography, CT, ultrasound, nuclear medicine, and lithotripsy.

Readers should note that the AHA Annual Survey of Hospitals gathers the number of hospitals that provide certain types of services involving medical technologies such as MRI or CT scans, rather than the number of devices in hospitals. For example, data for 1990 show 955 community hospitals offering MRI services. This figure does not reflect those facilities owning more than one device, nor hospitals offering a particular service on site, but sharing the use of a mobile device. In addition, because MRI services (and others) are now available in many nonhospital settings, the number of hospitals offering these services represent only a

Text Table 10 **Selected AIDS-Related Services Provided by Community Hospitals, 1989-90**

	1989		1990	
	Hospitals	Percent	Hospitals	Percent
Hospital-based				
General inpatient care	3,285	64.0%	3,413	67.5%
AIDS/ARC unit	109	2.1%	109	2.2%
Specialized outpatient program	257	5.0%	290	5.7%
HIV testing	2,597	50.6%	2,794	55.3%
Number of hospitals reporting	5,134		5,056	

portion of the number of MRI units now available in the United States (see text table 11)

Cardiac

An area of advancement has been in the treatment, care and diagnosis of cardiac care patients. Open-heart surgery facilities are now available in 16.8 percent of all community hospitals compared to 15.7 percent in 1989 and 12.2 percent in 1985. In 1990, 20.6 percent of community hospitals performed angioplasties compared to 18.3 percent in 1989. Cardiac catheterizations facilities are now available in 27.5 percent of hospitals compared to 24.7 percent in 1989 and 18.4 percent in 1985.

In addition to the surgical procedures mentioned above, 54.4 percent of community hospitals offer diagnostic procedures such as Non-invasive cardiac assessment services; (EKG, cardiac nuclear medicine) and 40.0 percent of hospitals provide some type of Cardiac Rehabilitation programs.

Diagnostic and Therapeutic

One of the largest growth areas over the decade has been with CT scanners. In 1985, 2,947 community hospitals reported CT Scanner services. Dramatically, 1990 figures show 3,544 hospitals with CT scanner services available. Another technological evaluation method, magnetic resonance imaging (MRI) has shown a steady increase in use since introduction. Currently, 18.2 percent of community hospitals reported providing MRI service. A diagnostic treatment method showing steady growth over the 1980s is megavoltage radiation therapy with a 9.0 percent increase since 1985.

Recognition of the importance of chemical and metabolic information on the early and effective treatment of disease will encourage the growth of nuclear medicine. Specifically, the 1990s should see increased use of single photon emission tomography (SPECT) for cardiac and brain imaging. In 1990, 934 hospitals reported providing SPECT services.

Transplants

Another medical advancement experiencing significant growth is organ/tissue transplants. This includes both deceased and live organ/tissue donors. Over the past five years, the number of hospitals equipped with the necessary staff and equipment to perform organ/tissue transplants has more than doubled, growing from 259 in 1985 to 526 in 1990.

Personnel Trends

Changes in Staffing Levels

Hospitals employed 3.4 million full-time equivalent (FTE) employees in 1990, maintaining a relatively sustained level of hospital employment. The number of FTEs increased at 3.5 percent rate over the 1989 level. Trends in hospitals' use of FTEs have been unpredictable throughout the 1980s, rising through 1982, declining in 1983 through 1985 during the initial years of PPS, then

Text Table 11 Trends in Selected Medical Technologies Provided by Community Hospitals, 1985 and 1989-90 (Number/Percentage of Reporting Hospitals with Selected Medical Technology)

	1985		1989		1990	
	No. of Hospitals	Percent	No. of Hospitals	Percent	No. of Hospitals	Percent
Angioplasty	—	—	940	18.3%	1,040	20.6%
Cardiac catheterization	978	18.4%	1,269	24.7%	1,390	27.5%
Cardiac rehabilitation	—	—	—	—	2,024	40.0%
CT scanner	2,947	55.5%	3,433	66.9%	3,544	70.1%
Lithotripsy (ESWL)	48	0.9%	321	6.3%	319	6.3%
Magnetic resonance imaging (MRI)	—	—	772	15.0%	919	18.2%
Megavoltage radiation therapy	912	17.2%	980	19.1%	994	19.7%
Non-invasive cardiac assessment	—	—	—	—	2,748	54.4%
Open-heart surgery	650	12.2%	807	15.7%	847	16.8%
Organ transplantation	259	4.9%	489	9.5%	526	10.4%
Single photon emission computerized tomography (SPECT)	—	—	—	—	934	18.5%
Number of hospitals reporting	5,313		5,134		5,056	

increasing slightly the rest of the decade (see text table 12).

Staffing Mix

Regardless of changes in total staffing levels, some continual trends in staffing mix have developed. Hospitals have slowly been changing the mix of FTEs employed. Specifically, hospitals now employ more registered nurses and fewer licensed practical nurses. The percentage of physicians and dentists and other hospital personnel has remained fairly constant. Allied health professions are expected to grow most rapidly in the 1990s.

Average Salary and Benefits

Increases in average salary and benefits has maintained a steady growth trend. The average annual salary for a community hospital employee in 1990 was $26,590 compared to $24,816 in 1989. This 7.1 percent increase exceeded the 6.1 percent change in the consumer price index from 1989 to 1990.[6] As employers, hospitals provided an average of $5,318 fringe benefits for each employee, a 9.3 percent increase over average benefits provided in 1989 (see text table 13).

Noncommunity Hospital Distribution Trends

The AHA reports data for noncommunity hospitals separately as these hospitals, in general, care for patients requiring longer hospital stays. The noncommunity hospital category includes psychiatric hospitals, hospitals for tuberculosis and other respiratory diseases, chronic disease hospitals, institutions for the mentally retarded, alcoholism and chemical dependency hospitals, and other long-term hospitals and hospital units, including the various armed services hospitals, veteran's hospitals, and Indian Health Service facilities.

The total number of noncommunity hospitals for 1990 was 1,265 the same as in 1989. During the past 10 years, noncommunity hospitals have grown from 1,137 in 1980 to 1,265 in 1990, an increase of 11.2 percent. Psychiatric hospitals have led the increase in noncommunity hospitals during this time period.

The increase in nonfederal psychiatric hospitals was 2.1 percent from 741 in 1989 to 757 in 1990. The total number

Text Table 12 **Trends in FTE Personnel in Community Hospitals, 1989-90**

	Full-time Equivalent Personnel (000s)[a]			Full-time Equivalent Personnel per 100 Adjusted Census[b]		
	1989	1990	Percent Change* 1989-90	1989	1990	Percent Change* 1989-90
Total community hospitals	3,303	3,420	3.5%	415	421	1.3%
Urban community hospitals	2,776	2,868	3.3%	438	445	1.6%
Rural community hospitals	527	551	4.6%	326	328	0.6%
Bed-size category						
6-24 Beds	11	11	−1.1%	434	437	0.8%
25-49	86	90	4.6%	398	398	0.1%
50-99	238	245	2.9%	347	350	0.8%
100-199	566	582	2.8%	369	373	1.1%
200-299	630	645	2.3%	403	404	0.2%
300-399	524	547	4.4%	436	441	1.2%
400-499	371	409	10.3%	435	446	2.4%
500 or more	878	892	1.6%	467	478	2.3%

[a] Excludes medical and dental residents (and interns) and other trainees.
[b] Adjusted census figures available for community hospitals only.
*Percent changes are based on actual figures, not rounded.

Text Table 13 **Average Salary and Benefits of Employees in Community Hospitals, 1980 and 1989-90**

				Percent Change	
	1980	1989	1990	1980-90	1989-90
Average Annual Salary	$13,010	$24,816	$26,590	104.4%	7.1%
Average Annual Benefits	2,551	4,864	5,318	108.5%	9.3%

Text Table 14 Trends Among Noncommunity Hospitals, 1980 and 1990

	Hospitals		Beds (000s)		Admissions (000s)		Average Length of Stay (Days)	
	1980	1990	1980	1990	1980	1990	1980	1990
Federal hospitals	361	337	117	98	2,044	1,759	17	15
Nonfederal psychiatric hospitals	534	757	215	160	566	721	118	66
Nonfederal TB and other respiratory disease hospitals	11	4	2	0	8	2	48	62
Long-term								
General and other special	157	131	39	25	76	88	160	88
Short-term								
Units of institutions	74	36	4	2	55	22	10	19

of United States noncommunity hospitals remained the same in 1990 at 1,265 as was reported in 1989. The total number of noncommunity hospitals had been rising since 1983 after several decades of decline.

Although the number of facilities stay the same, the number of beds in noncommunity hospitals is decreasing. Beds in noncommunity hospitals totaled 285,000 in 1990 approximately 92,000 fewer than the 377,000 beds reported in 1980. Overall admissions have declined over the decade but was offset by increasing admissions in psychiatric hospitals (see text table 14).

Nonfederal Psychiatric Hospitals

The changes in psychiatric hospitals in the past decade have run counter to some of the trends in other noncommunity hospitals and are influencing the aggregate noncommunity hospital statistics. Psychiatric hospitals have increased in number by 223 in the past 10 years, and admissions over the 10 year period rose 27 percent.

Similar to trends in other hospitals, the number of psychiatric hospital beds has declined by approximately 55,000 beds. The average length of stay in psychiatric hospitals has also been significantly reduced, falling from 118 days in 1980 to 66 days in 1990, almost a 44 percent reduction.

Federal Hospitals

The next largest category of noncommunity hospitals is federal hospitals, which are owned and operated by the federal government. Federal hospitals have experienced a decline in number, from 361 in 1980 to 337 in 1990. During the past 10 years, the number of beds in federal hospitals was reduced 16 percent, and admissions declined by almost 14 percent to approximately 1.7 million. Compared to 1980 federal facilities admitted 285,000 fewer patients than in 1990. The average length of stay in federal hospitals has been reduced slightly, from 17 days in 1980 to 15 days in 1990.

Footnotes

[1]The American Hospital Association's *Environmental Assessment 91/92* formed the basis for the discussion of the environmental factors that faced the nations' hospitals in 1990. For more information about this publication, please call Deborah Reczynski at (312) 280-6162.

[2]U.S. Department of Commerce, Bureau of the Census, *Current Population Reports, Series P-60, No. 175, Poverty in the U.S., 1990*, Government Printing Office, 1991, Table 1, pp.15.

[3]This number reflects the sum of hospitals that were reported to have closed as of the end of December of each year. Some of these facilities may have reopened in a following calendar year. In addition, while no longer acute care facilities, may continue to provide other health care services.

[4]See Revenue under the "Definitions of Terms" section, page xxiii.

[5]In 1988, the AHA's definition of trauma care center was changed to include only state-certified trauma care centers. Some of the reduction in the number of hospitals with trauma care centers may be the result of this change.

[6]The Consumer Price Index (CPI) study is conducted by the United States Bureau of Labor Statistics. The CPI measures price changes over time in the goods and services purchased by consumers.

Tables

1-4

Notes

Table 1

Table 1 presents hospital utilization, personnel, and financial data for each year from 1946 to the present. Please refer to Table 1 in the *Guide Issue of Hospitals, J.A.H.A.*, August 1, 1965, pages 448 and 449, for comparable data for each year from 1946 through 1964, and to Table 1 in *AHA Hospital Statistics, 1982 Edition,* for 1965 through 1969.

Table 4

In the 1981 edition, tables 4A and 4B presented utilization data of short-term hospitals and short-term units in hospitals, and long-term hospitals and long-term units in hospitals, respectively, by classification.

In the 1982 edition, tables 4A and 4B presented data on hospital units and nursing-home-type units operated by hospitals and community hospitals, respectively.

In the 1983 edition, two tables were added and the data presented as follows: Tables 4A and 4C presented data on the utilization, personnel, and finances in hospital units and nursing-home-type units operated by hospitals, by classification. Tables 4B and 4D presented data on the utilization, personnel, and finances in hospital units and nursing-home-type units operated by community hospitals, by state. For a definition of nursing-home-type unit, see "Definitions of Terms," p. xxiii.

Table

1

Trends in Utilization, Personnel, and Finances for Selected Years from 1946 through 1990

Data are for all AHA-registered hospitals in the United States. Data are estimated for nonreporting hospitals with the exception of newborn and outpatient data before 1972. Personnel data exclude residents, interns, and students from 1952 on; personnel data include full-time personnel and full-time equivalents for part-time personnel from 1954 on. As a result of the AHA Annual Survey validation process, the New York state expense data for 1976 were revised after the 1977 edition was published. The revised figures are included below. In order to provide trend data on a consistent basis, the 1970 and 1971 psychiatric and long-term data have been slightly modified. The 1982 FTE figures have been updated to provide the most accurate data possible.

CLASSIFICATION	YEAR	HOSPITALS	BEDS (in thousands)	ADMISSIONS (in thousands)	AVERAGE DAILY CENSUS (in thousands)	ADJUSTED AVERAGE DAILY CENSUS (in thousands)	OCCUPANCY, percent	AVERAGE LENGTH OF STAY, days	OUTPATIENT VISITS (in thousands)	NEWBORNS		FTE PERSONNEL		EXPENSES					
														LABOR			TOTAL		
										Bassinets	Births	Number (in thousands)	Per 100 Adjusted Census	PAYROLL Amount (in millions of dollars)	EMPLOYEE BENEFITS Amount (in millions of dollars)	Adjusted, per Inpatient Day (dollars)	Amount (in millions of dollars)	Adjusted, per Inpatient Stay (dollars)	Adjusted, per Inpatient Day (dollars)
Total United States	1946	6,125	1,436	15,675	1,142		79.5			85,585	2,135,327	830		$ 1,103			$ 1,963		
	1950	6,788	1,456	18,483	1,253		86.0			90,101	2,742,780	1,058		2,191			3,651		
	1955	6,956	1,604	21,073	1,363		85.0			98,823	3,476,753	1,301		3,582			5,594		
	1960	6,876	1,658	25,027	1,402		84.6			102,764	3,835,735	1,598		5,588			8,421		
	1965	7,123	1,704	28,812	1,403		82.3		125,793	101,287	3,565,344	1,952		8,551			12,948		
	1970	7,123	1,616	31,759	1,298		80.3		181,370	97,128	3,537,000	2,537		15,706			25,556		
	1971	7,097	1,556	32,664	1,237		79.5		199,725	94,344	3,464,513	2,589		17,635	$ 1,531		28,812		
	1972	7,061	1,550	33,265	1,209		78.0		219,182	92,960	3,231,875	2,671		19,530	1,925		32,667		
	1973	7,123	1,535	34,352	1,189		77.5		233,555	90,071	3,087,210	2,769		21,330	2,238		36,290		
	1974	7,174	1,513	35,506	1,167		77.2		250,481	88,269	3,043,386	2,919		23,821	2,611		41,406		
	1975	7,156	1,466	36,157	1,125		76.7		254,844	86,875	3,091,629	3,023		27,135	3,175		48,706		
	1976	7,082	1,434	36,776	1,090		76.0		270,951	85,284	3,067,063	3,108		30,438	3,848		56,005		
	1977	7,099	1,407	37,060	1,066		75.8		263,775	83,193	3,223,699	3,213		33,742	4,691		63,630		
	1978	7,015	1,381	37,243	1,042		75.5		263,606	80,650	3,250,373	3,280		37,196	5,378		70,927		
	1979	6,988	1,372	37,802	1,043		76.1		262,009	79,720	3,376,467	3,382		41,464	6,155		79,796		
	1980	6,965	1,365	38,892	1,060		77.7		262,951	79,842	3,500,043	3,492		46,970	7,221		91,886		
	1981	6,933	1,362	39,169	1,061		77.9		265,332	78,823	3,558,274	3,661		54,516	8,738		107,146		
	1982	6,915	1,360	39,095	1,053		77.4		313,667	77,998	3,615,751	3,746		62,015	10,420		123,219		
	1983	6,888	1,350	38,887	1,028		76.1		273,168	77,837	3,596,146	3,707		67,742	12,036		136,315		
	1984	6,872	1,339	37,938	970		72.5		276,566	77,845	3,563,106	3,630		71,007	13,005		144,114		
	1985	6,872	1,318	36,304	910		69.0		282,140	77,202	3,630,961	3,625		74,387	13,875		153,327		
	1986	6,841	1,290	35,219	883		68.4		294,634	76,002	3,680,178	3,647		78,589	14,400		165,194		
	1987	6,821	1,267	34,439	873		68.9		310,707	74,770	3,698,294	3,742		83,778	15,318		178,662		
	1988	6,780	1,248	34,107	863		69.2		336,208	72,568	3,794,369	3,839		91,841	16,990		196,704		
	1989	6,720	1,226	33,742	853		69.6		352,248	71,491	3,920,384	3,937		99,256	19,375		214,886		
	1990	6,649	1,213	33,774	844		69.5		368,184	70,539	4,046,704	4,063		108,719	21,797		234,870		
Federal	1946	404	236	1,593	166		70.3			2,376	37,273	162		247			373		
	1950	414	189	1,284	152		80.4			2,625	63,133	169		520			712		
	1955	428	183	1,415	157		85.8			4,070	157,197	192		666			837		
	1960	435	177	1,476	154		87.2			4,097	148,232	186		921			1,134		
	1965	443	174	1,640	150		86.1		30,393	4,170	145,098	199		1,264			1,568		
	1970	408	161	1,741	128		79.6		42,913	3,834	128,943	216		1,751			2,483		
	1971	407	148	1,788	123		83.2		46,504	3,796	126,228	225		1,962	133		2,821		
	1972	401	143	1,770	114		80.0		46,095	3,589	112,216	232		2,132	166		3,148		
	1973	397	142	1,865	112		79.0		47,948	3,202	100,013	238		2,384	179		3,524		
	1974	387	136	1,841	109		80.7		48,682	3,037	95,937	244		2,651	204		3,971		
	1975	382	132	1,913	107		80.7		51,957	3,018	92,971	256		2,928	244		4,540		
	1976	380	129	1,998	102		79.3		56,168	2,953	104,745	269		3,415	291		5,313		
	1977	377	124	2,018	98		79.6		53,142	2,949	105,897	278		3,949	325		6,163		
	1978	370	122	1,997	96		78.4		50,353	2,553	93,795	277		4,288	399		6,732		
	1979	361	117	1,986	92		78.2		51,239	2,440	89,302	273		4,566	424		7,266		
	1980	359	117	2,044	94		80.1		50,566	2,297	91,332	279		4,927	457		7,869		
	1981	348	116	2,032	91		79.0		52,555	2,246	92,561	283		5,380	502		8,606		
	1982	346	114	2,014	90		79.4		56,068	2,251	100,990	297		5,849	536		9,506		
	1983	342	113	2,055	91		80.5		52,317	2,358	105,517	286		6,460	673		10,679		
	1984	341	112	2,074	89		79.0		53,813	2,255	106,612	290		6,863	729		11,156		
	1985	343	112	2,103	85		76.3		52,342	2,269	108,400	299		7,624	776		12,335		
	1986	342	111	2,117	82		74.1		53,651	2,312	95,628	296		7,941	815		13,133		
	1987	342	110	2,085	81		73.7		55,558	2,252	95,868	297		8,198	964		13,668		
	1988	342	105	1,862	77		73.2		57,353	2,205	87,616	295		8,668	1,199		14,601		
	1989	340	101	1,811	74		73.4		56,987	2,049	89,313	288		8,699	1,307		15,091		
	1990	337	98	1,759	72		72.9		58,527	2,063	85,808	303		8,743	1,493		15,244		

Table 1 (Continued)

CLASSIFICATION	YEAR	HOSPITALS	BEDS (in thousands)	ADMISSIONS (in thousands)	AVERAGE DAILY CENSUS (in thousands)	ADJUSTED AVERAGE DAILY CENSUS (in thousands)	OCCUPANCY, percent	AVERAGE LENGTH OF STAY, days	OUTPATIENT VISITS (in thousands)	NEWBORNS Bassinets	NEWBORNS Births	FTE PERSONNEL Number (in thousands)	FTE PERSONNEL Per 100 Adjusted Census	EXPENSES LABOR PAYROLL Amount (in millions of dollars)	EXPENSES LABOR EMPLOYEE BENEFITS Amount (in millions of dollars)	EXPENSES LABOR Adjusted, per Inpatient Day (dollars)	EXPENSES TOTAL Amount (in millions of dollars)	EXPENSES TOTAL Adjusted, per Inpatient Stay (dollars)	EXPENSES TOTAL Adjusted, per Inpatient Day (dollars)
Nonfederal psychiatric	1946	476	568	202	517		91.0			414	656	99		$ 152			$ 262		
	1950	533	620	293	607		97.9			234	820	147		305			539		
	1955	542	707	312	677		95.8			119	326	188		537			923		
	1960	488	722	362	672		93.1			137	392	238		848			1,205		
	1965	483	685	491	607		88.6		1,003	105	364	274		1,241			1,662		
	1970	519	527	598	447		84.8		2,740	57	211	305		1,997			2,712		
	1971	513	469	602	393		83.8		2,988	32	87	285		2,077	$ 171		2,803		
	1972	529	457	585	378		82.8		4,139	30	79	307		2,312	223		3,134		
	1973	543	422	588	342		81.1		4,611	12	66	303		2,465	259		3,351		
	1974	543	383	595	307		80.0		5,240	20	57	308		2,669	304		3,708		
	1975	544	330	604	265		80.3		5,287	19	29	292		2,788	379		3,997		
	1976	528	291	598	230		79.1		5,496	19	12	285		2,887	413		4,175		
	1977	541	261	587	211		80.7		5,018	13	46	287		3,025	512		4,494		
	1978	526	235	580	190		80.9		5,602	5	8	278		3,174	537		4,723		
	1979	527	224	567	187		83.2		5,614	3	6	282		3,460	588		5,136		
	1980	534	215	566	183		85.2		4,630	1	10	275		3,826	714		5,791		
	1981	549	202	558	174		85.9		4,976	0	4	275		4,154	823		6,415		
	1982	558	195	568	168		86.1		5,392	0	0	277		4,474	874		7,047		
	1983	564	185	552	160		86.5		5,713	0	0	264		4,707	956		7,442		
	1984	579	175	578	151		86.3		5,206	0	0	260		4,819	1,025		7,699		
	1985	610	171	602	147		85.9		4,902	0	0	263		5,150	1,183		8,344		
	1986	634	167	607	143		85.7		5,427	0	1	263		5,540	1,285		9,120		
	1987	684	166	638	142		85.6		5,856	0	0	269		5,878	1,350		9,883		
	1988	726	166	688	140		84.6		5,623	0	1	281		6,532	1,425		10,855		
	1989	741	161	707	136		84.2		5,462	0	0	284		7,048	1,639		12,049		
	1990	757	160	721	130		81.1		5,398	5	177	280		7,429	1,728		12,905		
Non federal tuberculosis and other respiratory diseases	1946	412	75	85	55		73.3			510	1,733	36		48			91		
	1950	398	72	79	62		86.1			12	125	45		91			162		
	1955	347	70	87	56		80.0			104	5,245	48		133			208		
	1960	238	52	68	39		75.4			11	172	39		128			192		
	1965	178	37	52	26		70.0		489	8	78	29		116			165		
	1970	101	20	36	12		61.8		784	6	31	18		107			152		
	1971	94	18	34	11		60.7		790	7	8	16		106	11		153		
	1972	72	13	28	8		61.2		454	4	11	12		82	8		119		
	1973	63	10	26	6		61.9		429	0	6	11		78	8		114		
	1974	46	8	21	5		63.2		91	0	0	9		69	8		102		
	1975	36	6	17	3		57.7		100	0	3	7		58	7		93		
	1976	21	4	12	2		57.8		75	0	0	5		41	6		64		
	1977	19	3	12	2		60.4		35	0	0	5		44	7		70		
	1978	15	3	11	2		59.9		104	0	0	4		42	8		68		
	1979	12	2	8	1		61.8		34	0	0	3		38	7		62		
	1980	11	2	8	1		67.0		54	0	0	3		37	7		63		
	1981	11	2	8	1		66.5		44	0	0	3		40	8		67		
	1982	10	1	8	1		62.3		44	0	0	3		38	8		68		
	1983	8	1	7	1		67.5		43	0	0	2		34	9		62		
	1984	7	1	6	1		63.4		43	0	0	2		30	8		58		
	1985	7	1	6	1		64.1		35	0	0	2		37	10		72		
	1986	4	0	4	0		59.0		21	0	0	1		18	5		37		
	1987	5	1	3	0		63.0		20	0	0	1		21	6		42		
	1988	4	0	2	0		68.0		15	0	0	1		18	5		35		
	1989	4	0	2	0		70.3		17	0	0	1		20	5		38		
	1990	4	0	2	0		66.4		17	0	0	1		26	6		50		

Table **1** (Continued)

Trends in Utilization, Personnel, and Finances for Selected Years from 1946 through 1990

Data are for all AHA-registered hospitals in the United States. Data are estimated for nonreporting hospitals with the exception of newborn and outpatient data before 1972. Personnel data exclude residents, interns, and students from 1952 on; personnel data include full-time personnel and full-time equivalents for part-time personnel from 1954 on. As a result of the 1989 Annual Survey validation process, the New York state expense data for 1976 were revised after the 1977 edition was published. The revised figures are included below. In order to provide trend data on a consistent basis, the 1970 and 1971 psychiatric and long-term data have been slightly modified. The 1982 FTE figures have been updated to provide the most accurate data possible.

										NEWBORNS		FTE PERSONNEL		EXPENSES					
														LABOR			TOTAL		
CLASSIFICATION	YEAR	HOSPITALS	BEDS (in thousands)	ADMISSIONS (in thousands)	AVERAGE DAILY CENSUS (in thousands)	ADJUSTED AVERAGE DAILY CENSUS (in thousands)	OCCUPANCY, percent	AVERAGE LENGTH OF STAY, days	OUTPATIENT VISITS (in thousands)	Bassinets	Births	Number (in thousands)	Per 100 Adjusted Census	PAYROLL Amount (in millions of dollars)	EMPLOYEE BENEFITS Amount (in millions of dollars)	Adjusted, per Inpatient Day (dollars)	Amount (in millions of dollars)	Adjusted, per Inpatient Stay (dollars)	Adjusted, per Inpatient Day (dollars)
Nonfederal long-term general and other special	1946	389	83	139	63		75.9			1,298	8,162	28		$ 38			$ 68		
	1950	412	70	164	60		85.7			1,211	17,720	34		72			117		
	1955	402	76	158	65		85.5			662	9,534	47		128			192		
	1960	308	67	151	58		86.9			392	8,888	55		192			273		
	1965	283	66	166	56		85.3		1,277	222	6,434	65		287			406		
	1970	236	60	132	49		82.0		1,389	152	4,751	69		431			649		
	1971	218	54	97	45		83.4		1,020	65	585	63		438	$ 40		636		
	1972	216	54	106	45		83.0		1,511	22	123	63		485	52		718		
	1973	229	57	112	47		82.1		1,629	6	36	67		536	60		805		
	1974	221	54	106	45		82.5		1,630	4	50	69		571	65		873		
	1975	215	51	103	42		82.1		1,189	4	36	68		611	76		966		
	1976	197	49	100	40		82.7		1,487	5	1	66		657	86		1,051		
	1977	189	45	89	38		84.3		1,342	3	0	63		662	103		1,071		
	1978	169	41	80	35		84.0		1,085	2	0	58		658	106		1,056		
	1979	165	40	81	35		86.1		1,249	0	2	61		702	118		1,148		
	1980	157	39	76	33		85.9		949	5	2	56		722	129		1,193		
	1981	146	35	77	30		86.2		1,028	10	26	61		799	135		1,318		
	1982	138	34	76	30		87.9		1,274	8	0	59		888	170		1,503		
	1983	131	30	73	26		86.5		1,100	8	0	53		894	176		1,500		
	1984	131	30	78	27		88.7		1,030	3	27	54		975	202		1,651		
	1985	128	31	92	27		88.1		2,087	34	1,265	58		1,088	243		1,876		
	1986	133	30	81	27		88.8		1,264	2	19	56		1,171	255		1,997		
	1987	131	28	79	25		87.2		1,569	2	10	55		1,214	254		2,159		
	1988	129	27	75	24		87.3		1,780	2	4	54		1,283	269		2,271		
	1989	138	28	81	24		85.5		1,874	6	20	56		1,379	331		2,504		
	1990	131	25	88	21		85.6		1,551	28	2,073	55		1,519	362		2,744		
Total nonfederal short-term general and other special	1946	4,444	473	13,655	341		72.1	9.1		80,987	2,087,503	505		619			1,169		
	1950	5,031	505	16,663	372		73.7	8.1		86,019	2,660,982	662		1,203			2,120		
	1955	5,237	568	19,100	407		71.5	7.8		93,868	3,304,451	826		2,117			3,434		
(These data are totals of the data in the next three classifications)	1960	5,407	639	22,970	477		74.7	7.6		98,127	3,678,051	1,080		3,499			5,617		
	1965	5,736	741	26,463	563	620	76.0	7.8	92,631	96,782	3,413,370	1,386	224	5,644			9,147	$ 316.37	$ 40.56
	1970	5,859	848	29,252	662	727	78.0	8.2	133,545	93,079	3,403,064	1,929	265	11,421			19,560	604.59	73.73
	1971	5,865	867	30,142	665	736	76.7	8.0	148,423	90,444	3,337,605	1,999	272	13,053	1,176	$ 53.10	22,400	667.44	83.43
	1972	5,843	884	30,777	664	739	75.2	7.9	166,983	89,315	3,119,446	2,056	278	14,519	1,476	59.24	25,549	747.42	94.61
	1973	5,891	903	31,761	681	768	75.4	7.8	178,939	86,851	2,987,089	2,149	280	15,867	1,731	62.86	28,496	793.88	101.78
	1974	5,977	931	32,943	701	793	75.3	7.8	194,838	85,208	2,947,342	2,289	289	17,861	2,030	68.76	32,751	883.04	113.21
	1975	5,979	947	33,519	708	806	74.8	7.7	196,311	83,834	2,998,590	2,399	298	20,749	2,469	79.00	39,110	1,024.72	133.08
	1976	5,956	961	34,068	715	816	74.4	7.7	207,725	82,307	2,962,305	2,483	304	23,437	3,053	88.08	45,402	1,172.25	152.24
	1977	5,973	974	34,353	717	820	73.6	7.6	204,238	80,228	3,117,756	2,581	315	26,062	3,743	99.63	51,832	1,316.70	173.25
	1978	5,935	980	34,575	720	825	73.5	7.6	204,461	78,090	3,156,570	2,662	323	29,034	4,329	110.82	58,348	1,470.13	193.81
	1979	5,923	988	35,160	729	841	73.8	7.6	203,873	77,277	3,287,157	2,762	328	32,699	5,018	122.95	66,184	1,631.16	215.75
	1980	5,904	992	36,198	748	861	75.4	7.6	206,752	77,539	3,408,699	2,879	334	37,460	5,914	137.74	76,970	1,844.19	244.44
	1981	5,879	1,007	36,494	764	876	75.9	7.6	206,729	76,567	3,465,683	3,039	347	44,142	7,271	160.88	90,739	2,167.70	283.94
	1982	5,863	1,015	36,429	763	882	75.2	7.6	250,888	75,739	3,514,761	3,110	353	50,767	8,832	185.26	105,094	2,493.09	326.68
	1983	5,843	1,021	36,201	750	869	73.4	7.6	213,995	75,471	3,490,629	3,102	357	55,648	10,222	207.84	116,632	2,775.55	368.01
	1984	5,814	1,020	35,202	703	824	68.9	7.3	216,474	75,587	3,456,467	3,023	367	58,319	11,042	230.09	123,550	2,984.00	409.85
	1985	5,784	1,003	33,501	650	780	64.8	7.1	222,773	74,899	3,521,296	3,003	385	60,487	11,663	253.70	130,700	3,238.94	459.57
	1986	5,728	982	32,410	631	774	64.2	7.1	234,270	73,688	3,584,530	3,032	392	63,919	12,040	269.10	140,907	3,529.60	499.19
	1987	5,659	961	31,633	624	780	64.9	7.2	247,704	72,516	3,602,416	3,120	400	68,468	12,743	285.18	152,909	3,848.79	536.96
	1988	5,579	949	31,480	622	795	65.5	7.2	271,436	70,361	3,706,748	3,209	404	75,340	14,093	307.61	168,941	4,194.39	581.08
	1989	5,497	936	31,141	619	805	66.2	7.3	287,909	69,436	3,831,051	3,307	411	82,110	16,093	334.37	185,204	4,572.23	630.59
	1990	5,420	929	31,203	620	820	66.8	7.3	302,691	68,443	3,958,646	3,423	417	91,001	18,208	364.97	203,927	4,929.93	681.52

Table 1 (Continued)

CLASSIFICATION	YEAR	HOSPITALS	BEDS (in thousands)	ADMISSIONS (in thousands)	AVERAGE DAILY CENSUS (in thousands)	ADJUSTED AVERAGE DAILY CENSUS (in thousands)	OCCUPANCY, percent	AVERAGE LENGTH OF STAY, days	OUTPATIENT VISITS (in thousands)	NEWBORNS: Bassinets	NEWBORNS: Births	FTE PERSONNEL: Number (in thousands)	FTE PERSONNEL: Per 100 Adjusted Census	EXPENSES – LABOR: PAYROLL Amount (in millions of dollars)	EXPENSES – LABOR: EMPLOYEE BENEFITS Amount (in millions of dollars)	EXPENSES – LABOR: Adjusted, per Inpatient Day (dollars)	EXPENSES – TOTAL: Amount (in millions of dollars)	EXPENSES – TOTAL: Adjusted, per Inpatient Stay (dollars)	EXPENSES – TOTAL: Adjusted, per Inpatient Day (dollars)
Nongovernment not-for-profit short-term general and other special	1946	2,584	301	9,554	231		76.7	8.8		59,254	1,596,127	362		$ 431			$ 848		
	1950	2,871	332	11,629	247		74.4	7.7		62,465	2,010,434	473		848			1,523		
	1955	3,097	389	13,875	285		73.0	7.5		68,024	2,483,013	597		1,533			2,508		
	1960	3,291	446	16,788	341		76.6	7.4		71,689	2,748,229	792		2,561			4,139		
	1965	3,426	515	19,001	401		77.8	7.7	59,233	69,971	2,508,879	1,011		4,088			6,643		
	1970	3,386	592	20,948	474	518	80.1	8.2	90,992	64,910	2,491,938	1,387	268	8,340			14,163	$ 614.51	$ 74.94
	1971	3,363	604	21,515	477	523	79.0	8.1	103,016	63,346	2,445,819	1,438	275	9,532	$ 847	$ 54.43	16,344	693.20	85.58
	1972	3,326	617	21,875	478	527	77.4	8.0	112,039	62,016	2,242,747	1,474	280	10,494	1,066	59.93	18,384	762.40	95.30
	1973	3,320	629	22,488	489	545	77.8	7.9	120,273	60,325	2,134,201	1,535	282	11,442	1,249	63.80	20,418	810.86	102.64
	1974	3,381	650	23,374	506	568	77.8	7.9	131,394	58,877	2,113,205	1,634	288	12,858	1,458	69.15	23,494	896.57	113.49
	1975	3,364	659	23,735	510	575	77.4	7.8	132,368	57,496	2,131,057	1,714	298	14,961	1,760	79.71	27,965	1,039.82	133.31
	1976	3,368	671	24,098	517	586	77.1	7.9	141,781	56,448	2,100,994	1,793	306	17,157	2,223	90.36	32,796	1,208.07	152.92
	1977	3,371	680	24,284	519	589	76.3	7.8	139,045	54,902	2,197,940	1,863	316	19,138	2,698	101.62	37,523	1,362.19	174.64
	1978	3,360	684	24,443	521	594	76.1	7.8	142,617	53,417	2,219,710	1,927	324	21,337	3,141	112.99	42,262	1,513.58	195.07
	1979	3,350	690	24,885	528	604	76.5	7.7	140,525	52,865	2,308,669	2,000	331	24,043	3,608	125.62	47,969	1,681.70	217.93
	1980	3,339	693	25,576	542	621	78.2	7.7	142,864	52,665	2,389,604	2,087	336	27,652	4,254	140.44	55,815	1,900.40	245.67
	1981	3,356	706	25,955	555	636	78.5	7.8	143,953	52,308	2,455,208	2,213	348	32,785	5,281	164.01	66,288	2,223.39	285.61
	1982	3,354	712	25,908	554	633	77.8	7.8	176,838	51,572	2,483,516	2,266	355	37,775	6,403	189.93	76,850	2,570.80	330.40
	1983	3,363	718	25,837	544	628	75.8	7.7	151,444	51,655	2,465,781	2,272	361	41,554	7,463	213.76	85,675	2,865.06	373.62
	1984	3,366	717	25,246	512	598	71.4	7.4	153,928	51,497	2,446,699	2,223	371	43,614	8,079	236.17	90,883	3,072.45	415.23
	1985	3,364	708	24,188	476	570	67.2	7.2	160,002	51,430	2,507,449	2,217	389	45,242	8,578	258.92	96,239	3,308.28	463.00
	1986	3,338	690	23,492	461	563	66.8	7.2	168,284	50,891	2,547,292	2,242	398	47,784	8,841	275.37	103,581	3,558.16	503.73
	1987	3,289	673	22,946	455	556	67.6	7.2	178,089	50,139	2,557,414	2,299	406	51,113	9,242	291.99	112,397	3,911.98	543.75
	1988	3,256	668	22,946	456	577	68.2	7.3	195,864	48,864	2,654,140	2,374	411	56,477	10,231	315.95	124,770	4,267.14	590.95
	1989	3,233	661	22,798	455	585	68.8	7.3	209,641	48,336	2,751,862	2,455	420	61,815	11,747	344.86	136,941	4,638.20	641.99
	1990	3,202	657	22,883	455	597	69.3	7.3	221,175	47,472	2,833,587	2,534	425	68,467	13,345	375.61	150,693	4,995.12	691.86
Investor-owned (for-profit) short-term general and other special	1946	1,076	39	1,408	25		64.1	6.6		9,254	214,363	35		47			94		
	1950	1,218	42	1,661	26		61.9	5.6		9,607	230,816	41		72			143		
	1955	1,020	37	1,459	22		59.5	5.6		7,771	206,152	41		91			174		
	1960	856	37	1,550	24		65.4	5.7		6,537	187,703	48		143			275		
	1965	857	47	1,844	32		68.6	6.3	3,437	5,207	145,164	70		260			510		
	1970	769	53	2,031	38	41	72.2	6.8	4,698	4,415	145,491	97	238	546			1,068	485.52	71.40
	1971	750	54	2,088	38	41	71.0	6.6	4,858	3,831	125,852	100	245	612	54	45.08	1,214	537.50	81.44
	1972	738	57	2,161	39	42	68.7	6.6	7,842	3,967	126,945	105	249	697	65	49.79	1,407	606.61	91.91
	1973	757	63	2,334	43	47	68.3	6.7	7,593	3,916	129,139	117	249	799	83	51.96	1,689	665.91	99.39
	1974	775	70	2,553	47	52	67.5	6.7	8,667	3,892	127,192	133	257	952	105	56.21	2,046	729.30	108.85
	1975	775	73	2,646	48	53	65.9	6.6	7,713	4,062	141,392	139	263	1,114	131	64.56	2,561	876.48	132.80
	1976	752	76	2,734	50	54	64.8	6.6	8,048	4,044	144,751	147	272	1,276	156	72.54	3,085	1,031.91	156.35
	1977	751	80	2,849	52	57	64.6	6.6	8,355	4,140	160,248	159	279	1,492	207	81.95	3,669	1,168.13	176.99
	1978	732	81	2,880	52	57	63.8	6.5	8,911	4,122	166,499	165	290	1,651	237	91.38	4,180	1,318.60	202.36
	1979	727	83	2,963	53	59	63.9	6.6	9,289	4,110	174,843	174	297	1,930	306	104.78	4,820	1,477.33	225.87
	1980	730	87	3,165	57	62	65.2	6.5	9,696	4,439	199,722	189	304	2,319	354	117.45	5,847	1,676.75	257.12
	1981	729	88	3,239	58	63	66.4	6.5	9,961	4,523	207,405	203	322	2,769	449	140.32	6,856	1,952.56	299.02
	1982	748	91	3,316	60	66	65.5	6.6	13,193	4,736	219,675	212	320	3,250	580	159.24	8,177	2,224.75	340.03
	1983	757	94	3,299	59	66	63.1	6.5	10,389	5,039	228,883	213	323	3,631	703	181.44	9,208	2,517.53	385.42
	1984	786	100	3,314	57	64	57.0	6.3	11,090	5,807	242,088	214	334	3,985	777	203.59	10,251	2,748.51	438.30
	1985	805	104	3,242	54	63	52.1	6.1	12,378	6,117	266,839	221	350	4,338	852	226.14	11,486	3,033.06	500.48
	1986	834	107	3,231	54	65	50.7	6.1	14,896	6,305	291,112	229	354	4,641	885	235.03	12,987	3,341.79	552.40
	1987	828	106	3,157	54	66	51.1	6.2	16,566	6,391	306,492	242	367	5,029	984	250.04	14,067	3,617.19	585.01
	1988	790	104	3,090	53	66	50.9	6.2	17,926	6,254	308,828	249	379	5,527	1,128	277.97	15,545	4,022.77	649.33
	1989	769	102	3,071	53	67	51.7	6.3	19,341	6,354	325,711	261	390	6,064	1,312	302.88	17,240	4,406.20	707.90
	1990	749	101	3,066	53	69	52.8	6.4	20,110	6,261	340,555	273	397	6,732	1,493	328.44	18,822	4,727.27	751.55

Table 1 (Continued)

Trends in Utilization, Personnel, and Finances for Selected Years from 1946 through 1990

Data are for all AHA-registered hospitals in the United States. Data are estimated for nonreporting hospitals with the exception of newborn and outpatient data before 1972. Personnel data exclude residents, interns, and students from 1952 on; personnel data include full-time personnel and full-time equivalents for part-time personnel from 1954 on. As a result of the AHA Annual Survey validation process, the New York state expense data for 1976 were revised after the 1977 edition was published. The revised figures are included below. In order to provide trend data on a consistent basis, the 1970 and 1971 psychiatric and long-term data have been slightly modified. The 1982 FTE figures have been updated to provide the most accurate data possible.

CLASSIFICATION	YEAR	HOSPITALS	BEDS (in thousands)	ADMISSIONS (in thousands)	AVERAGE DAILY CENSUS (in thousands)	ADJUSTED AVERAGE DAILY CENSUS (in thousands)	OCCUPANCY, percent	AVERAGE LENGTH OF STAY, days	OUTPATIENT VISITS (in thousands)	NEWBORNS: Bassinets	NEWBORNS: Births	FTE PERSONNEL: Number (in thousands)	FTE PERSONNEL: Per 100 Adjusted Census	EXPENSES, LABOR: PAYROLL Amount (in millions of dollars)	EXPENSES, LABOR: EMPLOYEE BENEFITS Amount (in millions of dollars)	EXPENSES, LABOR: Adjusted, per Inpatient Day (dollars)	EXPENSES, TOTAL: Amount (in millions of dollars)	EXPENSES, TOTAL: Adjusted, per Inpatient Stay (dollars)	EXPENSES, TOTAL: Adjusted, per Inpatient Day (dollars)
State and local government short-term general and other special	1946	785	133	2,694	84		63.2	11.4		12,479	277,013	108		$ 140			$ 227		
	1950	942	131	3,374	99		75.6	10.7		13,947	419,732	148		282			454		
	1955	1,120	142	3,766	100		70.4	9.7		18,073	615,286	188		494			752		
	1960	1,260	156	4,632	112		71.6	8.8		19,901	742,119	241		796			1,203		
	1965	1,453	179	5,617	131		72.8	8.5	29,962	21,604	759,327	306		1,295			1,994		
	1970	1,704	204	6,273	149	168	73.2	8.7	37,854	23,754	765,635	444	264	2,535			4,328	$ 613.87	$ 70.56
	1971	1,752	209	6,540	150	172	71.6	8.3	40,550	23,267	765,934	461	269	2,910	$ 274	$ 50.95	4,842	641.92	77.34
	1972	1,779	209	6,741	147	169	70.2	8.0	47,103	23,332	749,754	477	282	3,328	345	59.41	5,758	745.04	93.13
	1973	1,814	211	6,939	149	176	70.6	7.8	51,072	22,610	723,749	497	283	3,626	398	62.82	6,389	777.97	99.74
	1974	1,821	211	7,016	148	174	70.2	7.7	54,777	22,439	706,945	522	300	4,052	467	71.18	7,211	874.64	113.59
	1975	1,840	215	7,138	150	178	69.7	7.6	56,230	22,276	726,141	546	307	4,674	577	81.01	8,584	1,006.32	132.41
	1976	1,836	214	7,237	148	175	69.2	7.5	57,896	21,815	716,560	543	310	5,004	674	85.22	9,520	1,115.10	148.68
	1977	1,851	214	7,220	146	174	68.3	7.4	56,838	21,186	759,568	559	321	5,432	839	98.64	10,640	1,238.54	167.37
	1978	1,843	215	7,253	148	175	68.7	7.4	54,933	20,551	770,361	571	327	6,046	951	109.75	11,906	1,384.88	186.77
	1979	1,846	214	7,312	148	179	69.1	7.4	54,060	20,302	803,645	588	329	6,726	1,103	119.88	13,395	1,524.24	205.10
	1980	1,835	212	7,458	150	178	70.7	7.4	54,192	20,435	819,373	602	339	7,489	1,305	135.40	15,308	1,724.04	235.69
	1981	1,794	213	7,299	151	177	71.2	7.6	52,816	19,736	803,070	622	352	8,588	1,541	156.92	17,594	2,061.68	272.57
	1982	1,761	212	7,205	150	178	70.7	7.6	60,857	19,431	811,570	632	355	9,742	1,850	178.16	20,067	2,337.39	308.44
	1983	1,723	209	7,064	146	175	70.0	7.6	52,163	18,777	795,965	618	354	10,463	2,056	196.45	21,749	2,570.73	341.30
	1984	1,662	203	6,642	134	162	65.9	7.4	51,457	18,283	767,680	586	362	10,720	2,186	218.06	22,415	2,769.28	378.71
	1985	1,616	191	6,071	120	147	62.8	7.2	50,394	17,352	747,008	565	385	10,906	2,234	245.24	22,975	3,073.41	428.78
	1986	1,556	185	5,687	116	146	62.6	7.4	51,091	16,492	746,126	560	385	11,494	2,315	259.89	24,338	3,395.57	458.07
	1987	1,542	182	5,530	115	148	63.1	7.6	53,049	15,986	738,510	578	391	12,326	2,517	274.79	26,445	3,720.06	489.57
	1988	1,533	178	5,444	113	152	63.8	7.6	57,646	15,243	743,780	587	385	13,336	2,735	288.71	28,627	3,990.35	514.28
	1989	1,495	172	5,271	112	154	64.8	7.7	58,926	14,746	753,478	592	385	14,231	3,034	308.09	31,024	4,388.56	553.60
	1990	1,469	171	5,254	112	155	65.3	7.8	61,407	14,710	784,504	617	399	15,802	3,370	340.09	34,413	4,769.19	610.45
Hospital units of institutions	1972	97	5	68	2		29.9		4,315	2	15	5		60	5		87		
	1973	102	5	90	2		31.8		5,870	5	27	7		85	8		124		
	1974	102	5	77	2		30.4		5,899	5	24	7		94	9		135		
	1975	104	5	85	2		36.7		5,639	5	38	7		97	11		148		
	1976	99	5	90	2		37.4		6,477	11	89	7		104	12		161		
	1977	92	5	80	2	6	37.3	8.1	5,530	5	6	8		118	13		186		
	1978	84	4	69	2	5	37.8	8.4	4,531	11	114	7	145	102	14	68.73	168	732.94	99.68
	1979	81	4	61	2	8	42.0	10.0	5,096	11	145	6	76	112	14	41.08	181	488.64	53.80
	1980	74	4	55	2	4	41.9	10.1	4,442	17	217	6	150	79	9	64.92	119	544.79	87.36
	1981	66	3	55	1	3	39.4	8.7	3,962	6	282	5	191	100	17	114.61	166	1,154.93	162.09
	1982	62	3	50	1	4	36.6	8.1	2,765	6	304	6	167	129	28	116.57	219	1,028.72	161.95
	1983	60	3	49	1	5	40.9	8.8	3,951	6	375	6	129	123	23	81.29	194	705.60	107.70
	1984	55	3	47	1	4	35.9	7.5	4,513	6	159	6	146	131	26	109.33	213	932.59	148.72
	1985	52	2	52	1	2	45.8	7.8	4,057	6	161	6	250	126	23	182.21	201	1,497.32	246.00
	1986	50	3	31	2	4	54.1	19.9	2,358	6	122	7	176	146	42	132.54	252	2,418.92	177.89
	1987	48	3	32	2	5	60.4	21.9	2,180	6	120	6	131	162	57	131.62	324	3,295.55	195.03
	1988	46	3	27	1	8	51.0	18.8	2,307	36	346	4	52	106	25	43.98	219	1,288.49	73.69
	1989	42	2	25	1	9	55.7	20.0	2,197	31	436	4	44	135	24	46.64	307	1,496.54	89.68
	1990	36	2	22	1	7	56.1	18.6	1,362	31	383	4	55	76	21	36.54	235	1,252.25	88.43

Table 1 (Continued)

CLASSIFICATION	YEAR	HOSPITALS	BEDS (in thousands)	ADMISSIONS (in thousands)	AVERAGE DAILY CENSUS (in thousands)	ADJUSTED AVERAGE DAILY CENSUS (in thousands)	OCCUPANCY, percent	AVERAGE LENGTH OF STAY, days	OUTPATIENT VISITS (in thousands)	NEWBORNS: Bassinets	NEWBORNS: Births	FTE PERSONNEL: Number (in thousands)	FTE PERSONNEL: Per 100 Adjusted Census	EXPENSES, LABOR: PAYROLL Amount (in millions of dollars)	EXPENSES, LABOR: EMPLOYEE BENEFITS Amount (in millions of dollars)	EXPENSES, LABOR: Adjusted, per Inpatient Day (dollars)	EXPENSES, TOTAL: Amount (in millions of dollars)	EXPENSES, TOTAL: Adjusted, per Inpatient Stay (dollars)	EXPENSES, TOTAL: Adjusted, per Inpatient Day (dollars)
Total community hospitals (These data are totals of the data in the next three classifications)	1972	5,746	879	30,709	663	734	75.4	7.9	162,668	89,313	3,119,431	2,051	279	$14,459	$ 1,471	$ 59.36	$ 25,462	$ 749.47	$ 94.87
	1973	5,789	898	31,671	680	760	75.7	7.8	173,068	86,846	2,987,062	2,142	282	15,782	1,724	63.21	28,372	799.03	102.44
	1974	5,875	926	32,866	700	787	75.6	7.8	188,940	85,203	2,947,318	2,282	290	17,767	2,021	68.89	32,617	885.69	113.55
	1975	5,875	942	33,435	706	798	75.0	7.7	190,672	83,829	2,998,552	2,392	300	20,653	2,458	79.37	38,962	1,030.34	133.81
	1976	5,857	956	33,979	713	810	74.6	7.7	201,247	82,296	2,962,216	2,475	306	23,333	3,041	88.31	45,240	1,176.25	152.76
	1977	5,881	969	34,273	715	814	73.8	7.6	198,708	80,223	3,117,750	2,573	316	25,944	3,730	99.96	51,647	1,322.25	173.98
	1978	5,851	975	34,506	718	821	73.6	7.6	201,931	78,079	3,156,456	2,655	324	28,932	4,315	111.06	58,180	1,474.41	194.34
	1979	5,842	984	35,099	727	833	73.9	7.6	198,778	77,266	3,287,012	2,756	331	32,587	5,004	123.78	66,004	1,641.67	217.34
	1980	5,830	988	36,143	747	857	75.6	7.6	202,310	77,522	3,408,482	2,873	335	37,379	5,905	138.06	76,851	1,851.04	245.12
	1981	5,813	1,003	36,438	763	873	76.0	7.6	202,768	76,561	3,465,401	3,033	347	44,042	7,253	161.03	90,572	2,171.20	284.33
	1982	5,801	1,012	36,379	762	878	75.3	7.6	248,124	75,733	3,514,457	3,103	353	50,638	8,804	185.55	104,876	2,500.52	327.37
	1983	5,783	1,018	36,152	749	864	73.5	7.6	210,044	75,465	3,490,254	3,096	358	55,525	10,199	208.56	116,438	2,789.18	369.49
	1984	5,759	1,017	35,155	702	820	69.0	7.3	211,961	75,581	3,456,308	3,017	368	58,188	11,016	230.67	123,336	2,995.38	411.10
	1985	5,732	1,001	33,449	649	777	64.8	7.1	218,716	74,893	3,521,135	2,997	386	60,361	11,640	253.90	130,499	3,244.74	460.19
	1986	5,678	978	32,379	629	770	64.3	7.1	231,912	73,682	3,584,408	3,025	393	63,773	11,998	269.79	140,654	3,532.51	500.81
	1987	5,611	958	31,601	622	776	64.9	7.2	245,524	72,510	3,602,296	3,114	401	68,306	12,687	286.08	152,585	3,850.16	538.96
	1988	5,533	947	31,453	620	787	65.5	7.2	269,129	70,325	3,706,402	3,205	407	75,234	14,068	310.33	168,722	4,206.73	586.33
	1989	5,455	933	31,116	618	796	66.2	7.2	285,712	69,405	3,830,615	3,303	415	81,975	16,069	337.75	184,898	4,587.87	636.96
	1990	5,384	927	31,181	619	813	66.8	7.2	301,329	68,412	3,958,263	3,420	421	90,925	18,187	367.91	203,693	4,946.68	686.83
Nongovernment not-for-profit community hospitals	1972	3,301	617	21,862	478	527	77.5	8.0	111,317	62,016	2,242,747	1,473	280	10,484	1,065	59.93	18,369	762.56	95.32
	1973	3,295	628	22,473	489	545	77.9	7.9	119,425	60,325	2,134,201	1,534	282	11,431	1,248	63.83	20,399	811.33	102.70
	1974	3,355	649	23,359	506	567	77.9	7.9	130,438	58,877	2,113,205	1,633	288	12,843	1,457	69.13	23,472	896.49	113.48
	1975	3,339	658	23,722	510	574	77.5	7.8	131,435	57,496	2,131,057	1,712	298	14,945	1,759	79.73	27,938	1,040.21	133.36
	1976	3,345	670	24,082	517	586	77.2	7.9	140,914	56,442	2,100,917	1,791	306	17,139	2,220	90.36	32,764	1,208.23	152.94
	1977	3,350	679	24,272	519	588	76.4	7.8	138,224	54,902	2,197,940	1,861	316	19,122	2,696	101.64	37,495	1,362.50	174.68
	1978	3,339	683	24,428	520	593	76.2	7.8	141,862	53,411	2,219,609	1,925	325	21,318	3,139	112.97	42,228	1,514.66	195.07
	1979	3,330	690	24,874	528	603	76.5	7.7	139,565	52,859	2,308,548	1,999	332	24,024	3,606	125.69	47,937	1,684.40	218.06
	1980	3,322	692	25,566	542	621	78.2	7.7	142,156	52,659	2,389,478	2,086	336	27,642	4,253	140.47	55,780	1,901.64	245.74
	1981	3,340	706	25,945	555	636	78.6	7.8	143,380	52,302	2,455,033	2,213	399	32,773	5,279	164.02	66,267	2,225.17	285.64
	1982	3,338	712	25,898	553	637	77.8	7.8	176,245	51,566	2,483,345	2,265	355	37,751	6,397	189.92	76,806	2,572.93	330.41
	1983	3,347	718	25,827	544	629	75.8	7.7	150,839	51,649	2,465,604	2,270	362	41,531	7,458	213.83	85,637	2,868.80	373.78
	1984	3,351	716	25,236	512	598	71.4	7.4	153,281	51,491	2,446,540	2,222	372	43,575	8,070	236.03	90,814	3,072.51	415.04
	1985	3,349	707	24,179	476	569	67.2	7.2	158,953	51,424	2,507,288	2,216	389	45,191	8,567	258.69	96,150	3,307.41	462.69
	1986	3,323	689	23,483	460	563	66.8	7.2	167,633	50,885	2,547,170	2,241	398	47,751	8,834	275.28	103,524	3,589.64	503.64
	1987	3,274	673	22,937	455	566	67.6	7.2	177,413	50,133	2,557,294	2,298	406	51,073	9,233	291.89	112,325	3,914.23	543.67
	1988	3,242	668	22,939	456	577	68.2	7.3	195,363	48,828	2,653,794	2,373	412	56,441	10,223	316.01	124,703	4,272.95	591.13
	1989	3,220	661	22,792	455	584	68.8	7.3	209,191	48,305	2,751,426	2,454	420	61,788	11,742	345.09	136,889	4,649.22	642.45
	1990	3,191	657	22,878	455	596	69.3	7.3	221,073	47,441	2,833,204	2,533	424	68,457	13,343	375.88	150,673	5,001.24	692.36
Investor-owned (for profit) community hospitals	1972	738	57	2,161	39	42	68.7	6.6	7,842	3,967	126,945	105	249	697	65	54.04	1,407	606.61	91.91
	1973	757	63	2,334	43	47	68.3	6.7	7,593	3,916	129,139	117	249	799	84	51.96	1,689	665.91	99.39
	1974	775	70	2,553	47	52	67.5	6.7	8,667	3,892	127,192	133	257	952	105	56.21	2,046	729.30	108.85
	1975	775	73	2,646	48	53	65.9	6.6	7,713	4,062	141,392	139	263	1,114	131	64.56	2,561	876.48	132.80
	1976	752	76	2,734	50	54	64.8	6.6	8,048	4,044	144,751	147	272	1,276	156	72.54	3,085	1,031.91	156.35
	1977	751	80	2,849	52	57	64.6	6.6	8,355	4,140	160,248	159	279	1,492	207	81.95	3,669	1,168.13	176.99
	1978	732	81	2,880	52	57	63.8	6.5	8,911	4,122	166,499	165	290	1,651	237	91.38	4,180	1,316.93	202.36
	1979	727	83	2,963	53	59	63.9	6.6	9,289	4,110	174,843	174	300	1,930	306	104.78	4,820	1,476.42	225.87
	1980	730	87	3,165	57	62	65.2	6.5	9,696	4,439	199,722	189	304	2,317	354	117.45	5,847	1,675.85	257.12
	1981	729	88	3,239	58	63	66.4	6.5	9,961	4,523	207,405	203	322	2,769	449	140.32	6,856	1,952.56	299.02
	1982	748	91	3,316	60	66	65.5	6.6	13,193	4,736	219,675	212	320	3,250	580	159.24	8,177	2,224.75	340.03
	1983	757	94	3,299	59	66	63.1	6.5	10,389	5,039	228,883	213	323	3,631	703	181.44	9,208	2,517.53	385.42
	1984	786	100	3,314	57	64	57.0	6.3	11,090	5,807	242,088	214	335	3,985	777	203.59	10,251	2,748.51	438.30
	1985	805	104	3,242	54	63	52.1	6.1	12,378	6,117	266,839	221	350	4,338	852	226.14	11,486	3,033.06	500.48
	1986	834	107	3,231	54	65	50.7	6.1	14,896	6,305	291,112	229	354	4,641	885	235.03	12,987	3,341.79	552.40
	1987	828	106	3,157	54	66	51.1	6.2	16,566	6,391	306,492	242	367	5,029	984	250.04	14,067	3,617.19	585.01
	1988	790	104	3,090	53	66	50.9	6.2	17,926	6,254	308,828	249	379	5,527	1,128	277.96	15,545	4,022.77	649.33
	1989	769	102	3,071	53	67	51.7	6.3	19,341	6,354	325,711	261	390	6,064	1,312	302.88	17,240	4,406.20	707.90
	1990	749	101	3,066	54	69	52.8	6.4	20,110	6,261	340,555	273	396	6,732	1,493	328.44	18,822	4,727.27	751.55
State and local government community hospitals	1972	1,707	205	6,686	146	165	71.0	8.0	43,510	23,330	749,739	473	286	3,278	341	59.95	5,686	753.52	94.19
	1973	1,737	207	6,864	148	168	71.4	7.8	46,050	22,605	723,722	491	292	3,553	391	64.32	6,284	799.19	102.46
	1974	1,745	207	6,953	147	169	71.0	7.7	49,835	22,434	706,921	516	305	3,973	460	71.96	7,099	887.35	115.24
	1975	1,761	210	7,067	148	171	70.4	7.6	51,525	22,271	726,103	540	316	4,593	568	82.73	8,463	1,030.86	135.64
	1976	1,760	210	7,163	146	170	69.8	7.5	52,286	21,810	716,548	537	315	4,919	665	86.22	9,391	1,132.50	151.00
	1977	1,780	210	7,152	145	168	68.9	7.4	52,128	21,181	759,562	552	328	5,330	828	100.17	10,483	1,261.85	170.52
	1978	1,780	211	7,198	146	171	69.2	7.4	51,157	20,546	770,348	565	331	5,963	939	110.92	11,772	1,399.49	189.17
	1979	1,785	211	7,262	146	171	69.5	7.4	49,924	20,297	803,621	583	341	6,633	1,092	123.56	13,247	1,561.04	211.89
	1980	1,778	209	7,413	149	174	71.1	7.3	50,459	20,424	819,282	598	343	7,420	1,297	136.81	15,204	1,750.13	238.63
	1981	1,744	210	7,255	150	174	71.6	7.6	49,427	19,736	802,963	618	354	8,500	1,526	157.57	17,449	2,071.57	274.25
	1982	1,715	210	7,165	149	175	71.1	7.6	58,685	19,431	811,437	627	320	9,637	1,827	179.55	19,893	2,364.09	311.56
	1983	1,679	207	7,025	145	170	70.4	7.6	48,816	18,777	795,767	613	360	10,363	2,037	199.59	21,593	2,621.28	347.56
	1984	1,622	201	6,606	133	158	66.2	7.3	47,590	18,283	767,680	581	368	10,629	2,169	221.34	22,271	2,823.13	385.17
	1985	1,578	189	6,028	119	145	62.9	7.2	47,386	17,352	747,008	561	387	10,832	2,222	247.13	22,863	3,106.14	432.84
	1986	1,521	182	5,665	114	142	62.7	7.4	49,383	16,492	746,126	555	391	11,381	2,280	264.05	24,143	3,404.69	466.17
	1987	1,509	180	5,507	113	144	63.1	7.5	51,544	15,986	738,510	573	399	12,204	2,470	279.75	26,192	3,717.77	499.33
	1988	1,501	175	5,424	112	145	63.9	7.6	55,840	15,243	743,780	583	403	13,266	2,717	302.34	28,474	4,033.67	538.63
	1989	1,466	170	5,253	110	145	64.9	7.7	57,179	14,746	753,478	589	406	14,123	3,014	324.24	30,769	4,430.12	582.15
	1990	1,444	169	5,236	111	148	65.3	7.7	60,146	14,710	784,504	614	415	15,736	3,351	354.10	34,198	4,837.76	634.45

Table

2A

Utilization, Personnel, and Finances in Short-Term Hospitals

If there are no hospitals within a given classification, that classification does not appear.

CLASSIFICATION	HOSPITALS	BEDS	ADMISSIONS	OCCUPANCY, percent	AVERAGE DAILY CENSUS	ADJUSTED AVERAGE DAILY CENSUS	AVG. STAY, days	SURGICAL OPERATIONS	OUTPATIENT VISITS	NEWBORNS		FTE PERSONNEL	EXPENSES (in thousands of dollars)			
													LABOR			
										Bassinets	Births		PAYROLL	EMPLOYEE BENEFITS	TOTAL	TOTAL
TOTAL	6,141	1,047,851	33,301,614	67.0	702,156			23,046,645	361,298,604	70,511	4,044,631	3,763,927	$100,698,689	$19,958,163	$120,656,852	$221,721,289
GENERAL	5,535	987,060	32,400,593	67.1	662,273			22,704,952	353,503,807	69,632	3,976,048	3,612,291	96,521,167	19,074,076	115,595,243	212,746,728
Nongovernment not-for-profit	3,085	645,658	22,578,707	69.3	447,374	586,299	7.2	16,303,818	217,540,873	46,993	2,790,499	2,481,475	66,990,543	13,059,595	80,050,137	147,588,310
6-24 beds	78	1,499	34,017	34.0	509	1,154	5.5	15,386	635,276	256	3,752	3,603	74,974	13,916	88,890	162,121
25-49	381	14,517	398,491	42.8	6,219	9,958	5.7	229,854	5,345,231	1,689	39,091	39,509	814,060	151,041	965,101	1,847,186
50-99	592	42,494	1,221,549	55.7	23,676	34,954	7.1	848,880	14,847,905	4,034	134,869	121,775	2,739,395	535,393	3,274,788	6,149,328
100-199	748	106,988	3,587,789	63.3	67,701	94,842	6.9	2,733,046	39,143,680	8,478	410,710	360,985	8,997,107	1,748,123	10,745,230	19,941,127
200-299	557	135,847	4,881,859	69.0	93,782	125,210	7.0	3,645,490	49,700,815	9,951	580,273	507,758	13,475,224	2,617,227	16,092,452	29,698,132
300-399	328	112,298	4,151,335	70.6	79,305	101,640	7.0	3,055,682	35,655,206	8,139	540,230	440,677	12,132,286	2,374,853	14,507,138	26,547,872
400-499	179	79,534	2,938,011	74.2	59,039	74,511	7.3	2,094,007	24,997,049	5,681	402,204	323,102	9,118,393	1,772,116	10,890,509	19,739,883
500 or more	222	152,481	5,365,656	76.8	117,143	144,030	8.0	3,681,473	47,215,711	8,765	679,370	684,066	19,639,103	3,846,926	23,486,029	43,502,661
Investor-owned (for-profit)	693	96,764	2,978,930	52.6	50,898	65,529	6.2	2,269,599	19,491,526	5,866	315,237	260,403	6,456,660	1,432,102	7,888,762	18,097,444
6-24 beds	13	244	6,190	33.2	81	181	4.5	6,985	36,522	5	84	543	14,339	2,803	17,142	34,238
25-49	69	2,689	72,908	39.6	1,066	1,521	5.3	37,706	568,189	162	4,353	6,133	122,474	25,669	148,142	315,694
50-99	195	14,546	449,188	46.1	6,711	9,160	5.4	313,235	3,403,513	931	42,959	36,883	863,497	193,590	1,057,086	2,420,047
100-199	269	37,033	1,150,941	51.9	19,216	25,445	6.1	900,005	8,376,542	2,475	126,634	100,228	2,468,433	572,456	3,040,889	7,023,193
200-299	98	23,165	704,940	55.6	12,891	15,941	6.7	542,248	3,880,422	1,227	71,357	61,114	1,595,500	349,432	1,944,932	4,441,487
300-399	30	9,719	294,615	57.3	5,572	6,756	6.9	237,001	1,512,435	579	34,933	27,939	719,447	146,534	865,981	1,980,824
400-499	13	5,706	177,734	53.5	3,055	3,717	6.3	138,626	1,107,724	321	20,545	15,585	390,836	80,701	471,538	1,102,742
500 or more	6	3,662	122,414	63.0	2,306	2,808	6.9	93,793	606,179	166	14,372	11,978	282,135	60,916	343,051	779,220
Local government	1,358	143,557	4,395,916	63.5	91,208	125,561	7.6	2,474,417	48,089,913	13,376	675,373	483,015	12,294,774	2,536,061	14,830,835	26,396,852
6-24 beds	134	2,653	53,072	30.8	818	1,306	5.6	18,649	799,472	356	3,690	6,026	111,771	21,373	133,145	243,876
25-49	437	16,445	369,581	39.1	6,433	9,779	6.3	153,944	4,252,688	1,800	33,936	36,446	695,028	133,192	828,220	1,507,363
50-99	399	27,983	704,414	53.7	15,040	21,894	7.8	423,047	7,780,148	2,846	85,014	69,022	1,397,965	276,203	1,674,168	3,084,664
100-199	225	31,238	851,779	65.5	20,454	28,513	8.8	550,544	8,852,704	2,634	117,418	85,098	1,897,009	381,266	2,278,275	4,220,911
200-299	72	17,781	663,688	65.1	11,580	15,617	6.4	437,197	5,917,965	1,922	106,232	64,876	1,714,551	362,958	2,077,509	3,847,046
300-399	33	11,209	429,671	70.5	7,902	11,678	6.7	245,527	4,074,466	909	67,611	46,914	1,235,138	262,492	1,497,630	2,737,596
400-499	22	9,961	390,864	77.3	7,701	9,963	7.2	204,151	4,937,744	929	76,596	46,556	1,467,021	304,033	1,771,054	3,059,519
500 or more	36	26,287	932,847	81.0	21,280	26,811	8.3	441,358	11,474,726	1,980	184,876	128,077	3,776,290	794,545	4,570,835	7,695,877
State government	94	24,225	816,499	74.4	18,019	25,940	8.1	540,677	12,547,533	1,334	109,131	121,671	3,220,730	755,671	3,976,402	7,418,453
6-24 beds	7	120	732	35.0	42	184	20.9	434	282,059	2	7	325	4,490	1,224	5,714	13,698
25-49	14	463	5,871	50.3	233	876	14.4	2,152	180,684	12	130	1,053	23,872	5,718	29,590	62,430
50-99	15	1,077	21,038	56.8	612	2,232	10.6	9,896	693,078	37	1,637	2,651	72,425	13,354	85,778	157,746
100-199	15	2,111	62,517	65.0	1,373	2,156	8.0	38,812	867,841	184	10,406	5,953	142,845	27,400	170,245	326,594
200-299	6	1,511	39,688	74.9	1,132	2,760	10.4	23,243	942,804	97	5,328	5,582	155,026	42,345	197,371	380,472
300-399	12	4,179	167,934	77.9	3,257	4,076	7.1	88,391	2,303,524	270	27,259	24,967	708,610	148,550	857,160	1,544,531
400-499	8	3,632	137,343	78.4	2,847	3,521	7.6	96,815	2,351,502	165	17,156	23,497	641,217	159,817	801,034	1,395,094
500 or more	17	11,132	381,376	76.6	8,523	10,135	8.2	280,934	4,926,041	567	47,208	57,643	1,472,246	357,263	1,829,509	3,537,888
Federal government	305	76,856	1,630,541	71.3	54,774			1,116,441	55,833,962	2,063	85,808	265,727	7,558,459	1,290,647	8,849,107	13,245,669
6-24 beds	42	713	40,641	47.4	338			28,241	3,115,714	183	4,841	8,615	159,494	32,662	192,156	240,655
25-49	54	1,907	99,650	48.5	924			54,995	6,120,407	433	13,681	16,014	342,860	73,695	416,555	546,300
50-99	33	2,215	106,027	50.2	1,112			58,158	5,930,127	367	15,558	15,539	359,217	60,222	419,440	583,164
100-199	52	7,833	267,242	65.9	5,163			180,462	10,711,360	582	23,824	39,699	996,806	154,166	1,150,972	1,868,024
200-299	29	7,074	190,166	70.5	4,987			130,721	5,797,454	187	9,436	25,454	801,657	104,096	905,752	1,420,457
300-399	27	9,534	218,816	72.4	6,904			181,959	6,569,334	95	5,966	34,334	1,011,555	173,840	1,185,395	1,777,747
400-499	17	7,790	177,278	74.6	5,812			103,236	5,662,248	120	9,913	26,334	833,547	116,262	949,809	1,343,125
500 or more	51	39,790	530,721	74.2	29,534			378,669	11,927,318	96	2,589	99,738	3,053,323	575,705	3,629,027	5,466,197
PSYCHIATRIC	412	40,535	451,265	64.8	26,247			2,593	2,450,193	5	177	70,842	2,016,493	434,723	2,451,215	4,284,330
Nongovernment not-for-profit	82	7,194	99,813	68.0	4,889			1,102	918,499	5	177	15,715	432,464	89,828	522,292	856,523
6-24 beds	4	95	1,326	80.0	76			0	25,454	0	0	245	8,148	1,556	9,703	16,206
25-49	14	537	8,626	64.2	345			0	201,981	0	0	1,314	34,693	6,799	41,492	66,233
50-99	44	3,203	45,037	63.2	2,024			1,094	457,550	5	177	6,448	170,991	35,496	206,487	344,484
100-199	15	2,129	31,025	72.2	1,538			8	134,945	0	0	4,129	111,293	23,358	134,651	228,806
200-299	5	1,230	13,799	73.7	906			0	98,569	0	0	3,579	107,340	22,619	129,958	200,794

Table 2A (Continued)

CLASSIFICATION	HOSPITALS	BEDS	ADMISSIONS	OCCUPANCY, percent	AVERAGE DAILY CENSUS	ADJUSTED AVERAGE DAILY CENSUS	AVG. STAY, days	SURGICAL OPERATIONS	OUTPATIENT VISITS	NEWBORNS Bassinets	NEWBORNS Births	FTE PERSONNEL	EXPENSES (in thousands of dollars) LABOR PAYROLL	EXPENSES LABOR EMPLOYEE BENEFITS	EXPENSES LABOR TOTAL	EXPENSES TOTAL
Investor-owned (for-profit)	292	25,228	288,411	60.8	15,341			1,491	602,988	0	0	39,374	$ 1,143,156	$ 242,535	$ 1,385,691	$ 2,648,545
6-24 beds	3	44	405	47.7	21			0	5,087	0	0	71	1,506	412	1,918	3,706
25-49	37	1,339	15,329	60.0	803			0	36,608	0	0	2,249	58,381	12,221	70,602	138,995
50-99	164	12,182	150,811	61.0	7,429			1,491	301,406	0	0	19,340	559,573	115,786	675,359	1,288,135
100-199	81	10,143	105,171	58.8	5,963			0	221,624	0	0	14,897	442,908	96,589	539,497	1,045,490
200-299	7	1,520	16,695	74.0	1,125			0	38,263	0	0	2,817	80,790	17,526	98,315	172,220
Local government	9	2,208	11,602	85.5	1,888			0	438,230	0	0	3,848	115,511	25,962	141,474	209,750
25-49 beds	2	83	724	43.4	36			0	3,047	0	0	140	3,102	463	3,564	6,229
50-99	3	211	2,060	74.4	157			0	87,384	0	0	571	17,795	4,410	22,205	30,680
200-299	1	267	1,878	86.5	231			0	22,888	0	0	373	15,392	3,565	18,957	28,763
300-399	1	382	1,483	87.2	333			0	60,116	0	0	720	23,979	7,109	31,088	41,595
400-499	1	432	1,442	95.1	411			0	33,939	0	0	592	11,994	2,420	14,413	22,892
500 or more	1	833	4,015	86.4	720			0	230,856	0	0	1,452	43,250	7,996	51,246	79,590
State government	28	5,566	49,513	70.5	3,923			0	467,730	0	0	11,462	312,003	74,021	386,024	548,344
25-49 beds	3	135	1,278	60.0	81			0	59,667	0	0	461	14,595	720	15,315	18,465
50-99	8	584	6,896	73.6	430			0	267,280	0	0	2,046	41,613	10,516	52,129	76,674
100-199	5	777	9,152	79.0	614			0	8,679	0	0	1,709	49,661	11,206	60,867	87,107
200-299	6	1,400	12,506	84.1	1,177			0	132,104	0	0	2,880	68,038	18,493	86,531	123,082
300-399	5	1,793	18,427	87.6	1,571			0	0	0	0	3,276	87,538	21,376	108,913	148,539
500 or more	1	877	1,254	05.7	50			0	0	0	0	1,090	50,557	11,711	62,268	94,477
Federal government	1	339	1,926	60.8	206			0	22,746	0	0	443	13,358	2,377	15,735	21,168
300-399 beds	1	339	1,926	60.8	206			0	22,746	0	0	443	13,358	2,377	15,735	21,168
TB AND OTHER RESPIRATORY DISEASES	1	115	1,211	69.6	80			1,806	15,790	0	0	322	6,993	866	7,859	12,019
State government	1	115	1,211	69.6	80			1,806	15,790	0	0	322	6,993	866	7,859	12,019
100-199 beds	1	115	1,211	69.6	80			1,806	15,790	0	0	322	6,993	866	7,859	12,019
ALL OTHER	193	20,141	448,545	67.3	13,556			337,294	5,328,814	874	68,406	80,472	2,154,036	448,498	2,602,535	4,678,212
Nongovernment not-for-profit	117	11,358	304,729	69.6	7,902			250,523	3,633,643	479	43,088	52,330	1,476,141	285,202	1,761,343	3,104,445
6-24 beds	6	103	3,523	39.8	41			11,403	37,793	0	0	659	14,773	3,674	18,447	31,778
25-49	28	1,052	20,515	53.8	556			22,939	454,090	0	0	5,864	110,080	22,393	132,473	243,542
50-99	43	3,001	56,696	60.3	1,810			50,467	885,508	0	0	10,693	264,633	54,205	318,838	555,410
100-199	30	3,975	122,969	68.9	2,740			96,302	1,452,007	231	23,366	20,638	618,591	120,185	738,777	1,286,895
200-299	5	1,168	33,371	87.8	1,026			22,278	251,256	50	5,992	4,704	149,681	27,955	177,636	303,104
300-399	3	928	47,880	73.1	678			33,666	392,924	198	13,730	5,680	146,510	25,733	172,243	304,913
500 or more	2	1,131	19,775	92.0	1,041			13,468	160,065	0	0	4,092	171,873	31,057	202,930	378,803
Investor-owned (for profit)	56	4,613	87,268	56.6	2,612			60,496	617,982	395	25,318	12,239	275,791	60,887	336,678	724,163
6-24 beds	2	35	550	05.7	2			4,335	47,046	0	0	163	5,477	873	6,350	10,813
25-49	11	404	4,296	46.5	188			5,397	61,331	14	38	973	21,361	3,850	25,211	54,978
50-99	24	1,675	26,549	58.0	371			11,955	213,410	112	6,573	4,548	97,803	21,395	119,198	248,712
100-199	18	2,280	46,710	59.3	1,352			31,764	291,028	212	13,390	5,941	135,571	31,252	166,822	372,113
200-299	1	219	9,163	45.2	99			7,045	5,167	57	5,317	614	15,580	3,517	19,097	37,548
Local government	8	1,962	8,628	79.6	1 562			1,767	57,610	0	0	3,183	71,723	18,680	90,403	147,873
6-24 beds	1	27	285	14.8	4			333	882	0	0	61	1,120	212	1,332	2,418
50-99	1	78	864	34.6	27			0	9,537	0	0	153	4,974	978	5,952	10,965
100-199	1	104	1,233	75.0	78			0	19,662	0	0	293	7,306	2,729	10,035	16,094
200-299	1	197	1,941	78.7	155			0	6,000	0	0	416	9,156	3,872	13,027	18,594
300-399	3	951	3,450	74.1	705			1,313	14,449	0	0	1,519	32,591	6,997	39,588	66,131
500 or more	1	605	855	98.0	593			121	7,080	0	0	741	16,576	3,893	20,470	33,671
State government	9	1,237	32,477	67.1	830			20,030	711,573	0	0	9,173	215,077	59,527	274,604	449,959
25-49 beds	4	137	1,887	61.3	84			366	58,798	0	0	438	10,021	2,811	12,832	19,387
50-99	1	66	1,020	34.8	23			788	15,090	0	0	202	5,884	1,379	7,263	12,739
100-199	3	521	12,333	64.7	337			11,212	157,384	0	0	3,094	63,700	12,635	76,335	141,287
500 or more	1	513	17,237	75.2	386			7,664	480,301	0	0	5,439	135,472	42,703	178,174	276,545
Federal government	3	971	15,443	66.9	650			4,478	308,006	0	0	3,547	115,305	24,202	139,506	251,772
100-199 beds	1	150	1,804	58.7	88			0	58,819	0	0	523	15,945	2,962	18,907	27,203
300-399	1	350	4,322	83.7	293			2,432	98,253	0	0	967	25,820	5,241	31,061	36,883
400-499	1	471	9,317	57.1	269			2,046	150,934	0	0	2,057	73,540	15,999	89,539	187,686

Table

2B

Utilization, Personnel, and Finances in Long-Term Hospitals

If there are no hospitals within a given classification, that classification does not appear.

CLASSIFICATION	HOSPITALS	BEDS	ADMISSIONS	OCCUPANCY, percent	AVERAGE DAILY CENSUS	ADJUSTED AVERAGE DAILY CENSUS	AVG. STAY, days	SURGICAL OPERATIONS	OUTPATIENT VISITS	NEWBORNS: Bassinets	NEWBORNS: Births	FTE PERSONNEL	EXPENSES (in thousands of dollars): LABOR: PAYROLL	LABOR: EMPLOYEE BENEFITS	LABOR: TOTAL	TOTAL
TOTAL	508	165,476	471,960	85.6	141,568			44,679	6,884,994	28	2,073	299,361	$ 8,019,883	$ 1,838,349	$ 9,858,232	$ 13,148,617
GENERAL	31	11,599	80,225	78.4	9,093			32,330	1,511,716	26	2,071	23,593	754,889	137,398	892,287	1,284,857
Nongovernment not-for-profit	9	1,018	12,286	78.5	799			5,775	182,763	22	2,046	2,619	56,954	10,790	67,744	117,491
6-24 beds	3	55	326	69.1	38			85	3,414	0	0	152	4,667	1,013	5,680	8,936
50-99	3	220	828	58.6	129			0	13,881	0	0	570	10,772	1,984	12,756	22,268
100-199	1	123	307	87.8	108			97	30,791	0	0	104	3,589	624	4,213	7,184
300-399	2	620	10,825	84.5	524			5,593	134,677	22	2,046	1,793	37,927	7,168	45,095	79,103
Investor-owned (for-profit)	1	56	223	60.7	34			362	513	0	0	125	4,752	1,031	5,783	9,099
50-99 beds	1	56	223	60.7	34			362	513	0	0	125	4,752	1,031	5,783	9,099
Local government	7	1,869	12,972	87.3	1,631			4,651	171,422	4	25	5,463	158,444	40,686	199,130	296,578
6-24 beds	1	23	56	87.0	20			0	1,170	0	0	17	431	45	475	825
25-49	1	26	156	73.1	19			0	2,978	0	0	47	2,206	479	2,685	4,225
50-99	2	149	773	78.5	117			306	6,361	4	25	258	6,691	1,406	8,097	12,812
100-199	1	186	985	79.0	147			110	22,980	0	0	563	15,783	3,425	19,207	30,221
400-499	1	440	4,176	100.0	440			3,393	90,051	0	0	2,601	77,759	20,675	98,435	150,824
500 or more	1	1,045	6,826	85.0	888			842	47,882	0	0	1,977	55,574	14,657	70,230	97,670
State government	3	616	2,401	75.3	464			1,235	37,982	0	0	1,135	33,315	7,165	40,480	53,612
100-199 beds	1	100	552	46.0	46			329	6,194	0	0	212	4,711	1,134	5,844	7,244
200-299	2	516	1,849	81.0	418			906	31,788	0	0	923	28,605	6,032	34,636	46,368
Federal government	11	8,040	52,343	76.7	6,165			20,307	1,119,036	0	0	14,251	501,424	77,725	579,149	808,078
100-199 beds	1	207	1,048	79.2	164			270	64,511	0	0	398	12,062	2,295	14,357	21,800
200-299	2	454	5,904	78.0	354			2,107	50,082	0	0	1,028	42,077	7,319	49,396	77,545
400-499	1	403	6,176	75.2	303			4,122	45,267	0	0	1,072	30,057	5,613	35,670	53,308
500 or more	7	6,976	39,215	76.6	5,344			13,808	959,176	0	0	11,753	417,229	62,498	479,727	655,425
PSYCHIATRIC	362	131,356	328,578	86.1	113,103			7,133	4,155,080	0	0	228,012	5,948,546	1,387,724	7,336,271	9,512,712
Nongovernment not-for-profit	45	5,218	22,745	76.5	3,994			0	360,240	0	0	12,151	347,647	71,804	419,451	641,525
6-24 beds	4	105	363	61.0	64			0	9,555	0	0	194	4,457	849	5,307	10,901
25-49	8	292	676	83.6	244			0	6,154	0	0	534	15,747	3,472	19,219	32,930
50-99	18	1,255	5,373	78.5	985			0	46,614	0	0	3,043	80,981	15,882	96,863	148,818
100-199	6	726	2,769	80.2	582			0	112,034	0	0	1,704	52,076	9,962	62,037	99,653
200-299	4	1,008	6,869	79.5	801			0	48,166	0	0	2,725	69,098	13,394	82,492	121,249
300-399	4	1,323	6,521	90.5	1,197			0	137,717	0	0	3,656	119,185	27,143	146,328	215,872
500 or more	1	509	174	23.8	121			0	0	0	0	295	6,103	1,102	7,205	12,103
Investor-owned (for-profit)	80	7,923	40,402	72.7	5,762			0	164,972	0	0	15,810	429,371	101,205	530,576	899,594
6-24 beds	1	20	69	60.0	12			0	1,820	0	0	37	937	172	1,109	2,076
25-49	15	573	2,688	75.0	430			0	7,565	0	0	1,188	28,678	6,635	35,313	66,537
50-99	30	2,249	11,124	70.2	1,579			0	45,865	0	0	4,414	136,612	29,218	165,830	290,550
100-199	33	4,747	24,464	73.2	3,474			0	99,990	0	0	9,449	245,338	60,845	306,183	511,942
300-399	1	334	2,057	79.9	267			0	9,732	0	0	722	17,807	4,335	22,141	28,489
Local government	4	2,435	4,143	87.6	2,132			0	46,523	0	0	3,820	154,525	42,674	197,199	245,043
100-199 beds	1	148	583	49.3	73			0	413	0	0	291	4,909	1,786	6,695	9,756
300-399	1	388	621	88.9	345			0	0	0	0	596	15,452	4,552	20,005	28,956
400-499	1	400	38	80.8	323			0	11,502	0	0	819	27,319	7,480	34,799	38,064
500 or more	1	1,499	2,901	92.8	1,391			0	34,608	0	0	2,114	106,844	28,856	135,701	168,265
State government	217	104,465	204,540	88.1	92,055			3,236	2,398,757	0	0	177,901	4,494,189	1,079,841	5,574,029	6,855,268
25-49 beds	4	159	750	89.9	143			0	25,220	0	0	309	9,967	2,466	12,433	20,488
50-99	16	1,162	4,600	77.8	904			0	191,685	0	0	3,357	82,055	18,507	100,562	139,067
100-199	29	4,557	16,591	83.4	3,802			21	243,500	0	0	9,403	269,097	64,889	333,986	467,016
200-299	22	5,516	20,524	90.8	5,009			357	120,530	0	0	10,770	259,577	57,034	316,611	400,153
300-399	42	14,887	45,690	89.9	13,381			0	399,198	0	0	27,966	723,229	170,533	893,762	1,117,347
400-499	28	13,306	18,009	87.3	11,619			46	131,077	0	0	20,565	531,853	142,856	674,709	811,707
500 or more	76	64,878	98,376	88.2	57,197			2,812	1,287,547	0	0	105,531	2,618,411	623,555	3,241,965	3,899,490

Table 2B (Continued)

CLASSIFICATION	HOSPITALS	BEDS	ADMISSIONS	OCCUPANCY, percent	AVERAGE DAILY CENSUS	ADJUSTED AVERAGE DAILY CENSUS	AVG. STAY, days	SURGICAL OPERATIONS	OUTPATIENT VISITS	NEWBORNS: Bassinets	NEWBORNS: Births	FTE PERSONNEL	EXPENSES (in thousands of dollars) LABOR: PAYROLL	LABOR: EMPLOYEE BENEFITS	LABOR: TOTAL	TOTAL
Federal government	16	11,315	56,748	81.0	9,160			3,897	1,184,588	0	0	18,330	$ 522,815	$ 92,200	$ 615,016	$ 871,283
300-399 beds	1	319	1,086	89.7	286			0	36,245	0	0	593	15,888	2,972	18,859	26,838
400-499	1	494	2,847	88.7	438			0	112,847	0	0	870	24,880	4,600	29,480	45,822
500 or more	14	10,502	52,815	80.3	8,436			3,897	1,035,496	0	0	16,867	482,047	84,629	566,676	798,622
TB AND OTHER RESPIRATORY DISEASES	3	355	638	65.4	232			233	1,073	0	0	942	19,072	4,742	23,815	38,429
Nongovernment not-for-profit	1	63	276	55.6	35			230	710	0	0	199	5,266	1,564	6,829	11,812
50-99 beds	1	63	276	55.6	35			230	710	0	0	199	5,266	1,564	6,829	11,812
State government	2	292	362	67.5	197			3	363	0	0	743	13,807	3,179	16,985	26,617
100-199 beds	2	292	362	67.5	197			3	363	0	0	743	13,807	3,179	16,985	26,617
ALL OTHER	112	22,166	62,519	86.3	19,140			4,983	1,217,125	2	2	46,814	1,297,375	308,484	1,605,859	2,312,619
Nongovernment not-for-profit	49	7,324	29,306	85.9	6,289			2,460	728,364	0	0	18,691	511,957	109,073	621,029	942,305
6-24 beds	1	12	72	66.7	8			0	10,107	0	0	137	3,918	690	4,608	6,504
25-49	6	241	1,384	68.5	165			279	51,635	0	0	738	21,126	3,591	24,717	41,541
50-99	22	1,758	9,419	84.1	1,479			1,946	455,990	0	0	6,634	178,717	34,359	213,076	332,063
100-199	7	1,021	5,941	81.8	835			7	69,249	0	0	3,439	97,584	23,771	121,355	184,798
200-299	7	1,638	9,824	88.3	1,447			228	126,662	0	0	4,301	120,426	24,631	145,057	207,615
300-399	4	1,361	2,191	81.9	1,115			0	14,721	0	0	2,108	54,714	13,644	68,357	108,754
500 or more	2	1,293	475	95.9	1,240			0	0	0	0	1,334	35,472	8,386	43,858	61,030
Investor-owned (for-profit)	17	1,197	7,783	75.9	909			112	221,930	0	0	3,625	101,375	23,268	124,643	205,959
25-49 beds	4	159	763	84.9	135			0	5,744	0	0	465	14,810	3,718	18,529	31,827
50-99	11	766	5,058	72.7	557			112	73,939	0	0	2,031	56,541	13,616	70,157	120,787
100-199	2	272	1,962	79.8	2[illegible]7			0	142,247	0	0	1,129	30,024	5,933	35,957	53,346
Local government	20	8,072	14,081	90.2	7,230			1,534	85,939	0	0	13,906	392,680	102,404	495,083	662,949
25-49 beds	1	36	156	75.0	27			182	3,088	0	0	95	2,605	911	3,516	4,664
50-99	2	170	856	85.3	145			42	9,062	0	0	507	14,425	3,130	17,555	27,622
100-199	7	1,016	2,970	82.9	842			128	4,974	0	0	1,934	50,866	10,941	61,807	94,507
300-399	2	632	684	86.2	545			0	0	0	0	816	16,724	2,467	19,190	28,140
400-499	1	408	1,752	94.6	386			0	0	0	0	816	28,881	8,662	37,543	50,792
500 or more	7	5,810	7,663	91.8	5,335			1,182	68,815	0	0	9,738	279,179	76,293	355,472	457,224
State government	25	4,839	9,292	82.2	3,980			877	122,139	2	2	9,419	259,873	68,046	327,919	455,687
6-24 beds	1	15	45	73.3	11			0	3,303	2	2	32	976	132	1,108	1,606
25-49	2	72	562	69.4	50			0	17,934	0	0	321	14,472	3,325	17,797	26,854
50-99	5	422	1,888	79.9	337			0	23,912	0	0	1,469	30,398	4,639	35,036	55,701
100-199	7	980	4,619	75.3	738			674	69,834	0	0	2,585	80,144	19,326	99,470	149,625
200-299	5	1,223	965	76.5	936			149	7,156	0	0	2,029	54,474	16,157	70,630	88,677
300-399	2	684	772	94.4	646			54	0	0	0	1,276	38,651	13,754	52,405	67,967
400-499	2	918	271	81.6	749			0	0	0	0	962	20,053	6,506	26,559	33,060
500 or more	1	525	170	97.7	513			0	0	0	0	745	20,706	4,207	24,913	32,196
Federal government	1	734	2,057	92.9	682			0	58,753	0	0	1,173	31,491	5,694	37,185	45,719
500 or more beds	1	734	2,057	92.9	682			0	58,753	0	0	1,173	31,491	5,694	37,185	45,719

Table

3

Utilization, Personnel Per Census, and Finances Per Inpatient Day

Expense components may not add to total expenses because of rounding to the nearest thousand.

CLASSIFICATION	HOSPITALS	BEDS	ADMISSIONS	OCCUPANCY, percent	AVERAGE DAILY CENSUS	ADJUSTED AVERAGE DAILY CENSUS	AVG. STAY, days	SURGICAL OPERATIONS	NEWBORNS			OUTPATIENT VISITS		
									Bassinets	Births	Days	Emergency	Other	Total
UNITED STATES	6,649	1,213,327	33,773,574	69.5	843,724			23,091,324	70,539	4,046,704	10,374,771	92,080,647	276,102,951	368,183,598
6-24 beds	301	5,763	141,672	36.2	2,085			85,851	804	12,376	34,449	812,468	4,202,206	5,014,674
25-49	1,095	41,266	1,006,291	44.1	18,191			507,814	4,110	91,229	207,390	4,348,468	13,114,571	17,463,039
50-99	1,633	117,585	2,832,567	56.4	66,323			1,722,009	8,336	286,812	673,809	10,004,788	25,755,680	35,760,468
100-199	1,562	219,772	6,315,029	62.8	137,922			4,545,600	14,796	725,748	1,792,749	20,400,801	50,778,344	71,179,145
200-299	830	201,734	6,615,629	68.4	138,056			4,811,969	13,491	783,935	1,980,128	18,791,024	48,387,067	67,178,091
300-399	503	172,230	5,410,306	72.6	125,032			3,851,618	10,212	691,775	1,759,063	13,134,141	38,301,602	51,435,743
400-499	276	123,895	3,865,258	75.4	93,392			2,646,442	7,216	526,414	1,346,379	8,979,614	30,652,270	39,631,884
500 or more	449	331,082	7,586,822	79.4	262,723			4,920,021	11,574	928,415	2,580,804	15,609,343	64,911,211	80,520,554
Federal	337	98,255	1,759,058	72.9	71,637			1,145,123	2,063	85,808	245,884	4,951,556	53,575,535	58,527,091
Psychiatric	17	11,654	58,674	80.4	9,366			3,897	0	0	0	6,374	1,200,960	1,207,334
General and other special	320	86,601	1,700,384	71.9	62,271			1,141,226	2,063	85,808	245,884	4,945,182	52,374,575	57,319,757
Nonfederal	6,312	1,115,072	32,014,516	69.2	772,087			21,946,201	68,476	3,960,896	10,128,887	87,129,091	222,527,416	309,656,507
Psychiatric	757	160,237	721,169	81.1	129,984			5,829	5	177	286	281,959	5,115,980	5,397,939
Nongovernment not-for-profit	127	12,412	122,558	71.6	8,883			1,102	5	177	286	38,007	1,240,732	1,278,739
Investor-owned (for-profit)	372	33,151	328,813	63.7	21,103			1,491	0	0	0	60,276	707,684	767,960
State and local government	258	114,674	269,798	87.2	99,998			3,236	0	0	0	183,676	3,167,564	3,351,240
TB and other respiratory diseases	4	470	1,849	66.4	312			2,039	0	0	0	0	16,863	16,863
Nongovernment not-for-profit	1	63	276	55.6	35			230	0	0	0	0	710	710
Investor-owned (for-profit)	0	0	0	00.0	0			0	0	0	0	0	0	0
State and local government	3	407	1,573	68.1	277			1,809	0	0	0	0	16,153	16,153
Long-term general and other special	131	24,991	88,344	85.6	21,386			17,006	28	2,073	6,010	64,630	1,486,422	1,551,052
Nongovernment not-for-profit	58	8,342	41,592	85.0	7,088			8,235	22	2,046	5,938	36,176	874,951	911,127
Investor-owned (for-profit)	18	1,253	8,006	75.3	943			474	0	0	0	866	221,577	222,443
State and local government	55	15,396	38,746	86.7	13,355			8,297	6	27	72	27,588	389,894	417,482
Short-term general and other special	5,420	929,374	31,203,154	66.8	620,405	820,033	7.3	21,921,327	68,443	3,958,646	10,122,591	86,782,502	215,908,151	302,690,653
6-24 beds	241	4,681	98,369	32.0	1,497	2,946	5.5	57,525	619	7,533	18,469	372,148	1,466,902	1,839,050
25-49	944	35,707	873,549	41.4	14,789	23,395	6.2	452,358	3,677	77,548	171,791	3,398,360	7,522,651	10,921,011
50-99	1,270	90,920	2,481,318	53.8	48,870	71,882	7.2	1,658,268	7,960	271,052	633,028	9,238,997	18,609,192	27,848,189
100-199	1,309	184,250	5,836,271	61.5	113,251	156,667	7.1	4,361,685	14,214	701,924	1,724,681	19,268,091	39,892,757	59,160,848
200-299	740	179,888	6,334,650	67.1	120,665	161,041	7.0	4,677,501	13,304	774,499	1,953,804	18,256,614	42,447,815	60,704,429
300-399	409	139,284	5,094,885	69.9	97,419	125,843	7.0	3,661,580	10,095	683,763	1,739,202	12,818,279	31,134,725	43,953,004
400-499	222	98,833	3,643,952	73.5	72,642	91,712	7.3	2,533,599	7,096	516,501	1,312,495	8,546,087	24,847,932	33,394,019
500 or more	285	195,811	6,840,160	77.3	151,272	186,547	8.1	4,518,811	11,478	925,826	2,569,121	14,883,926	49,986,177	64,870,103
Nongovernment not-for-profit	3,202	657,016	22,883,436	69.3	455,276	596,782	7.3	16,554,341	47,472	2,833,587	7,285,316	60,840,688	160,333,828	221,174,516
6-24 beds	84	1,602	37,540	34.3	550	1,242	5.4	26,789	256	3,752	10,906	131,977	541,092	673,069
25-49	409	15,569	419,006	43.6	6,785	10,850	5.9	252,793	1,689	39,091	84,828	1,702,549	4,096,772	5,799,321
50-99	635	45,495	1,278,245	56.0	25,486	37,352	7.3	899,347	4,034	134,869	317,269	4,905,583	10,827,830	15,733,413
100-199	778	110,963	3,710,758	63.5	70,441	98,321	6.9	2,829,348	8,709	434,076	1,062,976	12,562,821	28,032,866	40,595,687
200-299	562	137,015	4,915,230	69.2	94,808	126,441	7.0	3,667,768	10,001	586,265	1,514,181	14,156,147	35,795,924	49,952,071
300-399	331	113,226	4,199,215	70.6	79,983	102,497	7.0	3,089,348	8,337	553,960	1,427,884	10,427,333	25,620,797	36,048,130
400-499	179	79,534	2,938,011	74.2	59,039	74,511	7.3	2,094,007	5,681	402,204	1,031,070	6,456,628	18,540,421	24,997,049
500 or more	224	153,612	5,385,431	76.9	118,184	145,568	8.0	3,694,941	8,765	679,370	1,836,202	10,497,650	36,878,126	47,375,776
Investor-owned (for-profit)	749	101,377	3,066,198	52.8	53,510	68,744	6.4	2,330,095	6,261	340,555	805,571	8,002,054	12,107,454	20,109,508
6-24 beds	15	279	6,740	29.7	83	208	4.3	11,320	5	84	189	17,924	65,644	83,568
25-49	80	3,093	77,204	40.5	1,254	1,760	5.9	43,103	176	4,391	9,302	223,741	405,779	629,520
50-99	219	16,221	475,737	47.4	7,682	10,320	5.9	325,190	1,043	49,532	111,439	1,511,786	2,105,137	3,616,923
100-199	287	39,313	1,197,651	52.3	20,568	27,119	6.2	931,769	2,687	140,024	333,241	3,353,261	5,314,309	8,667,570
200-299	99	23,384	714,103	55.6	12,990	16,056	6.6	549,293	1,284	76,674	185,564	1,705,302	2,180,287	3,885,589
300-399	30	9,719	294,615	57.3	5,572	6,756	6.9	237,001	579	34,933	81,409	570,566	941,869	1,512,435
400-499	13	5,706	177,734	53.5	3,055	3,717	6.3	138,626	321	20,545	47,724	377,232	730,492	1,107,724
500 or more	6	3,662	122,414	63.0	2,306	2,808	6.9	93,793	166	14,372	36,703	242,242	363,937	606,179
State and local government	1,469	170,981	5,253,520	65.3	111,619	154,507	7.8	3,036,891	14,710	784,504	2,031,704	17,939,760	43,466,869	61,406,629
6-24 beds	142	2,800	54,089	30.9	864	1,496	5.8	19,416	358	3,697	7,374	222,247	860,166	1,082,413
25-49	455	17,045	377,339	39.6	6,750	10,785	6.5	156,462	1,812	34,066	77,661	1,472,070	3,020,100	4,492,170
50-99	416	29,204	727,336	53.8	15,702	24,210	7.9	433,731	2,883	86,651	204,320	2,821,628	5,676,225	8,497,853
100-199	244	33,974	927,862	65.5	22,242	31,227	8.7	600,568	2,818	127,824	328,464	3,352,009	6,545,582	9,897,591
200-299	79	19,489	705,317	66.0	12,867	18,544	6.7	460,440	2,019	111,560	254,059	2,395,165	4,471,604	6,866,769
300-399	48	16,339	601,055	72.6	11,864	16,590	7.2	335,231	1,179	94,870	229,909	1,820,380	4,572,059	6,392,439
400-499	30	13,593	528,207	77.6	10,548	13,484	7.3	300,966	1,094	93,752	233,701	1,712,227	5,577,019	7,289,246
500 or more	55	38,537	1,332,315	79.9	30,782	38,171	8.4	730,077	2,547	232,084	696,216	4,144,034	12,744,114	16,888,148
Hospital units of institutions	36	2,014	22,108	56.1	1,130	7,281	18.6	6,459	31	383	4,196	89,999	1,271,892	1,361,891
Community hospitals	5,384	927,360	31,181,046	66.8	619,275	812,752	7.2	21,914,868	68,412	3,958,263	10,118,395	86,692,503	214,636,259	301,328,762

Table 3 (Continued)

CLASSIFICATION	FULL-TIME EQUIVALENT PERSONNEL: TOTAL Number	TOTAL Per 100 Adjusted Census	RN Number	RN Per 100 Adjusted Census	LPN Number	LPN Per 100 Adjusted Census	EXPENSES: LABOR: PAYROLL Amount (in thousands)	EMPLOYEE BENEFITS Amount (in thousands)	LABOR TOTAL Amount (in thousands)	LABOR TOTAL Adjusted, per Admission	LABOR TOTAL Adjusted per Inpatient Day	OTHER Amount (in thousands)	TOTAL Amount (in thousands)	TOTAL Adjusted, per Admission	TOTAL Adjusted per Inpatient Day
UNITED STATES	**4,063,288**		**895,324**		**197,843**		**$108,718,572**	**$21,796,512**	**$130,515,084**			**$103,403,897**	**$234,869,906**		
6-24 beds	20,880		3,112		1,335		411,477	81,606	493,083			298,916	790,358		
25-49	114,291		20,056		8,621		2,360,135	463,171	2,823,306			2,216,015	5,055,866		
50-99	312,478		61,771		21,730		7,202,973	1,448,263	8,651,236			7,401,562	16,133,345		
100-199	675,463		149,928		40,321		16,834,154	3,393,302	20,227,456			17,723,493	38,260,572		
200-299	701,943		163,997		35,654		18,762,191	3,698,171	22,460,362			19,002,392	41,613,305		
300-399	626,962		145,886		28,051		17,176,408	3,421,669	20,598,077			16,198,975	36,909,265		
400-499	465,428		107,119		18,636		13,277,352	2,647,740	15,925,092			12,029,874	28,034,520		
500 or more	1,145,843		243,455		43,454		32,693,882	6,642,590	39,336,472			28,532,671	68,072,675		
Federal	**303,471**		**45,663**		**14,118**		**8,742,853**	**1,492,845**	**10,235,698**			**5,037,711**	**15,243,688**		
Psychiatric	18,773		2,458		824		536,173	94,577	630,750			261,673	892,451		
General and other special	284,698		43,205		13,324		8,206,680	1,398,267	9,604,947			4,776,038	14,351,237		
Nonfederal	**3,759,817**		**849,661**		**183,695**		**99,975,719**	**20,303,667**	**120,279,386**			**98,366,187**	**219,626,218**		
Psychiatric	280,081		32,343		12,031		7,428,866	1,727,870	9,156,736			3,699,476	12,904,591		
Nongovernment not-for-profit	27,866		4,151		436		780,111	161,632	941,743			550,068	1,498,048		
Investor-owned (for-profit)	55,184		9,196		1,714		1,572,527	343,740	1,916,267			1,599,715	3,548,139		
State and local government	197,031		18,996		9,381		5,076,228	1,222,498	6,298,726			1,549,694	7,858,404		
TB and other respiratory diseases	1,264		144		105		26,065	5,609	31,674			18,720	50,448		
Nongovernment not-for-profit	199		35		27		5,266	1,564	6,829			4,983	11,812		
Investor-owned (for-profit)	0		0		0		0	0	0			0	0		
State and local government	1,065		109		78		20,800	4,045	24,844			13,737	38,636		
Long-term general and other special	54,983		6,521		2,993		1,519,349	362,463	1,881,812			852,357	2,743,679		
Nongovernment not-for-profit	21,310		2,747		999		568,911	119,863	688,774			370,081	1,059,796		
Investor-owned (for-profit)	3,750		422		301		106,127	24,299	130,426			83,953	215,058		
State and local government	29,923		3,352		1,693		844,311	218,302	1,062,613			398,323	1,468,825		
Short-term general and other special	3,423,489	417	810,653	99	166,566	21	91,001,439	18,207,726	109,209,165	$2,640.12	$364.97	93,795,634	203,927,499	$4,929.93	$681.52
6-24 beds	11,380	387	2,070	70	1,095	37	226,943	44,076	271,019	1,362.22	252.57	225,622	498,942	2,507.83	464.98
25-49	90,416	387	16,885	72	7,806	33	1,796,894	344,675	2,141,569	1,554.94	251.07	1,895,432	4,050,580	2,941.03	474.87
50-99	245,927	342	51,928	72	13,359	27	5,446,576	1,096,495	6,543,071	1,758.80	249.59	6,038,526	12,639,610	3,397.57	482.15
100-199	582,230	372	136,449	87	36,573	23	14,330,561	2,896,045	17,226,606	2,123.51	301.47	15,814,256	33,328,214	4,108.33	583.25
200-299	645,064	401	155,960	97	32,968	20	17,114,718	3,407,306	20,522,024	2,445.58	349.15	18,054,661	38,726,382	4,614.97	658.86
300-399	547,696	435	135,514	108	24,373	19	14,974,583	2,965,158	17,939,741	2,745.47	390.58	15,104,875	33,181,867	5,078.09	722.42
400-499	408,740	446	98,969	108	15,745	17	11,617,468	2,316,667	13,934,135	3,029.30	416.31	11,286,792	25,297,239	5,499.65	755.80
500 or more	892,036	478	212,878	114	30,647	16	25,493,695	5,137,303	30,630,998	3,633.20	449.89	25,375,469	56,204,665	6,666.54	825.49
Nongovernment not-for-profit	2,533,805	425	609,054	102	111,276	19	68,466,684	13,344,797	81,811,481	2,711.86	375.61	68,331,592	150,692,755	4,995.12	691.86
6-24 beds	4,262	344	802	65	347	28	89,747	17,590	107,337	1,262.03	237.05	85,897	193,899	2,279.80	428.21
25-49	45,373	418	9,072	84	3,141	29	924,140	173,434	1,097,574	1,620.69	277.17	985,807	2,090,728	3,087.19	527.97
50-99	132,468	355	28,899	77	9,141	24	3,004,028	589,598	3,593,626	1,860.04	263.64	3,085,393	6,704,738	3,470.34	491.89
100-199	381,623	388	89,589	91	21,260	22	9,615,698	1,868,308	11,484,006	2,200.44	320.02	9,663,019	21,228,022	4,067.48	591.55
200-299	512,462	405	123,561	98	24,232	19	13,624,906	2,645,182	16,270,088	2,483.61	352.57	13,618,290	30,001,235	4,579.64	650.12
300-399	446,357	436	109,566	107	19,123	19	12,278,796	2,400,585	14,679,381	2,728.18	392.40	12,076,744	26,852,785	4,990.63	717.80
400-499	323,102	434	79,840	107	12,015	16	9,118,393	1,772,116	10,890,509	2,938.17	400.48	8,783,803	19,739,883	5,325.65	725.90
500 or more	688,158	473	167,725	115	22,017	15	19,810,977	3,877,983	23,688,960	3,580.27	445.87	20,032,640	43,881,464	6,632.10	825.93
Investor-owned (for-profit)	272,642	397	68,801	100	19,712	29	6,732,451	1,492,989	8,225,440	2,065.92	328.44	10,335,140	18,821,608	4,727.27	751.55
6-24 beds	706	353	156	78	75	38	19,816	3,676	23,492	1,087.32	317.56	20,878	45,051	2,085.22	609.00
25-49	7,106	404	1,165	66	744	42	143,834	29,519	173,353	1,535.30	271.55	195,023	370,672	3,282.84	580.64
50-99	41,431	401	8,808	85	3,697	36	961,300	214,984	1,176,284	1,811.71	313.40	1,466,335	2,668,759	4,110.41	711.04
100-199	106,169	392	27,248	101	7,653	28	2,604,003	603,708	3,207,711	2,018.46	324.97	3,994,470	7,395,306	4,653.52	749.20
200-299	61,728	385	16,689	104	4,119	26	1,611,080	352,950	1,964,029	2,217.38	335.13	2,489,830	4,479,034	5,056.82	764.27
300-399	27,939	414	7,513	111	1,823	27	719,447	146,534	865,981	2,427.89	351.33	1,104,775	1,980,824	5,553.49	803.63
400-499	15,585	420	4,054	109	963	26	390,836	80,701	471,538	2,174.56	347.62	629,635	1,102,742	5,085.44	812.96
500 or more	11,978	428	3,168	113	638	23	282,135	60,916	343,051	2,298.33	334.56	434,194	779,220	5,220.52	759.93
State and local government	617,042	399	132,798	86	37,578	24	15,802,304	3,369,940	19,172,244	2,657.01	340.09	15,128,902	34,413,137	4,769.19	610.45
6-24 beds	6,412	430	1,112	75	673	45	117,381	22,810	140,191	1,518.89	256.64	118,847	259,992	2,816.88	475.95
25-49	37,937	352	6,648	62	3,921	36	728,920	141,721	870,641	1,482.88	221.45	714,603	1,589,180	2,706.70	404.21
50-99	72,028	298	14,221	59	6,521	27	1,481,248	291,913	1,773,161	1,556.90	200.78	1,486,798	3,266,114	2,867.76	369.84
100-199	94,438	302	19,612	63	7,660	25	2,110,860	424,029	2,534,889	1,943.64	222.63	2,156,768	4,704,886	3,607.50	413.20
200-299	70,874	382	15,710	85	4,617	25	1,878,733	409,174	2,287,907	2,396.37	337.96	1,946,541	4,246,112	4,447.40	627.21
300-399	73,400	442	18,435	111	3,427	21	1,976,340	418,039	2,394,379	3,004.27	395.33	1,923,357	4,348,258	5,455.83	717.92
400-499	70,053	520	15,075	112	2,767	21	2,108,239	463,850	2,572,088	3,802.74	522.73	1,873,353	4,454,613	6,585.99	905.32
500 or more	191,900	503	41,985	110	7,992	21	5,400,584	1,198,404	6,598,987	3,963.18	473.68	4,908,635	11,543,981	6,933.01	828.63
Hospital units of institutions	3,970	55	726	10	633	9	76,046	21,028	97,074	517.48	36.54	137,519	234,909	1,252.25	88.43
Community hospitals	3,419,519	421	809,927	100	167,933	21	90,925,393	18,186,698	109,112,090	2,649.79	367.91	93,658,115	203,692,591	4,946.68	686.83

Table

4A

Utilization of Hospital Units and Nursing-Home-Type Units Operated by Hospitals

Separate nursing-home-type unit data are presented for only those hospitals that reported separate units. For the definition of a separate nursing-home-type unit, see Section E of the AHA Annual Survey on page 255. Note that the Total Facilities column in this series of tables corresponds to the Hospital Column in all other tables.

In tables 4A and 4B, the number of beds at the end of the reporting period has been used rather than the average number of beds for a 12-month period. Therefore, there is a difference between the total number of beds in tables 4A and 4B and the totals in other tables. In addition, internal transfers between the hospital unit and the nursing-home-type unit may be reflected in the admissions figures for both units of the facility. Therefore, the total admissions figures for Hospital Units and Nursing-Home-Type Units may be greater than the admissions figures for Total Facilities.

CLASSIFICATION	TOTAL FACILITIES				HOSPITAL UNITS				NURSING-HOME-TYPE UNITS			
	Facilities	Beds	Admissions	Inpatient Days	Units	Beds	Admissions	Inpatient Days	Units	Beds	Admissions	Inpatient Days
UNITED STATES	6,649	1,210,761	33,773,574	307,871,443	6,649	1,121,034	33,559,566	278,527,348	1,321	89,727	216,882	29,344,095
6-24 beds	301	5,701	141,672	757,399	301	5,597	141,502	722,221	8	104	170	35,178
25-49	1,095	41,006	1,006,291	6,636,239	1,095	39,200	1,003,320	6,060,577	89	1,806	2,971	575,662
50-99	1,633	117,574	2,832,567	24,167,419	1,633	105,433	2,812,312	20,176,555	331	12,141	20,739	3,990,864
100-199	1,562	219,500	6,315,029	50,307,197	1,562	198,533	6,269,084	43,405,174	383	20,967	47,966	6,902,023
200-299	830	202,014	6,615,629	50,387,554	830	190,308	6,575,443	46,661,048	177	11,706	40,186	3,726,506
300-399	503	172,289	5,410,306	45,632,571	503	163,748	5,370,450	42,886,852	112	8,541	40,019	2,745,719
400-499	276	123,467	3,865,258	34,088,579	276	117,455	3,848,579	32,107,629	65	6,012	16,679	1,980,950
500 or more	449	329,210	7,586,822	95,894,485	449	300,760	7,538,876	86,507,292	156	28,450	48,152	9,387,193
Federal	337	97,709	1,759,058	26,145,504	337	82,779	1,740,252	21,388,832	120	14,930	18,806	4,756,672
Psychiatric	17	11,542	58,674	3,418,801	17	9,357	57,151	2,746,859	16	2,185	1,523	671,942
General and other special	320	86,167	1,700,384	22,726,703	320	73,422	1,683,101	18,641,973	104	12,745	17,283	4,084,730
Nonfederal	6,312	1,113,052	32,014,516	281,725,939	6,312	1,038,255	31,819,314	257,138,516	1,201	74,797	198,076	24,587,423
Psychiatric	757	157,621	721,169	47,427,207	757	150,658	718,585	45,085,371	43	6,963	2,790	2,341,836
Nongovernment not-for-profit	127	12,313	122,558	3,240,558	127	11,789	122,297	3,057,029	5	524	261	183,529
Investor-owned (for-profit)	372	33,096	328,813	7,684,302	372	32,961	328,521	7,638,539	4	135	292	45,763
State and local government	258	112,212	269,798	36,502,347	258	105,908	267,767	34,389,803	34	6,304	2,237	2,112,544
TB and other respiratory diseases	4	470	1,849	113,912	4	470	1,849	113,912	0	0	0	0
Nongovernment not-for-profit	1	63	276	12,635	1	63	276	12,635	0	0	0	0
Investor-owned (for-profit)	0	0	0	0	0	0	0	0	0	0	0	0
State and local government	3	407	1,573	101,277	3	407	1,573	101,277	0	0	0	0
Long-term general and other special	131	24,897	88,344	7,801,569	131	17,813	71,397	5,410,824	28	7,084	16,947	2,390,745
Nongovernment not-for-profit	58	8,335	41,592	2,587,359	58	6,846	28,696	2,091,963	10	1,489	12,896	495,396
Investor-owned (for-profit)	18	1,249	8,006	339,093	18	1,164	7,839	324,000	2	85	167	15,093
State and local government	55	15,313	38,746	4,875,117	55	9,803	34,862	2,994,861	16	5,510	3,884	1,880,256
Short-term general and other special	5,420	930,064	31,203,154	226,383,251	5,420	869,314	31,027,483	206,528,409	1,130	60,750	178,339	19,854,842
6-24 beds	241	4,653	98,369	543,920	241	4,562	98,199	513,487	7	91	170	30,433
25-49	944	35,480	873,549	5,394,677	944	33,674	870,578	4,819,015	89	1,806	2,971	575,662
50-99	1,270	91,009	2,481,318	17,819,004	1,270	79,213	2,461,665	13,931,283	323	11,796	20,137	3,887,721
100-199	1,309	184,446	5,836,271	41,303,094	1,309	164,825	5,793,917	34,826,450	355	19,621	44,375	6,476,644
200-299	740	180,286	6,334,650	44,040,191	740	170,497	6,297,071	40,947,988	159	9,789	37,579	3,092,203
300-399	409	139,746	5,094,885	35,553,986	409	135,076	5,069,250	34,105,551	82	4,670	25,798	1,448,435
400-499	222	98,880	3,643,952	26,514,574	222	95,497	3,629,333	25,398,955	46	3,383	14,619	1,115,619
500 or more	285	195,564	6,840,160	55,213,805	285	185,970	6,807,470	51,985,680	69	9,594	32,690	3,228,125
Nongovernment not-for-profit	3,202	657,311	22,883,436	166,162,657	3,202	617,491	22,749,265	153,160,056	714	39,820	136,708	13,002,601
6-24 beds	84	1,584	37,540	200,879	84	1,580	37,503	200,096	1	4	37	783
25-49	409	15,420	419,006	2,476,468	409	14,840	418,004	2,290,705	33	580	1,002	185,763
50-99	635	45,581	1,278,245	9,298,319	635	39,209	1,267,861	7,175,951	168	6,372	10,737	2,122,368
100-199	778	110,974	3,710,758	25,709,550	778	100,325	3,684,770	22,244,406	206	10,649	28,009	3,465,144
200-299	562	137,264	4,915,230	34,601,587	562	129,177	4,883,739	32,011,896	135	8,087	31,491	2,589,691
300-399	331	113,556	4,199,215	29,189,842	331	109,779	4,176,621	28,008,976	71	3,777	22,757	1,180,866
400-499	179	79,509	2,938,011	21,547,580	179	76,615	2,925,007	20,599,263	40	2,894	13,004	948,317
500 or more	224	153,423	5,385,431	43,138,432	224	145,966	5,355,760	40,628,763	60	7,457	29,671	2,509,669
Investor-owned (for-profit)	749	101,737	3,066,198	19,494,671	749	100,064	3,055,659	19,057,879	66	1,673	10,539	436,792
6-24 beds	15	279	6,740	28,887	15	279	6,740	28,887	0	0	0	0
25-49	80	3,094	77,204	456,565	80	3,036	77,153	435,513	2	58	51	21,052
50-99	219	16,222	475,737	2,794,183	219	15,942	474,197	2,731,848	19	280	1,540	62,335
100-199	287	39,512	1,197,651	7,483,360	287	38,582	1,192,465	7,219,676	32	930	5,186	263,684
200-299	99	23,452	714,103	4,741,067	99	23,167	711,672	4,677,896	7	285	2,431	63,171
300-399	30	9,826	294,615	2,033,761	30	9,748	293,837	2,017,322	4	78	778	16,439
400-499	13	5,710	177,734	1,115,208	13	5,668	177,181	1,105,097	2	42	553	10,111
500 or more	6	3,642	122,414	841,640	6	3,642	122,414	841,640	0	0	0	0
State and local government	1,469	171,016	5,253,520	40,725,923	1,469	151,759	5,222,559	34,310,474	350	19,257	31,092	6,415,449
6-24 beds	142	2,790	54,089	314,154	142	2,703	53,956	284,504	6	87	133	29,650
25-49	455	16,966	377,339	2,461,644	455	15,798	375,421	2,092,797	54	1,168	1,918	368,847
50-99	416	29,206	727,336	5,726,502	416	24,062	719,607	4,023,484	136	5,144	7,860	1,703,018
100-199	244	33,960	927,862	8,110,184	244	25,918	916,682	5,362,368	117	8,042	11,180	2,747,816
200-299	79	19,570	705,317	4,697,537	79	18,153	701,660	4,258,196	17	1,417	3,657	439,341
300-399	48	16,364	601,055	4,330,383	48	15,549	598,792	4,079,253	7	815	2,263	251,130
400-499	30	13,661	528,207	3,851,786	30	13,214	527,145	3,694,595	4	447	1,062	157,191
500 or more	55	38,499	1,332,315	11,233,733	55	36,362	1,329,296	10,515,277	9	2,137	3,019	718,456
Hospital units of institutions	36	2,009	22,108	411,598	36	1,953	22,099	393,639	1	56	9	17,959
Community hospitals	5,384	928,055	31,181,046	225,971,653	5,384	867,361	31,005,384	206,134,770	1,129	60,694	178,330	19,836,883

4B

Utilization of Hospital Units and Nursing-Home-Type Units Operated by Community Hospitals, by State

CLASSIFICATION	TOTAL FACILITIES				HOSPITAL UNITS				NURSING-HOME-TYPE UNITS			
	Facilities	Beds	Admissions	Inpatient Days	Units	Beds	Admissions	Inpatient Days	Units	Beds	Admissions	Inpatient Days
UNITED STATES	5,384	928,055	31,181,046	225,971,653	5,384	867,361	31,005,384	206,134,770	1,129	60,694	178,330	19,836,883
6-24 beds	226	4,399	95,487	520,031	226	4,308	95,317	489,598	7	91	170	30,433
25-49	935	35,193	869,830	5,342,360	935	33,387	866,859	4,766,698	89	1,806	2,971	575,662
50-99	1,263	90,483	2,474,497	17,727,304	1,263	78,743	2,454,853	13,857,542	322	11,740	20,128	3,869,762
100-199	1,306	184,063	5,832,890	41,206,512	1,306	164,442	5,790,536	34,729,868	355	19,621	44,375	6,476,644
200-299	739	180,073	6,333,181	43,968,781	739	170,284	6,295,602	40,876,578	159	9,789	37,579	3,092,203
300-399	408	139,400	5,091,049	35,478,286	408	134,730	5,065,414	34,029,851	82	4,670	25,798	1,448,435
400-499	222	98,880	3,643,952	26,514,574	222	95,497	3,629,333	25,398,955	46	3,383	14,619	1,115,619
500 or more	285	195,564	6,840,160	55,213,805	285	185,970	6,807,470	51,985,680	69	9,594	32,690	3,228,125
CENSUS DIVISION 1, NEW ENGLAND	229	44,214	1,620,584	11,987,553	229	43,257	1,618,840	11,658,117	24	957	1,744	329,436
Connecticut	35	9,623	355,057	2,704,095	35	9,529	354,989	2,670,402	1	94	68	33,693
Maine	39	4,506	145,569	1,173,342	39	4,009	144,543	1,003,846	14	497	1,026	169,496
Massachusetts	101	21,725	810,991	5,921,378	101	21,725	810,991	5,921,378	0	0	0	0
New Hampshire	27	3,459	124,532	846,149	27	3,193	123,960	755,838	6	266	572	90,311
Rhode Island	12	3,176	126,730	921,295	12	3,176	126,730	921,295	0	0	0	0
Vermont	15	1,725	57,705	421,294	15	1,625	57,627	385,358	3	100	78	35,936
CENSUS DIVISION 2, MIDDLE ATLANTIC	568	156,218	5,249,072	45,750,807	568	147,402	5,234,748	42,719,666	116	8,816	16,298	3,031,141
New Jersey	95	28,889	1,131,509	8,438,916	95	28,210	1,130,652	8,231,641	8	679	857	207,275
New York	235	74,723	2,321,509	23,372,299	235	69,210	2,315,919	21,407,101	63	5,513	5,715	1,965,198
Pennsylvania	238	52,606	1,796,054	13,939,592	238	49,982	1,788,177	13,080,924	45	2,624	9,726	858,668
CENSUS DIVISION 3, SOUTH ATLANTIC	803	158,207	5,511,559	38,807,448	803	150,472	5,494,560	36,291,568	131	7,735	16,999	2,515,880
Delaware	8	2,006	84,090	560,406	8	2,006	84,090	560,406	0	0	0	0
District of Columbia	11	4,507	157,832	1,252,183	11	4,507	157,832	1,252,183	0	0	0	0
Florida	224	50,717	1,638,871	11,405,957	224	49,724	1,633,877	11,088,664	14	993	4,994	317,293
Georgia	163	25,699	888,048	6,120,975	163	23,221	885,725	5,291,146	27	2,478	2,323	829,829
Maryland	52	13,560	562,280	3,863,982	52	13,204	560,491	3,752,991	7	356	1,789	110,991
North Carolina	120	21,994	784,414	5,856,343	120	20,799	781,423	5,457,319	28	1,195	2,991	399,024
South Carolina	69	11,273	413,045	2,899,854	69	10,547	412,314	2,659,051	15	726	731	240,803
Virginia	97	20,031	706,240	4,918,759	97	18,698	703,906	4,507,916	25	1,333	2,334	410,843
West Virginia	59	8,420	276,739	1,928,989	59	7,766	274,902	1,721,892	15	654	1,837	207,097
CENSUS DIVISION 4, EAST NORTH CENTRAL	818	163,178	5,404,346	38,598,241	818	152,874	5,372,866	35,215,329	176	10,304	31,480	3,382,912
Illinois	210	45,812	1,499,435	11,053,001	210	42,393	1,482,217	9,987,747	67	3,419	17,218	1,065,254
Indiana	113	21,831	727,241	4,832,689	113	21,167	723,332	4,615,805	21	664	3,909	216,884
Michigan	176	33,877	1,069,361	8,116,557	176	31,397	1,065,422	7,273,915	30	2,480	3,939	842,642
Ohio	190	43,055	1,511,655	10,187,427	190	41,723	1,507,258	9,761,873	26	1,332	4,397	425,554
Wisconsin	129	18,603	596,654	4,408,567	129	16,194	594,637	3,575,989	32	2,409	2,017	832,578
CENSUS DIVISION 5, EAST SOUTH CENTRAL	464	71,036	2,322,816	16,159,889	464	66,772	2,316,487	14,709,578	85	4,264	6,329	1,450,311
Alabama	120	18,597	597,023	4,254,741	120	17,441	595,873	3,851,301	14	1,156	1,150	403,440
Kentucky	107	15,907	531,817	3,580,816	107	15,139	529,891	3,327,773	25	768	1,926	253,043
Mississippi	103	12,902	395,804	2,799,572	103	11,842	394,980	2,448,982	24	1,060	824	350,590
Tennessee	134	23,630	798,172	5,524,760	134	22,350	795,743	5,081,522	22	1,280	2,429	443,238
CENSUS DIVISION 6, WEST NORTH CENTRAL	742	86,810	2,335,033	19,621,868	742	73,600	2,296,690	15,240,111	264	13,210	39,037	4,381,757
Iowa	124	14,258	385,138	3,206,410	124	12,362	376,821	2,568,214	49	1,896	8,317	638,196
Kansas	138	11,761	304,551	2,393,809	138	10,479	299,857	2,003,828	44	1,282	4,700	389,981
Minnesota	152	19,406	529,744	4,735,154	152	14,760	522,981	3,135,911	65	4,646	6,813	1,599,243
Missouri	135	24,329	737,219	5,489,754	135	22,615	723,291	4,977,065	49	1,714	14,394	512,689
Nebraska	90	8,464	187,977	1,810,607	90	6,995	184,552	1,321,030	26	1,469	3,597	489,577
North Dakota	50	4,392	95,983	1,033,620	50	3,252	95,353	654,120	14	1,140	630	379,500
South Dakota	53	4,200	94,421	952,514	53	3,137	93,835	579,943	17	1,063	586	372,571
CENSUS DIVISION 7, WEST SOUTH CENTRAL	765	101,550	3,321,869	21,468,716	765	98,529	3,305,484	20,604,685	102	3,021	16,385	864,031
Arkansas	86	10,888	346,819	2,453,917	86	10,255	345,849	2,246,575	10	633	970	207,342
Louisiana	140	19,086	606,863	3,998,692	140	18,488	603,351	3,815,257	22	598	3,512	183,435
Oklahoma	111	12,356	381,928	2,617,927	111	12,029	379,469	2,515,966	11	327	2,459	101,961
Texas	428	59,220	1,986,259	12,398,180	428	57,757	1,976,815	12,026,887	59	1,463	9,444	371,293
CENSUS DIVISION 8, MOUNTAIN	355	42,254	1,425,988	9,331,969	355	37,248	1,408,552	7,723,355	104	5,006	17,436	1,608,614
Arizona	61	9,878	396,422	2,249,577	61	9,365	392,478	2,101,173	12	513	3,944	148,404
Colorado	69	10,426	334,781	2,409,593	69	8,851	326,157	1,916,022	20	1,575	8,624	493,571
Idaho	43	3,191	96,621	650,658	43	2,642	95,839	468,089	14	549	782	182,569
Montana	55	4,588	105,405	1,035,165	55	3,233	104,077	594,834	30	1,355	1,328	440,331
Nevada	21	3,417	115,995	741,705	21	3,337	115,866	716,876	3	80	129	24,829
New Mexico	37	4,203	153,319	879,852	37	3,926	152,488	785,815	5	277	831	94,037
Utah	42	4,399	175,472	944,509	42	4,245	174,199	892,913	9	154	1,273	51,596
Wyoming	27	2,152	47,973	420,910	27	1,649	47,448	247,633	11	503	525	173,277
CENSUS DIVISION 9, PACIFIC	640	104,588	3,989,779	24,245,162	640	97,207	3,957,157	21,972,361	127	7,381	32,622	2,272,801
Alaska	16	1,185	37,201	215,935	16	1,061	37,083	175,735	7	124	118	40,200
California	445	80,471	3,063,199	18,734,637	445	74,961	3,035,797	17,064,338	86	5,510	27,402	1,670,299
Hawaii	18	2,875	95,958	896,665	18	2,190	94,504	667,121	9	685	1,454	229,544
Oregon	70	8,102	301,903	1,671,563	70	7,494	299,634	1,483,301	12	608	2,269	188,262
Washington	91	11,955	491,518	2,726,362	91	11,501	490,139	2,581,866	13	454	1,379	144,496

Table

4C

Personnel and Finances in Hospital Units and Nursing-Home-Type Units Operated by Hospitals

In tables 4C and 4D, expenses for Hospital Units and Nursing-Home-Type Units may not add to Total Facilities because of rounding to the nearest thousand. Also, in these two tables, total payroll expense has been used, whereas in other tables, payroll expense excludes medical and dental residents, interns, and other trainees. Therefore, there is a difference between Payroll Expense in tables 4C and 4D and Payroll Expense as shown in other tables.

	TOTAL FACILITIES				HOSPITAL UNITS				NURSING-HOME-TYPE UNITS			
CLASSIFICATION	Facilities	FTEs	Payroll Expense	Total Expense	Units	FTEs	Payroll Expense	Total Expense	Units	FTEs	Payroll Expense	Total Expense
UNITED STATES	6,649	4,063,288	$110,925,804	$234,869,906	6,649	3,995,851	$109,064,960	$231,567,144	1,321	67,437	$1,822,091	$ 3,141,319
6-24 beds	301	20,880	412,521	790,358	301	20,758	410,300	787,193	8	122	2,221	3,165
25-49	1,095	114,291	2,365,625	5,055,866	1,095	112,747	2,342,680	5,015,275	89	1,544	21,710	37,639
50-99	1,633	312,478	7,216,820	16,133,345	1,633	303,643	7,056,552	15,850,710	331	8,835	152,352	267,525
100-199	1,562	675,463	16,934,786	38,260,572	1,562	659,800	16,629,823	37,725,733	383	15,663	299,504	523,174
200-299	830	701,943	18,944,806	41,613,305	830	692,095	18,702,620	41,166,149	177	9,848	242,186	447,156
300-399	503	626,962	17,487,566	36,909,265	503	620,330	17,251,157	36,464,885	112	6,632	212,268	395,579
400-499	276	465,428	13,590,094	28,034,520	276	460,133	13,403,041	27,728,493	65	5,295	187,053	306,027
500 or more	449	1,145,843	33,973,584	68,072,675	449	1,126,345	33,268,786	66,828,706	156	19,498	704,798	1,161,055
Federal	337	303,471	9,041,920	15,243,688	337	296,186	8,634,309	14,664,156	120	7,285	407,611	579,532
Psychiatric	17	18,773	538,253	892,451	17	17,758	457,360	775,485	16	1,015	80,894	116,966
General and other special	320	284,698	8,503,667	14,351,237	320	278,428	8,176,950	13,888,672	104	6,270	326,717	462,566
Nonfederal	6,312	3,759,817	101,883,883	219,626,218	6,312	3,699,665	100,430,651	216,902,987	1,201	60,152	1,414,480	2,561,787
Psychiatric	757	280,081	7,507,343	12,904,591	757	274,376	7,372,710	12,631,519	43	5,705	134,633	190,157
Nongovernment not-for-profit	127	27,866	788,910	1,498,048	127	27,449	780,217	1,481,810	5	417	8,693	16,238
Investor-owned (for-profit)	372	55,184	1,579,663	3,548,139	372	54,982	1,575,291	3,538,368	4	202	4,372	9,771
State and local government	258	197,031	5,138,770	7,858,404	258	191,945	5,017,202	7,611,341	34	5,086	121,568	164,149
TB and other respiratory diseases	4	1,264	26,065	50,448	4	1,264	26,065	50,448	0	0	0	0
Nongovernment not-for-profit	1	199	5,266	11,812	1	199	5,266	11,812	0	0	0	0
Investor-owned (for-profit)	0	0	0	0	0	0	0	0	0	0	0	0
State and local government	3	1,065	20,800	38,636	3	1,065	20,800	38,636	0	0	0	0
Long-term general and other special	131	54,983	1,535,475	2,743,679	131	49,414	1,257,382	2,299,153	28	5,569	278,093	444,527
Nongovernment not-for-profit	58	21,310	575,910	1,059,796	58	20,000	520,254	968,630	10	1,310	55,656	91,166
Investor-owned (for-profit)	18	3,750	106,288	215,058	18	3,684	104,185	211,195	2	66	2,102	3,863
State and local government	55	29,923	853,277	1,468,825	55	25,730	632,943	1,119,327	16	4,193	220,334	349,497
Short-term general and other special	5,420	3,423,489	92,815,000	203,927,499	5,420	3,374,611	91,774,494	201,921,867	1,130	48,878	1,001,754	1,927,103
6-24 beds	241	11,380	227,488	498,942	241	11,261	225,445	495,977	7	119	2,042	2,965
25-49	944	90,416	1,799,194	4,050,580	944	88,872	1,776,249	4,009,988	89	1,544	21,710	37,639
50-99	1,270	245,927	5,453,186	12,639,610	1,270	237,325	5,302,185	12,371,091	323	8,602	143,084	253,409
100-199	1,309	582,230	14,397,850	33,328,214	1,309	567,456	14,133,074	32,863,128	355	14,774	259,317	453,421
200-299	740	645,064	17,254,078	38,726,382	740	636,651	17,061,944	38,352,979	159	8,413	192,134	373,403
300-399	409	547,696	15,216,686	33,181,867	409	543,974	15,099,431	32,938,976	82	3,722	93,113	194,090
400-499	222	408,740	11,896,198	25,297,239	222	405,412	11,823,887	25,156,958	46	3,328	72,311	140,280
500 or more	285	892,036	26,570,321	56,204,665	285	883,660	26,352,278	55,732,770	69	8,376	218,042	471,896
Nongovernment not-for-profit	3,202	2,533,805	69,707,454	150,692,755	3,202	2,500,347	68,994,342	149,312,507	714	33,458	688,970	1,331,446
6-24 beds	84	4,262	90,219	193,899	84	4,225	90,045	193,485	1	37	174	414
25-49	409	45,373	925,781	2,090,728	409	44,727	917,299	2,074,675	33	646	8,482	16,053
50-99	635	132,468	3,008,645	6,704,738	635	127,776	2,923,984	6,555,684	168	4,692	84,661	149,054
100-199	778	381,623	9,672,452	21,228,022	778	373,631	9,521,932	20,975,544	206	7,992	150,519	252,478
200-299	562	512,462	13,732,997	30,001,235	562	505,424	13,583,238	29,710,011	135	7,038	149,759	291,225
300-399	331	446,357	12,428,307	26,852,785	331	443,163	12,324,503	26,630,144	71	3,194	79,663	173,840
400-499	179	323,102	9,292,547	19,739,883	179	320,439	9,232,528	19,622,252	40	2,663	60,019	117,631
500 or more	224	688,158	20,556,505	43,881,464	224	680,962	20,400,812	43,550,711	60	7,196	155,693	330,753
Investor-owned (for-profit)	749	272,642	6,745,387	18,821,608	749	271,107	6,719,228	18,763,694	66	1,535	26,159	57,914
6-24 beds	15	706	19,845	45,051	15	706	19,845	45,051	0	0	0	0
25-49	80	7,106	143,950	370,672	80	7,067	143,234	369,743	2	39	715	928
50-99	219	41,431	962,749	2,668,759	219	41,174	959,448	2,656,840	19	257	3,301	11,918
100-199	287	106,169	2,605,860	7,395,306	287	105,216	2,591,430	7,366,565	32	953	14,430	28,741
200-299	99	61,728	1,616,859	4,479,034	99	61,581	1,613,701	4,472,709	7	147	3,158	6,325
300-399	30	27,939	720,970	1,980,824	30	27,870	719,029	1,976,391	4	69	1,941	4,433
400-499	13	15,585	391,844	1,102,742	13	15,515	389,231	1,097,175	2	70	2,613	5,567
500 or more	6	11,978	283,310	779,220	6	11,978	283,310	779,220	0	0	0	0
State and local government	1,469	617,042	16,362,160	34,413,137	1,469	603,157	16,060,923	33,845,666	350	13,885	286,625	537,743
6-24 beds	142	6,412	117,423	259,992	142	6,330	115,555	257,441	6	82	1,868	2,551
25-49	455	37,937	729,463	1,589,180	455	37,078	715,715	1,565,570	54	859	12,513	20,658
50-99	416	72,028	1,481,792	3,266,114	416	68,375	1,418,753	3,158,567	136	3,653	55,122	92,436
100-199	244	94,438	2,119,538	4,704,886	244	88,609	2,019,712	4,521,018	117	5,829	94,367	172,203
200-299	79	70,874	1,904,223	4,246,112	79	69,646	1,865,005	4,170,260	17	1,228	39,218	75,853
300-399	48	73,400	2,067,408	4,348,258	48	72,941	2,055,899	4,332,441	7	459	11,509	15,817
400-499	30	70,053	2,211,807	4,454,613	30	69,458	2,202,128	4,437,531	4	595	9,680	17,082
500 or more	55	191,900	5,730,506	11,543,981	55	190,720	5,668,157	11,402,838	9	1,180	62,349	141,143
Hospital units of institutions	36	3,970	76,872	234,909	36	3,906	75,637	233,016	1	64	1,235	1,893
Community hospitals	5,384	3,419,519	92,738,128	203,692,591	5,384	3,370,705	91,698,857	201,688,851	1,129	48,814	1,000,519	1,925,210

4D

Personnel and Finances in Hospital Units and Nursing-Home-Type Units Operated by Community Hospitals, by State

CLASSIFICATION	TOTAL FACILITIES				HOSPITAL UNITS				NURSING-HOME-TYPE UNITS			
	Facilities	FTEs	Payroll Expense	Total Expense	Units	FTEs	Payroll Expense	Total Expense	Units	FTEs	Payroll Expense	Total Expense
UNITED STATES	5,384	3,419,519	$92,738,128	$203,692,591	5,384	3,370,705	$91,698,857	$201,688,851	1,129	48,814	$1,000,519	$1,925,210
6-24 beds	226	10,774	216,067	472,665	226	10,655	214,024	469,700	7	119	2,042	2,965
25-49	935	89,737	1,786,428	4,011,849	935	88,193	1,763,483	3,971,257	89	1,544	21,710	37,639
50-99	1,263	245,044	5,436,897	12,589,773	1,263	236,506	5,287,132	12,323,147	322	8,538	141,849	251,516
100-199	1,306	581,531	14,382,384	33,281,777	1,306	566,757	14,117,607	32,816,690	355	14,774	259,317	453,421
200-299	739	644,645	17,245,988	38,697,924	739	636,232	17,053,854	38,324,521	159	8,413	192,134	373,403
300-399	408	547,012	15,203,846	33,136,699	408	543,290	15,086,591	32,893,808	82	3,722	93,113	194,090
400-499	222	408,740	11,896,198	25,297,239	222	405,412	11,823,887	25,156,958	46	3,328	72,311	140,280
500 or more	285	892,036	26,570,321	56,204,665	285	883,660	26,352,278	55,732,770	69	8,376	218,042	471,896
CENSUS DIVISION 1, NEW ENGLAND	229	197,689	6,232,830	12,425,400	229	196,724	6,213,137	12,387,667	24	965	19,692	37,733
Connecticut	35	44,378	1,586,479	2,957,637	35	44,298	1,583,304	2,948,065	1	80	3,174	9,572
Maine	39	17,705	452,044	918,199	39	17,175	441,453	900,199	14	530	10,591	18,000
Massachusetts	101	100,945	3,202,320	6,543,022	101	100,945	3,202,320	6,543,022	0	0	0	0
New Hampshire	27	13,545	376,049	805,208	27	13,294	371,865	798,253	6	251	4,183	6,954
Rhode Island	12	14,699	439,594	844,596	12	14,699	439,594	844,596	0	0	0	0
Vermont	15	6,417	176,345	356,738	15	6,313	174,602	353,532	3	104	1,743	3,206
CENSUS DIVISION 2, MIDDLE ATLANTIC	568	628,648	19,030,573	38,182,676	568	621,833	18,860,131	37,851,302	116	6,815	170,442	331,374
New Jersey	95	107,790	3,217,938	6,504,894	95	107,425	3,210,032	6,488,327	8	365	7,907	16,567
New York	235	309,569	10,049,061	19,375,140	235	305,380	9,930,286	19,144,434	63	4,189	118,774	230,706
Pennsylvania	238	211,289	5,763,574	12,302,642	238	209,028	5,719,813	12,218,541	45	2,261	43,761	84,101
CENSUS DIVISION 3, SOUTH ATLANTIC	803	578,299	14,805,906	33,812,948	803	571,692	14,684,588	33,566,273	131	6,607	110,997	226,645
Delaware	8	10,010	274,962	574,402	8	10,010	274,962	574,402	0	0	0	0
District of Columbia	11	20,272	732,346	1,507,467	11	20,272	732,346	1,507,467	0	0	0	0
Florida	224	171,897	4,461,481	11,019,208	224	170,893	4,434,753	10,938,106	14	1,004	18,812	65,991
Georgia	163	89,408	2,165,544	5,000,289	163	87,510	2,138,318	4,949,522	27	1,898	24,822	45,848
Maryland	52	58,742	1,600,204	3,346,704	52	58,371	1,591,360	3,326,519	7	371	8,845	20,186
North Carolina	120	87,961	2,143,665	4,553,511	120	86,805	2,124,991	4,523,467	28	1,156	18,674	30,043
South Carolina	69	41,034	967,235	2,236,923	69	40,367	958,282	2,221,536	15	667	8,954	15,387
Virginia	97	71,193	1,815,654	4,084,237	97	70,247	1,793,589	4,050,666	25	946	22,065	33,572
West Virginia	59	27,782	644,814	1,490,207	59	27,217	635,987	1,474,588	15	565	8,827	15,618
CENSUS DIVISION 4, EAST NORTH CENTRAL	818	627,134	16,623,605	36,057,873	818	619,144	16,433,290	35,713,652	176	7,990	166,173	295,419
Illinois	210	173,511	4,718,994	10,254,113	210	170,663	4,660,877	10,147,108	67	2,848	58,117	107,005
Indiana	113	83,870	1,969,952	4,393,563	113	83,262	1,927,900	4,314,307	21	608	17,910	30,454
Michigan	176	135,162	3,809,333	8,210,713	176	133,554	3,779,003	8,158,330	30	1,608	30,330	52,383
Ohio	190	172,316	4,556,089	9,821,385	190	170,977	4,521,682	9,755,647	26	1,339	34,407	65,738
Wisconsin	129	62,275	1,569,237	3,378,099	129	60,688	1,543,828	3,338,260	32	1,587	25,410	39,839
CENSUS DIVISION 5, EAST SOUTH CENTRAL	464	223,715	4,996,429	11,853,113	464	220,418	4,943,761	11,744,121	85	3,297	49,612	102,246
Alabama	120	59,150	1,309,752	3,160,340	120	58,274	1,298,087	3,138,119	14	876	8,610	15,476
Kentucky	107	50,465	1,114,185	2,641,957	107	49,767	1,103,162	2,617,980	25	698	11,023	23,977
Mississippi	103	34,105	703,451	1,594,603	103	33,267	688,374	1,567,022	24	838	15,077	27,582
Tennessee	134	79,995	1,869,040	4,456,213	134	79,110	1,854,139	4,421,001	22	885	14,902	35,212
CENSUS DIVISION 6, WEST NORTH CENTRAL	742	268,978	6,608,963	14,407,136	742	259,019	6,432,278	14,078,199	264	9,959	176,684	328,936
Iowa	124	43,646	984,824	2,174,443	124	42,153	959,598	2,124,707	49	1,493	25,226	49,737
Kansas	138	34,946	788,786	1,710,015	138	34,028	772,514	1,681,321	44	918	16,272	28,694
Minnesota	152	55,553	1,625,370	3,375,761	152	52,328	1,566,872	3,269,995	65	3,225	58,498	105,766
Missouri	135	89,248	2,219,399	4,916,508	135	87,634	2,182,313	4,843,135	49	1,614	37,086	73,373
Nebraska	90	23,926	515,631	1,191,070	90	22,806	497,845	1,159,970	26	1,120	17,786	31,100
North Dakota	50	10,875	248,311	564,565	50	10,086	236,104	543,242	14	789	12,206	21,323
South Dakota	53	10,784	226,643	474,773	53	9,984	217,032	455,828	17	800	9,611	18,945
CENSUS DIVISION 7, WEST SOUTH CENTRAL	765	341,100	8,083,790	19,368,316	765	337,880	8,018,367	19,238,028	102	3,220	64,188	127,336
Arkansas	86	33,400	721,408	1,685,047	86	32,978	715,474	1,675,706	10	422	5,934	9,341
Louisiana	140	62,909	1,478,355	3,575,006	140	62,366	1,462,138	3,542,980	22	543	16,216	32,026
Oklahoma	111	41,565	896,294	2,091,066	111	41,023	888,386	2,072,881	11	542	7,908	18,185
Texas	428	203,226	4,987,733	12,017,198	428	201,513	4,952,369	11,946,462	59	1,713	34,130	67,784
CENSUS DIVISION 8, MOUNTAIN	355	145,195	3,809,654	8,954,950	355	141,389	3,739,188	8,824,113	104	3,806	70,467	130,837
Arizona	61	35,880	1,021,367	2,516,625	61	35,478	1,009,810	2,490,461	12	402	11,557	26,164
Colorado	69	39,157	1,074,644	2,322,897	69	38,039	1,056,933	2,292,719	20	1,118	17,711	30,178
Idaho	43	9,662	219,384	512,279	43	9,256	213,873	502,777	14	406	5,512	9,502
Montana	55	11,251	249,505	552,973	55	10,259	232,679	522,577	30	992	16,826	30,395
Nevada	21	11,406	320,261	790,498	21	11,341	319,536	789,391	3	65	725	1,107
New Mexico	37	14,381	357,016	897,073	37	14,165	353,391	889,922	5	216	3,625	7,151
Utah	42	17,994	448,820	1,092,626	42	17,789	440,375	1,076,421	9	205	8,446	16,205
Wyoming	27	5,464	118,655	269,979	27	5,062	112,591	259,844	11	402	6,064	10,135
CENSUS DIVISION 9, PACIFIC	640	408,761	12,546,378	28,630,179	640	402,606	12,374,116	28,285,497	127	6,155	172,262	344,683
Alaska	16	3,780	137,231	318,243	16	3,677	133,187	309,945	7	103	4,044	8,298
California	445	310,556	9,819,621	22,617,379	445	306,060	9,678,033	22,333,468	86	4,496	141,587	283,911
Hawaii	18	12,178	314,301	718,524	18	11,494	301,065	690,876	9	684	13,236	27,648
Oregon	70	33,007	876,376	1,912,802	70	32,497	868,324	1,897,308	12	510	8,052	15,494
Washington	91	49,240	1,398,850	3,063,232	91	48,878	1,393,507	3,053,901	13	362	5,343	9,332

Table

5

U.S. Census Divisions	States		
1 New England	Connecticut Maine	Massachusetts New Hampshire	Rhode Island Vermont
2 Middle Atlantic	New Jersey	New York	Pennsylvania
3 South Atlantic	Delaware District of Columbia Florida	Georgia Maryland North Carolina	South Carolina Virginia West Virginia
4 East North Central	Illinois Indiana	Michigan Ohio	Wisconsin
5 East South Central	Alabama Kentucky	Mississippi	Tennessee
6 West North Central	Iowa Kansas Minnesota	Missouri Nebraska	North Dakota South Dakota
7 West South Central	Arkansas Louisiana	Oklahoma	Texas
8 Mountain	Arizona Colorado Idaho	Montana Nevada New Mexico	Utah Wyoming
9 Pacific	Alaska California	Hawaii Oregon	Washington
U.S. Associated Areas	American Samoa Guam	Marshall Islands Puerto Rico	Virgin Islands

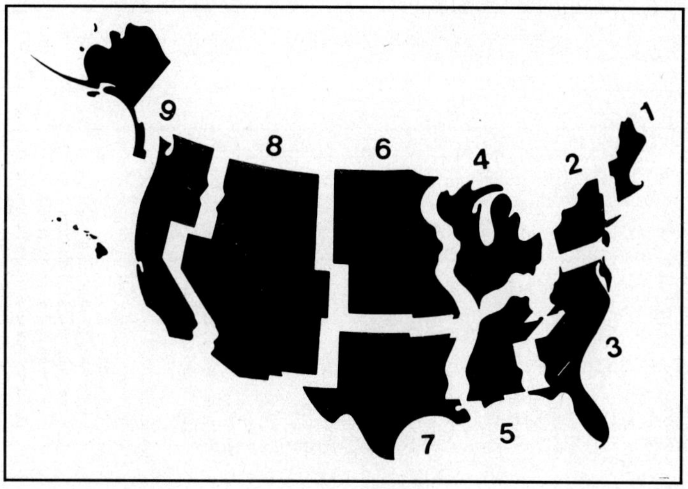

Table

5A

Utilization, Personnel, and Finances in U.S. Registered Hospitals

Excludes U.S.-associated areas, Puerto Rico, and nonregistered hospitals (see Tables 5D, 5E, and 14).

CLASSIFICATION	HOSPITALS	BEDS	ADMISSIONS	INPATIENT DAYS	ADJUSTED PATIENT DAYS	OCCUPANCY, percent	AVERAGE DAILY CENSUS	ADJUSTED AVERAGE DAILY CENSUS	AVERAGE STAY, days	SURGICAL OPERATIONS	OUTPATIENT VISITS: Emergency	OUTPATIENT VISITS: Other	OUTPATIENT VISITS: Total	NEWBORNS: Bassinets	NEWBORNS: Births
UNITED STATES	6,649	1,213,327	33,773,574	307,871,443		69.5	843,724			23,091,324	92,080,647	276,102,951	368,183,598	70,539	4,046,704
6-24 beds	301	5,763	141,672	757,399		36.2	2,085			85,851	812,468	4,202,206	5,014,674	804	12,376
25-49	1,095	41,266	1,006,291	6,636,239		44.1	18,191			507,814	4,348,468	13,114,571	17,463,039	4,110	91,229
50-99	1,633	117,585	2,832,567	24,167,419		56.4	66,323			1,722,009	10,004,788	25,755,680	35,760,468	8,336	286,812
100-199	1,562	219,772	6,315,029	50,307,197		62.8	137,922			4,545,600	20,400,801	50,778,344	71,179,145	14,796	725,748
200-299	830	201,734	6,615,629	50,387,554		68.4	138,056			4,811,969	18,791,024	48,387,067	67,178,091	13,491	783,935
300-399	503	172,230	5,410,306	45,632,571		72.6	125,032			3,851,618	13,134,141	38,301,602	51,435,743	10,212	691,775
400-499	276	123,895	3,865,258	34,088,579		75.4	93,392			2,646,442	8,979,614	30,652,270	39,631,884	7,216	526,414
500 or more	449	331,082	7,586,822	95,894,485		79.4	262,723			4,920,021	15,609,343	64,911,211	80,520,554	11,574	928,415
Psychiatric	774	171,891	779,843	50,846,008		81.1	139,350			9,726	288,333	6,316,940	6,605,273	5	177
Hospitals	756	160,634	778,549	47,000,528		80.2	128,817			9,659	283,964	6,302,735	6,586,699	5	177
Institutions for mentally retarded	18	11,257	1,294	3,845,480		93.6	10,533			67	4,369	14,205	18,574	0	0
General	5,566	998,659	32,480,818	244,990,722		67.2	671,366			22,737,282	91,331,000	263,684,523	355,015,523	69,658	3,978,119
Hospitals	5,523	995,681	32,448,665	244,311,846		67.2	669,504			22,725,345	91,173,821	261,949,921	353,123,742	69,627	3,977,736
Hospital units of institutions	43	2,978	32,153	678,876		62.5	1,862			11,937	157,179	1,734,602	1,891,781	31	383
TB and other respiratory diseases	4	470	1,849	113,912		66.4	312			2,039	0	16,863	16,863	0	0
Obstetrics and gynecology	12	1,894	95,525	396,840		57.4	1,087			60,690	57,967	222,979	280,946	664	55,347
Eye, ear, nose, and throat	12	669	32,145	78,036		31.8	213			79,215	78,334	458,909	537,243	0	0
Rehabilitation	142	12,688	113,313	3,395,173		73.6	9,337			5,308	29,179	2,296,677	2,325,856	0	0
Orthopedic	29	2,099	48,309	424,981		55.5	1,164			58,129	39,735	570,338	610,073	0	0
Chronic disease	32	10,869	15,082	3,582,080		90.3	9,811			1,034	4,571	118,071	122,642	0	0
All other	78	14,088	206,690	4,043,691		78.7	11,084			137,901	251,528	2,417,651	2,669,179	212	13,061
Federal	337	98,255	1,759,058	26,145,504		72.9	71,637			1,145,123	4,951,556	53,575,535	58,527,091	2,063	85,808
Psychiatric	17	11,654	58,674	3,418,801		80.4	9,366			3,897	6,374	1,200,960	1,207,334	0	0
General and other special	320	86,601	1,700,384	22,726,703		71.9	62,271			1,141,226	4,945,182	52,374,575	57,319,757	2,063	85,808
Nonfederal	6,312	1,115,072	32,014,516	281,725,939		69.2	772,087			21,946,201	87,129,091	222,527,416	309,656,507	68,476	3,960,896
Psychiatric	757	160,237	721,169	47,427,207		81.1	129,984			5,829	281,959	5,115,980	5,397,939	5	177
Hospitals	739	148,980	719,875	43,581,727		80.2	119,451			5,762	277,590	5,101,775	5,379,365	5	177
Institutions for mentally retarded	18	11,257	1,294	3,845,480		93.6	10,533			67	4,369	14,205	18,574	0	0
TB and other respiratory diseases	4	470	1,849	113,912		66.4	312			2,039	0	16,863	16,863	0	0
Long-term general and other special	131	24,991	88,344	7,801,569		85.6	21,386			17,006	64,630	1,486,422	1,551,052	28	2,073
Short-term general and other special	5,420	929,374	31,203,154	226,383,251		66.8	620,405			21,921,327	86,782,502	215,908,151	302,690,653	68,443	3,958,646
Hospital units of institutions	36	2,014	22,108	411,598		56.1	1,130			6,459	89,999	1,271,892	1,361,891	31	383
Community hospitals*	5,384	927,360	31,181,046	225,971,653	296,569,640	66.8	619,275	812,752	7.2	21,914,868	86,692,503	214,636,259	301,328,762	68,412	3,958,263
6-24 beds	226	4,427	95,487	520,031	897,849	32.3	1,431	2,465	5.4	56,792	341,976	1,128,661	1,470,637	594	7,228
25-49	935	35,420	869,830	5,342,360	8,211,239	41.3	14,645	22,521	6.1	451,130	3,390,541	7,421,297	10,811,838	3,677	77,548
50-99	1,263	90,394	2,474,497	17,727,304	25,543,455	53.8	48,617	70,040	7.2	1,656,801	9,214,121	18,368,107	27,582,228	7,954	270,974
100-199	1,306	183,867	5,832,890	41,206,512	56,877,191	61.5	112,987	155,941	7.1	4,360,405	19,256,694	39,683,061	58,939,755	14,214	701,924
200-299	739	179,670	6,333,181	43,968,781	58,182,567	67.1	120,469	159,411	6.9	4,677,159	18,255,185	42,305,601	60,560,786	13,304	774,499
300-399	408	138,938	5,091,049	35,478,286	45,300,397	70.0	97,212	124,115	7.0	3,660,171	12,803,973	30,895,423	43,699,396	10,095	683,763
400-499	222	98,833	3,643,952	26,514,574	33,470,716	73.5	72,642	91,712	7.3	2,533,599	8,546,087	24,847,932	33,394,019	7,096	516,501
500 or more	285	195,811	6,840,160	55,213,805	68,086,226	77.3	151,272	186,547	8.1	4,518,811	14,883,926	49,986,177	64,870,103	11,478	925,826
Nongovernment not-for-profit	3,191	656,755	22,878,443	166,143,064	217,624,139	69.3	455,221	596,275	7.3	16,553,917	60,817,572	160,255,808	221,073,380	47,441	2,833,204
Investor-owned (for-profit)	749	101,377	3,066,198	19,494,671	25,043,803	52.8	53,510	68,744	6.4	2,330,095	8,002,054	12,107,454	20,109,508	6,261	340,555
State and local government	1,444	169,228	5,236,405	40,333,918	53,901,698	65.3	110,544	147,733	7.7	3,030,856	17,872,877	42,272,997	60,145,874	14,710	784,504

*For information on community hospitals that excludes nursing-home-type data, refer to Hospital Units columns in tables 4A through 4D, pages 14 through 17.

CLASSIFICATION	FULL-TIME EQUIVALENT PERSONNEL: Physicians and Dentists	Registered Nurses	Licensed Practical Nurses	Other Salaried Personnel	Total Personnel	FULL-TIME EQUIVALENT TRAINEES: Medical and Dental Residents	Other Trainees	Total Trainees	EXPENSES — LABOR: Payroll (in thousands)	Employee Benefits (in thousands)	Total (in thousands)	Percent of Total	EXPENSES — TOTAL: Amount (in thousands)	Adjusted, per Admission	Adjusted, per Inpatient Day
UNITED STATES	63,775	895,324	197,843	2,906,346	4,063,288	77,477	6,278	83,755	$108,718,572	$21,796,512	$130,515,084	55.6	$234,869,906		
6-24 beds	796	3,112	1,336	15,636	20,880	15	6	21	411,477	81,606	493,083	62.4	790,358		
25-49	1,832	20,056	8,621	83,782	114,291	82	118	200	2,360,135	463,171	2,823,306	55.8	5,055,866		
50-99	3,270	61,771	21,730	225,707	312,478	471	213	684	7,202,973	1,448,263	8,651,236	53.6	16,133,345		
100-199	7,164	149,928	40,321	478,050	675,463	3,175	401	3,576	16,834,154	3,393,302	20,227,456	52.9	38,260,572		
200-299	7,280	163,997	35,694	494,972	701,943	6,073	813	6,886	18,762,191	3,698,171	22,460,362	54.0	41,613,305		
300-399	8,783	145,886	28,051	444,242	626,962	10,946	829	11,775	17,176,408	3,421,669	20,598,077	55.8	36,909,265		
400-499	7,450	107,119	18,636	332,223	465,428	11,437	836	12,273	13,277,352	2,647,740	15,925,092	56.8	28,034,520		
500 or more	27,200	243,455	43,454	831,734	1,145,843	45,278	3,062	48,340	32,693,882	6,642,590	39,336,472	57.8	68,072,675		
Psychiatric	6,661	34,801	12,855	244,537	298,854	1,049	728	1,777	7,965,039	1,822,447	9,787,486	70.9	13,797,042		
Hospitals	6,549	34,162	12,303	224,283	277,297	1,049	601	1,650	7,498,473	1,707,263	9,205,736	70.3	13,087,096		
Institutions for mentally retarded	112	639	552	20,254	21,557	0	127	127	466,567	115,184	581,750	81.9	709,946		
General	54,354	838,938	179,382	2,563,210	3,635,884	75,146	5,064	80,210	97,276,056	19,211,474	116,487,530	54.4	214,031,585		
Hospitals	53,917	837,954	178,637	2,559,152	3,629,660	75,139	5,057	80,196	97,150,160	19,179,475	116,329,635	54.4	213,710,190		
Hospital units of institutions	437	984	745	4,058	6,224	7	7	14	125,896	31,999	157,895	49.1	321,395		
TB and other respiratory diseases	29	144	105	986	1,264	0	0	0	26,065	5,609	31,674	62.8	50,448		
Obstetrics and gynecology	58	2,473	296	4,727	7,554	36	0	36	217,542	42,781	260,323	53.1	489,959		
Eye, ear, nose, and throat	94	568	84	3,165	3,911	129	0	129	93,183	22,712	115,895	52.4	221,359		
Rehabilitation	448	5,505	2,237	30,924	39,114	102	4	106	1,004,600	212,326	1,216,926	60.1	2,026,012		
Orthopedic	237	1,608	261	5,651	7,757	126	10	136	226,179	44,762	270,941	52.8	512,928		
Chronic disease	364	1,745	949	15,172	18,230	45	3	48	514,067	131,095	645,162	73.9	873,076		
All other	1,530	9,542	1,674	37,974	50,720	844	469	1,313	1,395,841	303,307	1,699,147	59.3	2,867,497		
Federal	19,067	45,663	14,148	224,593	303,471	11,208	1,410	12,618	8,742,853	1,492,845	10,235,698	67.1	15,243,688		
Psychiatric	613	2,458	824	14,878	18,773	33	41	74	536,173	94,577	630,750	70.7	892,451		
General and other special	18,454	43,205	13,324	209,715	284,698	11,175	1,369	12,544	8,206,680	1,398,267	9,604,947	66.9	14,351,237		
Nonfederal	44,708	849,661	183,695	2,681,753	3,759,817	66,269	4,868	71,137	99,975,719	20,303,667	120,279,386	54.8	219,626,218		
Psychiatric	6,048	32,343	12,031	229,659	280,081	1,016	687	1,703	7,428,866	1,727,870	9,156,736	71.0	12,904,591		
Hospitals	5,936	31,704	11,479	209,405	258,524	1,016	560	1,576	6,962,300	1,612,686	8,574,985	70.3	12,194,645		
Institutions for mentally retarded	112	639	552	20,254	21,557	0	127	127	466,567	115,184	581,750	81.9	709,946		
TB and other respiratory diseases	29	144	105	986	1,264	0	0	0	26,065	5,609	31,674	62.8	50,448		
Long-term general and other special	1,074	6,521	2,993	44,395	54,983	251	50	301	1,519,349	362,463	1,881,812	68.6	2,743,679		
Short-term general and other special	37,557	810,653	168,566	2,406,713	3,423,489	65,002	4,131	69,133	91,001,439	18,207,726	109,209,165	53.6	203,927,499		
Hospital units of institutions	295	726	633	2,316	3,970	7	7	14	76,046	21,028	97,074	41.3	234,909		
Community hospitals*	37,262	809,927	167,933	2,404,397	3,419,519	64,995	4,124	69,119	90,925,393	18,186,698	109,112,090	53.6	203,692,591	$4,946.68	$686.83
6-24 beds	60	1,953	1,020	7,741	10,774	9	6	15	215,736	41,617	257,353	54.4	472,665	2,701.48	526.44
25-49	283	16,765	7,689	65,000	89,737	54	109	163	1,784,626	340,896	2,125,522	53.0	4,011,849	2,967.27	488.58
50-99	1,106	51,766	19,243	172,929	245,044	259	73	332	5,430,287	1,091,853	6,522,140	51.8	12,589,773	3,460.68	492.88
100-199	3,589	136,360	36,487	405,095	581,531	2,268	276	2,544	14,315,210	2,891,902	17,207,112	51.7	33,281,777	4,108.64	585.15
200-299	4,799	155,860	32,860	451,126	644,645	4,648	646	5,294	17,106,628	3,404,984	20,511,613	53.0	38,697,924	4,618.31	665.11
300-399	5,449	135,376	24,242	381,945	547,012	8,436	513	8,949	14,961,743	2,961,474	17,923,217	54.1	33,136,699	5,096.11	731.49
400-499	4,911	98,969	15,745	289,115	408,740	9,871	481	10,352	11,617,468	2,316,667	13,934,135	55.1	25,297,239	5,499.65	755.80
500 or more	17,065	212,878	30,647	631,446	892,036	39,450	2,020	41,470	25,493,695	5,137,303	30,630,998	54.5	56,204,665	6,666.54	825.49
Nongovernment not-for-profit	26,538	608,965	111,238	1,786,621	2,533,362	44,180	2,793	46,973	68,456,825	13,343,094	81,799,919	54.3	150,673,249	5,001.24	692.36
Investor-owned (for-profit)	456	68,801	19,712	183,673	272,642	179	124	303	6,732,451	1,492,989	8,225,440	43.7	18,821,608	4,727.27	751.55
State and local government	10,268	132,161	36,983	434,103	613,515	20,636	1,207	21,843	15,736,117	3,350,615	19,086,732	55.8	34,197,734	4,837.76	634.45

*For information on community hospitals that excludes nursing-home-type data, refer to Hospital Units columns in tables 4A through 4D, pages 14 through 17.

Table
5B Census Division 1, New England

Utilization, Personnel, and Finances in U.S. Census Divisions

Excludes AHA nonregistered hospitals (see Table 14, page 240).

CLASSIFICATION	HOSPITALS	BEDS	ADMISSIONS	INPATIENT DAYS	ADJUSTED PATIENT DAYS	OCCUPANCY, percent	AVERAGE DAILY CENSUS	ADJUSTED AVERAGE DAILY CENSUS	AVERAGE STAY, days	SURGICAL OPERATIONS	OUTPATIENT VISITS			NEWBORNS	
											Emergency	Other	Total	Bassinets	Births
CENSUS DIVISION 1, NEW ENGLAND	341	65,760	1,744,359	18,501,224		77.1	50,694			1,250,324	5,895,771	16,344,349	22,240,120	3,432	201,198
6-24 beds	10	200	4,110	31,194		43.5	87			1,654	22,075	160,320	182,395	14	413
25-49	29	1,125	25,547	248,217		60.4	680			14,123	153,019	498,283	651,302	91	1,980
50-99	88	6,214	149,994	1,505,146		66.4	4,124			100,248	702,017	1,920,493	2,622,510	335	10,655
100-199	89	13,109	366,946	3,450,027		72.1	9,449			263,232	1,357,032	3,575,669	4,932,701	844	48,444
200-299	56	13,774	407,954	3,771,090		75.0	10,333			325,389	1,595,347	3,962,588	5,557,935	827	44,242
300-399	37	12,565	315,317	3,819,406		83.3	10,467			226,762	958,317	2,530,656	3,488,973	547	31,723
400-499	16	7,437	191,162	2,270,257		83.7	6,222			139,801	472,792	1,377,640	1,850,432	316	24,566
500 or more	16	11,336	283,329	3,405,887		82.3	9,332			179,115	635,172	2,318,700	2,953,872	458	39,175
Psychiatric	59	10,530	55,949	3,222,343		83.9	8,830			0	18,997	583,870	602,867	0	0
Hospitals	59	10,530	55,949	3,222,343		83.9	8,830			0	18,997	583,870	602,867	0	0
Institutions for mentally retarded	0	0	0	0		00.0	0			0	0	0	0	0	0
General	236	46,642	1,624,497	12,561,441		73.8	34,423			1,219,853	5,803,846	15,026,352	20,830,198	3,323	188,364
Hospitals	229	46,495	1,621,806	12,535,744		73.9	34,351			1,219,549	5,800,002	14,964,243	20,764,245	3,323	188,364
Hospital units of institutions	7	147	2,691	25,697		49.0	72			304	3,844	62,109	65,953	0	0
TB and other respiratory diseases	0	0	0	0		00.0	0			0	0	0	0	0	0
Obstetrics and gynecology	2	311	19,206	95,480		83.9	261			6,534	19,710	44,164	63,874	109	12,834
Eye, ear, nose, and throat	1	109	8,766	23,192		58.7	64			15,150	38,463	81,777	120,240	0	0
Rehabilitation	12	1,575	13,863	477,372		83.0	1,307			356	0	279,578	279,578	0	0
Orthopedic	1	60	690	10,767		48.3	29			573	0	8,481	8,481	0	0
Chronic disease	16	3,536	3,727	1,178,435		91.2	3,226			96	0	37,812	37,812	0	0
All other	14	2,997	17,661	932,194		85.2	2,554			7,762	14,755	282,315	297,070	0	0
Federal	14	4,815	53,271	1,292,981		73.6	3,543			34,749	126,312	1,861,777	1,988,089	10	315
Psychiatric	2	1,395	5,659	397,748		78.1	1,090			0	0	215,532	215,532	0	0
General and other special	12	3,420	47,612	895,233		71.7	2,453			34,749	126,312	1,646,245	1,772,557	10	315
Nonfederal	327	60,945	1,691,088	17,208,243		77.4	47,151			1,215,575	5,769,459	14,482,572	20,252,031	3,422	200,883
Psychiatric	57	9,135	50,290	2,824,595		84.7	7,740			0	18,997	368,338	387,335	0	0
Hospitals	57	9,135	50,290	2,824,595		84.7	7,740			0	18,997	368,338	387,335	0	0
Institutions for mentally retarded	0	0	0	0		00.0	0			0	0	0	0	0	0
TB and other respiratory diseases	0	0	0	0		00.0	0			0	0	0	0	0	0
Long-term general and other special	34	7,300	17,523	2,370,398		88.9	6,493			1,586	0	313,316	313,316	0	0
Short-term general and other special	236	44,510	1,623,275	12,013,250		74.0	32,918			1,213,989	5,750,462	13,800,918	19,551,380	3,422	200,883
Hospital units of institutions	7	147	2,691	25,697		49.0	72			304	3,844	62,109	65,953	0	0
Community hospitals*	229	44,363	1,620,584	11,987,553	16,557,977	74.0	32,846	45,371	7.4	1,213,665	5,746,618	13,738,809	19,485,427	3,422	200,883
6-24 beds	2	58	1,414	7,927	19,651	37.9	22	53	5.6	1,006	8,837	34,023	42,860	4	98
25-49	16	637	19,869	126,135	201,542	54.2	345	553	6.3	11,725	117,190	231,396	348,586	91	1,980
50-99	60	4,135	128,452	943,146	1,458,530	62.5	2,584	3,996	7.3	95,867	665,560	1,456,092	2,121,652	335	10,655
100-199	64	9,402	339,166	2,410,258	3,534,029	70.2	6,603	9,682	7.1	263,051	1,355,205	3,221,273	4,576,478	844	48,444
200-299	44	10,820	392,281	2,851,587	4,037,375	72.2	7,814	11,064	7.3	307,515	1,568,701	3,678,587	5,247,288	827	44,242
300-399	23	7,778	296,395	2,226,234	2,976,080	78.4	6,100	8,155	7.5	224,276	956,041	2,332,407	3,288,448	547	31,723
400-499	11	5,039	186,110	1,450,794	1,888,342	78.9	3,976	5,175	7.8	139,801	472,030	1,260,520	1,732,550	316	24,566
500 or more	9	6,494	256,897	1,971,472	2,442,428	83.2	5,402	6,693	7.7	170,444	603,054	1,524,511	2,127,565	458	39,175
Nongovernment not-for-profit	209	41,399	1,525,149	11,185,343	15,443,138	74.0	30,648	42,317	7.3	1,148,489	5,363,245	12,411,167	17,774,412	3,251	193,481
Investor-owned (for-profit)	5	575	16,506	164,259	216,498	78.3	450	592	10.0	7,785	47,899	143,700	191,599	30	1,633
State and local government	15	2,389	78,929	637,951	898,341	73.2	1,748	2,462	8.1	57,411	335,474	1,183,942	1,519,416	141	5,769

*For information on community hospitals that excludes nursing-home-type data, refer to Hospital Units columns in tables 4A through 4D, pages 14 through 17.

CLASSIFICATION	FULL-TIME EQUIVALENT PERSONNEL					FULL-TIME EQUIVALENT TRAINEES			EXPENSES						
									LABOR				TOTAL		
	Physicians and Dentists	Registered Nurses	Licensed Practical Nurses	Other Salaried Personnel	Total Personnel	Medical and Dental Residents	Other Trainees	Total Trainees	Payroll (in thousands)	Employee Benefits (in thousands)	Total (in thousands)	Percent of Total	Amount (in thousands)	Adjusted, per Admission	Adjusted, per Inpatient Day
CENSUS DIVISION 1, NEW ENGLAND	6,251	52,971	8,877	176,374	244,473	6,468	324	6,792	$ 7,452,710	$ 1,512,559	$ 8,965,270	60.4	$ 14,832,602		
6-24 beds	28	104	31	456	619	0	0	0	13,540	2,779	16,319	59.9	27,260		
25-49	88	781	204	3,064	4,137	0	1	1	110,539	19,006	129,545	64.5	200,876		
50-99	380	4,342	1,063	15,848	21,633	78	53	131	574,229	107,854	682,083	60.8	1,121,231		
100-199	684	10,045	2,000	34,187	46,916	359	14	373	1,357,464	271,257	1,628,721	60.7	2,682,308		
200-299	703	11,157	1,847	36,354	50,061	574	43	617	1,582,898	317,696	1,900,595	61.2	3,105,765		
300-399	1,239	10,350	1,667	34,271	47,527	1,627	96	1,723	1,530,938	315,853	1,846,791	61.6	2,998,525		
400-499	450	5,769	1,000	19,164	26,383	915	43	958	841,223	185,270	1,026,492	60.4	1,699,169		
500 or more	2,679	10,423	1,065	33,030	47,197	2,915	74	2,999	1,441,879	292,845	1,734,724	57.9	2,997,467		
Psychiatric	623	3,099	559	17,747	22,028	220	90	310	623,275	148,358	771,633	69.5	1,110,109		
Hospitals	623	3,099	559	17,747	22,028	220	90	310	623,275	148,358	771,633	69.5	1,110,109		
Institutions for mentally retarded	0	0	0	0	0	0	0	0	0	0	0	0.0	0		
General	5,140	46,672	7,139	141,717	200,668	6,080	210	6,290	6,221,496	1,231,843	7,453,338	59.0	12,632,561		
Hospitals	5,131	46,622	7,117	141,552	200,422	6,080	210	6,290	6,214,883	1,230,457	7,445,340	59.0	12,617,186		
Hospital units of institutions	9	50	22	165	246	0	0	0	6,613	1,386	7,999	52.0	15,375		
TB and other respiratory diseases	0	0	0	0	0	0	0	0	0	0	0	0.0	0		
Obstetrics and gynecology	45	503	29	1,259	1,836	36	0	36	56,902	12,247	69,149	63.9	108,172		
Eye, ear, nose, and throat	80	142	16	941	1,179	41	0	41	25,377	4,753	30,130	52.6	57,325		
Rehabilitation	87	565	227	4,064	4,943	2	0	2	140,763	29,408	170,170	66.0	257,999		
Orthopedic	5	45	2	88	140	4	0	4	3,708	728	4,436	53.7	8,269		
Chronic disease	99	757	474	4,718	6,048	0	1	1	175,064	41,594	216,658	73.2	296,136		
All other	172	1,188	431	5,840	7,631	85	23	108	206,126	43,629	249,756	69.0	362,032		
Federal	780	1,966	321	9,054	12,121	464	61	525	391,182	72,069	463,251	69.0	671,432		
Psychiatric	99	329	39	1,601	2,068	6	2	8	64,779	11,584	76,363	67.9	112,495		
General and other special	681	1,637	282	7,453	10,053	458	59	517	326,403	60,485	386,888	69.2	558,937		
Nonfederal	5,471	51,005	8,556	167,320	232,352	6,004	263	6,267	7,061,528	1,440,491	8,502,019	60.0	14,161,169		
Psychiatric	524	2,770	520	16,146	19,960	214	88	302	558,495	136,774	695,270	69.7	997,614		
Hospitals	524	2,770	520	16,146	19,960	214	88	302	558,495	136,774	695,270	69.7	997,614		
Institutions for mentally retarded	0	0	0	0	0	0	0	0	0	0	0	0.0	0		
TB and other respiratory diseases	0	0	0	0	0	0	0	0	0	0	0	0.0	0		
Long-term general and other special	276	1,813	1,048	11,320	14,457	17	7	24	421,882	95,090	516,972	71.5	722,780		
Short-term general and other special	4,671	46,422	6,988	139,854	197,935	5,773	168	5,941	6,081,151	1,208,627	7,289,778	58.6	12,440,774		
Hospital units of institutions	9	50	22	165	246	0	0	0	6,613	1,386	7,999	52.0	15,375		
Community hospitals*	4,662	46,372	6,966	139,689	197,689	5,773	168	5,941	6,074,538	1,207,241	7,281,779	58.6	12,425,400	$5,513.56	$750.42
6-24 beds	1	38	10	120	169	0	0	0	4,925	1,071	5,996	57.5	10,430	2,894.67	530.74
25-49	14	540	146	1,657	2,357	0	0	0	55,465	9,911	65,376	59.5	109,857	3,454.95	545.08
50-99	162	3,467	876	10,814	15,319	19	8	27	409,726	78,942	488,668	58.9	830,052	4,131.50	569.10
100-199	495	8,770	1,591	27,346	38,202	211	11	222	1,104,741	213,601	1,318,341	59.6	2,212,825	4,396.12	626.15
200-299	492	10,169	1,517	31,181	43,359	505	39	544	1,384,111	276,069	1,660,179	60.1	2,762,049	4,972.54	684.12
300-399	936	8,977	1,202	25,787	36,902	1,552	55	1,607	1,222,651	242,248	1,464,899	59.0	2,480,921	6,247.83	833.62
400-499	317	5,253	874	15,779	22,223	876	30	906	719,053	144,774	863,827	58.3	1,482,952	6,107.36	785.32
500 or more	2,245	9,158	750	27,005	39,158	2,610	25	2,635	1,173,865	240,626	1,414,491	55.8	2,536,315	7,961.24	1,038.44
Nongovernment not-for-profit	4,218	43,288	6,427	130,708	184,641	5,243	157	5,400	5,682,170	1,124,451	6,806,620	58.8	11,577,649	5,465.41	749.70
Investor-owned (for-profit)	10	411	78	1,446	1,945	0	0	0	43,976	10,752	54,728	46.0	119,047	4,977.50	549.88
State and local government	434	2,673	461	7,535	11,103	530	11	541	348,392	72,038	420,430	57.7	728,703	6,544.79	811.17

*For information on community hospitals that excludes nursing-home-type data, refer to Hospital Units columns in tables 4A through 4D, pages 14 through 17.

(continued on next page)

Table

5B (Continued) Census Division 2, Middle Atlantic

Utilization, Personnel, and Finances in U.S. Census Divisions

Excludes AHA nonregistered hospitals (see Table 14, page 240).

CLASSIFICATION	HOSPITALS	BEDS	ADMISSIONS	INPATIENT DAYS	ADJUSTED PATIENT DAYS	OCCUPANCY, percent	AVERAGE DAILY CENSUS	ADJUSTED AVERAGE DAILY CENSUS	AVERAGE STAY, days	SURGICAL OPERATIONS	OUTPATIENT VISITS Emergency	OUTPATIENT VISITS Other	OUTPATIENT VISITS Total	NEWBORNS Bassinets	NEWBORNS Births
CENSUS DIVISION 2, MIDDLE ATLANTIC	726	211,432	5,509,624	63,122,336		81.8	172,943			3,749,994	14,632,428	52,516,353	67,148,781	9,864	578,234
6-24 beds	10	156	5,170	24,058		41.7	65			12,661	43,194	270,652	313,846	10	379
25-49	35	1,298	26,422	305,242		64.6	838			14,071	112,997	544,156	657,153	43	1,230
50-99	101	7,513	181,231	1,905,848		69.5	5,222			120,452	689,936	2,785,355	3,475,291	400	13,822
100-199	168	24,237	674,896	6,497,656		73.4	17,800			500,641	2,217,936	6,761,502	8,979,438	1,108	43,816
200-299	157	37,166	1,212,673	10,512,295		77.5	28,807			910,425	3,492,672	10,208,094	13,700,766	2,336	115,869
300-399	77	26,334	837,393	7,762,737		80.8	21,270			570,054	2,138,520	6,623,830	8,762,350	1,766	94,324
400-499	65	29,428	876,981	9,101,805		84.7	24,935			571,951	2,062,554	7,374,198	9,436,752	1,666	109,910
500 or more	113	85,300	1,694,858	27,012,695		86.8	74,006			1,049,739	3,874,619	17,948,566	21,823,185	2,535	198,884
Psychiatric	103	37,072	110,133	11,855,306		87.6	32,481			755	116,383	2,432,100	2,548,483	0	0
Hospitals	101	36,223	110,085	11,561,938		87.4	31,677			752	115,968	2,430,912	2,546,880	0	0
Institutions for mentally retarded	2	849	48	293,368		94.7	804			3	415	1,188	1,603	0	0
General	560	161,819	5,236,798	47,373,712		80.2	129,797			3,622,457	14,376,998	48,151,052	62,528,050	9,638	562,272
Hospitals	553	161,494	5,234,054	47,301,054		80.3	129,599			3,621,106	14,359,910	48,037,821	62,397,731	9,638	562,272
Hospital units of institutions	7	325	2,744	72,658		60.9	198			1,351	17,088	113,231	130,319	0	0
TB and other respiratory diseases	0	0	0	0		00.0	0			0	0	0	0	0	0
Obstetrics and gynecology	2	371	21,475	91,217		67.1	249			13,370	24,599	46,975	71,574	159	11,799
Eye, ear, nose, and throat	3	238	15,789	39,441		45.4	108			36,271	26,740	202,353	229,093	0	0
Rehabilitation	30	3,085	32,442	912,953		81.0	2,498			444	3,460	875,955	879,415	0	0
Orthopedic	4	502	13,683	137,329		75.1	377			16,411	0	199,491	199,491	0	0
Chronic disease	4	2,914	4,966	1,002,473		94.3	2,747			0	0	9,157	9,157	0	0
All other	20	5,431	74,338	1,709,905		86.3	4,686			60,286	84,248	599,270	683,518	67	4,163
Federal	30	14,043	134,582	3,975,434		77.6	10,892			115,390	313,288	3,703,635	4,016,923	19	562
Psychiatric	3	2,433	10,521	702,610		79.1	1,925			0	1,821	226,788	228,609	0	0
General and other special	27	11,610	124,061	3,272,824		77.2	8,967			115,390	311,467	3,476,847	3,788,314	19	562
Nonfederal	696	197,389	5,375,042	59,146,902		82.1	162,051			3,634,604	14,319,140	48,812,718	63,131,858	9,845	577,672
Psychiatric	100	34,639	99,612	11,152,696		88.2	30,556			755	114,562	2,205,312	2,319,874	0	0
Hospitals	98	33,790	99,564	10,859,328		88.0	29,752			752	114,147	2,204,124	2,318,271	0	0
Institutions for mentally retarded	2	849	48	293,368		94.7	804			3	415	1,188	1,603	0	0
TB and other respiratory diseases	0	0	0	0		00.0	0			0	0	0	0	0	0
Long-term general and other special	23	6,831	25,172	2,190,637		87.9	6,002			2,033	19,251	507,828	527,079	0	0
Short-term general and other special	573	155,919	5,250,258	45,803,569		80.5	125,493			3,631,816	14,185,327	46,099,578	60,284,905	9,845	577,672
Hospital units of institutions	5	208	1,186	52,762		69.2	144			316	3,979	38,644	42,623	0	0
Community hospitals*	568	155,711	5,249,072	45,750,807	59,441,544	80.5	125,349	162,848	8.7	3,631,500	14,181,348	46,060,934	60,242,282	9,845	577,672
6-24 beds	4	61	1,475	6,399	16,166	27.9	17	44	4.3	10,656	1,899	30,051	31,950	0	0
25-49	22	840	22,294	187,670	320,427	61.3	515	877	8.4	13,348	94,640	395,039	489,679	43	1,230
50-99	70	5,184	153,422	1,265,689	1,843,660	66.9	3,467	5,047	8.2	115,426	644,595	1,787,026	2,431,621	391	13,639
100-199	137	19,815	633,605	5,217,154	7,285,956	72.1	14,293	19,963	8.2	495,816	2,163,224	6,028,973	8,192,197	1,108	43,816
200-299	144	34,097	1,181,563	9,582,923	12,892,469	77.0	26,259	35,320	8.1	908,710	3,456,232	9,798,518	13,254,750	2,336	115,869
300-399	69	23,457	824,165	6,810,560	8,646,968	79.6	18,663	23,689	8.3	567,297	2,090,112	6,237,966	8,328,078	1,766	94,324
400-499	52	23,275	851,591	7,094,508	9,020,877	83.5	19,436	24,717	8.3	562,569	2,001,962	6,771,849	8,773,811	1,666	109,910
500 or more	70	48,982	1,580,957	15,585,904	19,415,021	87.2	42,699	53,191	9.9	957,678	3,728,684	15,011,512	18,740,196	2,535	198,884
Nongovernment not-for-profit	510	138,827	4,792,452	40,484,679	52,819,381	79.9	110,921	144,704	8.4	3,405,556	12,440,634	40,057,113	52,497,747	8,996	520,136
Investor-owned (for-profit)	21	3,296	98,198	976,067	1,207,210	81.0	2,671	3,308	9.9	75,186	210,197	317,339	527,536	119	5,994
State and local government	37	13,588	358,422	4,290,061	5,414,953	86.5	11,757	14,836	12.0	150,758	1,530,517	5,686,482	7,216,999	730	51,542

*For information on community hospitals that excludes nursing-home-type data, refer to Hospital Units columns in tables 4A through 4D, pages 14 through 17.

CLASSIFICATION	FULL-TIME EQUIVALENT PERSONNEL					FULL-TIME EQUIVALENT TRAINEES			EXPENSES						
									LABOR				TOTAL		
	Physicians and Dentists	Registered Nurses	Licensed Practical Nurses	Other Salaried Personnel	Total Personnel	Medical and Dental Residents	Other Trainees	Total Trainees	Payroll (in thousands)	Employee Benefits (in thousands)	Total (in thousands)	Percent of Total	Amount (in thousands)	Adjusted, per Admission	Adjusted, per Inpatient Day
CENSUS DIVISION 2, MIDDLE ATLANTIC	17,735	158,928	29,997	532,257	738,917	21,793	786	22,579	$21,643,747	$ 4,314,811	$25,958,558	59.8	$ 43,392,067		
6-24 beds	61	167	47	938	1,213	0	0	0	17,532	3,571	21,103	60.8	34,702		
25-49	95	647	242	2,891	3,875	1	0	1	86,330	15,609	101,939	57.5	177,269		
50-99	422	4,722	1,577	18,499	25,220	68	34	102	601,820	119,346	721,166	58.9	1,225,038		
100-199	982	17,337	4,272	58,169	80,760	634	39	673	2,093,311	419,942	2,513,253	57.1	4,402,768		
200-299	1,697	30,858	6,475	93,938	132,968	1,153	30	1,183	3,603,946	696,873	4,300,819	58.2	7,384,984		
300-399	2,200	22,184	4,284	67,141	95,809	2,031	9	2,040	2,737,687	560,331	3,298,018	58.5	5,642,205		
400-499	2,527	25,073	4,131	80,072	111,803	3,215	136	3,351	3,316,588	672,294	3,988,881	60.2	6,627,435		
500 or more	9,751	57,940	8,969	210,609	287,269	14,691	538	15,229	9,186,533	1,826,845	11,013,378	61.5	17,897,666		
Psychiatric	2,141	7,707	2,613	54,066	66,527	272	120	392	1,874,203	412,818	2,287,021	78.5	2,914,040		
Hospitals	2,134	7,664	2,577	52,651	65,026	272	120	392	1,839,478	404,462	2,243,940	78.4	2,860,643		
Institutions for mentally retarded	7	43	36	1,415	1,501	0	0	0	34,725	8,356	43,081	80.7	53,397		
General	14,518	144,957	26,168	449,256	634,899	20,952	641	21,593	18,650,782	3,656,512	22,307,294	58.3	38,275,619		
Hospitals	14,475	144,862	26,102	448,596	634,035	20,952	635	21,587	18,633,597	3,652,436	22,286,033	58.3	38,244,055		
Hospital units of institutions	43	95	66	660	864	0	6	6	17,185	4,076	21,261	67.4	31,564		
TB and other respiratory diseases	0	0	0	0	0	0	0	0	0	0	0	0.0	0		
Obstetrics and gynecology	1	547	92	1,135	1,775	0	0	0	53,198	10,112	63,310	56.7	111,712		
Eye, ear, nose, and throat	6	201	22	1,277	1,506	64	0	64	38,941	12,311	51,252	56.5	90,736		
Rehabilitation	175	1,597	558	7,999	10,329	28	3	31	276,542	59,064	335,606	63.2	530,776		
Orthopedic	148	403	70	1,828	2,449	74	0	74	82,648	17,266	99,914	57.0	175,294		
Chronic disease	113	294	113	4,695	5,215	15	0	15	164,132	42,389	206,520	78.7	262,545		
All other	633	3,222	361	12,001	16,217	388	22	410	503,301	104,339	607,639	58.9	1,031,344		
Federal	1,764	4,838	1,389	24,351	32,342	1,030	193	1,223	1,045,063	162,824	1,207,887	70.6	1,710,014		
Psychiatric	136	508	185	3,276	4,105	9	20	29	113,520	20,477	133,997	72.1	185,821		
General and other special	1,628	4,330	1,204	21,075	28,237	1,021	173	1,194	931,543	142,347	1,073,890	70.5	1,524,193		
Nonfederal	15,971	154,090	28,608	507,906	706,575	20,763	593	21,356	20,598,683	4,151,987	24,750,671	59.4	41,682,052		
Psychiatric	2,005	7,199	2,428	50,790	62,422	263	100	363	1,760,683	392,342	2,153,024	78.9	2,728,219		
Hospitals	1,998	7,156	2,392	49,375	60,921	263	100	363	1,725,958	383,986	2,109,943	78.9	2,674,821		
Institutions for mentally retarded	7	43	36	1,415	1,501	0	0	0	34,725	8,356	43,081	80.7	53,397		
TB and other respiratory diseases	0	0	0	0	0	0	0	0	0	0	0	0.0	0		
Long-term general and other special	341	1,604	618	12,499	15,062	82	28	110	435,580	109,815	545,395	72.5	751,893		
Short-term general and other special	13,625	145,287	25,562	444,617	629,091	20,418	465	20,883	18,402,421	3,649,830	22,052,251	57.7	38,201,940		
Hospital units of institutions	9	35	33	366	443	0	6	6	9,576	2,297	11,874	61.6	19,264		
Community hospitals*	13,616	145,252	25,529	444,251	628,648	20,418	459	20,877	18,392,844	3,647,533	22,040,378	57.7	38,182,676	$5,570.55	$ 642.36
6-24 beds	6	70	27	280	383	0	0	0	7,678	1,473	9,151	55.7	16,414	2,780.69	1,015.37
25-49	34	480	196	1,979	2,689	1	0	1	56,434	9,502	65,936	56.8	116,148	3,462.88	362.48
50-99	95	3,710	1,359	12,066	17,230	46	4	50	399,345	78,048	477,393	55.6	858,154	3,642.93	465.46
100-199	670	15,850	3,954	49,421	69,895	589	32	621	1,787,646	356,238	2,143,884	56.0	3,829,899	4,263.54	525.65
200-299	1,418	29,618	6,150	86,832	124,018	991	24	1,015	3,344,178	639,742	3,983,920	57.5	6,926,169	4,355.65	537.23
300-399	2,018	21,444	4,071	62,426	89,959	2,007	8	2,015	2,555,334	522,709	3,078,044	57.4	5,361,430	5,136.26	620.04
400-499	2,035	23,511	3,443	71,387	100,376	3,010	21	3,031	2,957,810	588,786	3,546,596	58.5	6,067,189	5,611.96	672.57
500 or more	7,340	50,569	6,329	159,860	224,098	13,774	370	14,144	7,284,419	1,451,035	8,735,454	58.2	15,007,272	7,633.56	772.97
Nongovernment not-for-profit	10,115	130,783	22,381	390,316	553,595	16,290	407	16,697	15,938,672	3,139,040	19,077,712	57.0	33,471,893	5,334.43	633.70
Investor-owned (for-profit)	80	2,467	621	6,474	9,642	1	0	1	255,169	54,468	309,638	51.5	601,305	4,894.59	498.10
State and local government	3,421	12,002	2,527	47,461	65,411	4,127	52	4,179	2,199,004	454,025	2,653,028	64.6	4,109,477	8,995.46	758.91

*For information on community hospitals that excludes nursing-home-type data, refer to Hospital Units columns in tables 4A through 4D, pages 14 through 17.

(continued on next page)

Table

5B (Continued) Census Division 3, South Atlantic

Utilization, Personnel, and Finances in U.S. Census Divisions

Excludes AHA nonregistered hospitals (see Table 14, page 240).

CLASSIFICATION	HOSPITALS	BEDS	ADMISSIONS	INPATIENT DAYS	ADJUSTED PATIENT DAYS	OCCUPANCY, percent	AVERAGE DAILY CENSUS	ADJUSTED AVERAGE DAILY CENSUS	AVERAGE STAY, days	SURGICAL OPERATIONS	OUTPATIENT VISITS Emergency	OUTPATIENT VISITS Other	OUTPATIENT VISITS Total	NEWBORNS Bassinets	NEWBORNS Births
CENSUS DIVISION 3, SOUTH ATLANTIC	1,050	213,076	6,106,214	54,128,326		69.6	148,341			4,212,969	17,290,573	41,776,492	59,067,065	11,118	682,668
6-24 beds	20	379	10,115	59,546		43.3	164			12,392	68,677	366,810	435,487	18	428
25-49	127	5,000	124,441	899,824		49.2	2,462			60,246	652,240	1,851,272	2,503,512	270	6,065
50-99	252	18,041	442,660	3,843,491		58.4	10,538			249,552	1,730,327	4,488,556	6,218,883	953	30,807
100-199	282	38,710	1,171,157	9,072,040		64.3	24,879			868,980	4,013,774	8,064,797	12,078,571	2,564	120,495
200-299	149	35,976	1,150,926	8,709,867		66.3	23,869			829,703	3,287,607	7,051,389	10,338,996	2,105	117,626
300-399	92	31,700	1,065,161	8,392,073		72.5	22,998			780,979	2,701,378	6,470,826	9,172,204	1,793	125,871
400-499	40	17,831	613,179	4,625,401		71.1	12,674			441,345	1,492,146	3,303,530	4,795,676	1,125	84,141
500 or more	88	65,439	1,528,575	18,526,084		77.6	50,757			969,772	3,344,424	10,179,312	13,523,736	2,290	197,235
Psychiatric	152	34,074	168,401	9,710,704		78.1	26,609			3,479	29,456	644,098	673,554	0	0
Hospitals	149	31,675	168,161	8,869,342		76.7	24,305			3,433	27,022	635,846	662,868	0	0
Institutions for mentally retarded	3	2,399	240	841,362		96.0	2,304			46	2,434	8,252	10,686	0	0
General	840	172,945	5,856,145	42,892,219		68.0	117,552			4,137,646	17,233,848	40,170,461	57,404,309	11,009	672,146
Hospitals	830	172,250	5,844,867	42,757,445		68.0	117,182			4,134,192	17,191,284	39,768,807	56,960,091	11,003	672,068
Hospital units of institutions	10	695	11,278	134,774		53.2	370			3,454	42,564	401,654	444,218	6	78
TB and other respiratory diseases	1	100	234	25,519		70.0	70			3	0	0	0	0	0
Obstetrics and gynecology	2	402	19,443	75,004		51.2	206			14,641	675	25,039	25,714	109	10,522
Eye, ear, nose, and throat	5	159	4,040	7,699		13.2	21			19,368	6,719	137,391	144,110	0	0
Rehabilitation	25	1,905	15,584	541,363		77.8	1,483			534	366	306,397	306,763	0	0
Orthopedic	8	637	15,631	117,284		50.4	321			23,742	15,309	180,965	196,274	0	0
Chronic disease	6	1,143	3,111	344,304		82.5	943			147	4,200	30,558	34,758	0	0
All other	11	1,711	23,625	414,230		66.4	1,136			13,409	0	281,583	281,583	0	0
Federal	62	19,067	413,908	5,060,564		72.7	13,865			288,945	1,221,683	13,318,771	14,540,454	524	21,764
Psychiatric	2	1,602	9,136	500,813		85.6	1,372			1,801	5	146,701	146,706	0	0
General and other special	60	17,465	404,772	4,559,751		71.5	12,493			287,144	1,221,678	13,172,070	14,393,748	524	21,764
Nonfederal	988	194,009	5,692,306	49,067,762		69.3	134,476			3,924,024	16,068,890	28,457,721	44,526,611	10,594	660,904
Psychiatric	150	32,472	159,265	9,209,891		77.7	25,237			1,678	29,451	497,397	526,848	0	0
Hospitals	147	30,073	159,025	8,368,529		76.3	22,933			1,632	27,017	489,145	516,162	0	0
Institutions for mentally retarded	3	2,399	240	841,362		96.0	2,304			46	2,434	8,252	10,686	0	0
TB and other respiratory diseases	1	100	234	25,519		70.0	70			3	0	0	0	0	0
Long-term general and other special	25	3,081	12,379	899,413		80.0	2,465			355	4,586	191,720	196,306	0	0
Short-term general and other special	812	158,356	5,520,428	38,932,939		67.4	106,704			3,921,988	16,034,853	27,768,604	43,803,457	10,594	660,904
Hospital units of institutions	9	645	8,869	125,491		53.5	345			2,139	26,535	277,221	303,756	6	78
Community hospitals*	803	157,711	5,511,559	38,807,448	49,974,178	67.4	106,359	136,951	7.0	3,919,849	16,008,318	27,491,383	43,499,701	10,588	660,826
6-24 beds	14	265	6,791	35,631	65,593	37.0	98	177	5.2	5,330	14,479	84,721	99,200	2	14
25-49	98	3,924	102,430	638,527	969,728	44.5	1,746	2,658	6.2	53,666	504,349	838,438	1,342,787	211	4,126
50-99	163	11,530	343,609	2,241,374	3,215,970	53.3	6,146	8,818	6.5	233,666	1,458,987	2,080,009	3,538,996	841	26,691
100-199	231	32,036	1,056,841	7,429,309	10,124,283	63.6	20,377	27,759	7.0	810,870	3,638,999	5,150,412	8,789,411	2,388	113,584
200-299	130	31,361	1,083,157	7,479,267	9,634,358	65.4	20,496	26,397	6.9	806,637	3,107,267	5,003,271	8,110,538	2,023	113,348
300-399	78	26,557	998,769	6,859,872	8,695,301	70.8	18,799	23,822	6.9	731,879	2,659,897	4,842,614	7,502,511	1,744	123,445
400-499	34	15,060	563,711	3,915,915	4,897,570	71.3	10,731	13,421	6.9	412,540	1,441,928	2,338,810	3,780,738	1,115	83,426
500 or more	55	36,978	1,356,251	10,207,553	12,371,375	75.6	27,966	33,899	7.5	865,261	3,182,412	7,153,108	10,335,520	2,264	196,192
Nongovernment not-for-profit	416	92,910	3,384,492	23,941,720	30,809,664	70.6	65,602	84,414	7.1	2,500,323	9,290,763	17,561,008	26,851,771	6,476	410,332
Investor-owned (for-profit)	188	29,914	914,352	5,999,178	7,602,704	55.0	16,449	20,841	6.6	704,190	2,468,880	3,401,404	5,870,284	1,190	68,277
State and local government	199	34,887	1,212,715	8,866,550	11,561,810	69.7	24,308	31,696	7.3	715,336	4,248,675	6,528,971	10,777,646	2,922	182,217

*For information on community hospitals that excludes nursing home type data, refer to Hospital Units columns in tables 4A through 4D, pages 14 through 17.

CLASSIFICATION	FULL-TIME EQUIVALENT PERSONNEL: Physicians and Dentists	Registered Nurses	Licensed Practical Nurses	Other Salaried Personnel	Total Personnel	FULL-TIME EQUIVALENT TRAINEES: Medical and Dental Residents	Other Trainees	Total Trainees	EXPENSES — LABOR: Payroll (in thousands)	Employee Benefits (in thousands)	Total (in thousands)	Percent of Total	EXPENSES — TOTAL: Amount (in thousands)	Adjusted, per Admission	Adjusted, per Inpatient Day
CENSUS DIVISION 3, SOUTH ATLANTIC	9,536	159,037	37,046	506,901	712,520	11,870	901	12,771	$18,076,305	$ 3,604,277	$21,680,582	53.9	$ 40,192,797		
6-24 beds	95	259	157	1,512	2,023	3	0	3	39,892	9,557	49,449	66.7	74,154		
25-49	282	2,314	1,078	11,808	15,482	14	43	57	329,645	66,103	395,747	54.5	725,619		
50-99	773	9,558	3,209	36,692	50,232	59	39	98	1,131,660	225,928	1,357,588	52.2	2,602,189		
100-199	1,024	27,346	8,051	85,549	121,970	377	75	452	2,890,591	557,496	3,448,087	51.2	6,739,717		
200-299	943	27,482	6,358	82,330	117,113	622	95	717	2,926,736	557,694	3,484,431	51.0	6,829,503		
300-399	855	26,932	5,186	80,273	113,246	1,250	114	1,364	2,848,686	533,497	3,382,183	54.1	6,256,808		
400-499	1,282	15,705	2,832	46,916	66,735	1,382	135	1,517	1,908,459	357,644	2,266,103	54.5	4,154,534		
500 or more	4,282	49,441	10,175	161,821	225,719	8,163	400	8,563	6,000,636	1,296,359	7,296,995	57.0	12,810,274		
Psychiatric	1,099	6,495	2,644	48,367	58,605	134	32	166	1,471,069	362,238	1,833,307	67.3	2,725,199		
Hospitals	1,075	6,349	2,534	43,828	53,786	134	25	159	1,375,181	338,317	1,713,498	66.4	2,581,923		
Institutions for mentally retarded	24	146	110	4,539	4,819	0	7	7	95,888	23,921	119,809	83.6	143,276		
General	8,167	148,708	33,609	444,430	634,914	11,664	825	12,489	16,099,655	3,133,467	19,233,122	52.9	36,337,282		
Hospitals	8,073	148,473	33,450	443,473	633,469	11,664	825	12,489	16,072,423	3,126,296	19,198,719	53.0	36,255,617		
Hospital units of institutions	94	235	159	957	1,445	0	0	0	27,232	7,171	34,403	42.1	81,665		
TB and other respiratory diseases	4	12	12	199	227	0	0	0	3,159	888	4,046	67.3	6,009		
Obstetrics and gynecology	11	561	73	847	1,492	0	0	0	44,498	7,446	51,944	49.8	104,302		
Eye, ear, nose, and throat	3	128	24	601	756	0	0	0	18,747	3,593	22,341	49.7	44,935		
Rehabilitation	81	859	306	4,646	5,892	26	1	27	153,135	35,661	188,796	58.8	321,079		
Orthopedic	26	581	32	1,499	2,138	11	5	16	54,588	10,402	64,989	47.5	136,898		
Chronic disease	17	226	159	1,643	2,045	1	2	3	50,249	10,768	61,017	61.5	99,256		
All other	128	1,467	187	4,669	6,451	34	36	70	181,204	39,816	221,020	52.9	417,836		
Federal	4,451	9,923	2,886	52,117	69,377	2,641	217	2,858	1,872,181	306,841	2,179,022	65.4	3,331,302		
Psychiatric	89	356	149	1,985	2,579	8	2	10	72,003	13,863	85,866	60.5	141,883		
General and other special	4,362	9,567	2,737	50,132	66,798	2,633	215	2,848	1,800,178	292,978	2,093,156	65.6	3,189,419		
Nonfederal	5,085	149,114	34,160	454,784	643,143	9,229	684	9,913	16,204,123	3,297,437	19,501,560	52.9	36,861,495		
Psychiatric	1,010	6,139	2,495	46,382	56,026	126	30	156	1,399,066	348,375	1,747,441	67.6	2,583,316		
Hospitals	986	5,993	2,385	41,843	51,207	126	23	149	1,303,178	324,454	1,627,632	66.7	2,440,040		
Institutions for mentally retarded	24	146	110	4,539	4,819	0	7	7	95,888	23,921	119,809	83.6	143,276		
TB and other respiratory diseases	4	12	12	199	227	0	0	0	3,159	888	4,046	67.3	6,009		
Long-term general and other special	114	930	507	5,950	7,501	27	5	32	196,149	47,231	243,380	62.4	390,262		
Short-term general and other special	3,957	142,033	31,146	402,253	579,389	9,076	649	9,725	14,605,749	2,900,943	17,506,693	51.7	33,881,909		
Hospital units of institutions	66	192	147	685	1,090	0	0	0	19,795	5,863	25,658	37.2	68,961		
Community hospitals*	3,891	141,841	30,999	401,568	578,299	9,076	649	9,725	14,585,955	2,895,080	17,481,035	51.7	33,812,948	$4,737.15	$676.61
6-24 beds	11	150	89	596	846	3	0	3	18,198	3,928	22,126	57.2	38,686	2,337.08	589.78
25-49	41	1,791	900	8,369	11,101	14	39	53	220,129	42,310	262,439	50.8	516,811	3,205.33	532.94
50-99	182	7,202	2,602	23,689	33,675	40	11	51	735,834	145,960	881,794	49.9	1,765,401	3,549.74	548.95
100-199	206	24,365	7,280	69,073	100,924	114	58	172	2,336,317	459,695	2,796,012	49.6	5,636,004	3,896.68	556.68
200-299	371	25,926	5,768	73,460	105,525	358	76	434	2,600,314	503,909	3,104,223	49.8	6,237,522	4,465.32	647.42
300-399	297	25,258	4,674	69,253	99,482	593	78	671	2,551,322	464,764	3,016,086	52.6	5,728,840	4,519.64	658.84
400-499	822	14,097	2,503	41,264	58,686	1,220	124	1,344	1,646,033	315,255	1,961,288	53.7	3,653,165	5,178.75	745.91
500 or more	1,961	43,052	7,183	115,864	168,060	6,734	263	6,997	4,477,807	959,260	5,437,066	53.1	10,236,519	6,217.12	827.44
Nongovernment not-for-profit	2,001	90,961	17,235	255,014	365,211	4,879	410	5,289	9,416,667	1,773,278	11,189,945	53.3	21,005,151	4,795.61	681.77
Investor-owned (for-profit)	79	20,655	5,452	53,454	79,640	72	9	81	1,930,938	422,656	2,353,595	42.8	5,498,523	4,699.31	723.23
State and local government	1,811	30,225	8,312	93,100	133,448	4,125	230	4,355	3,238,350	699,146	3,937,495	53.9	7,309,274	4,603.74	632.19

*For information on community hospitals that excludes nursing-home-type data, refer to Hospital Units columns in tables 4A through 4D, pages 14 through 17.

(continued on next page)

Table

5B (Continued) Census Division 4, East North Central

Utilization, Personnel, and Finances in U.S. Census Divisions

Excludes AHA nonregistered hospitals (see Table 14, page 240).

CLASSIFICATION	HOSPI-TALS	BEDS	ADMISSIONS	INPATIENT DAYS	ADJUSTED PATIENT DAYS	OCCU-PANCY, percent	AVERAGE DAILY CENSUS	ADJUSTED AVERAGE DAILY CENSUS	AVERAGE STAY, days	SURGICAL OPERATIONS	OUTPATIENT VISITS			NEWBORNS	
											Emergency	Other	Total	Bassinets	Births
CENSUS DIVISION 4, EAST NORTH CENTRAL	959	201,518	5,688,411	49,495,209		67.3	135,621			4,150,634	15,885,060	53,449,077	69,334,137	12,783	658,953
6-24 beds	17	348	9,000	41,301		32.8	114			5,890	102,758	677,847	780,605	29	762
25-49	95	3,671	97,502	560,635		42.0	1,540			65,359	445,762	1,334,966	1,780,728	368	8,205
50-99	242	17,566	451,358	3,380,241		52.7	9,258			299,267	1,664,737	5,326,772	6,991,509	1,554	44,393
100-199	248	35,394	961,787	7,731,457		59.8	21,183			712,045	3,095,365	8,307,435	11,402,800	2,634	104,865
200-299	137	34,529	1,111,864	8,363,550		66.4	22,916			854,515	3,258,753	9,623,408	12,882,161	2,401	118,966
300-399	89	30,799	906,383	7,741,981		68.9	21,215			688,917	2,483,195	7,166,353	9,649,548	1,890	108,848
400-499	54	24,407	739,521	6,485,141		72.8	17,768			558,820	1,740,868	6,269,909	8,010,777	1,524	103,223
500 or more	77	54,804	1,410,996	15,190,903		76.0	41,627			965,821	3,093,622	14,742,387	17,836,009	2,383	169,691
Psychiatric	105	24,935	123,908	7,375,601		81.0	20,204			2,212	31,056	988,202	1,019,258	0	0
Hospitals	102	23,605	123,255	6,938,921		80.5	19,008			2,207	30,367	985,814	1,016,181	0	0
Institutions for mentally retarded	3	1,330	653	436,680		89.9	1,196			5	689	2,388	3,077	0	0
General	825	172,411	5,517,876	41,010,824		65.2	112,380			4,120,061	15,776,944	51,845,311	67,622,255	12,729	656,759
Hospitals	822	172,354	5,517,668	41,010,133		65.2	112,378			4,119,964	15,755,262	51,628,377	67,383,639	12,729	656,759
Hospital units of institutions	3	57	208	691		03.5	2			97	21,682	216,934	238,616	0	0
TB and other respiratory diseases	0	0	0	0		00.0	0			0	0	0	0	0	0
Obstetrics and gynecology	1	144	4,163	21,488		41.0	59			4,661	0	10,597	10,597	54	2,194
Eye, ear, nose, and throat	0	0	0	0		00.0	0			0	0	0	0	0	0
Rehabilitation	16	1,835	13,534	462,257		68.9	1,265			254	7,495	290,162	297,657	0	0
Orthopedic	1	60	1,576	13,158		60.0	36			1,357	0	15,549	15,549	0	0
Chronic disease	2	1,147	1,312	369,270		88.1	1,011			754	371	40,428	40,799	0	0
All other	9	986	26,042	242,611		67.5	666			21,335	69,194	258,828	328,022	0	0
Federal	28	13,251	160,535	3,638,447		75.2	9,969			86,831	256,774	4,452,023	4,708,797	74	2,345
Psychiatric	4	2,817	15,706	807,760		78.6	2,213			2,096	4,548	301,895	306,443	0	0
General and other special	24	10,434	144,829	2,830,687		74.3	7,756			84,735	252,226	4,150,128	4,402,354	74	2,345
Nonfederal	931	188,267	5,527,876	45,856,762		66.7	125,652			4,063,803	15,628,286	48,997,054	64,625,340	12,709	656,608
Psychiatric	101	22,118	108,202	6,567,841		81.3	17,991			116	26,508	686,307	712,815	0	0
Hospitals	98	20,788	107,549	6,131,161		80.8	16,795			111	25,819	683,919	709,738	0	0
Institutions for mentally retarded	3	1,330	653	436,680		89.9	1,196			5	689	2,388	3,077	0	0
TB and other respiratory diseases	0	0	0	0		00.0	0			0	0	0	0	0	0
Long-term general and other special	9	2,380	15,120	689,989		79.4	1,889			6,457	26,672	211,475	238,147	22	2,046
Short-term general and other special	821	163,769	5,404,554	38,598,932		64.6	105,772			4,057,230	15,575,106	48,099,272	63,674,378	12,687	654,562
Hospital units of institutions	3	57	208	691		03.5	2			97	21,682	216,934	238,616	0	0
Community hospitals*	818	163,712	5,404,346	38,598,241	52,104,001	64.6	105,770	142,774	7.1	4,057,133	15,553,424	47,882,338	63,435,762	12,687	654,562
6-24 beds	8	174	3,613	16,500	31,713	26.4	46	89	4.6	2,807	16,587	74,811	91,398	10	157
25-49	88	3,400	93,481	495,781	822,873	40.1	1,363	2,253	5.3	65,359	445,737	1,289,810	1,735,547	368	8,205
50-99	210	15,128	417,191	2,783,539	4,267,652	50.4	7,625	11,692	6.7	296,887	1,643,304	4,642,047	6,285,351	1,554	44,393
100-199	213	30,351	914,258	6,417,472	9,216,551	57.9	17,583	25,263	7.0	705,447	3,043,539	7,790,897	10,834,436	2,609	104,098
200-299	127	32,002	1,083,263	7,586,754	10,337,868	65.0	20,789	28,323	7.0	845,629	3,193,420	8,933,077	12,126,497	2,371	117,993
300-399	72	24,880	853,471	5,930,614	7,899,120	65.3	16,252	21,644	6.9	656,664	2,451,244	6,348,620	8,799,864	1,868	106,802
400-499	44	19,739	724,834	5,045,073	6,566,581	70.0	13,823	17,993	7.0	554,592	1,737,139	5,976,315	7,713,454	1,524	103,223
500 or more	56	38,038	1,314,235	10,322,508	12,961,643	74.4	28,289	35,517	7.9	929,748	3,022,454	12,826,761	15,849,215	2,383	169,691
Nongovernment not-for-profit	643	141,092	4,767,958	33,667,292	45,297,431	65.4	92,251	124,113	7.1	3,629,967	13,399,233	40,860,731	54,259,964	10,770	578,424
Investor-owned (for-profit)	20	2,196	60,670	421,706	550,133	52.9	1,162	1,516	7.0	46,598	174,091	312,155	486,246	157	7,004
State and local government	155	20,424	575,718	4,509,243	6,256,437	60.5	12,357	17,145	7.8	380,568	1,980,100	6,709,452	8,689,552	1,760	69,134

*For information on community hospitals that excludes nursing-home-type data, refer to Hospital Units columns in tables 4A through 4D, pages 14 through 17.

CLASSIFICATION	FULL-TIME EQUIVALENT PERSONNEL					FULL-TIME EQUIVALENT TRAINEES			EXPENSES						
									LABOR				TOTAL		
	Physicians and Dentists	Registered Nurses	Licensed Practical Nurses	Other Salaried Personnel	Total Personnel	Medical and Dental Residents	Other Trainees	Total Trainees	Payroll (in thousands)	Employee Benefits (in thousands)	Total (in thousands)	Percent of Total	Amount (in thousands)	Adjusted, per Admission	Adjusted, per Inpatient Day
CENSUS DIVISION 4, EAST NORTH CENTRAL	8,285	158,692	27,473	507,163	701,613	14,635	1,251	15,886	$18,437,198	$ 3,637,386	$22,074,583	55.6	$ 39,729,137		
6-24 beds	108	251	98	1,305	1,762	6	0	6	34,090	6,249	40,340	63.8	63,181		
25-49	44	2,150	668	8,051	10,913	17	7	24	229,009	44,008	273,017	54.3	502,766		
50-99	400	10,161	3,113	34,987	48,661	84	14	98	1,064,406	216,659	1,281,065	55.1	2,326,924		
100-199	600	23,786	5,052	77,036	106,474	612	32	644	2,581,293	513,085	3,094,378	54.5	5,679,817		
200-299	852	28,802	5,552	87,564	122,770	1,570	177	1,747	3,262,417	638,069	3,900,487	54.8	7,122,304		
300-399	1,215	25,509	4,426	80,014	111,164	1,483	129	1,612	2,919,391	553,207	3,472,598	56.3	6,172,794		
400-499	1,073	20,836	2,651	64,083	88,643	2,299	101	2,400	2,450,154	478,846	2,929,000	56.9	5,144,285		
500 or more	3,993	47,197	5,913	154,123	211,226	8,564	791	9,355	5,896,437	1,187,263	7,083,700	55.7	12,717,066		
Psychiatric	956	4,861	1,561	33,279	40,657	108	170	278	1,152,284	243,126	1,395,410	73.1	1,908,492		
Hospitals	947	4,789	1,486	30,962	38,184	108	170	278	1,100,453	230,049	1,330,502	72.8	1,826,583		
Institutions for mentally retarded	9	72	75	2,317	2,473	0	0	0	51,831	13,077	64,907	79.2	81,909		
General	7,158	151,734	25,386	464,238	648,516	14,391	1,072	15,463	16,983,326	3,327,702	20,311,028	54.6	37,219,456		
Hospitals	7,146	151,699	25,355	464,116	648,316	14,391	1,072	15,463	16,980,897	3,327,097	20,307,994	54.6	37,212,338		
Hospital units of institutions	12	35	31	122	200	0	0	0	2,429	605	3,034	42.6	7,118		
TB and other respiratory diseases	0	0	0	0	0	0	0	0	0	0	0	0.0	0		
Obstetrics and gynecology	0	136	1	244	381	0	0	0	7,420	1,672	9,092	43.0	21,123		
Eye, ear, nose, and throat	0	0	0	0	0	0	0	0	0	0	0	0.0	0		
Rehabilitation	50	817	283	4,489	5,639	21	0	21	143,097	31,924	175,021	62.0	282,266		
Orthopedic	14	78	0	160	252	5	0	5	3,364	664	4,028	53.7	7,502		
Chronic disease	84	173	98	1,851	2,206	29	0	29	50,582	15,714	66,296	69.2	95,790		
All other	23	893	144	2,902	3,962	81	9	90	97,124	16,583	113,707	58.5	194,508		
Federal	1,766	5,041	1,302	24,044	32,153	1,120	145	1,265	974,795	163,821	1,138,616	67.4	1,689,795		
Psychiatric	146	596	148	3,772	4,662	6	5	11	135,958	25,704	161,662	72.7	222,409		
General and other special	1,620	4,445	1,154	20,272	27,491	1,114	140	1,254	838,837	138,117	976,954	66.6	1,467,386		
Nonfederal	6,519	153,651	26,171	483,119	669,460	13,515	1,106	14,621	17,462,403	3,473,565	20,935,967	55.0	38,039,342		
Psychiatric	810	4,265	1,413	29,507	35,995	102	165	267	1,016,326	217,421	1,233,748	73.2	1,686,083		
Hospitals	801	4,193	1,338	27,190	33,522	102	165	267	964,496	204,345	1,168,840	72.9	1,604,174		
Institutions for mentally retarded	9	72	75	2,317	2,473	0	0	0	51,831	13,077	64,907	79.2	81,909		
TB and other respiratory diseases	0	0	0	0	0	0	0	0	0	0	0	0.0	0		
Long-term general and other special	137	751	249	4,994	6,131	78	10	88	149,078	36,756	185,834	64.5	288,268		
Short-term general and other special	5,572	148,635	24,509	448,618	627,334	13,335	931	14,266	16,296,998	3,219,388	19,516,386	54.1	36,064,991		
Hospital units of institutions	12	35	31	122	200	0	0	0	2,429	605	3,034	42.6	7,118		
Community hospitals*	5,560	148,600	24,478	448,496	627,134	13,335	931	14,266	16,294,569	3,218,782	19,513,352	54.1	36,057,873	$4,900.01	$692.04
6-24 beds	0	97	48	308	453	0	0	0	9,064	1,589	10,653	50.4	21,127	2,996.33	666.20
25-49	31	2,089	645	7,541	10,306	17	7	24	213,126	40,728	253,854	54.1	468,857	2,986.03	569.78
50-99	234	9,365	2,991	30,014	42,604	73	7	80	919,977	186,851	1,106,829	54.1	2,044,994	3,124.87	479.18
100-199	292	22,278	4,629	68,891	96,090	506	17	523	2,289,676	448,374	2,738,050	53.6	5,111,445	3,853.48	554.59
200-299	579	27,839	5,292	83,159	116,869	1,386	152	1,538	3,067,561	615,518	3,683,079	54.0	6,816,056	4,596.73	659.33
300-399	743	23,580	3,857	69,679	97,859	1,092	59	1,151	2,522,282	474,950	2,997,233	54.5	5,502,911	4,824.98	696.65
400-499	853	20,119	2,321	58,114	81,407	2,177	87	2,264	2,254,092	438,919	2,693,011	55.6	4,843,790	5,128.91	737.64
500 or more	2,828	43,233	4,695	130,790	181,546	8,084	602	8,686	5,018,790	1,011,853	6,030,643	53.6	11,248,692	6,833.69	867.84
Nongovernment not-for-profit	4,715	129,926	20,778	391,585	547,004	10,620	770	11,390	14,259,378	2,762,638	17,022,016	53.7	31,671,867	4,907.57	699.20
Investor-owned (for-profit)	8	1,522	376	4,372	6,278	20	2	22	141,736	27,369	169,105	45.3	373,667	4,681.48	679.23
State and local government	837	17,152	3,324	52,539	73,852	2,695	159	2,854	1,893,456	428,775	2,322,231	57.9	4,012,339	4,862.04	641.31

*For information on community hospitals that excludes nursing-home-type data, refer to Hospital Units columns in tables 4A through 4D, pages 14 through 17.

(continued on next page)

Table

5B (Continued) Census Division 5, East South Central

Utilization, Personnel, and Finances in U.S. Census Divisions

Excludes AHA nonregistered hospitals (see Table 14, page 240).

CLASSIFICATION	HOSPITALS	BEDS	ADMISSIONS	INPATIENT DAYS	ADJUSTED PATIENT DAYS	OCCUPANCY, percent	AVERAGE DAILY CENSUS	ADJUSTED AVERAGE DAILY CENSUS	AVERAGE STAY, days	SURGICAL OPERATIONS	OUTPATIENT VISITS			NEWBORNS	
											Emergency	Other	Total	Bassinets	Births
CENSUS DIVISION 5, EAST SOUTH CENTRAL	532	89,028	2,505,047	21,481,579		66.1	58,867			1,570,122	6,666,210	13,928,367	20,594,577	4,963	232,958
6-24 beds	9	180	4,287	23,277		36.1	65			1,507	17,204	67,086	84,290	0	0
25-49	80	3,082	89,072	543,259		48.4	1,491			29,527	348,919	804,394	1,153,313	183	3,919
50-99	181	13,314	334,638	2,492,188		51.3	6,835			154,345	1,231,431	1,925,600	3,157,031	879	24,515
100-199	132	18,213	518,025	4,046,012		60.9	11,088			341,537	1,732,454	3,843,666	5,576,120	1,255	49,015
200-299	48	11,603	376,961	2,645,445		62.5	7,247			242,964	910,513	1,764,153	2,674,666	760	32,394
300-399	30	10,056	330,716	2,581,901		70.4	7,075			246,086	774,181	1,537,757	2,311,938	620	33,986
400-499	19	8,356	288,323	2,247,589		73.7	6,158			177,896	658,410	1,277,640	1,936,050	501	31,733
500 or more	33	24,224	563,025	6,901,908		78.1	18,908			376,260	993,098	2,708,071	3,701,169	765	57,396
Psychiatric	42	10,312	50,157	3,182,208		84.6	8,721			0	6,871	170,879	177,750	0	0
Hospitals	42	10,312	50,157	3,182,208		84.6	8,721			0	6,871	170,879	177,750	0	0
Institutions for mentally retarded	0	0	0	0		00.0	0			0	0	0	0	0	0
General	474	77,156	2,439,111	17,907,404		63.6	49,071			1,558,541	6,650,083	13,569,766	20,219,849	4,909	231,074
Hospitals	473	77,051	2,437,947	17,884,432		63.6	49,008			1,558,114	6,645,742	13,497,146	20,142,888	4,909	231,074
Hospital units of institutions	1	105	1,164	22,972		60.0	63			427	4,341	72,620	76,961	0	0
TB and other respiratory diseases	0	0	0	0		00.0	0			0	0	0	0	0	0
Obstetrics and gynecology	1	111	3,342	13,040		32.4	36			2,808	418	618	1,036	40	1,846
Eye, ear, nose, and throat	1	91	1,434	2,707		07.7	7			3,962	6,412	10,761	17,173	0	0
Rehabilitation	9	636	7,399	169,528		73.1	465			1,382	1,261	138,371	139,632	0	0
Orthopedic	1	50	1,145	12,281		68.0	34			1,037	0	13,936	13,936	0	0
Chronic disease	2	585	363	182,565		85.5	500			20	0	0	0	0	0
All other	2	87	2,096	11,846		37.9	33			2,372	1,165	24,036	25,201	14	38
Federal	22	7,877	134,410	2,144,051		74.6	5,874			80,568	368,374	3,620,383	3,988,757	128	5,504
Psychiatric	1	702	4,245	224,638		87.6	615			0	0	58,274	58,274	0	0
General and other special	21	7,175	130,165	1,919,413		73.3	5,259			80,568	368,374	3,562,109	3,930,483	128	5,504
Nonfederal	510	81,151	2,370,637	19,337,528		65.3	52,993			1,489,554	6,297,836	10,307,984	16,605,820	4,835	227,454
Psychiatric	41	9,610	45,912	2,957,570		84.3	8,106			0	6,871	112,605	119,476	0	0
Hospitals	41	9,610	45,912	2,957,570		84.3	8,106			0	6,871	112,605	119,476	0	0
Institutions for mentally retarded	0	0	0	0		00.0	0			0	0	0	0	0	0
TB and other respiratory diseases	0	0	0	0		00.0	0			0	0	0	0	0	0
Long-term general and other special	4	656	745	197,097		82.3	540			20	316	12,702	13,018	0	0
Short-term general and other special	465	70,885	2,323,980	16,182,861		62.6	44,347			1,489,534	6,290,649	10,182,677	16,473,326	4,835	227,454
Hospital units of institutions	1	105	1,164	22,972		60.0	63			427	4,341	72,620	76,961	0	0
Community hospitals*	464	70,780	2,322,816	16,159,889	20,738,062	62.6	44,284	56,830	7.0	1,489,107	6,286,308	10,110,057	16,396,365	4,835	227,454
6-24 beds	8	173	3,570	21,021	37,300	34.1	59	102	5.9	1,068	11,499	10,514	22,013	0	0
25-49	72	2,794	79,959	476,799	694,144	46.8	1,308	1,905	6.0	24,331	295,017	411,181	706,198	168	3,052
50-99	161	11,863	315,539	2,170,016	3,007,682	50.2	5,951	8,248	6.9	149,362	1,147,622	1,614,365	2,761,987	837	23,613
100-199	119	16,510	485,237	3,599,451	4,899,019	59.7	9,864	13,426	7.4	332,589	1,607,708	2,509,709	4,117,417	1,202	46,303
200-299	42	10,000	349,829	2,221,016	2,909,449	60.8	6,084	7,970	6.3	237,527	879,414	1,483,840	2,363,254	760	32,394
300-399	25	8,345	306,129	2,051,633	2,527,671	67.4	5,622	6,925	6.7	235,195	739,179	1,053,844	1,793,023	602	32,963
400-499	17	7,410	279,461	1,957,978	2,347,192	72.4	5,364	6,432	7.0	174,046	648,026	1,139,736	1,787,762	501	31,733
500 or more	20	13,685	503,092	3,661,975	4,315,605	73.3	10,032	11,822	7.3	334,989	957,843	1,886,868	2,844,711	765	57,396
Nongovernment not-for-profit	195	35,837	1,242,094	8,597,888	10,882,393	65.7	23,555	29,815	6.9	818,011	3,010,906	5,517,079	8,527,985	2,289	113,119
Investor-owned (for-profit)	113	13,481	403,411	2,573,630	3,343,292	52.3	7,054	9,159	6.4	289,168	1,229,934	1,582,172	2,812,106	886	35,306
State and local government	156	21,462	677,311	4,988,371	6,512,377	63.7	13,675	17,856	7.4	381,928	2,045,468	3,010,806	5,056,274	1,660	79,029

*For information on community hospitals that excludes nursing-home-type data, refer to Hospital Units columns in tables 4A through 4D, pages 14 through 17.

CLASSIFICATION	FULL-TIME EQUIVALENT PERSONNEL					FULL-TIME EQUIVALENT TRAINEES			EXPENSES						
									LABOR				TOTAL		
	Physicians and Dentists	Registered Nurses	Licensed Practical Nurses	Other Salaried Personnel	Total Personnel	Medical and Dental Residents	Other Trainees	Total Trainees	Payroll (in thousands)	Employee Benefits (in thousands)	Total (in thousands)	Percent of Total	Amount (in thousands)	Adjusted, per Admission	Adjusted, per Inpatient Day
CENSUS DIVISION 5, EAST SOUTH CENTRAL	2,722	55,763	18,764	184,441	261,690	2,603	547	3,150	$ 5,942,385	$ 1,155,194	$ 7,097,579	52.1	$ 13,630,076		
6-24 beds	16	83	34	399	532	2	0	2	6,946	1,284	8,231	54.2	15,175		
25-49	104	1,454	904	6,753	9,215	2	30	32	159,096	32,099	191,195	55.1	346,921		
50-99	172	5,681	2,952	21,097	29,902	37	23	60	592,485	116,014	708,499	51.1	1,387,739		
100-199	383	9,748	4,328	33,409	47,868	38	20	58	1,009,029	205,732	1,214,761	49.7	2,446,342		
200-299	306	8,392	2,714	24,787	36,199	203	36	239	829,547	158,751	988,298	51.2	1,931,541		
300-399	254	8,077	1,859	23,052	33,242	448	185	633	788,596	152,782	941,379	50.8	1,852,970		
400-499	90	7,369	2,002	22,307	31,768	137	85	222	734,879	134,657	869,536	50.7	1,713,674		
500 or more	1,397	14,959	3,971	52,637	72,964	1,736	168	1,904	1,821,806	353,874	2,175,680	55.3	3,935,715		
Psychiatric	269	1,659	697	13,111	15,736	20	15	35	358,882	85,040	443,922	68.1	651,520		
Hospitals	269	1,659	697	13,111	15,736	20	15	35	358,882	85,040	443,922	68.1	651,520		
Institutions for mentally retarded	0	0	0	0	0	0	0	0	0	0	0	0.0	0		
General	2,437	53,238	17,821	167,679	241,175	2,550	506	3,056	5,501,367	1,052,081	6,553,448	51.2	12,800,019		
Hospitals	2,416	53,197	17,782	167,573	240,968	2,550	506	3,056	5,497,471	1,050,963	6,548,434	51.2	12,786,312		
Hospital units of institutions	21	41	39	106	207	0	0	0	3,897	1,118	5,015	36.6	13,707		
TB and other respiratory diseases	0	0	0	0	0	0	0	0	0	0	0	0.0	0		
Obstetrics and gynecology	0	93	6	108	207	0	0	0	4,521	685	5,206	39.8	13,090		
Eye, ear, nose, and throat	4	35	6	134	179	18	0	18	3,122	596	3,718	36.2	10,271		
Rehabilitation	2	422	106	1,623	2,153	10	0	10	48,785	9,103	57,888	56.1	103,252		
Orthopedic	1	34	1	140	176	4	0	4	3,347	660	4,006	53.7	7,463		
Chronic disease	4	21	28	620	673	0	0	0	14,853	5,575	20,428	75.9	26,921		
All other	5	261	99	1,026	1,391	1	26	27	7,509	1,454	8,963	51.1	17,539		
Federal	1,306	3,128	1,319	16,456	22,209	771	187	958	631,277	114,119	745,396	66.7	1,117,847		
Psychiatric	28	118	71	845	1,062	2	3	5	27,633	5,335	32,968	76.7	42,985		
General and other special	1,278	3,010	1,248	15,611	21,147	769	184	953	603,644	108,783	712,428	66.3	1,074,862		
Nonfederal	1,416	52,635	17,445	167,985	239,481	1,832	360	2,192	5,311,108	1,041,075	6,352,183	50.8	12,512,229		
Psychiatric	241	1,541	626	12,266	14,674	18	12	30	331,249	79,705	410,954	67.5	608,536		
Hospitals	241	1,541	626	12,266	14,674	18	12	30	331,249	79,705	410,954	67.5	608,536		
Institutions for mentally retarded	0	0	0	0	0	0	0	0	0	0	0	0.0	0		
TB and other respiratory diseases	0	0	0	0	0	0	0	0	0	0	0	0.0	0		
Long-term general and other special	7	43	38	797	885	0	0	0	19,166	6,461	25,628	69.5	36,873		
Short-term general and other special	1,168	51,051	16,781	154,922	223,922	1,814	348	2,162	4,960,693	954,909	5,915,602	49.8	11,866,820		
Hospital units of institutions	21	41	39	106	207	0	0	0	3,897	1,118	5,015	36.6	13,707		
Community hospitals*	1,147	51,010	16,742	154,816	223,715	1,814	348	2,162	4,956,796	953,791	5,910,587	49.9	11,853,113	$3,953.83	$571.56
6-24 beds	1	63	34	233	331	2	0	2	5,753	1,019	6,772	51.7	13,093	2,031.46	351.01
25-49	21	1,245	821	5,463	7,550	2	30	32	118,606	23,945	142,551	51.0	279,321	2,372.58	402.40
50-99	57	5,151	2,867	18,501	26,576	36	21	57	506,611	98,608	605,219	49.9	1,212,167	2,710.00	403.02
100-199	69	9,060	4,036	29,345	42,510	7	20	27	883,254	179,768	1,063,022	48.7	2,181,568	3,305.28	445.31
200-299	110	7,731	2,483	21,821	32,145	39	10	49	709,538	135,169	844,707	49.6	1,703,775	3,724.33	585.60
300-399	31	7,506	1,641	19,907	29,079	194	80	274	675,806	131,531	807,337	48.8	1,655,571	4,384.03	654.98
400-499	13	7,097	1,933	20,595	29,638	74	81	155	682,676	123,793	806,470	49.7	1,621,702	4,830.19	690.91
500 or more	845	13,157	2,927	38,957	55,886	1,460	106	1,566	1,374,551	259,958	1,634,509	51.3	3,185,916	5,349.64	738.23
Nongovernment not-for-profit	297	28,086	8,402	86,546	123,331	679	266	945	2,785,065	529,264	3,314,329	50.8	6,526,963	4,117.36	599.77
Investor-owned (for-profit)	15	8,478	2,774	22,473	33,740	6	26	32	758,747	166,756	925,504	43.2	2,143,836	4,071.80	641.23
State and local government	835	14,446	5,566	45,797	66,644	1,129	56	1,185	1,412,983	257,771	1,670,754	52.5	3,182,314	3,591.19	488.66

*For information on community hospitals that excludes nursing-home-type data, refer to Hospital Units columns in tables 4A through 4D, pages 14 through 17.

(continued on next page)

Table
5B (Continued) Census Division 6, West North Central

Utilization, Personnel, and Finances in U.S. Census Divisions

Excludes AHA nonregistered hospitals (see Table 14, page 240).

CLASSIFICATION	HOSPITALS	BEDS	ADMISSIONS	INPATIENT DAYS	ADJUSTED PATIENT DAYS	OCCUPANCY, percent	AVERAGE DAILY CENSUS	ADJUSTED AVERAGE DAILY CENSUS	AVERAGE STAY, days	SURGICAL OPERATIONS	OUTPATIENT VISITS			NEWBORNS	
											Emergency	Other	Total	Bassinets	Births
CENSUS DIVISION 6, WEST NORTH CENTRAL	846	108,967	2,529,769	25,730,847		64.7	70,500			1,840,423	5,666,556	19,513,171	25,179,727	6,988	270,717
6-24 beds	87	1,669	36,866	211,950		34.9	582			14,273	124,123	732,197	856,320	322	2,479
25-49	240	8,800	182,898	1,302,875		40.6	3,574			90,307	531,569	2,249,589	2,781,158	1,213	18,365
50-99	221	15,627	292,086	3,385,764		59.4	9,285			188,688	818,445	2,385,177	3,203,622	1,414	31,312
100-199	140	19,513	417,129	4,519,270		63.5	12,381			300,291	1,161,046	3,610,124	4,771,170	1,251	45,484
200-299	58	14,162	361,175	3,559,643		68.8	9,750			261,305	810,592	2,700,045	3,510,637	705	36,301
300-399	43	14,801	403,755	3,691,226		68.3	10,110			329,285	813,711	2,587,493	3,401,204	737	48,883
400-499	20	8,825	194,847	2,202,254		68.4	6,032			155,020	385,578	1,450,557	1,836,135	395	22,424
500 or more	37	25,570	641,013	6,857,865		73.5	18,786			501,254	1,021,492	3,797,989	4,819,481	951	65,469
Psychiatric	54	13,446	49,475	3,920,066		79.8	10,735			492	16,612	447,532	464,144	0	0
Hospitals	49	11,054	49,352	3,141,381		77.8	8,602			492	16,612	447,532	464,144	0	0
Institutions for mentally retarded	5	2,392	123	778,685		89.2	2,133			0	0	0	0	0	0
General	776	93,875	2,468,427	21,379,546		62.4	58,582			1,835,314	5,639,217	18,906,211	24,545,428	6,988	270,717
Hospitals	773	93,122	2,465,514	21,147,020		62.2	57,944			1,834,032	5,623,921	18,794,915	24,418,836	6,988	270,717
Hospital units of institutions	3	753	2,913	232,526		84.7	638			1,282	15,296	111,296	126,592	0	0
TB and other respiratory diseases	0	0	0	0		00.0	0			0	0	0	0	0	0
Obstetrics and gynecology	0	0	0	0		00.0	0			0	0	0	0	0	0
Eye, ear, nose, and throat	0	0	0	0		00.0	0			0	0	0	0	0	0
Rehabilitation	9	759	4,796	213,693		77.2	586			0	3,113	91,252	94,365	0	0
Orthopedic	2	90	2,552	18,651		56.7	51			1,748	4,137	14,400	18,537	0	0
Chronic disease	0	0	0	0		00.0	0			0	0	0	0	0	0
All other	5	797	4,519	198,891		68.5	546			2,869	3,477	53,776	57,253	0	0
Federal	41	8,700	146,466	2,230,592		70.3	6,114			98,886	331,380	3,807,533	4,138,913	155	4,870
Psychiatric	2	1,248	6,070	355,051		77.9	972			0	0	114,038	114,038	0	0
General and other special	39	7,452	140,396	1,875,541		69.0	5,142			98,886	331,380	3,693,495	4,024,875	155	4,870
Nonfederal	805	100,267	2,383,303	23,500,255		64.2	64,386			1,741,537	5,335,176	15,705,638	21,040,814	6,833	265,847
Psychiatric	52	12,198	43,405	3,565,015		80.0	9,763			492	16,612	333,494	350,106	0	0
Hospitals	47	9,806	43,282	2,786,330		77.8	7,630			492	16,612	333,494	350,106	0	0
Institutions for mentally retarded	5	2,392	123	778,685		89.2	2,133			0	0	0	0	0	0
TB and other respiratory diseases	0	0	0	0		00.0	0			0	0	0	0	0	0
Long-term general and other special	10	1,004	4,798	307,924		84.2	845			223	5,308	40,793	46,101	0	0
Short-term general and other special	743	87,065	2,335,100	19,627,316		61.8	53,778			1,740,822	5,313,256	15,331,351	20,644,607	6,833	265,847
Hospital units of institutions	1	18	67	5,448		83.3	15			0	0	0	0	0	0
Community hospitals*	742	87,047	2,335,033	19,621,868	26,104,823	61.8	53,763	71,532	8.4	1,740,822	5,313,256	15,331,351	20,644,607	6,833	265,847
6-24 beds	76	1,480	30,373	179,141	281,898	33.0	489	772	5.9	10,602	71,601	323,521	395,122	292	2,136
25-49	224	8,230	166,082	1,186,103	1,790,015	39.6	3,255	4,909	7.1	81,960	442,417	1,426,220	1,868,637	1,147	16,372
50-99	207	14,602	284,086	3,113,861	4,426,495	58.5	8,539	12,137	11.0	188,196	814,272	2,295,839	3,110,111	1,414	31,312
100-199	120	16,694	378,855	3,830,104	5,256,675	62.9	10,494	14,399	10.1	286,900	1,083,852	2,741,601	3,825,453	1,204	43,494
200-299	42	10,303	311,533	2,475,783	3,243,000	65.8	6,781	8,886	7.9	236,699	728,883	1,866,102	2,594,985	693	35,757
300-399	33	11,346	376,670	2,686,535	3,420,906	64.9	7,358	9,375	7.1	296,572	813,711	2,197,537	3,011,248	737	48,883
400-499	14	6,037	189,502	1,394,423	1,758,250	63.3	3,819	4,817	7.4	155,020	385,578	1,450,557	1,836,135	395	22,424
500 or more	26	18,355	597,932	4,755,918	5,927,584	71.0	13,028	16,237	8.0	484,873	972,942	3,029,974	4,002,916	951	65,469
Nongovernment not-for-profit	429	63,243	1,804,840	14,615,995	19,129,716	63.3	40,042	52,418	8.1	1,342,896	4,002,350	10,475,406	14,477,756	4,763	210,135
Investor-owned (for-profit)	22	3,611	99,328	672,636	873,035	51.0	1,840	2,391	6.8	80,510	212,939	577,279	790,218	246	13,252
State and local government	291	20,193	430,865	4,333,237	6,102,072	58.8	11,881	16,723	10.1	317,416	1,097,967	4,278,666	5,376,633	1,824	42,460

*For information on community hospitals that excludes nursing-home-type data, refer to Hospital Units columns in tables 4A through 4D, pages 14 through 17.

Table 5B (Continued) **U.S. Census Division 6, West North Central**

CLASSIFICATION	FULL-TIME EQUIVALENT PERSONNEL: Physicians and Dentists	Registered Nurses	Licensed Practical Nurses	Other Salaried Personnel	Total Personnel	FULL-TIME EQUIVALENT TRAINEES: Medical and Dental Residents	Other Trainees	Total Trainees	EXPENSES — LABOR: Payroll (in thousands)	Employee Benefits (in thousands)	Total (in thousands)	Percent of Total	EXPENSES — TOTAL: Amount (in thousands)	Adjusted, per Admission	Adjusted, per Inpatient Day
CENSUS DIVISION 6, WEST NORTH CENTRAL	3,255	70,620	14,807	228,721	317,403	3,824	589	4,413	$ 7,778,492	$ 1,443,439	$ 9,221,931	55.6	$ 16,589,676		
6-24 beds	109	737	283	3,243	4,372	0	6	6	78,855	14,894	93,749	59.8	156,736		
25-49	226	3,870	1,381	14,119	19,596	2	2	4	379,741	70,222	449,964	56.8	791,925		
50-99	121	7,010	2,252	25,153	34,536	23	19	42	700,340	123,852	824,192	55.2	1,491,919		
100-199	477	10,479	2,805	35,533	49,294	202	41	243	1,107,350	208,948	1,316,297	54.7	2,405,663		
200-299	489	9,701	2,150	31,494	43,834	465	86	551	1,079,458	187,413	1,266,870	55.0	2,301,794		
300-399	481	12,069	2,118	36,568	51,236	634	40	674	1,393,578	257,022	1,650,600	56.2	2,937,366		
400-499	380	7,096	982	22,381	30,839	739	191	930	752,719	145,193	897,912	57.6	1,559,316		
500 or more	972	19,658	2,836	60,230	83,696	1,759	204	1,963	2,286,451	435,896	2,722,347	55.1	4,944,957		
Psychiatric	425	2,438	1,049	19,956	23,868	90	141	231	598,745	131,453	730,198	76.0	960,790		
Hospitals	391	2,298	928	15,554	19,171	90	33	123	487,807	104,727	592,534	74.2	798,457		
Institutions for mentally retarded	34	140	121	4,402	4,697	0	108	108	110,938	26,726	137,664	84.8	162,333		
General	2,773	67,595	13,519	205,292	289,179	3,711	447	4,158	7,083,608	1,293,695	8,377,302	54.3	15,438,266		
Hospitals	2,736	67,499	13,464	204,479	288,178	3,711	447	4,158	7,058,708	1,287,822	8,346,530	54.2	15,392,960		
Hospital units of institutions	37	96	55	813	1,001	0	0	0	24,900	5,872	30,772	67.9	45,306		
TB and other respiratory diseases	0	0	0	0	0	0	0	0	0	0	0	0.0	0		
Obstetrics and gynecology	0	0	0	0	0	0	0	0	0	0	0	0.0	0		
Eye, ear, nose, and throat	0	0	0	0	0	0	0	0	0	0	0	0.0	0		
Rehabilitation	20	223	142	1,886	2,271	1	0	1	46,436	7,790	54,226	62.3	87,010		
Orthopedic	4	73	15	238	330	0	1	1	8,662	1,676	10,338	53.2	19,429		
Chronic disease	0	0	0	0	0	0	0	0	0	0	0	0.0	0		
All other	33	291	82	1,349	1,755	22	0	22	41,041	8,826	49,867	59.2	84,182		
Federal	1,298	3,773	1,187	17,508	23,766	694	198	892	665,755	122,941	788,696	66.1	1,193,915		
Psychiatric	42	252	96	1,446	1,836	0	9	9	56,314	5,557	61,871	80.2	77,136		
General and other special	1,256	3,521	1,091	16,062	21,930	694	189	883	609,441	117,384	726,825	65.1	1,116,779		
Nonfederal	1,957	66,847	13,620	211,213	293,637	3,130	391	3,521	7,112,737	1,320,498	8,433,235	54.8	15,395,761		
Psychiatric	383	2,186	953	18,510	22,032	90	132	222	542,431	125,895	668,327	75.6	883,654		
Hospitals	349	2,046	832	14,108	17,335	90	24	114	431,493	99,170	530,663	73.6	721,321		
Institutions for mentally retarded	34	140	121	4,402	4,697	0	108	108	110,938	26,726	137,664	84.8	162,333		
TB and other respiratory diseases	0	0	0	0	0	0	0	0	0	0	0	0.0	0		
Long-term general and other special	27	236	152	2,169	2,584	3	0	3	56,573	10,333	66,905	64.3	104,065		
Short-term general and other special	1,547	64,425	12,515	190,534	269,021	3,037	259	3,296	6,513,733	1,184,270	7,698,003	53.4	14,408,043		
Hospital units of institutions	0	6	4	33	43	0	0	0	550	206	756	83.4	907		
Community hospitals*	1,547	64,419	12,511	190,501	268,978	3,037	259	3,296	6,513,183	1,184,063	7,697,246	53.4	14,407,136	$4,611.03	$551.90
6-24 beds	14	579	253	2,218	3,064	0	6	6	54,148	8,807	62,955	54.8	114,798	2,364.08	407.23
25-49	29	3,512	1,309	12,191	17,041	0	2	2	320,825	55,188	376,013	54.7	687,064	2,688.53	383.83
50-99	85	6,664	2,124	23,223	32,096	5	13	18	637,473	112,823	750,296	54.9	1,366,127	3,230.98	308.62
100-199	235	9,462	2,462	30,340	42,499	145	7	152	952,901	176,488	1,129,389	53.8	2,100,020	3,993.28	399.50
200-299	117	8,367	1,654	23,590	33,728	182	35	217	816,153	136,461	952,614	51.8	1,838,464	4,512.30	566.90
300-399	226	11,122	1,740	30,753	43,841	525	26	551	1,185,689	214,737	1,400,426	54.0	2,593,454	5,410.92	758.12
400-499	312	6,784	782	18,314	26,192	739	83	822	642,010	120,725	762,735	54.5	1,398,309	5,845.28	795.28
500 or more	529	17,929	2,187	49,872	70,517	1,441	87	1,528	1,903,984	358,835	2,262,819	52.5	4,308,901	5,778.21	726.92
Nongovernment not-for-profit	1,115	49,907	8,918	142,835	202,776	1,530	181	1,711	5,062,327	886,555	5,948,882	53.4	11,136,382	4,682.62	582.15
Investor-owned (for-profit)	38	2,338	649	7,940	10,965	31	11	42	215,520	49,947	265,468	43.6	608,719	4,669.92	697.24
State and local government	394	12,174	2,944	39,725	55,237	1,476	67	1,543	1,235,336	247,561	1,482,897	55.7	2,662,035	4,322.16	436.25

*For information on community hospitals that excludes nursing-home-type data, refer to Hospital Units columns in tables 4A through 4D, pages 14 through 17.

(continued on next page)

Table

5B (Continued) Census Division 7, West South Central

Utilization, Personnel, and Finances in U.S. Census Divisions

Excludes AHA nonregistered hospitals (see Table 14, page 240).

CLASSIFICATION	HOSPITALS	BEDS	ADMISSIONS	INPATIENT DAYS	ADJUSTED PATIENT DAYS	OCCUPANCY, percent	AVERAGE DAILY CENSUS	ADJUSTED AVERAGE DAILY CENSUS	AVERAGE STAY, days	SURGICAL OPERATIONS	OUTPATIENT VISITS: Emergency	OUTPATIENT VISITS: Other	OUTPATIENT VISITS: Total	NEWBORNS: Bassinets	NEWBORNS: Births
CENSUS DIVISION 7, WEST SOUTH CENTRAL	943	130,846	3,691,880	28,957,707		60.7	79,450			2,357,567	9,129,170	22,968,011	32,097,181	8,923	459,011
6-24 beds	61	1,158	27,896	126,262		29.7	344			13,812	159,696	657,211	816,907	153	2,465
25-49	237	8,970	216,035	1,261,761		38.6	3,465			81,904	737,341	1,578,246	2,315,587	805	16,926
50-99	243	17,353	405,650	3,139,993		49.9	8,663			235,920	1,193,251	1,912,748	3,105,999	1,213	45,134
100-199	217	30,281	853,241	6,195,147		56.2	17,024			569,658	2,396,293	4,543,806	6,940,099	2,350	110,461
200-299	75	18,200	585,306	4,139,656		62.3	11,340			430,798	1,471,788	2,935,254	4,407,042	1,485	66,352
300-399	47	16,000	503,433	3,979,165		68.1	10,901			351,840	1,042,119	2,312,177	3,354,296	1,081	78,344
400-499	22	9,929	293,684	2,443,311		67.4	6,695			198,236	606,600	1,650,107	2,256,707	571	37,218
500 or more	41	28,955	806,635	7,672,412		72.6	21,018			475,399	1,522,082	7,378,462	8,900,544	1,265	102,111
Psychiatric	120	16,552	104,718	4,162,997		69.1	11,430			1,482	32,720	477,687	510,407	5	177
Hospitals	120	16,552	104,718	4,162,997		69.1	11,430			1,482	32,720	477,687	510,407	5	177
Institutions for mentally retarded	0	0	0	0		00.0	0			0	0	0	0	0	0
General	777	109,813	3,503,879	23,816,435		59.5	65,298			2,310,875	9,022,558	21,579,051	30,601,609	8,666	442,591
Hospitals	773	109,715	3,503,235	23,813,464		59.5	65,290			2,310,591	9,015,209	21,448,182	30,463,391	8,641	442,286
Hospital units of institutions	4	98	644	2,971		08.2	8			284	7,349	130,869	138,218	25	305
TB and other respiratory diseases	1	115	1,211	29,224		69.6	80			1,806	0	15,790	15,790	0	0
Obstetrics and gynecology	3	488	24,432	91,254		51.2	250			15,933	12,565	85,506	98,071	173	13,377
Eye, ear, nose, and throat	1	39	744	1,962		12.8	5			2,520	0	25,952	25,952	0	0
Rehabilitation	28	2,023	17,679	413,653		58.0	1,174			838	10,229	139,532	149,761	0	0
Orthopedic	4	251	5,825	46,894		51.4	129			5,544	2,348	52,299	54,647	0	0
Chronic disease	1	418	205	113,429		74.4	311			0	0	0	0	0	0
All other	8	1,147	33,187	281,859		67.4	773			18,569	48,750	592,194	640,944	79	2,866
Federal	42	11,854	264,156	3,184,552		73.6	8,726			164,328	734,367	7,299,129	8,033,496	384	14,138
Psychiatric	1	799	4,325	250,599		86.0	687			0	0	78,741	78,741	0	0
General and other special	41	11,055	259,831	2,933,953		72.7	8,039			164,328	734,367	7,220,388	7,954,755	384	14,138
Nonfederal	901	118,992	3,427,724	25,773,155		59.4	70,724			2,193,239	8,394,803	15,668,882	24,063,685	8,539	444,873
Psychiatric	119	15,753	100,393	3,912,398		68.2	10,743			1,482	32,720	398,946	431,666	5	177
Hospitals	119	15,753	100,393	3,912,398		68.2	10,743			1,482	32,720	398,946	431,666	5	177
Institutions for mentally retarded	0	0	0	0		00.0	0			0	0	0	0	0	0
TB and other respiratory diseases	1	115	1,211	29,224		69.6	80			1,806	0	15,790	15,790	0	0
Long-term general and other special	12	1,328	3,607	359,846		75.3	1,000			760	1,696	27,927	29,623	0	0
Short-term general and other special	769	101,796	3,322,513	21,471,687		57.9	58,901			2,189,191	8,360,387	15,226,219	23,586,606	8,534	444,696
Hospital units of institutions	4	98	644	2,971		08.2	8			284	7,349	130,869	138,218	25	305
Community hospitals*	765	101,698	3,321,869	21,468,716	27,555,732	57.9	58,893	75,594	6.5	2,188,907	8,353,038	15,095,350	23,448,388	8,509	444,391
6-24 beds	49	979	21,108	98,923	166,849	27.6	270	460	4.7	9,466	77,838	161,176	239,014	103	1,315
25-49	214	8,073	199,215	1,071,125	1,555,863	36.5	2,943	4,274	5.4	76,127	644,277	970,819	1,615,096	733	15,348
50-99	174	12,368	351,769	2,127,370	2,905,984	47.3	5,852	7,989	6.0	227,914	1,062,790	1,356,366	2,419,156	1,130	41,579
100-199	179	24,869	787,810	4,945,520	6,544,424	54.7	13,596	17,988	6.3	550,455	2,226,257	3,009,354	5,235,611	2,274	107,609
200-299	67	16,318	540,483	3,588,840	4,513,338	60.2	9,831	12,363	6.6	384,903	1,383,011	2,007,855	3,390,866	1,447	63,882
300-399	38	12,956	475,839	3,044,787	3,817,942	64.4	8,341	10,460	6.4	327,908	1,016,100	1,857,552	2,873,652	1,081	78,344
400-499	17	7,772	270,938	1,830,418	2,225,102	64.5	5,015	6,097	6.8	187,372	545,318	1,025,853	1,571,171	546	35,749
500 or more	27	18,363	674,707	4,761,733	5,826,230	71.0	13,045	15,963	7.1	424,762	1,397,447	4,706,375	6,103,822	1,195	100,565
Nongovernment not-for-profit	247	48,578	1,702,152	11,328,925	14,207,597	63.9	31,038	38,918	6.7	1,180,639	3,753,960	6,775,958	10,529,918	3,439	194,797
Investor-owned (for-profit)	209	26,190	754,042	4,605,201	5,902,646	48.4	12,681	16,262	6.1	562,223	1,727,729	2,289,154	4,016,883	2,047	103,763
State and local government	309	26,930	865,675	5,534,590	7,445,489	56.3	15,174	20,414	6.4	446,045	2,871,349	6,030,238	8,901,587	3,023	145,831

*For information on community hospitals that excludes nursing-home-type data, refer to Hospital Units columns in tables 4A through 4D, pages 14 through 17.

CLASSIFICATION	FULL-TIME EQUIVALENT PERSONNEL: Physicians and Dentists	Registered Nurses	Licensed Practical Nurses	Other Salaried Personnel	Total Personnel	FULL-TIME EQUIVALENT TRAINEES: Medical and Dental Residents	Other Trainees	Total Trainees	EXPENSES: LABOR: Payroll (in thousands)	Employee Benefits (in thousands)	Total (in thousands)	Percent of Total	TOTAL: Amount (in thousands)	Adjusted, per Admission	Adjusted, per Inpatient Day
CENSUS DIVISION 7, WEST SOUTH CENTRAL	3,805	82,666	32,776	291,770	411,017	6,688	976	7,664	$ 9,849,875	$ 1,915,540	$11,765,415	51.3	$ 22,941,628		
6-24 beds	121	535	388	2,687	3,731	0	0	0	78,852	16,110	94,961	62.5	151,917		
25-49	211	3,313	2,701	15,375	21,600	13	18	31	400,991	75,071	476,061	53.1	897,267		
50-99	233	7,788	4,484	28,967	41,472	34	1	35	935,852	194,355	1,130,207	50.0	2,262,306		
100-199	502	17,780	7,649	58,984	84,915	352	46	398	1,976,741	414,754	2,391,495	48.1	4,970,849		
200-299	379	13,366	5,150	42,370	61,265	400	126	526	1,517,122	278,166	1,795,288	49.2	3,649,108		
300-399	364	11,387	4,207	38,830	54,788	1,080	129	1,209	1,333,524	265,241	1,598,764	51.4	3,109,728		
400-499	261	6,738	2,097	22,269	31,365	312	63	375	813,605	141,371	954,976	53.1	1,798,564		
500 or more	1,734	21,759	6,100	82,288	111,881	4,497	593	5,090	2,793,189	530,473	3,323,662	54.5	6,101,889		
Psychiatric	439	3,820	1,343	22,949	28,551	106	40	146	743,443	156,533	899,976	61.9	1,453,540		
Hospitals	439	3,820	1,343	22,949	28,551	106	40	146	743,443	156,533	899,976	61.9	1,453,540		
Institutions for mentally retarded	0	0	0	0	0	0	0	0	0	0	0	0.0	0		
General	2,957	76,064	30,479	256,127	365,627	6,379	608	6,987	8,707,800	1,662,790	10,370,590	50.4	20,584,538		
Hospitals	2,942	76,022	30,453	256,023	365,440	6,379	608	6,987	8,703,957	1,661,802	10,365,759	50.4	20,576,405		
Hospital units of institutions	15	42	26	104	187	0	0	0	3,842	988	4,830	59.4	8,133		
TB and other respiratory diseases	14	44	26	238	322	0	0	0	6,993	866	7,859	65.4	12,019		
Obstetrics and gynecology	0	592	77	999	1,668	0	0	0	45,367	9,356	54,723	47.2	115,987		
Eye, ear, nose, and throat	1	41	15	141	198	6	0	6	4,396	938	5,335	49.5	10,780		
Rehabilitation	23	668	472	3,969	5,132	13	0	13	121,151	24,437	145,587	49.9	291,683		
Orthopedic	13	156	89	747	1,005	8	0	8	22,929	4,208	27,137	49.8	54,508		
Chronic disease	4	11	19	371	405	0	0	0	6,913	1,048	7,961	69.7	11,416		
All other	354	1,270	256	6,229	8,109	176	328	504	190,883	55,364	246,247	60.5	407,159		
Federal	2,588	5,788	2,204	29,413	39,993	1,899	162	2,061	1,110,303	207,637	1,317,940	64.6	2,041,561		
Psychiatric	43	154	89	1,139	1,425	2	0	2	36,720	6,708	43,429	70.4	61,715		
General and other special	2,545	5,634	2,115	28,274	38,568	1,897	162	2,059	1,073,583	200,928	1,274,511	64.4	1,979,846		
Nonfederal	1,217	76,878	30,572	262,357	371,024	4,789	814	5,603	8,739,572	1,707,904	10,447,475	50.0	20,900,067		
Psychiatric	396	3,666	1,254	21,810	27,126	104	40	144	706,723	149,825	856,547	61.5	1,391,824		
Hospitals	396	3,666	1,254	21,810	27,126	104	40	144	706,723	149,825	856,547	61.5	1,391,824		
Institutions for mentally retarded	0	0	0	0	0	0	0	0	0	0	0	0.0	0		
TB and other respiratory diseases	14	44	26	238	322	0	0	0	6,993	866	7,859	65.4	12,019		
Long-term general and other special	12	228	167	1,882	2,289	0	0	0	59,855	11,429	71,283	59.5	119,775		
Short-term general and other special	795	72,940	29,125	238,427	341,287	4,685	774	5,459	7,966,001	1,545,784	9,511,786	49.1	19,376,449		
Hospital units of institutions	15	42	26	104	187	0	0	0	3,842	988	4,830	59.4	8,133		
Community hospitals*	780	72,898	29,099	238,323	341,100	4,685	774	5,459	7,962,159	1,544,797	9,506,955	49.1	19,368,316	$4,508.20	$702.88
6-24 beds	8	369	339	1,505	2,221	0	0	0	42,385	8,313	50,698	54.0	93,885	2,550.47	562.70
25-49	48	2,881	2,563	13,060	18,552	8	18	26	340,302	62,144	402,445	51.5	780,942	2,681.08	501.94
50-99	50	6,084	3,969	22,065	32,168	21	1	22	650,175	136,346	786,521	47.5	1,656,239	3,411.42	569.94
100-199	87	15,883	7,175	49,625	72,770	268	43	311	1,642,069	344,589	1,986,659	46.6	4,261,640	4,065.72	651.19
200-299	28	12,544	4,811	38,230	55,613	229	112	341	1,335,102	251,163	1,586,265	47.8	3,320,705	4,877.43	735.75
300-399	90	10,553	3,800	33,050	47,493	820	108	928	1,141,795	227,856	1,369,651	49.6	2,761,386	4,617.99	723.27
400-499	24	6,040	1,815	18,386	26,265	135	7	142	651,903	117,259	769,162	49.7	1,548,233	4,707.22	695.80
500 or more	445	18,544	4,627	62,402	86,018	3,204	485	3,689	2,158,429	397,126	2,555,555	51.7	4,945,286	5,981.52	848.80
Nongovernment not-for-profit	233	40,100	14,262	127,701	182,296	1,439	338	1,777	4,309,847	804,747	5,114,595	50.4	10,150,163	4,722.57	714.42
Investor-owned (for-profit)	32	15,592	6,173	43,687	65,484	16	33	49	1,564,961	361,467	1,926,427	42.7	4,513,659	4,620.81	764.68
State and local government	515	17,206	8,664	66,935	93,320	3,230	403	3,633	2,087,351	378,582	2,465,933	52.4	4,704,494	4,020.46	631.86

*For information on community hospitals that excludes nursing-home-type data, refer to Hospital Units columns in tables 4A through 4D, pages 14 through 17.

(continued on next page)

Table

5B (Continued) Census Division 8, Mountain

Utilization, Personnel, and Finances in U.S. Census Divisions

Excludes AHA nonregistered hospitals (see Table 14, page 240).

CLASSIFICATION	HOSPITALS	BEDS	ADMISSIONS	INPATIENT DAYS	ADJUSTED PATIENT DAYS	OCCUPANCY, percent	AVERAGE DAILY CENSUS	ADJUSTED AVERAGE DAILY CENSUS	AVERAGE STAY, days	SURGICAL OPERATIONS	OUTPATIENT VISITS			NEWBORNS	
											Emergency	Other	Total	Bassinets	Births
CENSUS DIVISION 8, MOUNTAIN	464	55,155	1,630,425	12,739,934		63.3	34,904			1,125,550	4,548,409	15,844,845	20,393,254	4,046	233,444
6-24 beds	47	897	24,766	135,952		41.9	376			12,077	149,746	805,970	955,716	177	3,892
25-49	124	4,631	118,620	791,058		46.7	2,164			62,085	697,383	2,196,174	2,893,557	612	16,705
50-99	122	8,613	194,162	1,902,572		60.6	5,216			103,118	584,562	2,082,139	2,666,701	693	30,802
100-199	82	11,005	337,897	2,334,679		58.1	6,397			250,511	1,027,766	3,382,006	4,409,772	873	45,782
200-299	45	10,949	397,399	2,603,384		65.1	7,131			329,245	989,338	2,436,043	3,425,381	760	59,965
300-399	25	8,555	233,284	2,195,064		70.3	6,012			145,726	485,240	1,929,618	2,414,858	401	28,216
400-499	10	4,451	161,918	1,147,886		70.6	3,144			122,182	337,381	2,081,136	2,418,517	289	25,807
500 or more	9	6,054	162,379	1,629,339		73.7	4,464			100,606	276,993	931,759	1,208,752	241	22,275
Psychiatric	58	7,235	42,844	2,063,157		78.1	5,648			650	11,167	293,622	304,789	0	0
Hospitals	56	6,673	42,831	1,862,155		76.4	5,098			650	11,167	293,622	304,789	0	0
Institutions for mentally retarded	2	562	13	201,002		97.9	550			0	0	0	0	0	0
General	395	47,204	1,577,453	10,516,398		61.0	28,817			1,119,354	4,535,777	15,406,210	19,941,987	4,026	230,669
Hospitals	395	47,204	1,577,453	10,516,398		61.0	28,817			1,119,354	4,535,777	15,406,210	19,941,987	4,026	230,669
Hospital units of institutions	0	0	0	0		00.0	0			0	0	0	0	0	0
TB and other respiratory diseases	0	0	0	0		00.0	0			0	0	0	0	0	0
Obstetrics and gynecology	1	67	3,464	9,357		38.8	26			2,743	0	10,080	10,080	20	2,775
Eye, ear, nose, and throat	0	0	0	0		00.0	0			0	0	0	0	0	0
Rehabilitation	7	475	4,343	114,238		65.7	312			1,500	0	98,540	98,540	0	0
Orthopedic	2	69	1,011	12,056		47.8	33			1,303	0	14,355	14,355	0	0
Chronic disease	0	0	0	0		00.0	0			0	0	0	0	0	0
All other	1	105	1,310	24,728		64.8	68			0	1,465	22,038	23,503	0	0
Federal	50	6,157	163,846	1,483,934		66.0	4,066			105,697	755,454	5,436,316	6,191,770	318	13,930
Psychiatric	2	658	3,012	179,582		74.8	492			0	0	58,991	58,991	0	0
General and other special	48	5,499	160,834	1,304,352		65.0	3,574			105,697	755,454	5,377,325	6,132,779	318	13,930
Nonfederal	414	48,998	1,466,579	11,256,000		62.9	30,838			1,019,853	3,792,955	10,408,529	14,201,484	3,728	219,514
Psychiatric	56	6,577	39,832	1,883,575		78.4	5,156			650	11,167	234,631	245,798	0	0
Hospitals	54	6,015	39,819	1,682,573		76.6	4,606			650	11,167	234,631	245,798	0	0
Institutions for mentally retarded	2	562	13	201,002		97.9	550			0	0	0	0	0	0
TB and other respiratory diseases	0	0	0	0		00.0	0			0	0	0	0	0	0
Long-term general and other special	3	183	759	40,456		60.1	110			1,500	398	5,379	5,777	0	0
Short-term general and other special	355	42,238	1,425,988	9,331,969		60.5	25,572			1,017,703	3,781,390	10,168,519	13,949,909	3,728	219,514
Hospital units of institutions	0	0	0	0		00.0	0			0	0	0	0	0	0
Community hospitals*	355	42,238	1,425,988	9,331,969	12,452,759	60.5	25,572	34,129	6.5	1,017,703	3,781,390	10,168,519	13,949,909	3,728	219,514
6-24 beds	34	654	13,981	83,936	150,358	35.6	233	412	6.0	7,320	57,280	210,426	267,706	133	2,650
25-49	99	3,712	85,122	608,101	962,887	44.8	1,663	2,640	7.1	48,549	349,322	917,107	1,266,429	483	12,141
50-99	82	5,640	144,996	1,218,222	1,729,376	59.3	3,344	4,747	8.4	87,940	452,778	985,432	1,438,210	611	25,630
100-199	70	9,374	304,177	1,973,044	2,705,609	57.7	5,407	7,410	6.5	221,750	945,084	2,654,700	3,599,784	825	43,706
200-299	41	10,062	392,692	2,314,144	3,008,085	63.0	6,339	8,243	5.9	326,815	989,338	2,350,294	3,339,632	760	59,965
300-399	16	5,344	205,518	1,277,649	1,591,584	65.5	3,500	4,360	6.2	135,502	452,454	1,401,990	1,854,444	401	28,216
400-499	7	3,159	131,853	794,979	991,824	68.9	2,177	2,718	6.0	94,071	258,664	934,811	1,193,475	274	24,931
500 or more	6	4,293	147,649	1,061,894	1,313,036	67.8	2,909	3,599	7.2	95,756	276,470	713,759	990,229	241	22,275
Nongovernment not-for-profit	196	27,024	971,646	6,120,342	8,072,968	62.1	16,777	22,132	6.3	707,000	2,368,692	6,344,428	8,713,120	2,272	147,438
Investor-owned (for-profit)	37	5,941	199,958	1,178,385	1,556,067	54.3	3,228	4,261	5.9	168,753	543,938	1,587,712	2,131,650	526	28,330
State and local government	122	9,273	254,384	2,033,242	2,823,724	60.0	5,567	7,736	8.0	141,950	868,760	2,236,379	3,105,139	930	43,746

*For information on community hospitals that excludes nursing-home-type data, refer to Hospital Units columns in tables 4A through 4D, pages 14 through 17.

CLASSIFICATION	FULL-TIME EQUIVALENT PERSONNEL					FULL-TIME EQUIVALENT TRAINEES			EXPENSES						
									LABOR				TOTAL		
	Physicians and Dentists	Registered Nurses	Licensed Practical Nurses	Other Salaried Personnel	Total Personnel	Medical and Dental Residents	Other Trainees	Total Trainees	Payroll (in thousands)	Employee Benefits (in thousands)	Total (in thousands)	Percent of Total	Amount (in thousands)	Adjusted, per Admission	Adjusted, per Inpatient Day
CENSUS DIVISION 8, MOUNTAIN	3,195	42,149	7,680	129,617	182,641	1,445	182	1,627	$ 4,726,850	$ 941,644	$ 5,668,494	52.9	$ 10,707,441		
6-24 beds	169	553	168	2,676	3,566	4	0	4	76,497	13,232	89,728	68.6	130,750		
25-49	458	2,522	707	10,636	14,323	15	9	24	298,640	62,374	361,014	58.1	621,462		
50-99	324	4,357	949	16,175	21,805	39	26	65	513,457	100,172	613,629	54.2	1,132,802		
100-199	385	7,854	1,791	24,259	34,289	75	26	101	875,097	170,903	1,046,000	50.0	2,091,334		
200-299	963	11,043	1,314	28,845	42,165	90	82	172	1,106,692	213,079	1,319,771	50.6	2,607,564		
300-399	379	6,821	1,038	21,025	29,263	487	25	512	820,835	172,896	993,731	54.7	1,816,178		
400-499	331	3,901	903	12,093	17,228	497	12	509	493,627	106,469	600,096	54.9	1,093,960		
500 or more	186	5,098	810	13,908	20,002	238	2	240	542,005	102,519	644,525	53.1	1,213,392		
Psychiatric	163	1,587	440	11,086	13,276	31	22	53	330,178	74,058	404,236	64.3	629,006		
Hospitals	156	1,538	378	9,742	11,814	31	10	41	304,864	66,536	371,400	63.2	587,359		
Institutions for mentally retarded	7	49	62	1,344	1,462	0	12	12	25,314	7,522	32,836	78.8	41,647		
General	2,953	40,175	7,123	116,168	166,419	1,406	159	1,565	4,301,942	851,757	5,153,700	52.0	9,903,800		
Hospitals	2,953	40,175	7,123	116,168	166,419	1,406	159	1,565	4,301,942	851,757	5,153,700	52.0	9,903,800		
Hospital units of institutions	0	0	0	0	0	0	0	0	0	0	0	0.0	0		
TB and other respiratory diseases	0	0	0	0	0	0	0	0	0	0	0	0.0	0		
Obstetrics and gynecology	1	41	18	135	195	0	0	0	5,636	1,263	6,898	44.3	15,574		
Eye, ear, nose, and throat	0	0	0	0	0	0	0	0	0	0	0	0.0	0		
Rehabilitation	6	211	86	1,147	1,450	1	0	1	40,458	7,353	47,811	56.3	84,897		
Orthopedic	9	33	10	149	201	7	0	7	5,805	1,157	6,962	53.7	12,977		
Chronic disease	0	0	0	0	0	0	0	0	0	0	0	0.0	0		
All other	63	102	3	932	1,100	0	1	1	42,831	6,056	48,887	79.9	61,188		
Federal	1,756	3,849	1,375	17,750	24,730	458	65	523	640,135	119,913	760,048	66.5	1,143,012		
Psychiatric	30	145	47	814	1,036	0	0	0	29,245	5,349	34,594	72.1	48,007		
General and other special	1,726	3,704	1,328	16,936	23,694	458	65	523	610,890	114,564	725,454	66.3	1,095,005		
Nonfederal	1,439	38,300	6,305	111,867	157,911	987	117	1,104	4,086,715	821,731	4,908,446	51.3	9,564,429		
Psychiatric	133	1,442	393	10,272	12,240	31	22	53	300,933	68,709	369,641	63.6	580,999		
Hospitals	126	1,393	331	8,928	10,778	31	10	41	275,619	61,187	336,806	62.4	539,352		
Institutions for mentally retarded	7	49	62	1,344	1,462	0	12	12	25,314	7,522	32,836	78.8	41,647		
TB and other respiratory diseases	0	0	0	0	0	0	0	0	0	0	0	0.0	0		
Long-term general and other special	2	68	37	369	476	1	0	1	13,895	2,373	16,268	57.1	28,480		
Short-term general and other special	1,304	36,790	5,875	101,226	145,195	955	95	1,050	3,771,887	750,649	4,522,537	50.5	8,954,950		
Hospital units of institutions	0	0	0	0	0	0	0	0	0	0	0	0.0	0		
Community hospitals*	1,304	36,790	5,875	101,226	145,195	955	95	1,050	3,771,887	750,649	4,522,537	50.5	8,954,950	$4,680.06	$719.11
6-24 beds	16	298	116	1,156	1,586	4	0	4	32,732	6,871	39,604	53.8	73,659	2,980.96	489.89
25-49	36	1,779	516	6,744	9,075	3	9	12	184,956	38,383	223,339	51.8	430,749	3,053.40	447.35
50-99	14	3,067	732	10,093	13,906	0	7	7	308,693	58,624	367,317	50.7	724,688	3,472.58	419.05
100-199	144	7,171	1,485	21,010	29,810	61	7	68	751,439	149,282	900,722	48.6	1,853,703	4,363.65	685.13
200-299	917	10,869	1,225	27,177	40,188	76	60	136	1,058,672	202,639	1,261,311	49.9	2,527,886	4,944.58	840.36
300-399	60	5,774	763	15,130	21,727	252	10	262	617,913	130,223	748,136	51.9	1,441,341	5,612.13	905.60
400-499	64	3,222	425	8,686	12,397	333	2	335	375,947	82,230	458,177	53.3	859,490	5,208.53	866.58
500 or more	53	4,610	613	11,230	16,506	226	0	226	441,535	82,398	523,932	50.2	1,043,433	5,762.82	794.67
Nongovernment not-for-profit	1,189	25,587	3,378	68,124	98,278	492	49	541	2,636,358	507,286	3,143,644	51.7	6,085,754	4,707.28	753.84
Investor-owned (for-profit)	5	4,747	1,120	12,692	18,564	8	0	8	462,511	102,815	565,327	42.3	1,335,354	4,978.80	858.16
State and local government	110	6,456	1,377	20,410	28,353	455	46	501	673,018	140,548	813,566	53.0	1,533,843	4,352.82	543.20

*For information on community hospitals that excludes nursing-home-type data, refer to Hospital Units columns in tables 4A through 4D, pages 14 through 17.

(continued on next page)

Table
5B (Continued) Census Division 9, Pacific

Utilization, Personnel, and Finances in U.S. Census Divisions

Excludes AHA nonregistered hospitals (see Table 14, page 240).

CLASSIFICATION	HOSPITALS	BEDS	ADMISSIONS	INPATIENT DAYS	ADJUSTED PATIENT DAYS	OCCUPANCY, percent	AVERAGE DAILY CENSUS	ADJUSTED AVERAGE DAILY CENSUS	AVERAGE STAY, days	SURGICAL OPERATIONS	OUTPATIENT VISITS Emergency	OUTPATIENT VISITS Other	OUTPATIENT VISITS Total	NEWBORNS Bassinets	NEWBORNS Births
CENSUS DIVISION 9, PACIFIC	788	137,545	4,367,845	33,714,281		67.2	92,404			2,833,741	12,366,470	39,762,286	52,128,756	8,422	729,521
6-24 beds	40	776	19,462	103,859		37.1	288			11,585	124,995	464,113	589,108	81	1,558
25-49	128	4,689	125,754	723,368		42.2	1,977			90,192	669,238	2,057,491	2,726,729	525	17,834
50-99	183	13,344	380,788	2,612,176		53.8	7,182			270,419	1,390,082	2,928,840	4,318,922	895	55,372
100-199	204	29,310	1,013,951	6,460,909		60.5	17,721			738,705	3,399,135	8,689,339	12,088,474	1,917	157,386
200-299	105	25,375	1,011,371	6,082,624		65.7	16,663			627,625	2,974,414	7,706,093	10,680,507	2,112	192,220
300-399	63	21,420	814,864	5,469,018		70.0	14,984			511,969	1,737,480	7,142,892	8,880,372	1,377	141,580
400-499	30	13,231	505,643	3,564,935		73.8	9,764			281,191	1,223,285	5,867,553	7,090,838	829	87,392
500 or more	35	29,400	496,012	8,697,392		81.0	23,825			302,055	847,841	4,905,965	5,753,806	686	76,179
Psychiatric	81	17,735	74,258	5,353,626		82.8	14,692			656	25,071	278,950	304,021	0	0
Hospitals	78	14,010	74,041	4,059,243		79.6	11,146			643	24,240	276,573	300,813	0	0
Institutions for mentally retarded	3	3,725	217	1,294,383		95.2	3,546			13	831	2,377	3,208	0	0
General	683	116,794	4,256,632	27,532,743		64.6	75,446			2,813,181	12,291,729	39,030,109	51,321,838	8,370	723,527
Hospitals	675	115,996	4,246,121	27,346,156		64.6	74,935			2,808,443	12,246,714	38,404,220	50,650,934	8,370	723,527
Hospital units of institutions	8	798	10,511	186,587		64.0	511			4,738	45,015	625,889	670,904	0	0
TB and other respiratory diseases	2	255	404	59,169		63.5	162			230	0	1,073	1,073	0	0
Obstetrics and gynecology	0	0	0	0		00.0	0			0	0	0	0	0	0
Eye, ear, nose, and throat	1	33	1,372	3,035		24.2	8			1,944	0	675	675	0	0
Rehabilitation	6	395	3,673	90,116		62.5	247			0	3,255	76,890	80,145	0	0
Orthopedic	6	380	6,196	56,561		40.5	154			6,414	17,941	70,862	88,803	0	0
Chronic disease	1	1,126	1,398	391,604		95.3	1,073			17	0	116	116	0	0
All other	8	827	23,912	227,427		75.2	622			11,299	28,474	303,611	332,085	52	5,994
Federal	48	12,491	287,884	3,134,949		68.8	8,588			169,729	843,924	10,075,968	10,919,892	451	22,380
Psychiatric	0	0	0	0		00.0	0			0	0	0	0	0	0
General and other special	48	12,491	287,884	3,134,949		68.8	8,588			169,729	843,924	10,075,968	10,919,892	451	22,380
Nonfederal	740	125,054	4,079,961	30,579,332		67.0	83,816			2,664,012	11,522,546	29,686,318	41,208,864	7,971	707,141
Psychiatric	81	17,735	74,258	5,353,626		82.8	14,692			656	25,071	278,950	304,021	0	0
Hospitals	78	14,010	74,041	4,059,243		79.6	11,146			643	24,240	276,573	300,813	0	0
Institutions for mentally retarded	3	3,725	217	1,294,383		95.2	3,546			13	831	2,377	3,208	0	0
TB and other respiratory diseases	2	255	404	59,169		63.5	162			230	0	1,073	1,073	0	0
Long-term general and other special	11	2,228	8,241	745,809		91.7	2,042			4,072	6,403	175,282	181,685	6	27
Short-term general and other special	646	104,836	3,997,058	24,420,728		63.8	66,920			2,659,054	11,491,072	29,231,013	40,722,085	7,965	707,114
Hospital units of institutions	6	736	7,279	175,566		65.4	481			2,892	22,269	473,495	495,764	0	0
Community hospitals*	640	104,100	3,989,779	24,245,162	31,640,564	63.8	66,439	86,723	6.1	2,656,162	11,468,803	28,757,518	40,226,321	7,965	707,114
6-24 beds	31	583	13,162	70,553	128,321	33.8	197	356	5.4	8,537	81,956	199,418	281,374	50	858
25-49	102	3,810	101,378	552,119	893,760	39.6	1,507	2,452	5.4	76,065	497,592	941,287	1,438,879	433	15,094
50-99	136	9,944	335,433	1,864,087	2,688,106	51.4	5,109	7,366	5.6	261,543	1,324,213	2,150,931	3,475,144	841	53,462
100-199	173	24,816	932,941	5,384,200	7,310,645	59.5	14,770	20,051	5.8	693,527	3,192,826	6,576,142	9,768,968	1,760	150,870
200-299	102	24,707	998,380	5,868,467	7,606,625	65.1	16,076	20,845	5.9	622,724	2,948,919	7,184,057	10,132,976	2,087	191,049
300-399	54	18,275	754,093	4,590,402	5,724,825	68.8	12,577	15,685	6.1	484,878	1,625,235	4,622,893	6,248,128	1,349	139,063
400-499	26	11,342	445,952	3,030,486	3,774,978	73.2	8,301	10,342	6.8	253,588	1,055,442	3,949,481	5,004,923	759	80,539
500 or more	16	10,623	408,440	2,884,848	3,513,304	74.4	7,902	9,626	7.1	255,300	742,620	3,133,309	3,875,929	686	76,179
Nongovernment not-for-profit	346	67,845	2,687,660	16,200,880	20,961,851	65.4	44,387	57,444	6.0	1,821,036	7,187,789	20,252,918	27,440,707	5,185	465,342
Investor-owned (for-profit)	134	16,173	519,733	2,903,609	3,792,218	49.3	7,975	10,414	5.6	395,682	1,386,447	1,896,539	3,282,986	1,060	76,996
State and local government	160	20,082	782,386	5,140,673	6,886,495	70.1	14,077	18,865	6.6	439,444	2,894,567	6,608,061	9,502,628	1,720	164,776

*For information on community hospitals that excludes nursing-home-type data, refer to Hospital Units columns in tables 4A through 4D, pages 14 through 17.

CLASSIFICATION	FULL-TIME EQUIVALENT PERSONNEL					FULL-TIME EQUIVALENT TRAINEES			EXPENSES						
									LABOR				TOTAL		
	Physicians and Dentists	Registered Nurses	Licensed Practical Nurses	Other Salaried Personnel	Total Personnel	Medical and Dental Residents	Other Trainees	Total Trainees	Payroll (in thousands)	Employee Benefits (in thousands)	Total (in thousands)	Percent of Total	Amount (in thousands)	Adjusted, per Admission	Adjusted, per Inpatient Day
CENSUS DIVISION 9, PACIFIC	8,991	114,498	20,423	349,102	493,014	8,151	722	8,873	$14,811,010	$ 3,271,662	$18,082,672	55.0	$ 32,854,482		
6-24 beds	89	423	130	2,420	3,062	0	0	0	65,273	13,931	79,204	58.0	136,483		
25-49	324	3,005	736	11,085	15,150	18	8	26	366,145	78,680	444,824	56.2	791,760		
50-99	445	8,152	2,131	28,289	39,017	49	4	53	1,088,724	244,082	1,332,806	51.6	2,583,198		
100-199	2,127	25,553	4,373	70,924	102,977	526	108	634	2,943,278	631,186	3,574,464	52.2	6,841,775		
200-299	948	23,196	4,134	67,290	95,568	996	138	1,134	2,853,374	650,429	3,503,803	52.4	6,680,742		
300-399	1,796	22,557	3,266	63,068	90,687	1,906	102	2,008	2,803,173	610,840	3,414,013	55.8	6,122,691		
400-499	1,056	14,632	2,038	42,938	60,664	1,941	70	2,011	1,966,098	425,997	2,392,095	56.4	4,243,583		
500 or more	2,206	16,980	3,615	63,088	85,889	2,715	292	3,007	2,724,945	616,517	3,341,462	61.3	5,454,250		
Psychiatric	546	3,135	1,949	23,976	29,606	68	98	166	812,960	208,824	1,021,784	70.7	1,444,346		
Hospitals	515	2,946	1,801	17,739	23,001	68	98	166	665,089	173,241	838,331	68.9	1,216,962		
Institutions for mentally retarded	31	189	148	6,237	6,605	0	0	0	147,871	35,583	183,453	80.7	227,383		
General	8,251	109,795	18,138	318,303	454,487	8,013	596	8,609	13,726,080	3,001,627	16,727,707	54.2	30,840,044		
Hospitals	8,045	109,405	17,791	317,172	452,413	8,006	595	8,601	13,686,282	2,990,844	16,677,126	54.3	30,721,517		
Hospital units of institutions	206	390	347	1,131	2,074	7	1	8	39,798	10,783	50,581	42.7	118,527		
TB and other respiratory diseases	11	88	67	549	715	0	0	0	15,914	3,855	19,768	61.0	32,421		
Obstetrics and gynecology	0	0	0	0	0	0	0	0	0	0	0	0.0	0		
Eye, ear, nose, and throat	0	21	1	71	93	0	0	0	2,599	520	3,119	42.7	7,313		
Rehabilitation	4	143	57	1,101	1,305	0	0	0	34,233	7,587	41,820	62.4	67,051		
Orthopedic	17	205	42	802	1,066	13	4	17	41,128	8,001	49,129	54.2	90,589		
Chronic disease	43	263	58	1,274	1,638	0	0	0	52,275	14,007	66,282	81.8	81,011		
All other	119	848	111	3,026	4,104	57	24	81	125,821	27,241	153,062	52.5	291,708		
Federal	3,358	7,357	2,165	33,900	46,780	2,131	182	2,313	1,412,160	222,682	1,634,842	69.7	2,344,809		
Psychiatric	0	0	0	0	0	0	0	0	0	0	0	0.0	0		
General and other special	3,358	7,357	2,165	33,900	46,780	2,131	182	2,313	1,412,160	222,682	1,634,842	69.7	2,344,809		
Nonfederal	5,633	107,141	18,258	315,202	446,234	6,020	540	6,560	13,398,850	3,048,980	16,447,830	53.9	30,509,673		
Psychiatric	546	3,135	1,949	23,976	29,606	68	98	166	812,960	208,824	1,021,784	70.7	1,444,346		
Hospitals	515	2,946	1,801	17,739	23,001	68	98	166	665,089	173,241	838,331	68.9	1,216,962		
Institutions for mentally retarded	31	189	148	6,237	6,605	0	0	0	147,871	35,583	183,453	80.7	227,383		
TB and other respiratory diseases	11	88	67	549	715	0	0	0	15,914	3,855	19,768	61.0	32,421		
Long-term general and other special	158	848	177	4,415	5,598	43	0	43	167,172	42,976	210,147	69.8	301,284		
Short-term general and other special	4,918	103,070	16,065	286,262	410,315	5,909	442	6,351	12,402,805	2,793,325	15,196,130	52.9	28,731,623		
Hospital units of institutions	163	325	331	735	1,554	7	1	8	29,344	8,564	37,909	37.4	101,443		
Community hospitals*	4,755	102,745	15,734	285,527	408,761	5,902	441	6,343	12,373,461	2,784,761	15,158,221	52.9	28,630,179	$5,462.70	$ 904.86
6-24 beds	3	289	104	1,325	1,721	0	0	0	40,852	8,546	49,398	54.5	90,573	3,575.73	705.83
25-49	29	2,448	593	7,996	11,066	9	4	13	274,783	58,785	333,569	53.6	622,099	3,821.03	696.05
50-99	227	7,056	1,723	22,464	31,470	19	1	20	862,453	195,651	1,058,103	49.6	2,131,952	4,392.04	793.11
100-199	1,391	23,521	3,875	60,044	88,831	367	81	448	2,567,165	563,868	3,131,033	51.4	6,094,673	4,810.09	833.67
200-299	767	22,797	3,960	65,676	93,200	882	138	1,020	2,791,000	644,316	3,435,315	52.3	6,565,298	5,062.10	863.10
300-399	1,048	21,162	2,494	55,966	80,670	1,401	89	1,490	2,488,950	552,455	3,041,405	54.2	5,610,846	5,958.53	980.09
400-499	471	12,846	1,649	36,590	51,556	1,307	46	1,353	1,687,944	384,926	2,072,870	54.2	3,822,408	6,860.69	1,012.56
500 or more	819	12,626	1,336	35,466	50,247	1,917	82	1,999	1,660,314	376,214	2,036,528	55.2	3,692,330	7,316.30	1,050.96
Nongovernment not-for-profit	2,655	70,327	9,457	193,791	276,230	3,008	215	3,223	8,366,340	1,815,836	10,182,176	53.5	19,047,426	5,450.19	908.67
Investor-owned (for-profit)	189	12,591	2,469	31,135	46,384	25	43	68	1,358,892	296,757	1,655,649	45.6	3,627,498	5,311.41	956.56
State and local government	1,911	19,827	3,808	60,601	86,147	2,869	183	3,052	2,648,229	672,168	3,320,397	55.8	5,955,255	5,600.98	864.77

*For information on community hospitals that excludes nursing-home-type data, refer to Hospital Units columns in tables 4A through 4D, pages 14 through 17.

Table

5C Alabama

Utilization, Personnel, and Finances in States

Excludes AHA nonregistered hospitals (see Table 14, page 240).

CLASSIFICATION	HOSPITALS	BEDS	ADMISSIONS	INPATIENT DAYS	ADJUSTED PATIENT DAYS	OCCUPANCY, percent	AVERAGE DAILY CENSUS	ADJUSTED AVERAGE DAILY CENSUS	AVERAGE STAY, days	SURGICAL OPERATIONS	OUTPATIENT VISITS Emergency	OUTPATIENT VISITS Other	OUTPATIENT VISITS Total	NEWBORNS Bassinets	NEWBORNS Births
ALABAMA	138	23,552	639,880	5,704,845		66.4	15,627			394,335	1,719,490	3,981,836	5,701,326	1,420	60,465
6-24 beds	3	62	1,278	6,120		27.4	17			594	5,520	5,030	10,550	0	0
25-49	15	573	17,945	79,513		37.7	216			7,138	78,570	307,617	386,187	38	1,231
50-99	50	3,726	91,647	651,891		47.9	1,784			47,092	341,261	709,610	1,050,871	238	7,449
100-199	35	4,675	124,079	1,052,448		61.7	2,885			85,716	464,312	858,506	1,322,818	275	9,296
200-299	15	3,679	122,442	837,529		62.4	2,294			77,072	296,446	791,752	1,088,198	289	10,730
300-399	7	2,432	94,250	602,546		67.9	1,652			61,195	196,340	229,500	425,840	241	13,905
400-499	4	1,828	62,418	496,306		74.3	1,359			33,398	149,965	283,247	433,212	132	6,783
500 or more	9	6,577	125,821	1,978,492		82.4	5,420			82,130	187,076	796,574	983,650	207	11,071
Psychiatric	11	3,355	12,475	1,046,226		85.4	2,865			0	1,275	78,331	79,606	0	0
Hospitals	11	3,355	12,475	1,046,226		85.4	2,865			0	1,275	78,331	79,606	0	0
Institutions for mentally retarded	0	0	0	0		00.0	0			0	0	0	0	0	0
General	123	19,886	623,001	4,590,591		63.2	12,576			390,373	1,711,803	3,823,237	5,535,040	1,420	60,465
Hospitals	123	19,886	623,001	4,590,591		63.2	12,576			390,373	1,711,803	3,823,237	5,535,040	1,420	60,465
Hospital units of institutions	0	0	0	0		00.0	0			0	0	0	0	0	0
TB and other respiratory diseases	0	0	0	0		00.0	0			0	0	0	0	0	0
Obstetrics and gynecology	0	0	0	0		00.0	0			0	0	0	0	0	0
Eye, ear, nose, and throat	1	91	1,434	2,707		07.7	7			3,962	6,412	10,761	17,173	0	0
Rehabilitation	3	220	2,970	65,321		81.4	179			0	0	69,507	69,507	0	0
Orthopedic	0	0	0	0		00.0	0			0	0	0	0	0	0
Chronic disease	0	0	0	0		00.0	0			0	0	0	0	0	0
All other	0	0	0	0		00.0	0			0	0	0	0	0	0
Federal	8	2,261	34,627	628,516		76.1	1,721			18,970	98,275	933,852	1,032,127	37	1,348
Psychiatric	1	702	4,245	224,638		87.6	615			0	0	58,274	58,274	0	0
General and other special	7	1,559	30,382	403,878		70.9	1,106			18,970	98,275	875,578	973,853	37	1,348
Nonfederal	130	21,291	605,253	5,076,329		65.3	13,906			375,365	1,621,215	3,047,984	4,669,199	1,383	59,117
Psychiatric	10	2,653	8,230	821,588		84.8	2,250			0	1,275	20,057	21,332	0	0
Hospitals	10	2,653	8,230	821,588		84.8	2,250			0	1,275	20,057	21,332	0	0
Institutions for mentally retarded	0	0	0	0		00.0	0			0	0	0	0	0	0
TB and other respiratory diseases	0	0	0	0		00.0	0			0	0	0	0	0	0
Long-term general and other special	0	0	0	0		00.0	0			0	0	0	0	0	0
Short-term general and other special	120	18,638	597,023	4,254,741		62.5	11,656			375,365	1,619,940	3,027,927	4,647,867	1,383	59,117
Hospital units of institutions	0	0	0	0		00.0	0			0	0	0	0	0	0
Community hospitals*	120	18,638	597,023	4,254,741	5,374,854	62.5	11,656	14,727	7.1	375,365	1,619,940	3,027,927	4,647,867	1,383	59,117
6-24 beds	3	62	1,278	6,120	16,471	27.4	17	45	4.8	594	5,520	5,030	10,550	0	0
25-49	13	498	12,011	61,095	80,118	33.3	166	220	5.1	2,915	42,390	76,418	118,808	29	604
50-99	43	3,175	84,064	549,566	749,398	47.4	1,504	2,053	6.5	45,202	315,634	492,819	808,453	220	7,039
100-199	32	4,341	117,391	997,207	1,334,093	63.0	2,734	3,657	8.5	84,501	437,508	641,930	1,079,438	265	8,985
200-299	13	3,199	111,962	719,871	917,654	61.6	1,972	2,514	6.4	71,635	285,507	628,127	913,634	289	10,730
300-399	7	2,432	94,250	602,546	723,636	67.9	1,652	1,981	6.4	61,195	196,340	229,500	425,840	241	13,905
400-499	4	1,828	62,418	496,306	584,835	74.3	1,359	1,603	8.0	33,398	149,965	283,247	433,212	132	6,783
500 or more	5	3,103	113,649	822,030	968,649	72.6	2,252	2,654	7.2	75,925	187,076	670,856	857,932	207	11,071
Nongovernment not-for-profit	39	7,256	240,682	1,630,318	2,043,729	61.5	4,465	5,598	6.8	154,516	508,552	1,531,687	2,040,239	545	21,387
Investor-owned (for-profit)	32	3,943	117,859	812,323	1,034,915	56.5	2,227	2,835	6.9	85,589	395,298	432,726	828,024	204	8,898
State and local government	49	7,439	238,482	1,812,100	2,296,210	66.7	4,964	6,294	7.6	135,260	716,090	1,063,514	1,779,604	634	28,832

*For information on community hospitals that excludes nursing-home-type data, refer to Hospital Units columns in tables 4A through 4D, pages 14 through 17.

CLASSIFICATION	FULL-TIME EQUIVALENT PERSONNEL					FULL-TIME EQUIVALENT TRAINEES			EXPENSES: LABOR				EXPENSES: TOTAL		
	Physicians and Dentists	Registered Nurses	Licensed Practical Nurses	Other Salaried Personnel	Total Personnel	Medical and Dental Residents	Other Trainees	Total Trainees	Payroll (in thousands)	Employee Benefits (in thousands)	Total (in thousands)	Percent of Total	Amount (in thousands)	Adjusted, per Admission	Adjusted, per Inpatient Day
ALABAMA	1,142	14,921	5,043	47,382	68,488	871	61	932	$ 1,554,753	$ 302,414	$ 1,857,167	51.3	$ 3,622,866		
6-24 beds	0	16	9	67	92	0	0	0	2,559	490	3,050	52.8	5,778		
25-49	58	267	190	1,242	1,757	0	1	1	39,771	7,802	47,572	63.7	74,665		
50-99	84	1,688	783	5,930	8,485	18	2	20	181,192	34,063	215,255	52.2	412,368		
100-199	49	2,651	900	8,564	12,164	11	0	11	260,135	52,162	312,297	48.3	646,205		
200-299	168	2,836	798	7,800	11,602	146	15	161	286,536	56,200	342,736	50.1	683,896		
300-399	12	2,425	572	6,106	9,115	167	25	192	201,904	36,662	238,566	45.4	525,231		
400-499	6	1,434	530	4,613	6,583	72	0	72	145,444	28,744	174,189	53.9	323,114		
500 or more	765	3,604	1,261	13,060	18,690	457	18	475	437,212	86,291	523,502	55.0	951,608		
Psychiatric	88	442	229	3,829	4,588	3	8	11	118,843	27,377	146,220	70.3	208,015		
Hospitals	88	442	229	3,829	4,588	3	8	11	118,843	27,377	146,220	70.3	208,015		
Institutions for mentally retarded	0	0	0	0	0	0	0	0	0	0	0	0.0	0		
General	1,048	14,263	4,793	42,928	63,032	850	53	903	1,417,298	271,257	1,688,554	50.1	3,369,749		
Hospitals	1,048	14,263	4,793	42,928	63,032	850	53	903	1,417,298	271,257	1,688,554	50.1	3,369,749		
Hospital units of institutions	0	0	0	0	0	0	0	0	0	0	0	0.0	0		
TB and other respiratory diseases	0	0	0	0	0	0	0	0	0	0	0	0.0	0		
Obstetrics and gynecology	0	0	0	0	0	0	0	0	0	0	0	0.0	0		
Eye, ear, nose, and throat	4	35	6	134	179	18	0	18	3,122	596	3,718	36.2	10,271		
Rehabilitation	2	181	15	491	689	0	0	0	15,491	3,184	18,675	53.6	34,831		
Orthopedic	0	0	0	0	0	0	0	0	0	0	0	0.0	0		
Chronic disease	0	0	0	0	0	0	0	0	0	0	0	0.0	0		
All other	0	0	0	0	0	0	0	0	0	0	0	0.0	0		
Federal	322	726	439	4,325	5,812	125	27	152	170,315	31,785	202,100	67.9	297,496		
Psychiatric	28	118	71	845	1,062	2	3	5	27,633	5,335	32,968	76.7	42,985		
General and other special	294	608	368	3,480	4,750	123	24	147	142,682	26,450	169,132	66.5	254,511		
Nonfederal	820	14,195	4,604	43,057	62,676	746	34	780	1,384,438	270,629	1,655,067	49.8	3,325,370		
Psychiatric	60	324	158	2,984	3,526	1	5	6	91,210	22,042	113,252	68.6	165,030		
Hospitals	60	324	158	2,984	3,526	1	5	6	91,210	22,042	113,252	68.6	165,030		
Institutions for mentally retarded	0	0	0	0	0	0	0	0	0	0	0	0.0	0		
TB and other respiratory diseases	0	0	0	0	0	0	0	0	0	0	0	0.0	0		
Long-term general and other special	0	0	0	0	0	0	0	0	0	0	0	0.0	0		
Short-term general and other special	760	13,871	4,446	40,073	59,150	745	29	774	1,293,228	248,587	1,541,815	48.8	3,160,340		
Hospital units of institutions	0	0	0	0	0	0	0	0	0	0	0	0.0	0		
Community hospitals*	760	13,871	4,446	40,073	59,150	745	29	774	1,293,228	248,587	1,541,815	48.8	3,160,340	$4,174.75	$ 587.99
6-24 beds	0	16	9	67	92	0	0	0	2,559	490	3,050	52.8	5,778	1,714.66	350.82
25-49	1	161	132	637	931	0	1	1	17,903	3,242	21,146	50.7	41,726	2,597.97	520.81
50-99	28	1,539	769	5,002	7,338	18	2	20	145,375	26,984	172,359	50.6	340,950	2,897.07	454.97
100-199	13	2,535	876	7,992	11,416	6	0	6	234,578	47,796	282,374	47.9	589,791	3,760.08	442.09
200-299	67	2,581	662	6,656	9,966	28	1	29	231,183	45,847	277,030	48.2	575,215	4,045.46	626.83
300-399	12	2,425	572	6,106	9,115	167	25	192	201,904	36,662	238,566	45.4	525,231	4,645.39	725.82
400-499	6	1,434	530	4,613	6,583	72	0	72	145,444	28,744	174,189	53.9	323,114	4,382.88	552.49
500 or more	633	3,180	896	9,000	13,709	454	0	454	314,280	58,822	373,102	49.2	758,533	5,658.08	783.08
Nongovernment not-for-profit	97	5,709	1,610	16,514	23,930	122	1	123	528,889	94,941	623,829	49.0	1,271,968	4,190.64	622.38
Investor-owned (for-profit)	4	2,664	725	6,761	10,154	1	25	26	238,903	53,329	292,233	43.9	666,201	4,413.91	643.73
State and local government	659	5,498	2,111	16,798	25,066	622	3	625	525,436	100,317	625,753	51.2	1,222,170	4,039.51	532.26

*For information on community hospitals that excludes nursing-home-type data, refer to Hospital Units columns in Tables 4A through 4D, pages 14 through 17.

(continued on next page)

Table

5C (Continued) Alaska

Utilization, Personnel, and Finances in States

Excludes AHA nonregistered hospitals (see Table 14, page 240).

CLASSIFICATION	HOSPITALS	BEDS	ADMISSIONS	INPATIENT DAYS	ADJUSTED PATIENT DAYS	OCCUPANCY, percent	AVERAGE DAILY CENSUS	ADJUSTED AVERAGE DAILY CENSUS	AVERAGE STAY, days	SURGICAL OPERATIONS	OUTPATIENT VISITS Emergency	OUTPATIENT VISITS Other	OUTPATIENT VISITS Total	NEWBORNS Bassinets	NEWBORNS Births
ALASKA	27	1,976	59,266	375,086		51.9	1,025			35,442	238,978	1,062,435	1,301,413	217	11,018
6-24 beds	6	114	2,799	17,385		42.1	48			1,037	16,079	97,208	113,287	27	419
25-49	8	274	7,047	50,950		50.4	138			2,676	41,519	148,426	189,945	38	1,361
50-99	7	466	15,217	86,371		50.6	236			7,402	55,912	309,829	365,741	47	2,391
100-199	4	543	15,462	112,610		56.7	308			11,239	65,727	348,449	414,176	63	3,136
200-299	1	238	6,462	31,675		36.6	87			5,665	24,475	43,531	68,006	18	1,445
300-399	1	341	12,279	76,095		61.0	208			7,423	35,266	114,992	150,258	24	2,266
400-499	0	0	0	0		00.0	0			0	0	0	0	0	0
500 or more	0	0	0	0		00.0	0			0	0	0	0	0	0
Psychiatric	3	274	1,958	59,502		59.5	163			0	583	6,057	6,640	0	0
Hospitals	3	274	1,958	59,502		59.5	163			0	583	6,057	6,640	0	0
Institutions for mentally retarded	0	0	0	0		00.0	0			0	0	0	0	0	0
General	24	1,702	57,308	315,584		50.6	862			35,442	238,395	1,056,378	1,294,773	217	11,018
Hospitals	24	1,702	57,308	315,584		50.6	862			35,442	238,395	1,056,378	1,294,773	217	11,018
Hospital units of institutions	0	0	0	0		00.0	0			0	0	0	0	0	0
TB and other respiratory diseases	0	0	0	0		00.0	0			0	0	0	0	0	0
Obstetrics and gynecology	0	0	0	0		00.0	0			0	0	0	0	0	0
Eye, ear, nose, and throat	0	0	0	0		00.0	0			0	0	0	0	0	0
Rehabilitation	0	0	0	0		00.0	0			0	0	0	0	0	0
Orthopedic	0	0	0	0		00.0	0			0	0	0	0	0	0
Chronic disease	0	0	0	0		00.0	0			0	0	0	0	0	0
All other	0	0	0	0		00.0	0			0	0	0	0	0	0
Federal	8	508	20,107	99,649		53.5	272			11,693	99,095	753,218	852,313	88	3,652
Psychiatric	0	0	0	0		00.0	0			0	0	0	0	0	0
General and other special	8	508	20,107	99,649		53.5	272			11,693	99,095	753,218	852,313	88	3,652
Nonfederal	19	1,468	39,159	275,437		51.3	753			23,749	139,883	309,217	449,100	129	7,366
Psychiatric	3	274	1,958	59,502		59.5	163			0	583	6,057	6,640	0	0
Hospitals	3	274	1,958	59,502		59.5	163			0	583	6,057	6,640	0	0
Institutions for mentally retarded	0	0	0	0		00.0	0			0	0	0	0	0	0
TB and other respiratory diseases	0	0	0	0		00.0	0			0	0	0	0	0	0
Long-term general and other special	0	0	0	0		00.0	0			0	0	0	0	0	0
Short-term general and other special	16	1,194	37,201	215,935		49.4	590			23,749	139,300	303,160	442,460	129	7,366
Hospital units of institutions	0	0	0	0		00.0	0			0	0	0	0	0	0
Community hospitals*	16	1,194	37,201	215,935	297,512	49.4	590	816	5.8	23,749	139,300	303,160	442,460	129	7,366
6-24 beds	4	84	1,128	12,976	21,208	42.9	36	58	11.5	455	5,466	21,212	26,678	17	206
25-49	6	209	5,273	39,146	57,667	50.7	106	158	7.4	1,753	25,689	60,603	86,292	32	1,129
50-99	3	200	6,610	34,534	53,893	47.0	94	148	5.2	3,640	29,003	41,855	70,858	22	1,140
100-199	1	122	5,449	21,509	31,599	48.4	59	87	3.9	4,813	19,401	20,967	40,368	16	1,180
200-299	1	238	6,462	31,675	38,756	36.6	87	106	4.9	5,665	24,475	43,531	68,006	18	1,445
300-399	1	341	12,279	76,095	94,389	61.0	208	259	6.2	7,423	35,266	114,992	150,258	24	2,266
400-499	0	0	0	0	0	00.0	0	0	0.0	0	0	0	0	0	0
500 or more	0	0	0	0	0	00.0	0	0	0.0	0	0	0	0	0	0
Nongovernment not-for-profit	7	707	25,075	144,362	200,174	55.7	394	549	5.8	16,074	93,618	214,106	307,724	72	4,995
Investor-owned (for-profit)	1	238	6,462	31,675	38,756	36.6	87	106	4.9	5,665	24,475	43,531	68,006	18	1,445
State and local government	8	249	5,664	39,898	58,582	43.8	109	161	7.0	2,010	21,207	45,523	66,730	39	926

*For information on community hospitals that excludes nursing-home-type data, refer to Hospital Units columns in tables 4A through 4D, pages 14 through 17.

CLASSIFICATION	FULL-TIME EQUIVALENT PERSONNEL: Physicians and Dentists	Registered Nurses	Licensed Practical Nurses	Other Salaried Personnel	Total Personnel	FULL-TIME EQUIVALENT TRAINEES: Medical and Dental Residents	Other Trainees	Total Trainees	EXPENSES – LABOR: Payroll (in thousands)	Employee Benefits (in thousands)	Total (in thousands)	Percent of Total	EXPENSES – TOTAL: Amount (in thousands)	Adjusted, per Admission	Adjusted, per Inpatient Day
ALASKA	266	1,691	219	5,173	7,349	10	15	25	$ 242,730	$ 47,266	$ 289,996	57.4	$ 504,895		
6-24 beds	23	66	11	485	585	0	0	0	15,355	3,348	18,703	64.9	28,827		
25-49	30	171	19	672	892	0	0	0	25,836	6,180	32,017	61.2	52,293		
50-99	73	265	82	1,199	1,619	0	0	0	50,866	10,239	61,105	61.4	99,498		
100-199	140	554	74	1,527	2,295	10	15	25	75,492	11,228	86,721	61.9	140,026		
200-299	0	166	5	413	584	0	0	0	25,632	5,424	31,056	43.5	71,419		
300-399	0	469	28	877	1,374	0	0	0	49,549	10,846	60,395	53.5	112,832		
400-499	0	0	0	0	0	0	0	0	0	0	0	0.0	0		
500 or more	0	0	0	0	0	0	0	0	0	0	0	0.0	0		
Psychiatric	11	97	8	356	472	0	0	0	18,851	1,637	20,488	75.5	27,135		
Hospitals	11	97	8	356	472	0	0	0	18,851	1,637	20,488	75.5	27,135		
Institutions for mentally retarded	0	0	0	0	0	0	0	0	0	0	0	0.0	0		
General	255	1,594	211	4,817	6,877	10	15	25	223,879	45,629	269,508	56.4	477,760		
Hospitals	255	1,594	211	4,817	6,877	10	15	25	223,879	45,629	269,508	56.4	477,760		
Hospital units of institutions	0	0	0	0	0	0	0	0	0	0	0	0.0	0		
TB and other respiratory diseases	0	0	0	0	0	0	0	0	0	0	0	0.0	0		
Obstetrics and gynecology	0	0	0	0	0	0	0	0	0	0	0	0.0	0		
Eye, ear, nose, and throat	0	0	0	0	0	0	0	0	0	0	0	0.0	0		
Rehabilitation	0	0	0	0	0	0	0	0	0	0	0	0.0	0		
Orthopedic	0	0	0	0	0	0	0	0	0	0	0	0.0	0		
Chronic disease	0	0	0	0	0	0	0	0	0	0	0	0.0	0		
All other	0	0	0	0	0	0	0	0	0	0	0	0.0	0		
Federal	239	502	120	2,236	3,097	10	15	25	86,777	15,082	101,859	63.9	159,517		
Psychiatric	0	0	0	0	0	0	0	0	0	0	0	0.0	0		
General and other special	239	502	120	2,236	3,097	10	15	25	86,777	15,082	101,859	63.9	159,517		
Nonfederal	27	1,189	99	2,937	4,252	0	0	0	155,953	32,184	188,137	54.5	345,378		
Psychiatric	11	97	8	356	472	0	0	0	18,851	1,637	20,488	75.5	27,135		
Hospitals	11	97	8	356	472	0	0	0	18,851	1,637	20,488	75.5	27,135		
Institutions for mentally retarded	0	0	0	0	0	0	0	0	0	0	0	0.0	0		
TB and other respiratory diseases	0	0	0	0	0	0	0	0	0	0	0	0.0	0		
Long-term general and other special	0	0	0	0	0	0	0	0	0	0	0	0.0	0		
Short-term general and other special	16	1,092	91	2,581	3,780	0	0	0	137,102	30,547	167,649	52.7	318,243		
Hospital units of institutions	0	0	0	0	0	0	0	0	0	0	0	0.0	0		
Community hospitals*	16	1,092	91	2,581	3,780	0	0	0	137,102	30,547	167,649	52.7	318,243	$6,249.37	$1,069.68
6-24 beds	0	33	6	129	168	0	0	0	5,283	1,111	6,394	56.6	11,298	6,146.73	532.71
25-49	9	132	10	438	589	0	0	0	18,967	4,722	23,689	59.0	40,142	5,237.06	696.10
50-99	7	120	25	443	595	0	0	0	19,335	4,555	23,890	54.6	43,745	4,256.22	811.71
100-199	0	172	17	281	470	0	0	0	18,337	3,888	22,225	57.3	38,807	4,847.86	1,228.11
200-299	0	166	5	413	584	0	0	0	25,632	5,424	31,056	43.5	71,419	9,032.36	1,842.78
300-399	0	469	28	877	1,374	0	0	0	49,549	10,846	60,395	53.5	112,832	7,408.05	1,195.39
400-499	0	0	0	0	0	0	0	0	0	0	0	0.0	0	0.00	0.00
500 or more	0	0	0	0	0	0	0	0	0	0	0	0.0	0	0.00	0.00
Nongovernment not-for-profit	16	828	61	1,750	2,655	0	0	0	93,162	21,120	114,282	55.0	207,656	5,993.13	1,037.38
Investor-owned (for-profit)	0	166	5	413	584	0	0	0	25,632	5,424	31,056	43.5	71,419	9,032.36	1,842.78
State and local government	0	98	25	418	541	0	0	0	18,308	4,003	22,311	57.0	39,169	4,680.75	668.61

*For information on community hospitals that excludes nursing-home-type data, refer to Hospital Units columns in tables 4A through 4D, pages 14 through 17.

(continued on next page)

Table

5C (Continued) Arizona

Utilization, Personnel, and Finances in States

Excludes AHA nonregistered hospitals (see Table 14, page 240).

CLASSIFICATION	HOSPI-TALS	BEDS	ADMISSIONS	INPATIENT DAYS	ADJUSTED PATIENT DAYS	OCCU-PANCY, percent	AVERAGE DAILY CENSUS	ADJUSTED AVERAGE DAILY CENSUS	AVERAGE STAY, days	SURGICAL OPERATIONS	OUTPATIENT VISITS: Emergency	OUTPATIENT VISITS: Other	OUTPATIENT VISITS: Total	NEWBORNS: Bassinets	NEWBORNS: Births
ARIZONA	91	13,432	459,092	3,118,745		63.6	8,544			271,844	1,288,766	3,298,020	4,586,786	900	65,962
6-24 beds	4	77	2,738	11,074		40.3	31			1,096	24,196	165,547	189,743	10	258
25-49	21	836	28,395	137,102		44.9	375			15,756	302,280	506,956	809,236	121	4,196
50-99	25	1,886	50,072	397,337		57.6	1,087			23,862	151,038	628,585	779,623	150	7,077
100-199	19	2,722	105,045	585,391		59.0	1,605			59,940	293,077	534,222	827,299	193	13,218
200-299	9	2,256	94,906	524,742		63.7	1,438			74,806	235,792	432,013	667,805	166	18,041
300-399	6	1,944	65,325	439,937		62.0	1,205			40,024	114,594	257,765	372,359	66	3,552
400-499	2	884	25,673	240,937		74.7	660			8,985	62,013	227,634	289,647	48	4,833
500 or more	5	2,827	86,938	782,225		75.8	2,143			47,375	105,776	545,298	651,074	146	14,787
Psychiatric	14	1,411	10,979	393,195		76.2	1,075			0	1,021	38,351	39,372	0	0
Hospitals	14	1,411	10,979	393,195		76.2	1,075			0	1,021	38,351	39,372	0	0
Institutions for mentally retarded	0	0	0	0		00.0	0			0	0	0	0	0	0
General	77	12,021	448,113	2,725,550		62.1	7,469			271,844	1,287,745	3,259,669	4,547,414	900	65,962
Hospitals	77	12,021	448,113	2,725,550		62.1	7,469			271,844	1,287,745	3,259,669	4,547,414	900	65,962
Hospital units of institutions	0	0	0	0		00.0	0			0	0	0	0	0	0
TB and other respiratory diseases	0	0	0	0		00.0	0			0	0	0	0	0	0
Obstetrics and gynecology	0	0	0	0		00.0	0			0	0	0	0	0	0
Eye, ear, nose, and throat	0	0	0	0		00.0	0			0	0	0	0	0	0
Rehabilitation	0	0	0	0		00.0	0			0	0	0	0	0	0
Orthopedic	0	0	0	0		00.0	0			0	0	0	0	0	0
Chronic disease	0	0	0	0		00.0	0			0	0	0	0	0	0
All other	0	0	0	0		00.0	0			0	0	0	0	0	0
Federal	16	2,048	51,691	475,973		63.7	1,304			23,344	354,674	1,456,986	1,811,660	124	5,182
Psychiatric	0	0	0	0		00.0	0			0	0	0	0	0	0
General and other special	16	2,048	51,691	475,973		63.7	1,304			23,344	354,674	1,456,986	1,811,660	124	5,182
Nonfederal	75	11,384	407,401	2,642,772		63.6	7,240			248,500	934,092	1,841,034	2,775,126	776	60,780
Psychiatric	14	1,411	10,979	393,195		76.2	1,075			0	1,021	38,351	39,372	0	0
Hospitals	14	1,411	10,979	393,195		76.2	1,075			0	1,021	38,351	39,372	0	0
Institutions for mentally retarded	0	0	0	0		00.0	0			0	0	0	0	0	0
TB and other respiratory diseases	0	0	0	0		00.0	0			0	0	0	0	0	0
Long-term general and other special	0	0	0	0		00.0	0			0	0	0	0	0	0
Short-term general and other special	61	9,973	396,422	2,249,577		61.8	6,165			248,500	933,071	1,802,683	2,735,754	776	60,780
Hospital units of institutions	0	0	0	0		00.0	0			0	0	0	0	0	0
Community hospitals*	61	9,973	396,422	2,249,577	2,902,911	61.8	6,165	7,953	5.7	248,500	933,071	1,802,683	2,735,754	776	60,780
6-24 beds	1	22	384	1,665	2,735	22.7	5	7	4.3	156	674	1,901	2,575	0	0
25-49	13	515	15,300	72,516	125,414	38.6	199	343	4.7	9,027	61,794	172,611	234,405	62	2,220
50-99	12	936	31,875	187,094	262,959	54.7	512	720	5.9	19,422	82,337	184,566	266,903	107	4,866
100-199	17	2,465	97,157	524,927	678,477	58.4	1,440	1,857	5.4	57,071	270,091	415,850	685,941	181	12,481
200-299	9	2,256	94,906	524,742	679,047	63.7	1,438	1,862	5.5	74,806	235,792	432,013	667,805	166	18,041
300-399	5	1,585	59,074	367,875	447,662	63.6	1,008	1,227	6.2	37,071	114,594	103,194	217,788	66	3,552
400-499	1	478	21,864	129,316	179,626	74.1	354	492	5.9	7,772	62,013	155,008	217,021	48	4,833
500 or more	3	1,716	75,862	441,442	526,991	70.5	1,209	1,445	5.8	43,175	105,776	337,540	443,316	146	14,787
Nongovernment not-for-profit	46	7,899	323,151	1,823,617	2,317,674	63.3	4,998	6,351	5.6	207,599	727,632	1,371,877	2,099,509	594	50,580
Investor-owned (for-profit)	8	1,132	36,445	195,349	251,503	47.3	535	689	5.4	27,717	91,002	114,852	205,854	81	2,855
State and local government	7	942	36,826	230,611	333,734	67.1	632	913	6.3	13,184	114,437	315,954	430,391	101	7,345

*For information on community hospitals that include nursing-home type data, refer to Hospital Units columns in tables 4A through 4D, pages 14 through 17.

Table 5C (Continued) Arizona

CLASSIFICATION	FULL-TIME EQUIVALENT PERSONNEL					FULL-TIME EQUIVALENT TRAINEES			EXPENSES: LABOR				EXPENSES: TOTAL		
	Physicians and Dentists	Registered Nurses	Licensed Practical Nurses	Other Salaried Personnel	Total Personnel	Medical and Dental Residents	Other Trainees	Total Trainees	Payroll (in thousands)	Employee Benefits (in thousands)	Total (in thousands)	Percent of Total	Amount (in thousands)	Adjusted, per Admission	Adjusted, per Inpatient Day
ARIZONA	716	11,119	1,625	32,054	45,514	612	18	630	$ 1,266,112	$ 240,881	$ 1,506,993	50.4	$ 2,989,020		
6-24 beds	44	84	25	496	649	0	0	0	12,278	1,796	14,074	89.4	15,749		
25-49	180	524	146	2,546	3,396	11	0	11	76,340	16,498	92,838	61.0	152,277		
50-99	131	1,123	172	3,831	5,257	0	0	0	133,916	26,251	160,168	53.0	302,177		
100-199	111	2,396	359	5,973	8,839	65	4	69	241,746	42,178	283,925	46.4	612,115		
200-299	19	2,257	194	6,061	8,531	21	0	21	237,573	49,181	286,754	46.7	613,509		
300-399	59	1,627	228	3,948	5,862	100	12	112	193,684	35,224	228,908	50.1	457,185		
400-499	24	418	72	1,622	2,136	211	0	211	78,083	13,608	91,690	54.6	167,933		
500 or more	148	2,690	429	7,577	10,844	204	2	206	292,491	56,145	348,636	52.2	668,073		
Psychiatric	11	373	53	1,791	2,228	0	0	0	59,721	12,716	72,437	54.6	132,781		
Hospitals	11	373	53	1,791	2,228	0	0	0	59,721	12,716	72,437	54.6	132,781		
Institutions for mentally retarded	0	0	0	0	0	0	0	0	0	0	0	0.0	0		
General	705	10,746	1,572	30,263	43,286	612	18	630	1,206,391	228,165	1,434,555	50.2	2,856,239		
Hospitals	705	10,746	1,572	30,263	43,286	612	18	630	1,206,391	228,165	1,434,555	50.2	2,856,239		
Hospital units of institutions	0	0	0	0	0	0	0	0	0	0	0	0.0	0		
TB and other respiratory diseases	0	0	0	0	0	0	0	0	0	0	0	0.0	0		
Obstetrics and gynecology	0	0	0	0	0	0	0	0	0	0	0	0.0	0		
Eye, ear, nose, and throat	0	0	0	0	0	0	0	0	0	0	0	0.0	0		
Rehabilitation	0	0	0	0	0	0	0	0	0	0	0	0.0	0		
Orthopedic	0	0	0	0	0	0	0	0	0	0	0	0.0	0		
Chronic disease	0	0	0	0	0	0	0	0	0	0	0	0.0	0		
All other	0	0	0	0	0	0	0	0	0	0	0	0.0	0		
Federal	573	1,190	368	5,275	7,406	107	18	125	198,770	36,771	235,540	69.4	339,614		
Psychiatric	0	0	0	0	0	0	0	0	0	0	0	0.0	0		
General and other special	573	1,190	368	5,275	7,406	107	18	125	198,770	36,771	235,540	69.4	339,614		
Nonfederal	143	9,929	1,257	26,779	38,108	505	0	505	1,067,342	204,110	1,271,453	48.0	2,649,406		
Psychiatric	11	373	53	1,791	2,228	0	0	0	59,721	12,716	72,437	54.6	132,781		
Hospitals	11	373	53	1,791	2,228	0	0	0	59,721	12,716	72,437	54.6	132,781		
Institutions for mentally retarded	0	0	0	0	0	0	0	0	0	0	0	0.0	0		
TB and other respiratory diseases	0	0	0	0	0	0	0	0	0	0	0	0.0	0		
Long-term general and other special	0	0	0	0	0	0	0	0	0	0	0	0.0	0		
Short-term general and other special	132	9,556	1,204	24,988	35,880	505	0	505	1,007,621	191,394	1,199,015	47.6	2,516,625		
Hospital units of institutions	0	0	0	0	0	0	0	0	0	0	0	0.0	0		
Community hospitals*	132	9,556	1,204	24,988	35,880	505	0	505	1,007,621	191,394	1,199,015	47.6	2,516,625	$4,877.48	$ 866.93
6-24 beds	0	8	5	40	53	0	0	0	937	179	1,116	55.2	2,022	3,205.19	739.48
25-49	14	286	56	1,117	1,473	0	0	0	32,074	7,045	39,119	48.3	80,958	2,992.88	645.52
50-99	4	692	107	2,024	2,827	0	0	0	68,782	13,754	82,536	47.9	172,162	3,829.47	654.71
100-199	44	2,258	306	5,468	8,076	61	0	61	218,239	38,903	257,142	45.4	565,863	4,472.30	834.02
200-299	19	2,257	194	6,061	8,531	21	0	21	237,573	49,181	286,754	46.7	613,509	4,965.03	903.48
300-399	0	1,410	182	3,197	4,789	18	0	18	160,387	28,790	189,176	48.6	389,483	5,385.93	870.04
400-499	2	331	49	1,161	1,543	211	0	211	60,044	10,000	70,044	49.3	142,163	4,681.03	791.44
500 or more	49	2,314	305	5,920	8,588	194	0	194	229,586	43,542	273,127	49.6	550,466	6,078.94	1,044.55
Nongovernment not-for-profit	119	8,024	880	20,337	29,360	282	0	282	831,325	159,563	990,889	47.9	2,067,803	4,978.69	892.19
Investor-owned (for-profit)	4	840	136	2,240	3,220	8	0	8	79,028	17,463	96,491	43.0	224,287	4,755.67	891.79
State and local government	9	692	188	2,411	3,300	215	0	215	97,268	14,368	111,636	49.7	224,535	4,198.87	672.80

*For information on community hospitals that excludes nursing-home-type data, refer to Hospital Units columns in tables 4A through 4D, pages 14 through 17.

(continued on next page)

Table

5C (Continued) Arkansas

Utilization, Personnel, and Finances in States

Excludes AHA nonregistered hospitals (see Table 14, page 240).

CLASSIFICATION	HOSPITALS	BEDS	ADMISSIONS	INPATIENT DAYS	ADJUSTED PATIENT DAYS	OCCUPANCY, percent	AVERAGE DAILY CENSUS	ADJUSTED AVERAGE DAILY CENSUS	AVERAGE STAY, days	SURGICAL OPERATIONS	OUTPATIENT VISITS Emergency	OUTPATIENT VISITS Other	OUTPATIENT VISITS Total	NEWBORNS Bassinets	NEWBORNS Births
ARKANSAS	**96**	**12,867**	**375,428**	**3,043,456**		**64.8**	**8,344**			**225,697**	**955,373**	**1,779,199**	**2,734,572**	**833**	**34,951**
6-24 beds	4	67	2,329	11,921		47.8	32			1,052	17,875	82,998	100,873	13	539
25-49	19	737	19,680	101,571		38.1	281			7,402	66,321	95,491	161,812	56	814
50-99	32	2,217	54,924	407,960		50.6	1,121			21,494	175,896	346,771	522,667	208	5,529
100-199	24	3,215	94,005	728,410		62.1	1,996			55,534	247,834	373,547	621,381	230	10,687
200-299	6	1,354	51,454	359,264		72.7	984			35,204	167,642	280,004	447,646	58	2,840
300-399	6	1,867	58,607	469,580		68.9	1,287			37,619	127,239	220,827	348,066	144	8,682
400-499	2	949	30,660	250,170		72.3	686			28,265	85,149	58,086	143,235	90	3,668
500 or more	3	2,461	63,769	714,580		79.5	1,957			39,127	67,417	321,475	388,892	34	2,192
Psychiatric	6	645	4,381	192,386		82.0	529			0	0	4,568	4,568	0	0
Hospitals	6	645	4,381	192,386		82.0	529			0	0	4,568	4,568	0	0
Institutions for mentally retarded	0	0	0	0		00.0	0			0	0	0	0	0	0
General	86	11,911	367,720	2,773,637		63.8	7,602			225,658	955,373	1,752,061	2,707,434	833	34,951
Hospitals	86	11,911	367,720	2,773,637		63.8	7,602			225,658	955,373	1,752,061	2,707,434	833	34,951
Hospital units of institutions	0	0	0	0		00.0	0			0	0	0	0	0	0
TB and other respiratory diseases	0	0	0	0		00.0	0			0	0	0	0	0	0
Obstetrics and gynecology	0	0	0	0		00.0	0			0	0	0	0	0	0
Eye, ear, nose, and throat	0	0	0	0		00.0	0			0	0	0	0	0	0
Rehabilitation	4	311	3,327	77,433		68.5	213			39	0	22,570	22,570	0	0
Orthopedic	0	0	0	0		00.0	0			0	0	0	0	0	0
Chronic disease	0	0	0	0		00.0	0			0	0	0	0	0	0
All other	0	0	0	0		00.0	0			0	0	0	0	0	0
Federal	4	1,379	24,228	397,153		78.8	1,087			13,472	58,859	500,716	559,575	24	691
Psychiatric	0	0	0	0		00.0	0			0	0	0	0	0	0
General and other special	4	1,379	24,228	397,153		78.8	1,087			13,472	58,859	500,716	559,575	24	691
Nonfederal	92	11,488	351,200	2,646,303		63.2	7,257			212,225	896,514	1,278,483	2,174,997	809	34,260
Psychiatric	6	645	4,381	192,386		82.0	529			0	0	4,568	4,568	0	0
Hospitals	6	645	4,381	192,386		82.0	529			0	0	4,568	4,568	0	0
Institutions for mentally retarded	0	0	0	0		00.0	0			0	0	0	0	0	0
TB and other respiratory diseases	0	0	0	0		00.0	0			0	0	0	0	0	0
Long-term general and other special	0	0	0	0		00.0	0			0	0	0	0	0	0
Short-term general and other special	86	10,843	346,819	2,453,917		62.0	6,728			212,225	896,514	1,273,915	2,170,429	809	34,260
Hospital units of institutions	0	0	0	0		00.0	0			0	0	0	0	0	0
Community hospitals*	86	10,843	346,819	2,453,917	3,158,232	62.0	6,728	8,651	7.1	212,225	896,514	1,273,915	2,170,429	809	34,260
6-24 beds	3	56	1,471	9,578	15,923	46.4	26	44	6.5	413	5,455	12,049	17,504	5	55
25-49	19	737	19,680	101,571	159,810	38.1	281	436	5.2	7,402	66,321	95,491	161,812	56	814
50-99	26	1,828	49,638	310,928	418,729	46.7	854	1,150	6.3	20,326	150,911	187,305	338,216	192	5,322
100-199	23	3,050	90,923	685,760	898,977	61.6	1,879	2,462	7.5	53,382	240,451	323,234	563,685	230	10,687
200-299	6	1,354	51,454	359,264	460,054	72.7	984	1,259	7.0	35,204	167,642	280,004	447,646	58	2,840
300-399	5	1,561	57,574	369,323	469,642	64.8	1,012	1,286	6.4	37,619	127,239	220,827	348,066	144	8,682
400-499	2	949	30,660	250,170	312,342	72.3	686	856	8.2	28,265	85,149	58,086	143,235	90	3,668
500 or more	2	1,308	45,419	367,323	422,755	76.9	1,006	1,158	8.1	29,614	53,346	96,919	150,265	34	2,192
Nongovernment not-for-profit	42	7,022	231,472	1,702,054	2,163,173	66.4	4,665	5,922	7.4	155,040	610,162	830,786	1,440,948	451	19,753
Investor-owned (for-profit)	15	1,477	47,656	282,563	348,674	52.5	776	957	5.9	26,593	85,986	138,621	224,607	159	6,699
State and local government	29	2,344	67,691	469,300	646,385	54.9	1,287	1,772	6.9	30,592	200,366	304,508	504,874	199	7,808

CLASSIFICATION	FULL-TIME EQUIVALENT PERSONNEL					FULL-TIME EQUIVALENT TRAINEES			EXPENSES						
									LABOR				TOTAL		
	Physicians and Dentists	Registered Nurses	Licensed Practical Nurses	Other Salaried Personnel	Total Personnel	Medical and Dental Residents	Other Trainees	Total Trainees	Payroll (in thousands)	Employee Benefits (in thousands)	Total (in thousands)	Percent of Total	Amount (in thousands)	Adjusted, per Admission	Adjusted, per Inpatient Day
ARKANSAS	235	7,768	4,288	26,089	38,380	422	70	492	$ 857,002	$ 159,571	$ 1,016,573	52.2	$ 1,948,142		
6-24 beds	17	52	15	248	332	0	0	0	9,307	1,624	10,930	63.5	17,206		
25-49	5	258	261	1,239	1,763	0	0	0	30,083	5,098	35,181	53.8	65,416		
50-99	32	858	622	3,521	5,033	0	1	1	99,024	18,681	117,704	51.8	227,059		
100-199	25	1,447	1,162	5,526	8,160	21	1	22	156,889	31,027	187,916	47.2	398,440		
200-299	8	1,515	597	4,525	6,645	0	46	46	140,613	23,667	164,280	52.9	310,652		
300-399	14	1,250	629	3,594	5,487	261	1	262	144,362	29,094	173,456	52.2	332,058		
400-499	0	630	284	2,092	3,006	0	2	2	65,443	12,936	78,378	53.1	147,562		
500 or more	134	1,758	718	5,344	7,954	140	19	159	211,281	37,446	248,727	55.3	449,749		
Psychiatric	17	179	60	889	1,145	3	1	4	29,658	6,743	36,401	63.2	57,636		
Hospitals	17	179	60	889	1,145	3	1	4	29,658	6,743	36,401	63.2	57,636		
Institutions for mentally retarded	0	0	0	0	0	0	0	0	0	0	0	0.0	0		
General	217	7,488	4,150	24,632	36,487	406	69	475	812,410	150,180	962,590	51.9	1,854,408		
Hospitals	217	7,488	4,150	24,632	36,487	406	69	475	812,410	150,180	962,590	51.9	1,854,408		
Hospital units of institutions	0	0	0	0	0	0	0	0	0	0	0	0.0	0		
TB and other respiratory diseases	0	0	0	0	0	0	0	0	0	0	0	0.0	0		
Obstetrics and gynecology	0	0	0	0	0	0	0	0	0	0	0	0.0	0		
Eye, ear, nose, and throat	0	0	0	0	0	0	0	0	0	0	0	0.0	0		
Rehabilitation	1	101	78	568	748	13	0	13	14,934	2,648	17,582	48.7	36,099		
Orthopedic	0	0	0	0	0	0	0	0	0	0	0	0.0	0		
Chronic disease	0	0	0	0	0	0	0	0	0	0	0	0.0	0		
All other	0	0	0	0	0	0	0	0	0	0	0	0.0	0		
Federal	198	585	234	2,818	3,835	140	20	160	110,809	21,279	132,088	64.3	205,460		
Psychiatric	0	0	0	0	0	0	0	0	0	0	0	0.0	0		
General and other special	198	585	234	2,818	3,835	140	20	160	110,809	21,279	132,088	64.3	205,460		
Nonfederal	37	7,183	4,054	23,271	34,545	282	50	332	746,193	138,292	884,485	50.8	1,742,682		
Psychiatric	17	179	60	889	1,145	3	1	4	29,658	6,743	36,401	63.2	57,636		
Hospitals	17	179	60	889	1,145	3	1	4	29,658	6,743	36,401	63.2	57,636		
Institutions for mentally retarded	0	0	0	0	0	0	0	0	0	0	0	0.0	0		
TB and other respiratory diseases	0	0	0	0	0	0	0	0	0	0	0	0.0	0		
Long-term general and other special	0	0	0	0	0	0	0	0	0	0	0	0.0	0		
Short-term general and other special	20	7,004	3,994	22,382	33,400	279	49	328	716,536	131,549	848,084	50.3	1,685,047		
Hospital units of institutions	0	0	0	0	0	0	0	0	0	0	0	0.0	0		
Community hospitals*	20	7,004	3,994	22,382	33,400	279	49	328	716,536	131,549	848,084	50.3	1,685,047	$3,729.58	$ 533.54
6-24 beds	0	29	10	76	115	0	0	0	2,946	501	3,447	54.4	6,340	2,630.83	398.19
25-49	5	258	261	1,239	1,763	0	0	0	30,083	5,098	35,181	53.8	65,416	2,147.11	409.34
50-99	3	708	585	2,845	4,141	0	1	1	78,243	14,601	92,844	50.8	182,820	2,663.11	436.61
100-199	1	1,374	1,140	5,172	7,687	13	0	13	143,302	28,458	171,760	46.1	372,300	3,093.37	414.14
200-299	8	1,515	597	4,525	6,645	0	46	46	140,613	23,667	164,280	52.9	310,652	4,697.59	675.25
300-399	0	1,187	606	3,099	4,892	258	0	258	128,048	25,123	153,171	50.1	305,958	4,179.75	651.47
400-499	0	630	284	2,092	3,006	0	2	2	65,443	12,936	78,378	53.1	147,562	3,850.08	472.44
500 or more	3	1,303	511	3,334	5,151	8	0	8	127,857	21,165	149,023	50.7	293,999	5,624.73	695.44
Nongovernment not-for-profit	13	5,149	2,596	15,626	23,384	21	48	69	506,376	87,975	594,352	50.8	1,169,341	3,915.19	540.57
Investor-owned (for-profit)	6	763	538	2,374	3,681	0	0	0	75,602	19,681	95,284	42.3	225,103	3,757.85	645.60
State and local government	1	1,092	860	4,382	6,335	258	1	259	134,557	23,892	158,449	54.5	290,603	3,116.85	449.58

*For information on community hospitals that excludes nursing-home-type data, refer to Hospital Units columns in tables 4A through 4D, pages 14 through 17.

(continued on next page)

Table

5C (Continued) California

Utilization, Personnel, and Finances in States

Excludes AHA nonregistered hospitals (see Table 14, page 240).

CLASSIFICATION	HOSPITALS	BEDS	ADMISSIONS	INPATIENT DAYS	ADJUSTED PATIENT DAYS	OCCUPANCY, percent	AVERAGE DAILY CENSUS	ADJUSTED AVERAGE DAILY CENSUS	AVERAGE STAY, days	SURGICAL OPERATIONS	OUTPATIENT VISITS Emergency	OUTPATIENT VISITS Other	OUTPATIENT VISITS Total	NEWBORNS Bassinets	NEWBORNS Births
CALIFORNIA	548	105,381	3,316,969	25,956,575		67.5	71,155			2,062,025	9,125,587	28,279,763	37,405,350	6,187	581,109
6-24 beds	19	377	9,059	53,537		39.5	149			6,115	74,419	280,726	355,145	29	716
25-49	63	2,288	62,187	361,239		43.2	989			45,249	355,194	1,177,721	1,532,915	199	7,802
50-99	131	9,743	279,740	1,864,705		52.7	5,134			193,864	933,041	1,972,805	2,905,846	594	40,784
100-199	153	21,903	749,190	4,804,642		60.2	13,184			532,252	2,415,243	6,579,268	8,994,511	1,350	122,369
200-299	84	20,258	793,257	4,782,295		64.7	13,102			458,984	2,353,033	5,322,849	7,675,882	1,668	153,600
300-399	48	16,275	633,771	4,101,238		69.0	11,237			392,307	1,334,959	4,720,334	6,055,293	1,090	116,887
400-499	21	9,252	363,207	2,514,651		74.4	6,886			183,894	896,062	3,843,049	4,739,111	619	69,145
500 or more	29	25,285	426,558	7,474,268		81.0	20,474			249,360	763,636	4,383,011	5,146,647	638	69,806
Psychiatric	64	14,150	56,878	4,199,880		81.5	11,532			656	19,827	240,724	260,551	0	0
Hospitals	61	10,425	56,661	2,905,497		76.6	7,986			643	18,996	238,347	257,343	0	0
Institutions for mentally retarded	3	3,725	217	1,294,383		95.2	3,546			13	831	2,377	3,208	0	0
General	469	89,037	3,240,360	21,152,345		65.1	57,968			2,049,013	9,080,330	27,716,763	36,797,093	6,187	581,109
Hospitals	462	88,270	3,230,129	20,966,534		65.1	57,459			2,044,675	9,035,718	27,097,632	36,133,350	6,187	581,109
Hospital units of institutions	7	767	10,231	185,811		66.4	509			4,338	44,612	619,131	663,743	0	0
TB and other respiratory diseases	1	63	276	12,635		55.6	35			230	0	710	710	0	0
Obstetrics and gynecology	0	0	0	0		00.0	0			0	0	0	0	0	0
Eye, ear, nose, and throat	1	33	1,372	3,035		24.2	8			1,944	0	675	675	0	0
Rehabilitation	5	309	3,218	65,282		57.9	179			0	3,255	46,265	49,520	0	0
Orthopedic	3	270	4,135	37,645		38.1	103			4,850	15,283	53,208	68,491	0	0
Chronic disease	1	1,126	1,398	391,604		95.3	1,073			17	0	116	116	0	0
All other	4	393	9,332	94,149		65.4	257			5,315	6,892	221,302	228,194	0	0
Federal	29	8,679	183,214	2,226,270		70.3	6,099			109,565	481,653	6,348,907	6,830,560	262	11,262
Psychiatric	0	0	0	0		00.0	0			0	0	0	0	0	0
General and other special	29	8,679	183,214	2,226,270		70.3	6,099			109,565	481,653	6,348,907	6,830,560	262	11,262
Nonfederal	519	96,702	3,133,755	23,730,305		67.3	65,056			1,952,460	8,643,934	21,930,856	30,574,790	5,925	569,847
Psychiatric	64	14,150	56,878	4,199,880		81.5	11,532			656	19,827	240,724	260,551	0	0
Hospitals	61	10,425	56,661	2,905,497		76.6	7,986			643	18,996	238,347	257,343	0	0
Institutions for mentally retarded	3	3,725	217	1,294,383		95.2	3,546			13	831	2,377	3,208	0	0
TB and other respiratory diseases	1	63	276	12,635		55.6	35			230	0	710	710	0	0
Long-term general and other special	4	1,753	6,403	608,363		95.0	1,666			3,507	3,937	133,817	137,754	0	0
Short-term general and other special	450	80,736	3,070,198	18,909,427		64.2	51,823			1,948,067	8,620,170	21,555,605	30,175,775	5,925	569,847
Hospital units of institutions	5	705	6,999	174,790		67.9	479			2,492	21,866	466,737	488,603	0	0
Community hospitals*	445	80,031	3,063,199	18,734,637	24,076,492	64.2	51,344	65,990	6.1	1,945,575	8,598,304	21,088,868	29,687,172	5,925	569,847
6-24 beds	13	229	4,475	28,825	56,609	35.4	81	158	6.4	3,649	42,836	94,487	137,323	10	231
25-49	45	1,678	45,458	236,281	363,903	38.4	645	995	5.2	36,188	244,761	407,650	652,411	134	6,225
50-99	98	7,314	248,757	1,343,574	1,895,727	50.3	3,682	5,195	5.4	189,056	896,730	1,505,235	2,401,965	569	40,150
100-199	131	18,684	689,951	4,029,966	5,388,403	59.2	11,061	14,785	5.8	500,901	2,280,757	5,091,387	7,372,144	1,255	118,449
200-299	82	19,795	781,077	4,641,292	5,978,248	64.2	12,715	16,381	5.9	454,083	2,327,538	4,800,813	7,128,351	1,643	152,429
300-399	43	14,568	601,964	3,661,349	4,530,617	68.9	10,032	12,413	6.1	378,311	1,293,080	3,386,274	4,679,354	1,090	116,887
400-499	19	8,334	333,339	2,221,403	2,728,593	73.0	6,083	7,475	6.7	169,404	831,278	2,884,424	3,715,702	586	65,670
500 or more	14	9,429	358,178	2,571,947	3,134,392	74.7	7,045	8,588	7.2	213,983	681,324	2,918,598	3,599,922	638	69,806
Nongovernment not-for-profit	237	50,321	1,980,635	12,083,586	15,346,375	65.8	33,110	42,051	6.1	1,274,859	5,091,092	14,140,251	19,231,343	3,737	358,420
Investor-owned (for-profit)	119	14,604	468,047	2,613,317	3,377,835	49.2	7,178	9,280	5.6	355,262	1,166,596	1,608,428	2,775,024	978	72,921
State and local government	89	15,106	614,517	4,037,734	5,352,282	73.2	11,056	14,659	6.6	315,454	2,340,616	5,340,189	7,680,805	1,210	138,506

CLASSIFICATION	FULL-TIME EQUIVALENT PERSONNEL					FULL-TIME EQUIVALENT TRAINEES			EXPENSES: LABOR				EXPENSES: TOTAL		
	Physicians and Dentists	Registered Nurses	Licensed Practical Nurses	Other Salaried Personnel	Total Personnel	Medical and Dental Residents	Other Trainees	Total Trainees	Payroll (in thousands)	Employee Benefits (in thousands)	Total (in thousands)	Percent of Total	Amount (in thousands)	Adjusted, per Admission	Adjusted, per Inpatient Day
CALIFORNIA	6,372	84,249	15,748	265,121	371,490	6,734	600	7,334	$11,370,661	$ 2,599,330	$13,969,990	54.4	$ 25,677,627		
6-24 beds	63	202	69	1,301	1,635	0	0	0	29,569	6,730	36,299	57.0	63,651		
25-49	212	1,325	441	5,800	7,778	10	6	16	180,198	40,458	220,656	55.2	400,090		
50-99	328	5,687	1,600	20,259	27,874	38	4	42	802,892	183,977	986,869	50.6	1,951,528		
100-199	1,250	18,365	3,366	52,475	75,456	506	84	590	2,211,866	490,312	2,702,178	51.4	5,257,268		
200-299	882	17,572	3,479	52,362	74,295	878	103	981	2,265,801	539,007	2,804,807	52.4	5,353,804		
300-399	984	16,550	2,498	46,882	66,914	1,149	101	1,250	2,087,567	469,566	2,557,134	54.4	4,701,676		
400-499	716	10,155	1,456	30,726	43,053	1,579	41	1,620	1,396,527	326,244	1,722,771	55.1	3,128,637		
500 or more	1,937	14,393	2,839	55,316	74,485	2,574	261	2,835	2,396,241	543,035	2,939,277	61.0	4,820,971		
Psychiatric	399	2,268	1,402	19,326	23,395	64	97	161	644,143	164,452	808,594	69.5	1,163,884		
Hospitals	368	2,079	1,254	13,089	16,790	64	97	161	496,272	128,869	625,141	66.8	936,501		
Institutions for mentally retarded	31	189	148	6,237	6,605	0	0	0	147,871	35,583	183,453	80.7	227,383		
General	5,810	80,908	14,146	241,147	342,011	6,605	476	7,081	10,527,512	2,387,638	12,915,150	53.6	24,099,070		
Hospitals	5,614	80,536	13,808	240,058	340,016	6,598	476	7,074	10,488,864	2,377,185	12,866,049	53.6	23,984,590		
Hospital units of institutions	196	372	338	1,089	1,995	7	0	7	38,648	10,453	49,101	42.9	114,480		
TB and other respiratory diseases	0	35	27	137	199	0	0	0	5,266	1,564	6,829	57.8	11,812		
Obstetrics and gynecology	0	0	0	0	0	0	0	0	0	0	0	0.0	0		
Eye, ear, nose, and throat	0	21	1	71	93	0	0	0	2,599	520	3,119	42.7	7,313		
Rehabilitation	1	114	44	885	1,044	0	0	0	26,936	6,003	32,939	62.1	53,077		
Orthopedic	11	129	34	524	698	9	3	12	30,946	5,985	36,931	53.7	68,712		
Chronic disease	43	263	58	1,274	1,638	0	0	0	52,275	14,007	66,282	81.8	81,011		
All other	108	511	36	1,757	2,412	56	24	80	80,985	19,160	100,145	52.0	192,747		
Federal	2,273	4,729	1,343	22,880	31,225	1,584	111	1,695	880,168	145,738	1,025,906	66.9	1,533,398		
Psychiatric	0	0	0	0	0	0	0	0	0	0	0	0.0	0		
General and other special	2,273	4,729	1,343	22,880	31,225	1,584	111	1,695	880,168	145,738	1,025,906	66.9	1,533,398		
Nonfederal	4,099	79,520	14,405	242,241	340,265	5,150	489	5,639	10,490,493	2,453,592	12,944,084	53.6	24,144,229		
Psychiatric	399	2,268	1,402	19,326	23,395	64	97	161	644,143	164,452	808,594	69.5	1,163,884		
Hospitals	368	2,079	1,254	13,089	16,790	64	97	161	496,272	128,869	625,141	66.8	936,501		
Institutions for mentally retarded	31	189	148	6,237	6,605	0	0	0	147,871	35,583	183,453	80.7	227,383		
TB and other respiratory diseases	0	35	27	137	199	0	0	0	5,266	1,564	6,829	57.8	11,812		
Long-term general and other special	147	735	118	3,640	4,640	41	0	41	141,411	37,967	179,378	70.7	253,758		
Short-term general and other special	3,553	76,482	12,858	219,138	312,031	5,045	392	5,437	9,699,674	2,249,609	11,949,283	52.6	22,714,775		
Hospital units of institutions	153	307	322	693	1,475	7	0	7	28,194	8,234	36,428	37.4	97,397		
Community hospitals*	3,400	76,175	12,536	218,445	310,556	5,038	392	5,430	9,671,480	2,241,375	11,912,854	52.7	22,617,379	$5,708.83	$ 939.40
6-24 beds	0	107	52	584	743	0	0	0	16,195	3,715	19,910	54.0	36,876	3,784.51	651.42
25-49	2	942	338	3,596	4,878	3	3	6	123,663	27,984	151,646	52.2	290,657	4,180.72	798.72
50-99	194	4,900	1,313	16,216	22,623	8	1	9	644,238	148,398	792,636	48.7	1,627,940	4,626.38	858.74
100-199	753	17,130	3,007	44,966	65,856	363	73	436	1,961,501	446,767	2,408,268	50.7	4,746,318	5,144.10	880.84
200-299	703	17,234	3,349	51,066	72,352	764	103	867	2,214,359	534,245	2,748,604	52.3	5,253,713	5,214.35	878.80
300-399	528	15,734	2,081	42,966	61,309	845	89	934	1,920,242	432,672	2,352,914	53.9	4,367,820	5,853.26	964.07
400-499	421	9,166	1,313	27,184	38,084	1,210	41	1,251	1,296,039	301,418	1,597,457	54.1	2,950,202	7,189.57	1,081.22
500 or more	799	10,962	1,083	31,867	44,711	1,845	82	1,927	1,495,244	346,174	1,841,418	55.1	3,343,852	7,533.12	1,066.83
Nongovernment not-for-profit	1,747	50,131	7,091	143,152	202,121	2,639	169	2,808	6,312,805	1,417,107	7,729,912	53.2	14,518,420	5,748.15	946.05
Investor-owned (for-profit)	183	11,205	2,251	27,451	41,090	10	43	53	1,214,695	269,668	1,484,363	45.6	3,256,149	5,347.80	963.98
State and local government	1,470	14,839	3,194	47,842	67,345	2,389	180	2,569	2,143,980	554,599	2,698,579	55.7	4,842,810	5,854.52	904.81

*For information on community hospitals that excludes nursing-home-type data, refer to Hospital Units columns in tables 4A through 4D, pages 14 through 17.

(continued on next page)

Table
5C (Continued) Colorado

Utilization, Personnel, and Finances in States

Excludes AHA nonregistered hospitals (see Table 14, page 240).

CLASSIFICATION	HOSPITALS	BEDS	ADMISSIONS	INPATIENT DAYS	ADJUSTED PATIENT DAYS	OCCUPANCY, percent	AVERAGE DAILY CENSUS	ADJUSTED AVERAGE DAILY CENSUS	AVERAGE STAY, days	SURGICAL OPERATIONS	OUTPATIENT VISITS			NEWBORNS	
											Emergency	Other	Total	Bassinets	Births
COLORADO	86	13,621	388,681	3,341,043		67.2	9,157			304,852	1,022,152	4,491,994	5,514,146	879	52,084
6-24 beds	7	142	2,345	12,823		24.6	35			859	8,760	38,785	47,545	32	332
25-49	18	691	17,877	120,014		47.5	328			12,077	66,462	241,545	308,007	90	2,666
50-99	22	1,531	29,137	341,316		61.4	940			19,063	91,073	424,552	515,625	107	4,061
100-199	12	1,598	44,715	358,485		61.5	983			39,957	162,339	661,807	824,146	121	5,158
200-299	14	3,465	131,031	843,769		66.7	2,311			122,607	337,902	1,051,487	1,389,389	280	21,050
300-399	8	2,714	69,996	722,771		73.0	1,980			41,875	163,596	717,494	881,090	135	8,542
400-499	2	941	40,093	255,548		74.4	700			37,375	72,075	1,017,881	1,089,956	59	6,136
500 or more	3	2,539	53,487	686,317		74.0	1,880			31,039	119,945	338,443	458,388	55	4,139
Psychiatric	10	1,915	10,801	575,220		82.3	1,576			650	2,178	94,165	96,343	0	0
Hospitals	10	1,915	10,801	575,220		82.3	1,576			650	2,178	94,165	96,343	0	0
Institutions for mentally retarded	0	0	0	0		00.0	0			0	0	0	0	0	0
General	72	11,331	374,347	2,676,786		64.8	7,337			302,702	1,018,509	4,343,152	5,361,661	879	52,084
Hospitals	72	11,331	374,347	2,676,786		64.8	7,337			302,702	1,018,509	4,343,152	5,361,661	879	52,084
Hospital units of institutions	0	0	0	0		00.0	0			0	0	0	0	0	0
TB and other respiratory diseases	0	0	0	0		00.0	0			0	0	0	0	0	0
Obstetrics and gynecology	0	0	0	0		00.0	0			0	0	0	0	0	0
Eye, ear, nose, and throat	0	0	0	0		00.0	0			0	0	0	0	0	0
Rehabilitation	3	270	2,223	64,309		65.2	176			1,500	0	32,639	32,639	0	0
Orthopedic	0	0	0	0		00.0	0			0	0	0	0	0	0
Chronic disease	0	0	0	0		00.0	0			0	0	0	0	0	0
All other	1	105	1,310	24,728		64.8	68			0	1,465	22,038	23,503	0	0
Federal	6	1,549	43,482	427,445		75.7	1,172			40,328	148,117	1,790,395	1,938,512	68	2,905
Psychiatric	1	319	1,086	104,265		89.7	286			0	0	36,245	36,245	0	0
General and other special	5	1,230	42,396	323,180		72.0	886			40,328	148,117	1,754,150	1,902,267	68	2,905
Nonfederal	80	12,072	345,199	2,913,598		66.1	7,985			264,524	874,035	2,701,599	3,575,634	811	49,179
Psychiatric	9	1,596	9,715	470,955		80.8	1,290			650	2,178	57,920	60,098	0	0
Hospitals	9	1,596	9,715	470,955		80.8	1,290			650	2,178	57,920	60,098	0	0
Institutions for mentally retarded	0	0	0	0		00.0	0			0	0	0	0	0	0
TB and other respiratory diseases	0	0	0	0		00.0	0			0	0	0	0	0	0
Long-term general and other special	2	160	703	33,050		56.3	90			1,500	0	4,607	4,607	0	0
Short-term general and other special	69	10,316	334,781	2,409,593		64.0	6,605			262,374	871,857	2,639,072	3,510,929	811	49,179
Hospital units of institutions	0	0	0	0		00.0	0			0	0	0	0	0	0
Community hospitals*	69	10,316	334,781	2,409,593	3,203,958	64.0	6,605	8,790	7.2	262,374	871,857	2,639,072	3,510,929	811	49,179
6-24 beds	7	142	2,345	12,823	23,957	24.6	35	66	5.5	859	8,760	38,785	47,545	32	332
25-49	18	691	17,877	120,014	183,364	47.5	328	503	6.7	12,077	66,462	241,545	308,007	90	2,666
50-99	13	825	19,638	179,556	271,691	60.2	497	755	9.1	12,516	62,644	143,266	205,910	90	3,371
100-199	9	1,146	30,971	271,647	358,398	65.0	745	981	8.8	23,148	102,643	215,135	317,778	85	3,819
200-299	14	3,465	131,031	843,769	1,118,872	66.7	2,311	3,066	6.4	122,607	337,902	1,051,487	1,389,389	280	21,050
300-399	5	1,670	59,328	397,482	506,522	65.2	1,089	1,388	6.7	37,942	159,596	474,960	634,556	135	8,542
400-499	1	488	23,758	124,647	151,851	69.9	341	416	5.2	22,836	14,428	145,693	160,121	44	5,260
500 or more	2	1,889	49,833	459,655	589,303	66.6	1,259	1,615	9.2	30,389	119,422	328,201	447,623	55	4,139
Nongovernment not-for-profit	35	7,129	242,688	1,733,745	2,287,032	66.7	4,755	6,275	7.1	200,402	571,070	1,973,217	2,544,287	525	35,210
Investor-owned (for-profit)	5	1,120	35,348	237,523	296,476	58.1	651	812	6.7	31,105	89,867	193,626	283,493	80	4,616
State and local government	29	2,067	56,745	438,325	620,450	58.0	1,199	1,703	7.7	30,867	210,920	472,229	683,149	206	9,353

*For information on community hospitals that excludes nursing home type data, refer to Hospital Units columns in tables 4A through 4D, pages 14 through 17.

CLASSIFICATION	FULL-TIME EQUIVALENT PERSONNEL: Physicians and Dentists	Registered Nurses	Licensed Practical Nurses	Other Salaried Personnel	Total Personnel	FULL-TIME EQUIVALENT TRAINEES: Medical and Dental Residents	Other Trainees	Total Trainees	EXPENSES, LABOR: Payroll (in thousands)	Employee Benefits (in thousands)	Total (in thousands)	Percent of Total	EXPENSES, TOTAL: Amount (in thousands)	Adjusted, per Admission	Adjusted, per Inpatient Day
COLORADO	1,510	11,284	1,739	34,765	49,298	548	40	588	$ 1,317,593	$ 238,388	$ 1,555,981	55.3	$ 2,812,031		
6-24 beds	0	62	23	265	350	0	0	0	6,411	1,058	7,469	54.5	13,701		
25-49	0	463	126	1,570	2,159	0	0	0	42,961	7,833	50,794	52.9	96,036		
50-99	71	786	146	3,058	4,061	1	11	12	95,094	17,851	112,945	53.7	210,327		
100-199	180	1,149	256	4,527	6,112	8	1	9	168,374	28,713	197,088	57.6	341,976		
200-299	873	4,124	273	10,363	15,633	47	17	64	418,543	72,652	491,195	53.0	926,797		
300-399	170	2,302	270	6,712	9,454	198	1	199	280,245	54,132	334,377	56.1	596,283		
400-499	178	847	419	3,162	4,606	260	10	270	112,828	21,952	134,780	56.5	238,679		
500 or more	38	1,551	226	5,108	6,923	34	0	34	193,137	34,197	227,334	58.6	388,231		
Psychiatric	59	449	121	2,805	3,434	4	0	4	100,164	19,607	119,772	69.2	172,990		
Hospitals	59	449	121	2,805	3,434	4	0	4	100,164	19,607	119,772	69.2	172,990		
Institutions for mentally retarded	0	0	0	0	0	0	0	0	0	0	0	0.0	0		
General	1,386	10,618	1,567	30,372	43,943	543	39	582	1,148,965	208,284	1,357,248	53.8	2,525,035		
Hospitals	1,386	10,618	1,567	30,372	43,943	543	39	582	1,148,965	208,284	1,357,248	53.8	2,525,035		
Hospital units of institutions	0	0	0	0	0	0	0	0	0	0	0	0.0	0		
TB and other respiratory diseases	0	0	0	0	0	0	0	0	0	0	0	0.0	0		
Obstetrics and gynecology	0	0	0	0	0	0	0	0	0	0	0	0.0	0		
Eye, ear, nose, and throat	0	0	0	0	0	0	0	0	0	0	0	0.0	0		
Rehabilitation	2	115	48	656	821	1	0	1	25,633	4,441	30,074	56.9	52,818		
Orthopedic	0	0	0	0	0	0	0	0	0	0	0	0.0	0		
Chronic disease	0	0	0	0	0	0	0	0	0	0	0	0.0	0		
All other	63	102	3	932	1,100	0	1	1	42,831	6,056	48,887	79.9	61,188		
Federal	458	896	623	4,864	6,841	273	20	293	156,357	29,633	185,990	59.0	315,327		
Psychiatric	18	55	21	499	593	0	0	0	15,888	2,972	18,859	70.3	26,838		
General and other special	440	841	602	4,365	6,248	273	20	293	140,470	26,661	167,131	57.9	288,489		
Nonfederal	1,052	10,388	1,116	29,901	42,457	275	20	295	1,161,236	208,755	1,369,991	54.9	2,496,704		
Psychiatric	41	394	100	2,306	2,841	4	0	4	84,277	16,635	100,912	69.0	146,152		
Hospitals	41	394	100	2,306	2,841	4	0	4	84,277	16,635	100,912	69.0	146,152		
Institutions for mentally retarded	0	0	0	0	0	0	0	0	0	0	0	0.0	0		
TB and other respiratory diseases	0	0	0	0	0	0	0	0	0	0	0	0.0	0		
Long-term general and other special	2	65	36	356	459	1	0	1	13,464	2,329	15,793	57.1	27,655		
Short-term general and other special	1,009	9,929	980	27,239	39,157	270	20	290	1,063,495	189,791	1,253,286	54.0	2,322,897		
Hospital units of institutions	0	0	0	0	0	0	0	0	0	0	0	0.0	0		
Community hospitals*	1,009	9,929	980	27,239	39,157	270	20	290	1,063,495	189,791	1,253,286	54.0	2,322,897	$5,208.83	$ 725.01
6-24 beds	0	62	23	265	350	0	0	0	6,411	1,058	7,469	54.5	13,701	3,308.63	571.90
25-49	0	463	126	1,570	2,159	0	0	0	42,961	7,833	50,794	52.9	96,036	3,375.24	523.74
50-99	0	526	93	1,478	2,097	0	1	1	45,762	8,127	53,888	50.5	106,696	3,686.28	392.71
100-199	82	895	99	3,306	4,382	0	1	1	127,096	21,831	148,927	56.8	262,264	6,065.72	731.77
200-299	873	4,124	273	10,363	15,633	47	17	64	418,543	72,652	491,195	53.0	926,797	5,365.40	828.33
300-399	36	1,861	179	4,843	6,919	95	1	96	206,103	40,737	246,840	53.4	462,560	6,098.19	913.21
400-499	14	559	34	1,327	1,934	96	0	96	61,047	10,875	71,923	60.5	118,965	4,110.30	783.43
500 or more	4	1,439	153	4,087	5,683	32	0	32	155,572	26,678	182,250	54.3	335,880	5,277.15	569.96
Nongovernment not-for-profit	949	7,537	600	19,885	28,971	180	19	199	788,269	132,153	920,422	55.2	1,667,595	5,173.96	729.15
Investor-owned (for-profit)	0	718	119	2,538	3,375	0	0	0	97,241	20,885	118,125	43.7	270,505	6,060.78	912.40
State and local government	60	1,674	261	4,816	6,811	90	1	91	177,986	36,753	214,739	55.8	384,798	4,869.81	620.19

*For information on community hospitals that excludes nursing-home-type data, refer to Hospital Units columns in tables 4A through 4D, pages 14 through 17.

(continued on next page)

Table

5C (Continued) Connecticut

Utilization, Personnel, and Finances in States

Excludes AHA nonregistered hospitals (see Table 14, page 240).

CLASSIFICATION	HOSPITALS	BEDS	ADMISSIONS	INPATIENT DAYS	ADJUSTED PATIENT DAYS	OCCUPANCY, percent	AVERAGE DAILY CENSUS	ADJUSTED AVERAGE DAILY CENSUS	AVERAGE STAY, days	SURGICAL OPERATIONS	OUTPATIENT VISITS Emergency	OUTPATIENT VISITS Other	OUTPATIENT VISITS Total	NEWBORNS Bassinets	NEWBORNS Births
CONNECTICUT	63	14,533	377,463	4,246,303		80.1	11,637			270,179	1,270,172	3,551,731	4,821,903	742	50,428
6-24 beds	3	53	365	8,133		43.4	23			11	416	15,939	16,355	0	0
25-49	6	231	3,676	55,673		66.2	153			2,119	28,938	234,109	263,047	0	0
50-99	12	857	18,250	216,099		69.2	593			11,551	70,172	212,053	282,225	26	806
100-199	12	1,672	38,832	413,131		67.6	1,131			27,903	170,958	585,297	756,255	111	4,949
200-299	11	2,683	100,923	721,480		73.7	1,978			80,595	443,914	1,163,413	1,607,327	244	14,468
300-399	7	2,361	56,675	743,890		86.3	2,038			37,158	181,131	564,092	745,223	118	7,131
400-499	7	3,268	68,185	1,040,986		87.3	2,852			48,569	147,574	277,946	425,520	104	9,404
500 or more	5	3,408	90,557	1,046,911		84.2	2,869			62,273	227,069	498,882	725,951	139	13,670
Psychiatric	17	2,610	8,127	830,129		87.2	2,275			0	8,254	208,272	216,526	0	0
Hospitals	17	2,610	8,127	830,129		87.2	2,275			0	8,254	208,272	216,526	0	0
Institutions for mentally retarded	0	0	0	0		00.0	0			0	0	0	0	0	0
General	38	10,151	362,390	2,856,644		77.1	7,828			268,382	1,261,870	3,228,480	4,490,350	742	50,428
Hospitals	36	10,107	361,652	2,847,110		77.2	7,801			268,371	1,261,870	3,214,877	4,476,747	742	50,428
Hospital units of institutions	2	44	738	9,534		61.4	27			11	0	13,603	13,603	0	0
TB and other respiratory diseases	0	0	0	0		00.0	0			0	0	0	0	0	0
Obstetrics and gynecology	0	0	0	0		00.0	0			0	0	0	0	0	0
Eye, ear, nose, and throat	0	0	0	0		00.0	0			0	0	0	0	0	0
Rehabilitation	1	121	1,057	38,954		88.4	107			0	0	18,325	18,325	0	0
Orthopedic	0	0	0	0		00.0	0			0	0	0	0	0	0
Chronic disease	2	336	742	103,645		84.5	284			54	0	17,934	17,934	0	0
All other	5	1,315	5,147	416,931		86.9	1,143			1,743	48	78,720	78,768	0	0
Federal	3	728	10,787	193,777		73.1	532			4,142	44,592	351,456	396,048	0	0
Psychiatric	0	0	0	0		00.0	0			0	0	0	0	0	0
General and other special	3	728	10,787	193,777		73.1	532			4,142	44,592	351,456	396,048	0	0
Nonfederal	60	13,805	366,676	4,052,526		80.4	11,105			266,037	1,225,580	3,200,275	4,425,855	742	50,428
Psychiatric	17	2,610	8,127	830,129		87.2	2,275			0	8,254	208,272	216,526	0	0
Hospitals	17	2,610	8,127	830,129		87.2	2,275			0	8,254	208,272	216,526	0	0
Institutions for mentally retarded	0	0	0	0		00.0	0			0	0	0	0	0	0
TB and other respiratory diseases	0	0	0	0		00.0	0			0	0	0	0	0	0
Long-term general and other special	6	1,524	2,754	508,768		91.5	1,395			61	0	37,835	37,835	0	0
Short-term general and other special	37	9,671	355,795	2,713,629		76.9	7,435			265,976	1,217,326	2,954,168	4,171,494	742	50,428
Hospital units of institutions	2	44	738	9,534		61.4	27			11	0	13,603	13,603	0	0
Community hospitals*	35	9,627	355,057	2,704,095	3,586,130	77.0	7,408	9,825	7.6	265,965	1,217,326	2,940,565	4,157,891	742	50,428
6-24 beds	0	0	0	0	0	00.0	0	0	0.0	0	0	0	0	0	0
25-49	0	0	0	0	0	00.0	0	0	0.0	0	0	0	0	0	0
50-99	6	465	15,645	107,432	158,655	63.4	295	434	6.9	11,551	70,172	99,624	169,796	26	806
100-199	7	1,007	34,526	229,106	317,234	62.3	627	869	6.6	27,896	170,346	502,124	672,470	111	4,949
200-299	11	2,683	100,923	721,480	1,048,210	73.7	1,978	2,873	7.1	80,595	443,914	1,163,413	1,607,327	244	14,468
300-399	4	1,377	53,855	409,869	544,179	81.5	1,122	1,490	7.6	37,104	181,131	530,432	711,563	118	7,131
400-499	4	1,806	66,869	542,656	671,598	82.3	1,486	1,840	8.1	48,569	146,812	273,673	420,485	104	9,404
500 or more	3	2,289	83,239	693,552	846,254	83.0	1,900	2,319	8.3	60,250	204,951	371,299	576,250	139	13,670
Nongovernment not-for-profit	34	9,395	349,123	2,647,202	3,500,155	77.2	7,252	9,589	7.6	262,289	1,202,377	2,608,731	3,811,108	722	49,984
Investor-owned (for-profit)	0	0	0	0	0	00.0	0	0	0.0	0	0	0	0	0	0
State and local government	1	232	5,934	56,893	85,975	67.2	156	236	9.6	3,676	14,949	331,834	346,783	20	444

*For information on community hospitals that excludes nursing home type data, refer to Hospital Units columns in tables 4A through 4D, pages 14 through 17.

CLASSIFICATION	FULL-TIME EQUIVALENT PERSONNEL: Physicians and Dentists	Registered Nurses	Licensed Practical Nurses	Other Salaried Personnel	Total Personnel	FULL-TIME EQUIVALENT TRAINEES: Medical and Dental Residents	Other Trainees	Total Trainees	EXPENSES – LABOR: Payroll (in thousands)	Employee Benefits (in thousands)	Total (in thousands)	Percent of Total	EXPENSES – TOTAL: Amount (in thousands)	Adjusted, per Admission	Adjusted, per Inpatient Day
CONNECTICUT	1,266	12,077	1,744	40,434	55,521	1,540	118	1,658	$ 1,869,310	$ 406,953	$ 2,276,263	64.8	$ 3,510,387		
6-24 beds	2	12	4	64	82	0	0	0	1,857	277	2,134	62.0	3,441		
25-49	59	152	38	971	1,220	0	1	1	38,933	5,259	44,192	75.3	58,686		
50-99	114	690	89	2,676	3,569	45	31	76	102,382	22,189	124,570	66.8	186,411		
100-199	162	1,276	245	4,418	6,101	75	2	77	190,647	40,746	231,393	65.4	353,555		
200-299	235	2,710	374	8,974	12,293	164	10	174	438,709	96,652	535,362	64.7	827,559		
300-399	161	1,670	266	6,155	8,252	172	6	178	284,916	62,016	346,932	66.0	525,906		
400-499	260	2,207	344	8,221	11,032	335	25	360	358,742	91,275	450,017	64.7	695,768		
500 or more	273	3,360	384	8,955	12,972	749	43	792	453,123	88,540	541,663	63.1	859,062		
Psychiatric	228	863	145	4,772	6,008	107	44	151	166,641	47,489	214,131	73.5	291,189		
Hospitals	228	863	145	4,772	6,008	107	44	151	166,641	47,489	214,131	73.5	291,189		
Institutions for mentally retarded	0	0	0	0	0	0	0	0	0	0	0	0.0	0		
General	946	10,687	1,399	32,674	45,706	1,366	61	1,427	1,590,938	337,768	1,928,706	63.5	3,038,663		
Hospitals	943	10,673	1,394	32,647	45,657	1,366	61	1,427	1,589,601	337,412	1,927,013	63.5	3,034,483		
Hospital units of institutions	3	14	5	27	49	0	0	0	1,337	356	1,693	40.5	4,180		
TB and other respiratory diseases	0	0	0	0	0	0	0	0	0	0	0	0.0	0		
Obstetrics and gynecology	0	0	0	0	0	0	0	0	0	0	0	0.0	0		
Eye, ear, nose, and throat	0	0	0	0	0	0	0	0	0	0	0	0.0	0		
Rehabilitation	7	35	31	335	408	1	0	1	13,839	4,204	18,043	77.1	23,390		
Orthopedic	0	0	0	0	0	0	0	0	0	0	0	0.0	0		
Chronic disease	16	96	67	447	626	0	0	0	20,221	2,248	22,468	82.4	27,283		
All other	69	396	102	2,206	2,773	66	13	79	77,671	15,244	92,915	71.5	129,862		
Federal	145	400	60	1,784	2,389	106	14	120	77,395	14,807	92,202	68.0	135,673		
Psychiatric	0	0	0	0	0	0	0	0	0	0	0	0.0	0		
General and other special	145	400	60	1,784	2,389	106	14	120	77,395	14,807	92,202	68.0	135,673		
Nonfederal	1,121	11,677	1,684	38,650	53,132	1,434	104	1,538	1,791,915	392,146	2,184,061	64.7	3,374,715		
Psychiatric	228	863	145	4,772	6,008	107	44	151	166,641	47,489	214,131	73.5	291,189		
Hospitals	228	863	145	4,772	6,008	107	44	151	166,641	47,489	214,131	73.5	291,189		
Institutions for mentally retarded	0	0	0	0	0	0	0	0	0	0	0	0.0	0		
TB and other respiratory diseases	0	0	0	0	0	0	0	0	0	0	0	0.0	0		
Long-term general and other special	47	313	168	2,169	2,697	2	6	8	76,150	15,347	91,496	75.2	121,708		
Short-term general and other special	846	10,501	1,371	31,709	44,427	1,325	54	1,379	1,549,124	329,310	1,878,434	63.4	2,961,817		
Hospital units of institutions	3	14	5	27	49	0	0	0	1,337	356	1,693	40.5	4,180		
Community hospitals*	843	10,487	1,366	31,682	44,378	1,325	54	1,379	1,547,787	328,954	1,876,742	63.5	2,957,637	$ 6,237.82	$ 824.74
6-24 beds	0	0	0	0	0	0	0	0	0	0	0	0.0	0	0.00	0.00
25-49	0	0	0	0	0	0	0	0	0	0	0	0.0	0	0.00	0.00
50-99	43	452	68	1,581	2,144	1	5	6	74,083	16,390	90,474	66.6	135,933	5,881.22	856.78
100-199	103	1,002	154	2,861	4,120	8	0	8	133,848	28,376	162,224	63.5	255,311	5,294.93	804.80
200-299	235	2,710	374	8,974	12,293	164	10	174	438,709	96,652	535,362	64.7	827,559	5,649.21	789.50
300-399	100	1,392	204	4,749	6,445	149	0	149	224,906	49,860	274,765	64.2	428,277	5,979.85	787.01
400-499	175	1,871	252	6,085	8,383	296	14	310	281,417	61,093	342,510	61.6	556,284	6,694.07	828.30
500 or more	187	3,060	314	7,432	10,993	707	25	732	394,825	76,582	471,407	62.5	754,274	7,423.74	891.31
Nongovernment not-for-profit	842	10,218	1,366	30,798	43,224	1,302	54	1,356	1,510,025	317,697	1,827,722	63.7	2,867,286	6,163.83	819.19
Investor-owned (for-profit)	0	0	0	0	0	0	0	0	0	0	0	0.0	0	0.00	0.00
State and local government	1	269	0	884	1,154	23	0	23	37,762	11,258	49,020	54.3	90,351	10,075.92	1,050.90

*For information on community hospitals that excludes nursing-home-type data, refer to Hospital Units columns in tables 4A through 4D, pages 14 through 17.

(continued on next page)

Table

5C (Continued) Delaware

Utilization, Personnel, and Finances in States

Excludes AHA nonregistered hospitals (see Table 14, page 240).

CLASSIFICATION	HOSPITALS	BEDS	ADMISSIONS	INPATIENT DAYS	ADJUSTED PATIENT DAYS	OCCUPANCY, percent	AVERAGE DAILY CENSUS	ADJUSTED AVERAGE DAILY CENSUS	AVERAGE STAY, days	SURGICAL OPERATIONS	OUTPATIENT VISITS Emergency	OUTPATIENT VISITS Other	OUTPATIENT VISITS Total	NEWBORNS Bassinets	NEWBORNS Births
DELAWARE	13	2,837	92,111	808,848		78.1	2,216			80,506	269,623	898,816	1,168,439	149	11,647
6-24 beds	0	0	0	0		00.0	0			0	0	0	0	0	0
25-49	1	31	1,375	4,149		35.5	11			867	13,660	120,407	134,067	10	388
50-99	4	284	6,088	73,002		70.4	200			5,899	19,279	56,474	75,753	0	0
100-199	4	583	26,582	160,585		75.6	441			18,409	103,226	274,447	377,673	63	3,216
200-299	1	290	3,392	68,718		64.8	188			1,779	1,390	66,792	68,182	0	0
300-399	2	725	15,404	235,422		89.0	645			17,701	39,372	134,321	173,693	12	1,293
400-499	0	0	0	0		00.0	0			0	0	0	0	0	0
500 or more	1	924	39,270	266,972		79.1	731			35,851	92,696	246,375	339,071	64	6,750
Psychiatric	3	510	3,254	175,575		94.3	481			0	0	0	0	0	0
Hospitals	3	510	3,254	175,575		94.3	481			0	0	0	0	0	0
Institutions for mentally retarded	0	0	0	0		00.0	0			0	0	0	0	0	0
General	10	2,327	88,857	633,273		74.6	1,735			80,506	269,623	898,816	1,168,439	149	11,647
Hospitals	10	2,327	88,857	633,273		74.6	1,735			80,506	269,623	898,816	1,168,439	149	11,647
Hospital units of institutions	0	0	0	0		00.0	0			0	0	0	0	0	0
TB and other respiratory diseases	0	0	0	0		00.0	0			0	0	0	0	0	0
Obstetrics and gynecology	0	0	0	0		00.0	0			0	0	0	0	0	0
Eye, ear, nose, and throat	0	0	0	0		00.0	0			0	0	0	0	0	0
Rehabilitation	0	0	0	0		00.0	0			0	0	0	0	0	0
Orthopedic	0	0	0	0		00.0	0			0	0	0	0	0	0
Chronic disease	0	0	0	0		00.0	0			0	0	0	0	0	0
All other	0	0	0	0		00.0	0			0	0	0	0	0	0
Federal	2	321	4,767	72,867		62.0	199			2,646	15,050	187,199	202,249	10	388
Psychiatric	0	0	0	0		00.0	0			0	0	0	0	0	0
General and other special	2	321	4,767	72,867		62.0	199			2,646	15,050	187,199	202,249	10	388
Nonfederal	11	2,516	87,344	735,981		80.2	2,017			77,860	254,573	711,617	966,190	139	11,259
Psychiatric	3	510	3,254	175,575		94.3	481			0	0	0	0	0	0
Hospitals	3	510	3,254	175,575		94.3	481			0	0	0	0	0	0
Institutions for mentally retarded	0	0	0	0		00.0	0			0	0	0	0	0	0
TB and other respiratory diseases	0	0	0	0		00.0	0			0	0	0	0	0	0
Long-term general and other special	0	0	0	0		00.0	0			0	0	0	0	0	0
Short-term general and other special	8	2,006	84,090	560,406		76.6	1,536			77,860	254,573	711,617	966,190	139	11,259
Hospital units of institutions	0	0	0	0		00.0	0			0	0	0	0	0	0
Community hospitals*	8	2,006	84,090	560,406	745,334	76.6	1,536	2,043	6.7	77,860	254,573	711,617	966,190	139	11,259
6-24 beds	0	0	0	0	0	00.0	0	0	0.0	0	0	0	0	0	0
25-49	0	0	0	0	0	00.0	0	0	0.0	0	0	0	0	0	0
50-99	2	166	4,713	39,307	55,527	65.1	108	153	8.3	5,899	19,279	56,474	75,753	0	0
100-199	4	583	26,582	160,585	238,710	75.6	441	654	6.0	18,409	103,226	274,447	377,673	63	3,216
200-299	0	0	0	0	0	00.0	0	0	0.0	0	0	0	0	0	0
300-399	1	333	13,525	93,542	126,140	76.9	256	346	6.9	17,701	39,372	134,321	173,693	12	1,293
400-499	0	0	0	0	0	00.0	0	0	0.0	0	0	0	0	0	0
500 or more	1	924	39,270	266,972	324,957	79.1	731	890	6.8	35,851	92,696	246,375	339,071	64	6,750
Nongovernment not-for-profit	8	2,006	84,090	560,406	745,334	76.6	1,536	2,043	6.7	77,860	254,573	711,617	966,190	139	11,259
Investor-owned (for-profit)	0	0	0	0	0	00.0	0	0	0.0	0	0	0	0	0	0
State and local government	0	0	0	0	0	00.0	0	0	0.0	0	0	0	0	0	0

CLASSIFICATION	FULL-TIME EQUIVALENT PERSONNEL: Physicians and Dentists	Registered Nurses	Licensed Practical Nurses	Other Salaried Personnel	Total Personnel	FULL-TIME EQUIVALENT TRAINEES: Medical and Dental Residents	Other Trainees	Total Trainees	EXPENSES — LABOR: Payroll (in thousands)	Employee Benefits (in thousands)	Total (in thousands)	Percent of Total	EXPENSES — TOTAL: Amount (in thousands)	Adjusted, per Admission	Adjusted, per Inpatient Day
DELAWARE	187	2,949	476	8,281	11,893	244	1	245	$ 316,290	$ 66,529	$ 382,819	57.9	$ 661,059		
6-24 beds	0	0	0	0	0	0	0	0	0	0	0	0.0	0		
25-49	29	29	11	253	322	0	0	0	5,227	1,109	6,336	74.2	8,542		
50-99	55	295	27	1,115	1,492	11	0	11	37,971	8,079	46,050	55.8	82,496		
100-199	23	716	164	1,929	2,832	0	0	0	64,656	13,020	77,676	54.5	142,444		
200-299	45	121	20	463	649	32	1	33	20,633	3,602	24,235	62.3	38,920		
300-399	35	431	70	1,471	2,007	27	0	27	51,047	10,880	61,926	60.6	102,158		
400-499	0	0	0	0	0	0	0	0	0	0	0	0.0	0		
500 or more	0	1,357	184	3,050	4,591	174	0	174	136,757	29,839	166,596	58.1	286,499		
Psychiatric	12	91	33	776	912	12	0	12	20,850	5,000	25,849	66.0	39,195		
Hospitals	12	91	33	776	912	12	0	12	20,850	5,000	25,849	66.0	39,195		
Institutions for mentally retarded	0	0	0	0	0	0	0	0	0	0	0	0.0	0		
General	175	2,858	443	7,505	10,981	232	1	233	295,440	61,529	356,970	57.4	621,863		
Hospitals	175	2,858	443	7,505	10,981	232	1	233	295,440	61,529	356,970	57.4	621,863		
Hospital units of institutions	0	0	0	0	0	0	0	0	0	0	0	0.0	0		
TB and other respiratory diseases	0	0	0	0	0	0	0	0	0	0	0	0.0	0		
Obstetrics and gynecology	0	0	0	0	0	0	0	0	0	0	0	0.0	0		
Eye, ear, nose, and throat	0	0	0	0	0	0	0	0	0	0	0	0.0	0		
Rehabilitation	0	0	0	0	0	0	0	0	0	0	0	0.0	0		
Orthopedic	0	0	0	0	0	0	0	0	0	0	0	0.0	0		
Chronic disease	0	0	0	0	0	0	0	0	0	0	0	0.0	0		
All other	0	0	0	0	0	0	0	0	0	0	0	0.0	0		
Federal	74	150	31	716	971	32	1	33	25,860	4,712	30,571	64.4	47,462		
Psychiatric	0	0	0	0	0	0	0	0	0	0	0	0.0	0		
General and other special	74	150	31	716	971	32	1	33	25,860	4,712	30,571	64.4	47,462		
Nonfederal	113	2,799	445	7,565	10,922	212	0	212	290,431	61,817	352,248	57.4	613,597		
Psychiatric	12	91	33	776	912	12	0	12	20,850	5,000	25,849	66.0	39,195		
Hospitals	12	91	33	776	912	12	0	12	20,850	5,000	25,849	66.0	39,195		
Institutions for mentally retarded	0	0	0	0	0	0	0	0	0	0	0	0.0	0		
TB and other respiratory diseases	0	0	0	0	0	0	0	0	0	0	0	0.0	0		
Long-term general and other special	0	0	0	0	0	0	0	0	0	0	0	0.0	0		
Short-term general and other special	101	2,708	412	6,789	10,010	200	0	200	269,581	56,818	326,398	56.8	574,402		
Hospital units of institutions	0	0	0	0	0	0	0	0	0	0	0	0.0	0		
Community hospitals*	101	2,708	412	6,789	10,010	200	0	200	269,581	56,818	326,398	56.8	574,402	$5,111.88	$ 770.66
6-24 beds	0	0	0	0	0	0	0	0	0	0	0	0.0	0	0.00	0.00
25-49	0	0	0	0	0	0	0	0	0	0	0	0.0	0	0.00	0.00
50-99	55	246	20	937	1,258	11	0	11	32,062	7,185	39,247	57.1	68,688	10,018.63	1,237.01
100-199	23	716	164	1,929	2,832	0	0	0	64,656	13,020	77,676	54.5	142,444	3,608.64	596.72
200-299	0	0	0	0	0	0	0	0	0	0	0	0.0	0	0.00	0.00
300-399	23	389	44	873	1,329	15	0	15	36,105	6,774	42,879	55.9	76,771	4,209.40	608.62
400-499	0	0	0	0	0	0	0	0	0	0	0	0.0	0	0.00	0.00
500 or more	0	1,357	184	3,050	4,591	174	0	174	136,757	29,839	166,596	58.1	286,499	5,993.83	881.65
Nongovernment not-for-profit	101	2,708	412	6,789	10,010	200	0	200	269,581	56,818	326,398	56.8	574,402	5,111.88	770.66
Investor-owned (for-profit)	0	0	0	0	0	0	0	0	0	0	0	0.0	0	0.00	0.00
State and local government	0	0	0	0	0	0	0	0	0	0	0	0.0	0	0.00	0.00

*For information on community hospitals that excludes nursing-home-type data, refer to Hospital Units columns in tables 4A through 4D, pages 14 through 17.

(continued on next page)

5C (Continued) District of Columbia

Utilization, Personnel, and Finances in States

Excludes AHA nonregistered hospitals (see Table 14, page 240).

CLASSIFICATION	HOSPITALS	BEDS	ADMISSIONS	INPATIENT DAYS	ADJUSTED PATIENT DAYS	OCCUPANCY, percent	AVERAGE DAILY CENSUS	ADJUSTED AVERAGE DAILY CENSUS	AVERAGE STAY, days	SURGICAL OPERATIONS	OUTPATIENT VISITS: Emergency	OUTPATIENT VISITS: Other	OUTPATIENT VISITS: Total	NEWBORNS: Bassinets	NEWBORNS: Births
DISTRICT OF COLUMBIA	17	8,041	199,743	2,320,639		79.1	6,358			131,101	446,606	1,809,633	2,256,239	338	21,707
6-24 beds	0	0	0	0		00.0	0			0	0	0	0	0	0
25-49	0	0	0	0		00.0	0			0	0	0	0	0	0
50-99	2	161	1,692	42,942		73.3	118			2,720	10,585	7,898	18,483	0	0
100-199	2	343	11,308	84,469		67.6	232			7,596	0	44,138	44,138	52	5,205
200-299	2	480	13,466	141,540		80.8	388			8,017	53,235	202,768	256,003	0	0
300-399	2	744	27,029	206,796		76.1	566			25,106	42,190	89,627	131,817	41	3,455
400-499	4	1,914	60,465	533,693		76.4	1,463			44,824	213,449	356,284	569,733	162	7,484
500 or more	5	4,399	85,783	1,311,199		81.6	3,591			42,838	127,147	1,108,918	1,236,065	83	5,563
Psychiatric	2	1,700	5,162	571,715		92.1	1,566			0	1,973	34,112	36,085	0	0
Hospitals	2	1,700	5,162	571,715		92.1	1,566			0	1,973	34,112	36,085	0	0
Institutions for mentally retarded	0	0	0	0		00.0	0			0	0	0	0	0	0
General	12	5,918	183,188	1,637,128		75.8	4,485			123,505	444,633	1,731,383	2,176,016	286	16,502
Hospitals	12	5,918	183,188	1,637,128		75.8	4,485			123,505	444,633	1,731,383	2,176,016	286	16,502
Hospital units of institutions	0	0	0	0		00.0	0			0	0	0	0	0	0
TB and other respiratory diseases	0	0	0	0		00.0	0			0	0	0	0	0	0
Obstetrics and gynecology	1	183	10,280	38,961		58.5	107			7,596	0	20,547	20,547	52	5,205
Eye, ear, nose, and throat	0	0	0	0		00.0	0			0	0	0	0	0	0
Rehabilitation	1	160	1,028	45,508		78.1	125			0	0	23,591	23,591	0	0
Orthopedic	0	0	0	0		00.0	0			0	0	0	0	0	0
Chronic disease	1	80	85	27,327		93.8	75			0	0	0	0	0	0
All other	0	0	0	0		00.0	0			0	0	0	0	0	0
Federal	2	1,544	35,636	423,906		75.2	1,161			12,511	60,528	863,998	924,526	26	1,043
Psychiatric	0	0	0	0		00.0	0			0	0	0	0	0	0
General and other special	2	1,544	35,636	423,906		75.2	1,161			12,511	60,528	863,998	924,526	26	1,043
Nonfederal	15	6,497	164,107	1,896,733		80.0	5,197			118,590	386,078	945,635	1,331,713	312	20,664
Psychiatric	2	1,700	5,162	571,715		92.1	1,566			0	1,973	34,112	36,085	0	0
Hospitals	2	1,700	5,162	571,715		92.1	1,566			0	1,973	34,112	36,085	0	0
Institutions for mentally retarded	0	0	0	0		00.0	0			0	0	0	0	0	0
TB and other respiratory diseases	0	0	0	0		00.0	0			0	0	0	0	0	0
Long-term general and other special	2	240	1,113	72,835		83.3	200			0	0	23,591	23,591	0	0
Short-term general and other special	11	4,557	157,832	1,252,183		75.3	3,431			118,590	384,105	887,932	1,272,037	312	20,664
Hospital units of institutions	0	0	0	0		00.0	0			0	0	0	0	0	0
Community hospitals*	11	4,557	157,832	1,252,183	1,514,470	75.3	3,431	4,149	7.9	118,590	384,105	887,932	1,272,037	312	20,664
6-24 beds	0	0	0	0	0	00.0	0	0	0.0	0	0	0	0	0	0
25-49	0	0	0	0	0	00.0	0	0	0.0	0	0	0	0	0	0
50-99	1	81	1,607	15,615	18,059	53.1	43	49	9.7	2,720	10,585	7,898	18,483	0	0
100-199	1	183	10,280	38,961	50,867	58.5	107	139	3.8	7,596	0	20,547	20,547	52	5,205
200-299	1	279	11,205	77,590	96,986	76.3	213	266	6.9	8,017	53,118	201,408	254,526	0	0
300-399	2	744	27,029	206,796	248,135	76.1	566	680	7.7	25,106	42,190	89,627	131,817	41	3,455
400-499	4	1,914	60,465	533,693	669,784	76.4	1,463	1,835	8.8	44,824	213,449	356,284	569,733	162	7,484
500 or more	2	1,356	47,246	379,528	430,639	76.6	1,039	1,180	8.0	30,327	64,763	212,168	276,931	57	4,520
Nongovernment not-for-profit	10	4,075	143,788	1,130,975	1,352,494	76.0	3,099	3,705	7.9	101,799	304,207	772,052	1,076,259	240	18,497
Investor-owned (for-profit)	0	0	0	0	0	00.0	0	0	0.0	0	0	0	0	0	0
State and local government	1	482	14,044	121,208	161,976	68.9	332	444	8.6	16,791	79,898	115,880	195,778	72	2,167

*For information on community hospitals that exclude nursing home type data, refer to Hospital Units columns in tables 4A through 4D, pages 14 through 17.

CLASSIFICATION	FULL-TIME EQUIVALENT PERSONNEL: Physicians and Dentists	Registered Nurses	Licensed Practical Nurses	Other Salaried Personnel	Total Personnel	FULL-TIME EQUIVALENT TRAINEES: Medical and Dental Residents	Other Trainees	Total Trainees	EXPENSES — LABOR: Payroll (in thousands)	Employee Benefits (in thousands)	Total (in thousands)	Percent of Total	EXPENSES — TOTAL: Amount (in thousands)	Adjusted, per Admission	Adjusted, per Inpatient Day
DISTRICT OF COLUMBIA	1,337	6,336	826	22,522	31,021	1,563	101	1,664	$ 1,033,609	$ 202,876	$ 1,236,485	59.0	$ 2,096,508		
6-24 beds	0	0	0	0	0	0	0	0	0	0	0	0.0	0		
25-49	0	0	0	0	0	0	0	0	0	0	0	0.0	0		
50-99	4	87	29	37	491	0	2	2	14,050	2,558	16,607	56.4	29,465		
100-199	29	437	21	1,192	1,679	24	0	24	50,477	11,162	61,639	54.8	112,401		
200-299	0	578	33	1,958	2,569	79	0	79	79,896	16,492	96,388	51.1	188,509		
300-399	16	604	38	1,584	2,242	58	0	58	84,410	14,683	99,092	57.0	173,750		
400-499	514	1,807	327	5,675	8,323	513	1	514	291,487	52,989	344,476	56.1	614,436		
500 or more	774	2,823	378	11,742	15,717	889	98	987	513,290	104,993	618,283	63.2	977,946		
Psychiatric	55	269	134	2,084	2,542	4	0	4	118,339	31,050	149,389	73.3	203,842		
Hospitals	55	269	134	2,084	2,542	4	0	4	118,339	31,050	149,389	73.3	203,842		
Institutions for mentally retarded	0	0	0	0	0	0	0	0	0	0	0	0.0	0		
General	1,249	5,583	651	19,078	26,561	1,535	99	1,634	857,238	159,423	1,016,661	57.5	1,766,970		
Hospitals	1,249	5,583	651	19,078	26,561	1,535	99	1,634	857,238	159,423	1,016,661	57.5	1,766,970		
Hospital units of institutions	0	0	0	0	0	0	0	0	0	0	0	0.0	0		
TB and other respiratory diseases	0	0	0	0	0	0	0	0	0	0	0	0.0	0		
Obstetrics and gynecology	11	311	20	536	878	0	0	0	28,919	3,928	32,847	49.2	66,755		
Eye, ear, nose, and throat	0	0	0	0	0	0	0	0	0	0	0	0.0	0		
Rehabilitation	18	126	1	656	801	24	0	24	21,558	7,234	28,792	63.1	45,646		
Orthopedic	0	0	0	0	0	0	0	0	0	0	0	0.0	0		
Chronic disease	4	47	20	168	239	0	2	2	7,556	1,240	8,796	66.2	13,295		
All other	0	0	0	0	0	0	0	0	0	0	0	0.0	0		
Federal	626	858	124	5,559	7,167	473	66	539	176,522	36,341	212,863	65.2	326,258		
Psychiatric	0	0	0	0	0	0	0	0	0	0	0	0.0	0		
General and other special	626	858	124	5,559	7,167	473	66	539	176,522	36,341	212,863	65.2	326,258		
Nonfederal	711	5,478	702	16,963	23,854	1,090	35	1,125	857,087	166,535	1,023,622	57.8	1,770,250		
Psychiatric	55	269	134	2,084	2,542	4	0	4	118,339	31,050	149,389	73.3	203,842		
Hospitals	55	269	134	2,084	2,542	4	0	4	118,339	31,050	149,389	73.3	203,842		
Institutions for mentally retarded	0	0	0	0	0	0	0	0	0	0	0	0.0	0		
TB and other respiratory diseases	0	0	0	0	0	0	0	0	0	0	0	0.0	0		
Long-term general and other special	22	173	21	824	1,040	24	2	26	29,113	8,474	37,588	63.8	58,941		
Short-term general and other special	634	5,036	547	14,055	20,272	1,062	33	1,095	709,635	127,011	836,646	55.5	1,507,467		
Hospital units of institutions	0	0	0	0	0	0	0	0	0	0	0	0.0	0		
Community hospitals*	634	5,036	547	14,055	20,272	1,062	33	1,095	709,635	127,011	836,646	55.5	1,507,467	$ 7,875.55	$ 995.38
6-24 beds	0	0	0	0	0	0	0	0	0	0	0	0.0	0	0.00	0.00
25-49	0	0	0	0	0	0	0	0	0	0	0	0.0	0	0.00	0.00
50-99	0	40	9	203	252	0	0	0	6,494	1,317	7,811	48.3	16,170	8,698.36	895.41
100-199	11	311	20	536	878	0	0	0	28,919	3,928	32,847	49.2	66,755	4,973.90	1,312.34
200-299	0	511	30	1,600	2,141	79	0	79	68,401	14,298	82,699	54.1	152,932	10,919.02	1,576.84
300-399	16	604	38	1,584	2,242	58	0	58	84,410	14,683	99,092	57.0	173,750	5,335.00	700.22
400-499	514	1,807	327	5,675	8,323	513	1	514	291,487	52,989	344,476	56.1	614,436	8,095.45	917.37
500 or more	93	1,763	123	4,457	6,436	412	32	444	229,924	39,796	269,720	55.8	483,423	9,009.34	1,122.57
Nongovernment not-for-profit	469	4,658	445	12,697	18,269	882	33	915	648,825	116,906	765,731	55.5	1,379,461	7,990.25	1,019.94
Investor-owned (for-profit)	0	0	0	0	0	0	0	0	0	0	0	0.0	0	0.00	0.00
State and local government	165	378	102	1,358	2,003	180	0	180	60,810	10,104	70,914	55.4	128,006	6,820.46	790.28

*For information on community hospitals that excludes nursing-home-type data, refer to Hospital Units columns in tables 4A through 4D, pages 14 through 17.

(continued on next page)

Table

5C (Continued) Florida

Utilization, Personnel, and Finances in States

Excludes AHA nonregistered hospitals (see Table 14, page 240).

CLASSIFICATION	HOSPITALS	BEDS	ADMISSIONS	INPATIENT DAYS	ADJUSTED PATIENT DAYS	OCCUPANCY, percent	AVERAGE DAILY CENSUS	ADJUSTED AVERAGE DAILY CENSUS	AVERAGE STAY, days	SURGICAL OPERATIONS	OUTPATIENT VISITS: Emergency	OUTPATIENT VISITS: Other	OUTPATIENT VISITS: Total	NEWBORNS: Bassinets	NEWBORNS: Births
FLORIDA	288	62,736	1,769,204	14,581,049		63.7	39,962			1,187,758	4,673,858	10,657,613	15,331,471	2,646	190,345
6-24 beds	3	61	2,647	12,462		55.7	34			1,433	25,788	111,944	137,732	0	0
25-49	27	1,078	23,106	174,917		44.3	478			17,863	90,327	332,933	423,260	22	679
50-99	65	4,601	99,691	926,321		55.3	2,545			54,574	373,421	1,056,020	1,429,441	169	6,596
100-199	82	11,186	325,672	2,336,886		57.3	6,405			244,037	990,234	2,668,425	3,658,659	465	26,810
200-299	46	10,960	343,499	2,355,519		58.9	6,455			232,977	852,278	1,320,139	2,172,417	470	34,354
300-399	24	8,540	264,766	1,951,185		62.6	5,348			186,468	688,810	1,546,380	2,235,190	382	29,824
400-499	14	6,022	196,842	1,445,691		65.8	3,961			131,032	535,839	783,565	1,319,404	270	19,696
500 or more	27	20,288	512,981	5,378,068		72.6	14,736			319,374	1,117,161	2,838,207	3,955,368	868	72,386
Psychiatric	44	7,227	34,102	1,846,555		70.0	5,061			249	11,421	222,067	233,488	0	0
Hospitals	44	7,227	34,102	1,846,555		70.0	5,061			249	11,421	222,067	233,488	0	0
Institutions for mentally retarded	0	0	0	0		00.0	0			0	0	0	0	0	0
General	227	54,004	1,704,486	12,325,668		62.6	33,780			1,163,624	4,654,185	10,118,125	14,772,310	2,589	185,028
Hospitals	226	53,851	1,702,339	12,291,282		62.6	33,686			1,162,789	4,647,210	9,981,348	14,628,558	2,589	185,028
Hospital units of institutions	1	153	2,147	34,386		61.4	94			835	6,975	136,777	143,752	0	0
TB and other respiratory diseases	1	100	234	25,519		70.0	70			3	0	0	0	0	0
Obstetrics and gynecology	1	219	9,163	36,043		45.2	99			7,045	675	4,492	5,167	57	5,317
Eye, ear, nose, and throat	1	38	1,678	3,394		23.7	9			8,233	6,395	84,202	90,597	0	0
Rehabilitation	9	754	7,569	233,800		85.0	641			357	366	118,249	118,615	0	0
Orthopedic	1	60	1,487	15,122		68.3	41			1,003	0	11,158	11,158	0	0
Chronic disease	1	73	386	21,080		79.5	58			43	816	785	1,601	0	0
All other	3	261	10,099	73,868		77.8	203			7,201	0	98,535	98,535	0	0
Federal	13	4,368	91,165	1,171,088		73.5	3,209			79,460	266,879	2,996,367	3,263,246	144	5,040
Psychiatric	0	0	0	0		00.0	0			0	0	0	0	0	0
General and other special	13	4,368	91,165	1,171,088		73.5	3,209			79,460	266,879	2,996,367	3,263,246	144	5,040
Nonfederal	275	58,368	1,678,039	13,409,961		63.0	36,753			1,108,298	4,406,979	7,661,246	12,068,225	2,502	185,305
Psychiatric	44	7,227	34,102	1,846,555		70.0	5,061			249	11,421	222,067	233,488	0	0
Hospitals	44	7,227	34,102	1,846,555		70.0	5,061			249	11,421	222,067	233,488	0	0
Institutions for mentally retarded	0	0	0	0		00.0	0			0	0	0	0	0	0
TB and other respiratory diseases	1	100	234	25,519		70.0	70			3	0	0	0	0	0
Long-term general and other special	5	294	2,685	97,544		91.2	268			63	816	56,644	57,460	0	0
Short-term general and other special	225	50,747	1,641,018	11,440,343		61.8	31,354			1,107,983	4,394,742	7,382,535	11,777,277	2,502	185,305
Hospital units of institutions	1	153	2,147	34,386		61.4	94			835	6,975	136,777	143,752	0	0
Community hospitals*	224	50,594	1,638,871	11,405,957	14,328,466	61.8	31,260	39,258	7.0	1,107,148	4,387,767	7,245,758	11,633,525	2,502	185,305
6-24 beds	2	46	1,761	9,136	15,469	54.3	25	42	5.2	0	1,477	3,719	5,196	0	0
25-49	20	812	20,654	114,561	191,575	38.4	312	524	5.5	17,863	87,051	266,661	353,712	22	679
50-99	36	2,525	69,564	443,033	608,598	48.3	1,219	1,673	6.4	49,218	279,177	382,405	661,582	115	4,950
100-199	65	9,187	285,267	1,920,259	2,535,848	57.3	5,263	6,945	6.7	224,358	837,087	1,225,640	2,062,727	375	23,416
200-299	45	10,760	341,355	2,312,291	2,852,259	58.9	6,337	7,814	6.8	232,977	852,278	1,320,139	2,172,417	470	34,354
300-399	23	8,056	264,632	1,804,164	2,271,998	61.4	4,945	6,223	6.8	186,468	688,810	1,546,380	2,235,190	382	29,824
400-499	13	5,579	190,472	1,321,875	1,630,070	64.9	3,622	4,467	6.9	124,364	535,839	722,187	1,258,026	270	19,696
500 or more	20	13,629	465,166	3,480,638	4,222,649	70.0	9,537	11,570	7.5	271,900	1,106,048	1,778,627	2,884,675	868	72,386
Nongovernment not-for-profit	98	24,886	853,549	5,944,016	7,531,946	65.4	16,285	20,629	7.0	581,496	2,256,202	4,390,222	6,646,424	1,405	103,501
Investor-owned (for-profit)	93	17,576	508,206	3,425,843	4,272,304	53.5	9,397	11,713	6.7	377,185	1,266,338	1,698,313	2,964,651	468	28,659
State and local government	33	8,132	277,116	2,036,098	2,524,216	68.6	5,578	6,916	7.3	148,467	865,227	1,157,223	2,022,450	629	53,145

*For information on community hospitals that excludes nursing-home-type data, refer to Hospital Units columns in tables 4A through 4D, pages 14 through 17.

Table 5C (Continued) **Florida**

CLASSIFICATION	FULL-TIME EQUIVALENT PERSONNEL					FULL-TIME EQUIVALENT TRAINEES			EXPENSES						
									LABOR				TOTAL		
	Physicians and Dentists	Registered Nurses	Licensed Practical Nurses	Other Salaried Personnel	Total Personnel	Medical and Dental Residents	Other Trainees	Total Trainees	Payroll (in thousands)	Employee Benefits (in thousands)	Total (in thousands)	Percent of Total	Amount (in thousands)	Adjusted, per Admission	Adjusted, per Inpatient Day
FLORIDA	1,758	47,290	10,059	142,367	201,474	2,015	172	2,187	$ 5,164,921	$ 1,106,523	$ 6,271,444	50.6	$ 12,401,501		
6-24 beds	30	51	67	309	457	0	0	0	14,711	3,685	18,396	84.8	21,700		
25-49	16	468	167	2,274	2,925	1	3	4	65,867	13,660	79,527	46.1	172,374		
50-99	181	2,399	687	9,180	12,447	11	14	25	295,057	69,581	364,638	50.3	724,873		
100-199	387	7,956	1,751	25,082	35,176	150	14	164	865,324	178,609	1,043,933	46.9	2,226,045		
200-299	92	8,994	1,628	22,600	33,314	91	4	95	862,662	173,616	1,036,278	45.9	2,256,142		
300-399	51	6,992	1,375	19,601	28,019	53	0	53	710,599	141,899	852,498	49.9	1,708,888		
400-499	97	4,853	1,079	14,400	20,429	260	22	282	549,786	111,128	660,913	50.8	1,302,180		
500 or more	904	15,577	3,305	48,921	68,707	1,449	115	1,564	1,800,916	414,345	2,215,261	55.5	3,989,301		
Psychiatric	223	1,445	402	10,716	12,786	8	8	16	277,738	60,061	337,798	63.0	535,925		
Hospitals	223	1,445	402	10,716	12,786	8	8	16	277,738	60,061	337,798	63.0	535,925		
Institutions for mentally retarded	0	0	0	0	0	0	0	0	0	0	0	0.0	0		
General	1,515	44,638	9,425	127,425	183,003	1,979	161	2,140	4,751,929	1,017,035	5,768,963	50.0	11,546,549		
Hospitals	1,498	44,599	9,388	127,300	182,785	1,979	161	2,140	4,746,362	1,015,427	5,761,789	50.0	11,522,873		
Hospital units of institutions	17	39	37	125	218	0	0	0	5,567	1,608	7,175	30.3	23,676		
TB and other respiratory diseases	4	12	12	199	227	0	0	0	3,159	888	4,046	67.3	6,009		
Obstetrics and gynecology	0	250	53	311	614	0	0	0	15,580	3,517	19,097	50.9	37,548		
Eye, ear, nose, and throat	0	54	0	378	432	0	0	0	9,209	1,974	11,183	48.5	23,043		
Rehabilitation	5	262	121	1,380	1,768	0	0	0	45,873	11,012	56,885	52.2	108,920		
Orthopedic	6	62	4	122	194	4	3	7	3,864	759	4,623	53.7	8,616		
Chronic disease	2	25	11	183	221	0	0	0	6,194	1,344	7,538	63.6	11,861		
All other	3	542	31	1,653	2,229	24	0	24	51,376	9,934	61,310	49.8	123,031		
Federal	970	2,183	651	11,607	15,411	506	67	573	430,278	72,189	502,467	66.7	753,816		
Psychiatric	0	0	0	0	0	0	0	0	0	0	0	0.0	0		
General and other special	970	2,183	651	11,607	15,411	506	67	573	430,278	72,189	502,467	66.7	753,816		
Nonfederal	788	45,107	9,408	130,760	186,063	1,509	105	1,614	4,734,644	1,034,334	5,768,978	49.5	11,647,686		
Psychiatric	223	1,445	402	10,716	12,786	8	8	16	277,738	60,061	337,798	63.0	535,925		
Hospitals	223	1,445	402	10,716	12,786	8	8	16	277,738	60,061	337,798	63.0	535,925		
Institutions for mentally retarded	0	0	0	0	0	0	0	0	0	0	0	0.0	0		
TB and other respiratory diseases	4	12	12	199	227	0	0	0	3,159	888	4,046	67.3	6,009		
Long-term general and other special	6	114	95	720	935	0	0	0	24,602	7,568	32,169	51.2	62,868		
Short-term general and other special	555	43,536	8,899	119,125	172,115	1,501	97	1,598	4,429,146	965,818	5,394,964	48.9	11,042,884		
Hospital units of institutions	17	39	37	125	218	0	0	0	5,567	1,608	7,175	30.3	23,676		
Community hospitals*	538	43,497	8,862	119,000	171,897	1,501	97	1,598	4,423,579	964,210	5,387,789	48.9	11,019,208	$5,312.36	$ 769.04
6-24 beds	3	33	13	128	177	0	0	0	4,069	1,622	5,690	67.1	8,476	2,860.55	547.92
25-49	1	397	152	1,711	2,261	1	0	1	49,117	9,470	58,587	43.7	134,018	3,569.62	699.56
50-99	13	1,639	515	5,030	7,197	10	3	13	170,684	41,068	211,753	47.5	446,228	4,570.79	733.21
100-199	56	7,065	1,575	19,333	28,029	54	10	64	694,187	148,879	843,066	45.1	1,870,574	4,941.60	737.65
200-299	89	8,947	1,625	22,343	33,004	91	4	95	855,796	172,263	1,028,059	45.9	2,240,924	5,280.50	785.67
300-399	26	6,925	1,346	18,888	27,185	53	0	53	693,012	138,166	831,178	49.5	1,679,751	5,037.22	739.33
400-499	63	4,725	1,040	13,804	19,632	260	21	281	527,946	106,939	634,885	50.2	1,264,484	5,375.98	775.72
500 or more	287	13,766	2,596	37,763	54,412	1,032	59	1,091	1,428,767	345,803	1,774,570	52.6	3,374,754	5,977.92	799.20
Nongovernment not-for-profit	223	24,293	4,323	67,717	96,556	729	51	780	2,468,225	489,918	2,958,143	50.6	5,850,568	5,354.00	776.77
Investor-owned (for-profit)	34	12,057	2,907	29,788	44,786	29	9	38	1,135,504	244,894	1,380,398	42.5	3,249,003	5,107.25	760.48
State and local government	281	7,147	1,632	21,495	30,555	743	37	780	819,850	229,398	1,049,248	54.7	1,919,637	5,558.40	760.49

*For information on community hospitals that excludes nursing-home-type data, refer to Hospital Units columns in tables 4A through 4D, pages 14 through 17.

(continued on next page)

Table

5C (Continued) Georgia

Utilization, Personnel, and Finances in States

Excludes AHA nonregistered hospitals (see Table 14, page 240).

CLASSIFICATION	HOSPITALS	BEDS	ADMISSIONS	INPATIENT DAYS	ADJUSTED PATIENT DAYS	OCCUPANCY, percent	AVERAGE DAILY CENSUS	ADJUSTED AVERAGE DAILY CENSUS	AVERAGE STAY, days	SURGICAL OPERATIONS	OUTPATIENT VISITS: Emergency	OUTPATIENT VISITS: Other	OUTPATIENT VISITS: Total	NEWBORNS: Bassinets	NEWBORNS: Births
GEORGIA	203	34,681	989,479	8,594,215		67.9	23,555			626,828	3,041,183	6,195,292	9,236,475	2,063	109,673
6-24 beds	7	134	2,847	17,002		35.1	47			3,626	12,003	38,591	50,594	10	102
25-49	39	1,486	40,061	229,054		42.1	626			14,825	205,732	291,210	496,942	113	2,634
50-99	49	3,374	75,246	654,959		53.3	1,797			34,635	280,738	541,129	821,867	193	5,129
100-199	54	7,340	232,762	1,788,866		66.8	4,903			164,121	749,669	1,186,903	1,936,572	538	25,726
200-299	18	4,406	132,477	1,036,183		64.5	2,841			90,150	361,679	1,107,428	1,469,107	221	11,434
300-399	17	5,604	180,529	1,553,166		75.9	4,256			109,832	532,738	669,671	1,202,409	365	18,708
400-499	6	2,806	101,313	721,843		70.5	1,978			63,667	171,355	810,706	982,061	247	17,094
500 or more	13	9,531	224,244	2,593,142		74.6	7,107			145,972	727,269	1,549,654	2,276,923	376	28,846
Psychiatric	27	5,948	37,849	1,652,826		76.1	4,529			536	3,646	73,029	76,675	0	0
Hospitals	27	5,948	37,849	1,652,826		76.1	4,529			536	3,646	73,029	76,675	0	0
Institutions for mentally retarded	0	0	0	0		00.0	0			0	0	0	0	0	0
General	171	28,358	945,288	6,864,664		66.3	18,815			618,442	3,037,537	6,094,827	9,132,364	2,063	109,673
Hospitals	168	28,167	941,763	6,819,772		66.4	18,692			616,842	3,018,614	5,921,981	8,940,595	2,063	109,673
Hospital units of institutions	3	191	3,525	44,892		64.4	123			1,600	18,923	172,846	191,769	0	0
TB and other respiratory diseases	0	0	0	0		00.0	0			0	0	0	0	0	0
Obstetrics and gynecology	0	0	0	0		00.0	0			0	0	0	0	0	0
Eye, ear, nose, and throat	0	0	0	0		00.0	0			0	0	0	0	0	0
Rehabilitation	3	211	1,502	58,121		75.8	160			0	0	18,182	18,182	0	0
Orthopedic	1	100	3,209	15,684		43.0	43			3,688	0	5,625	5,625	0	0
Chronic disease	0	0	0	0		00.0	0			0	0	0	0	0	0
All other	1	64	1,631	2,920		12.5	8			4,162	0	3,629	3,629	0	0
Federal	9	2,931	61,420	740,823		69.3	2,030			52,570	231,980	2,018,660	2,250,640	64	3,457
Psychiatric	0	0	0	0		00.0	0			0	0	0	0	0	0
General and other special	9	2,931	61,420	740,823		69.3	2,030			52,570	231,980	2,018,660	2,250,640	64	3,457
Nonfederal	194	31,750	928,059	7,853,392		67.8	21,525			574,258	2,809,203	4,176,632	6,985,835	1,999	106,216
Psychiatric	27	5,948	37,849	1,652,826		76.1	4,529			536	3,646	73,029	76,675	0	0
Hospitals	27	5,948	37,849	1,652,826		76.1	4,529			536	3,646	73,029	76,675	0	0
Institutions for mentally retarded	0	0	0	0		00.0	0			0	0	0	0	0	0
TB and other respiratory diseases	0	0	0	0		00.0	0			0	0	0	0	0	0
Long-term general and other special	2	161	1,046	43,982		75.2	121			0	0	9,013	9,013	0	0
Short-term general and other special	165	25,641	889,164	6,156,584		65.8	16,875			573,722	2,805,557	4,094,590	6,900,147	1,999	106,216
Hospital units of institutions	2	141	1,116	35,609		69.5	98			285	2,894	48,413	51,307	0	0
Community hospitals*	163	25,500	888,048	6,120,975	7,937,120	65.8	16,777	21,747	6.9	573,437	2,802,663	4,046,177	6,848,840	1,999	106,216
6-24 beds	6	114	2,380	15,640	22,210	37.7	43	59	6.6	925	8,354	13,324	21,678	2	14
25-49	34	1,311	37,193	173,717	255,800	36.2	475	702	4.7	13,745	187,224	206,926	394,150	105	2,404
50-99	34	2,286	63,035	370,921	522,766	44.6	1,019	1,432	5.9	33,035	261,101	326,526	587,627	193	5,129
100-199	49	6,755	221,973	1,650,384	2,202,620	67.0	4,524	6,038	7.4	152,672	707,612	850,379	1,557,991	516	24,376
200-299	13	3,253	112,151	731,031	935,058	61.6	2,003	2,560	6.5	80,212	299,467	466,273	765,740	205	10,360
300-399	14	4,554	169,995	1,216,353	1,544,623	73.2	3,333	4,232	7.2	109,832	532,738	669,671	1,202,409	365	18,708
400-499	4	1,902	79,056	488,608	600,536	70.4	1,339	1,645	6.2	54,087	129,468	228,920	358,388	237	16,379
500 or more	9	5,325	202,265	1,474,321	1,853,507	75.9	4,041	5,079	7.3	128,929	676,699	1,284,158	1,960,857	376	28,846
Nongovernment not-for-profit	39	8,625	323,629	2,281,050	2,798,680	72.5	6,254	7,669	7.0	226,967	802,839	1,160,071	1,962,910	661	33,811
Investor-owned (for-profit)	39	4,593	148,868	884,909	1,147,844	52.8	2,426	3,145	5.9	110,690	391,641	575,419	967,060	264	13,827
State and local government	85	12,282	415,551	2,955,016	3,990,596	65.9	8,097	10,933	7.1	235,780	1,608,183	2,310,687	3,918,870	1,074	58,578

*For information on community hospitals that excludes nursing-home-type data, refer to Hospital Units columns in tables 4A through 4D, pages 14 through 17.

Table 5C (Continued) **Georgia**

CLASSIFICATION	FULL-TIME EQUIVALENT PERSONNEL					FULL-TIME EQUIVALENT TRAINEES			EXPENSES						
									LABOR				TOTAL		
	Physicians and Dentists	Registered Nurses	Licensed Practical Nurses	Other Salaried Personnel	Total Personnel	Medical and Dental Residents	Other Trainees	Total Trainees	Payroll (in thousands)	Employee Benefits (in thousands)	Total (in thousands)	Percent of Total	Amount (in thousands)	Adjusted, per Admission	Adjusted, per Inpatient Day
GEORGIA	1,369	22,558	6,997	79,982	110,906	1,973	109	2,082	$ 2,702,392	$ 534,934	$ 3,237,326	53.5	$ 6,046,028		
6-24 beds	34	79	27	503	643	3	0	3	7,699	1,335	9,034	56.9	15,869		
25-49	30	553	376	2,837	3,796	3	3	6	75,628	14,427	90,055	51.4	175,329		
50-99	74	1,388	680	5,947	8,089	1	4	5	174,449	33,761	208,210	48.8	426,957		
100-199	68	5,040	1,582	15,505	22,195	45	0	45	503,932	98,602	602,534	50.2	1,201,064		
200-299	109	2,549	932	9,867	13,457	36	8	44	324,717	61,695	386,412	49.1	786,241		
300-399	73	4,790	1,209	13,329	19,401	48	41	89	473,012	94,979	567,990	54.6	1,039,849		
400-499	266	2,142	423	7,598	10,429	170	36	206	305,604	53,038	358,642	57.3	626,445		
500 or more	715	6,017	1,768	24,396	32,896	1,667	17	1,684	837,352	177,097	1,014,448	57.2	1,774,274		
Psychiatric	163	1,003	542	8,492	10,200	17	4	21	244,961	68,625	313,586	63.2	495,945		
Hospitals	163	1,003	542	8,492	10,200	17	4	21	244,961	68,625	313,586	63.2	495,945		
Institutions for mentally retarded	0	0	0	0	0	0	0	0	0	0	0	0.0	0		
General	1,197	21,358	6,395	70,406	99,356	1,956	105	2,061	2,430,548	460,284	2,890,833	52.8	5,475,480		
Hospitals	1,155	21,274	6,347	69,931	98,707	1,956	105	2,061	2,418,827	457,644	2,876,471	52.8	5,451,053		
Hospital units of institutions	42	84	48	475	649	0	0	0	11,721	2,641	14,362	58.8	24,427		
TB and other respiratory diseases	0	0	0	0	0	0	0	0	0	0	0	0.0	0		
Obstetrics and gynecology	0	0	0	0	0	0	0	0	0	0	0	0.0	0		
Eye, ear, nose, and throat	0	0	0	0	0	0	0	0	0	0	0	0.0	0		
Rehabilitation	9	112	38	801	960	0	0	0	19,029	4,223	23,253	55.1	42,197		
Orthopedic	0	65	13	214	292	0	0	0	4,998	1,115	6,112	29.2	20,907		
Chronic disease	0	0	0	0	0	0	0	0	0	0	0	0.0	0		
All other	0	20	9	69	98	0	0	0	2,856	686	3,542	30.8	11,500		
Federal	634	1,361	678	7,568	10,241	553	19	572	304,483	36,304	340,787	67.6	503,869		
Psychiatric	0	0	0	0	0	0	0	0	0	0	0	0.0	0		
General and other special	634	1,361	678	7,568	10,241	553	19	572	304,483	36,304	340,787	67.6	503,869		
Nonfederal	735	21,197	6,319	72,414	100,665	1,420	90	1,510	2,397,909	498,629	2,896,539	52.3	5,542,160		
Psychiatric	163	1,003	542	8,492	10,200	17	4	21	244,961	68,625	313,586	63.2	495,945		
Hospitals	163	1,003	542	8,492	10,200	17	4	21	244,961	68,625	313,586	63.2	495,945		
Institutions for mentally retarded	0	0	0	0	0	0	0	0	0	0	0	0.0	0		
TB and other respiratory diseases	0	0	0	0	0	0	0	0	0	0	0	0.0	0		
Long-term general and other special	7	87	27	642	763	0	0	0	15,547	3,079	18,627	54.5	34,203		
Short-term general and other special	565	20,107	5,750	63,280	89,702	1,403	86	1,489	2,137,401	426,926	2,564,326	51.2	5,012,012		
Hospital units of institutions	14	41	36	203	294	0	0	0	4,284	1,333	5,617	47.9	11,723		
Community hospitals*	551	20,066	5,714	63,077	89,408	1,403	86	1,489	2,133,117	425,592	2,558,709	51.2	5,000,289	$4,302.95	$ 629.99
6-24 beds	2	42	25	196	265	3	0	3	4,289	575	4,865	49.0	9,921	2,954.30	446.67
25-49	1	481	357	2,379	3,218	3	3	6	62,958	11,877	74,836	51.2	146,193	2,651.40	571.51
50-99	10	1,002	561	3,769	5,342	0	0	0	110,348	20,327	130,675	46.7	279,835	3,105.62	535.30
100-199	20	4,794	1,502	14,218	20,534	37	0	37	462,021	92,950	554,971	49.8	1,113,607	3,717.40	505.58
200-299	2	2,212	772	7,397	10,383	0	8	8	230,847	46,610	277,456	45.1	614,598	4,275.20	657.28
300-399	23	4,569	1,088	11,677	17,357	43	41	84	423,271	80,237	503,508	52.9	951,193	4,402.06	615.81
400-499	19	1,703	235	5,381	7,338	35	26	61	201,764	43,168	244,932	53.3	459,652	4,704.58	765.40
500 or more	474	5,263	1,174	18,060	24,971	1,282	8	1,290	637,619	129,847	767,466	53.8	1,425,292	5,559.92	768.97
Nongovernment not-for-profit	158	8,354	1,840	25,766	36,118	461	30	491	888,408	184,749	1,073,158	51.9	2,066,563	5,125.33	738.41
Investor-owned (for-profit)	3	2,753	919	8,192	11,867	16	0	16	274,398	64,940	339,337	42.0	808,244	4,150.97	704.14
State and local government	390	8,959	2,955	29,119	41,423	926	56	982	970,311	175,903	1,146,214	53.9	2,125,483	3,767.64	532.62

*For information on community hospitals that excludes nursing-home-type data, refer to Hospital Units columns in tables 4A through 4D, pages 14 through 17.

(continued on next page)

Table
5C (Continued) Hawaii

Utilization, Personnel, and Finances in States

Excludes AHA nonregistered hospitals (see Table 14, page 240).

CLASSIFICATION	HOSPITALS	BEDS	ADMISSIONS	INPATIENT DAYS	ADJUSTED PATIENT DAYS	OCCUPANCY, percent	AVERAGE DAILY CENSUS	ADJUSTED AVERAGE DAILY CENSUS	AVERAGE STAY, days	SURGICAL OPERATIONS	OUTPATIENT VISITS Emergency	OUTPATIENT VISITS Other	OUTPATIENT VISITS Total	NEWBORNS Bassinets	NEWBORNS Births
HAWAII	26	4,093	118,199	1,241,579		83.0	3,399			71,303	325,820	2,362,145	2,687,965	260	19,842
6-24 beds	2	29	143	7,030		65.5	19			0	1,418	3,567	4,985	4	9
25-49	6	196	2,727	43,098		59.7	117			1,917	12,496	19,041	31,537	21	358
50-99	3	231	3,935	67,056		79.7	184			2,078	7,809	57,903	65,712	10	642
100-199	7	1,077	29,539	327,821		83.3	897			18,799	83,467	149,678	233,145	62	3,612
200-299	5	1,175	38,368	371,716		86.6	1,018			21,175	85,010	1,224,041	1,309,051	91	9,548
300-399	0	0	0	0		00.0	0			0	0	0	0	0	0
400-499	3	1,385	43,487	424,858		84.0	1,164			27,334	135,620	907,915	1,043,535	72	5,673
500 or more	0	0	0	0		00.0	0			0	0	0	0	0	0
Psychiatric	1	205	811	73,154		97.6	200			0	0	0	0	0	0
Hospitals	1	205	811	73,154		97.6	200			0	0	0	0	0	0
Institutions for mentally retarded	0	0	0	0		00.0	0			0	0	0	0	0	0
General	18	3,136	102,009	958,154		83.7	2,624			65,060	304,238	2,246,935	2,551,173	208	13,848
Hospitals	18	3,136	102,009	958,154		83.7	2,624			65,060	304,238	2,246,935	2,551,173	208	13,848
Hospital units of institutions	0	0	0	0		00.0	0			0	0	0	0	0	0
TB and other respiratory diseases	1	192	128	46,534		66.1	127			0	0	363	363	0	0
Obstetrics and gynecology	0	0	0	0		00.0	0			0	0	0	0	0	0
Eye, ear, nose, and throat	0	0	0	0		00.0	0			0	0	0	0	0	0
Rehabilitation	1	86	455	24,834		79.1	68			0	0	30,625	30,625	0	0
Orthopedic	1	40	216	5,625		37.5	15			259	0	1,913	1,913	0	0
Chronic disease	0	0	0	0		00.0	0			0	0	0	0	0	0
All other	4	434	14,580	133,278		84.1	365			5,984	21,582	82,309	103,891	52	5,994
Federal	1	483	20,237	130,482		73.9	357			9,420	103,059	764,598	867,657	37	3,378
Psychiatric	0	0	0	0		00.0	0			0	0	0	0	0	0
General and other special	1	483	20,237	130,482		73.9	357			9,420	103,059	764,598	867,657	37	3,378
Nonfederal	25	3,610	97,962	1,111,097		84.3	3,042			61,883	222,761	1,597,547	1,820,308	223	16,464
Psychiatric	1	205	811	73,154		97.6	200			0	0	0	0	0	0
Hospitals	1	205	811	73,154		97.6	200			0	0	0	0	0	0
Institutions for mentally retarded	0	0	0	0		00.0	0			0	0	0	0	0	0
TB and other respiratory diseases	1	192	128	46,534		66.1	127			0	0	363	363	0	0
Long-term general and other special	5	326	1,065	94,744		79.4	259			259	886	36,684	37,570	2	2
Short-term general and other special	18	2,887	95,958	896,665		85.1	2,456			61,624	221,875	1,560,500	1,782,375	221	16,462
Hospital units of institutions	0	0	0	0		00.0	0			0	0	0	0	0	0
Community hospitals*	18	2,887	95,958	896,665	1,126,889	85.1	2,456	3,089	9.3	61,624	221,875	1,560,500	1,782,375	221	16,462
6-24 beds	1	14	98	2,845	2,845	57.1	8	8	29.0	0	575	1,107	1,682	2	7
25-49	5	156	2,511	37,473	54,926	65.4	102	151	14.9	1,658	12,496	17,128	29,624	21	358
50-99	1	61	3,249	17,755	22,194	80.3	49	61	5.5	2,078	7,809	26,586	34,395	10	642
100-199	5	784	29,293	245,654	312,024	85.7	672	854	8.4	18,799	83,424	148,321	231,745	62	3,612
200-299	4	970	37,557	298,562	378,147	84.3	818	1,037	7.9	21,175	85,010	1,224,041	1,309,051	91	9,548
300-399	0	0	0	0	0	00.0	0	0	0.0	0	0	0	0	0	0
400-499	2	902	23,250	294,376	356,753	89.5	807	978	12.7	17,914	32,561	143,317	175,878	35	2,295
500 or more	0	0	0	0	0	00.0	0	0	0.0	0	0	0	0	0	0
Nongovernment not-for-profit	10	2,136	67,496	671,681	871,121	86.1	1,840	2,388	10.0	44,027	148,451	1,472,587	1,621,038	159	12,815
Investor-owned (for-profit)	1	159	7,644	54,921	72,584	94.3	150	199	7.2	4,442	27,088	40,038	67,126	0	0
State and local government	7	592	20,818	170,063	183,184	78.7	466	502	8.2	13,155	46,336	47,875	94,211	62	3,647

*For information on community hospitals that excludes nursing-home-type data, refer to Hospital Units columns in tables 4A through 4D, pages 14 through 17.

CLASSIFICATION	FULL-TIME EQUIVALENT PERSONNEL: Physicians and Dentists	Registered Nurses	Licensed Practical Nurses	Other Salaried Personnel	Total Personnel	FULL-TIME EQUIVALENT TRAINEES: Medical and Dental Residents	Other Trainees	Total Trainees	EXPENSES: LABOR: Payroll (in thousands)	Employee Benefits (in thousands)	Total (in thousands)	Percent of Total	TOTAL: Amount (in thousands)	Adjusted, per Admission	Adjusted, per Inpatient Day
HAWAII	226	3,374	808	12,027	16,435	198	7	205	$ 472,456	$ 75,536	$ 547,992	58.1	$ 943,048		
6-24 beds	0	13	4	43	60	0	0	0	1,650	213	1,863	64.1	2,909		
25-49	1	96	42	364	503	2	0	2	13,081	2,396	15,477	56.7	27,310		
50-99	5	125	41	476	647	0	0	0	17,851	3,096	20,947	60.2	34,810		
100-199	14	758	227	2,750	3,749	0	0	0	92,052	18,912	110,964	53.1	208,834		
200-299	24	1,027	265	4,046	5,362	28	2	30	115,282	22,101	137,383	54.4	252,317		
300-399	0	0	0	0	0	0	0	0	0	0	0	0.0	0		
400-499	182	1,355	229	4,348	6,114	168	5	173	232,540	28,817	261,357	62.7	416,867		
500 or more	0	0	0	0	0	0	0	0	0	0	0	0.0	0		
Psychiatric	2	61	44	318	425	0	0	0	10,933	1,352	12,285	80.0	15,352		
Hospitals	2	61	44	318	425	0	0	0	10,933	1,352	12,285	80.0	15,352		
Institutions for mentally retarded	0	0	0	0	0	0	0	0	0	0	0	0.0	0		
General	198	2,865	629	9,748	13,440	195	7	202	395,348	61,492	456,839	58.0	787,652		
Hospitals	198	2,865	629	9,748	13,440	195	7	202	395,348	61,492	456,839	58.0	787,652		
Hospital units of institutions	0	0	0	0	0	0	0	0	0	0	0	0.0	0		
TB and other respiratory diseases	11	53	40	412	516	0	0	0	10,648	2,291	12,939	62.8	20,609		
Obstetrics and gynecology	0	0	0	0	0	0	0	0	0	0	0	0.0	0		
Eye, ear, nose, and throat	0	0	0	0	0	0	0	0	0	0	0	0.0	0		
Rehabilitation	3	29	13	216	261	0	0	0	7,297	1,583	8,881	63.6	13,973		
Orthopedic	1	29	7	64	101	2	0	2	3,394	736	4,131	63.6	6,499		
Chronic disease	0	0	0	0	0	0	0	0	0	0	0	0.0	0		
All other	11	337	75	1,269	1,692	1	0	1	44,836	8,081	52,917	53.5	98,962		
Federal	179	510	181	1,746	2,616	168	0	168	118,452	6,649	125,101	81.3	153,849		
Psychiatric	0	0	0	0	0	0	0	0	0	0	0	0.0	0		
General and other special	179	510	181	1,746	2,616	168	0	168	118,452	6,649	125,101	81.3	153,849		
Nonfederal	47	2,864	627	10,281	13,819	30	7	37	354,004	68,887	422,891	53.6	789,198		
Psychiatric	2	61	44	318	425	0	0	0	10,933	1,352	12,285	80.0	15,352		
Hospitals	2	61	44	318	425	0	0	0	10,933	1,352	12,285	80.0	15,352		
Institutions for mentally retarded	0	0	0	0	0	0	0	0	0	0	0	0.0	0		
TB and other respiratory diseases	11	53	40	412	516	0	0	0	10,648	2,291	12,939	62.8	20,609		
Long-term general and other special	8	83	46	563	700	2	0	2	19,070	3,602	22,672	65.3	34,714		
Short-term general and other special	26	2,667	497	8,988	12,178	28	7	35	313,353	61,641	374,994	52.2	718,524		
Hospital units of institutions	0	0	0	0	0	0	0	0	0	0	0	0.0	0		
Community hospitals*	26	2,667	497	8,988	12,178	28	7	35	313,353	61,641	374,994	52.2	718,524	$ 6,048.48	$ 637.62
6-24 beds	0	7	0	21	28	0	0	0	674	81	755	58.0	1,303	13,293.58	457.92
25-49	0	67	35	300	402	0	0	0	9,687	1,659	11,347	54.5	20,811	5,626.12	378.89
50-99	0	77	6	154	237	0	0	0	6,946	1,032	7,978	53.6	14,876	3,663.06	670.26
100-199	1	705	187	2,183	3,076	0	0	0	77,609	15,952	93,561	51.5	181,552	5,063.78	581.85
200-299	22	966	221	3,728	4,937	28	2	30	104,349	20,749	125,098	52.8	236,964	4,999.46	626.65
300-399	0	0	0	0	0	0	0	0	0	0	0	0.0	0	0.00	0.00
400-499	3	845	48	2,602	3,498	0	5	5	114,088	22,168	136,256	51.8	263,018	9,500.38	737.26
500 or more	0	0	0	0	0	0	0	0	0	0	0	0.0	0	0.00	0.00
Nongovernment not-for-profit	25	2,044	294	7,181	9,544	28	7	35	248,026	50,000	298,026	53.3	559,018	6,462.64	641.72
Investor-owned (for-profit)	0	216	63	703	982	0	0	0	21,168	4,767	25,935	43.0	60,259	5,965.07	830.20
State and local government	1	407	140	1,104	1,652	0	0	0	44,160	6,874	51,034	51.4	99,246	4,472.16	541.78

*For information on community hospitals that excludes nursing-home-type data, refer to Hospital Units columns in tables 4A through 4D, pages 14 through 17.

(continued on next page)

Table
5C (Continued) Idaho

Utilization, Personnel, and Finances in States
Excludes AHA nonregistered hospitals (see Table 14, page 240).

CLASSIFICATION	HOSPITALS	BEDS	ADMISSIONS	INPATIENT DAYS	ADJUSTED PATIENT DAYS	OCCUPANCY, percent	AVERAGE DAILY CENSUS	ADJUSTED AVERAGE DAILY CENSUS	AVERAGE STAY, days	SURGICAL OPERATIONS	OUTPATIENT VISITS Emergency	OUTPATIENT VISITS Other	OUTPATIENT VISITS Total	NEWBORNS Bassinets	NEWBORNS Births
IDAHO	50	3,893	103,428	861,915		60.7	2,362			75,730	299,461	943,573	1,243,034	326	15,541
6-24 beds	10	194	5,511	30,693		43.8	85			3,043	27,943	133,365	161,308	39	746
25-49	14	493	9,013	85,326		47.3	233			4,095	31,391	97,047	128,438	57	981
50-99	12	810	16,247	174,271		59.0	478			8,055	51,147	109,972	161,119	76	2,779
100-199	10	1,394	37,668	314,349		61.8	861			33,431	110,332	364,397	474,729	93	5,827
200-299	4	1,002	34,989	257,276		70.4	705			27,106	78,648	238,792	317,440	61	5,208
300-399	0	0	0	0		00.0	0			0	0	0	0	0	0
400-499	0	0	0	0		00.0	0			0	0	0	0	0	0
500 or more	0	0	0	0		00.0	0			0	0	0	0	0	0
Psychiatric	5	491	1,724	159,532		89.0	437			0	0	0	0	0	0
Hospitals	4	286	1,716	84,570		81.1	232			0	0	0	0	0	0
Institutions for mentally retarded	1	205	8	74,962		100.0	205			0	0	0	0	0	0
General	44	3,352	101,032	691,876		56.6	1,896			75,730	299,461	918,881	1,218,342	326	15,541
Hospitals	44	3,352	101,032	691,876		56.6	1,896			75,730	299,461	918,881	1,218,342	326	15,541
Hospital units of institutions	0	0	0	0		00.0	0			0	0	0	0	0	0
TB and other respiratory diseases	0	0	0	0		00.0	0			0	0	0	0	0	0
Obstetrics and gynecology	0	0	0	0		00.0	0			0	0	0	0	0	0
Eye, ear, nose, and throat	0	0	0	0		00.0	0			0	0	0	0	0	0
Rehabilitation	1	50	672	10,507		58.0	29			0	0	24,692	24,692	0	0
Orthopedic	0	0	0	0		00.0	0			0	0	0	0	0	0
Chronic disease	0	0	0	0		00.0	0			0	0	0	0	0	0
All other	0	0	0	0		00.0	0			0	0	0	0	0	0
Federal	2	202	5,083	51,725		70.3	142			5,925	14,649	173,726	188,375	10	338
Psychiatric	0	0	0	0		00.0	0			0	0	0	0	0	0
General and other special	2	202	5,083	51,725		70.3	142			5,925	14,649	173,726	188,375	10	338
Nonfederal	48	3,691	98,345	810,190		60.1	2,220			69,805	284,812	769,847	1,054,659	316	15,203
Psychiatric	5	491	1,724	159,532		89.0	437			0	0	0	0	0	0
Hospitals	4	286	1,716	84,570		81.1	232			0	0	0	0	0	0
Institutions for mentally retarded	1	205	8	74,962		100.0	205			0	0	0	0	0	0
TB and other respiratory diseases	0	0	0	0		00.0	0			0	0	0	0	0	0
Long-term general and other special	0	0	0	0		00.0	0			0	0	0	0	0	0
Short-term general and other special	43	3,200	96,621	650,658		55.7	1,783			69,805	284,812	769,847	1,054,659	316	15,203
Hospital units of institutions	0	0	0	0		00.0	0			0	0	0	0	0	0
Community hospitals*	43	3,200	96,621	650,658	936,588	55.7	1,783	2,568	6.7	69,805	284,812	769,847	1,054,659	316	15,203
6-24 beds	8	152	3,589	20,892	34,383	38.2	58	94	5.8	1,986	13,294	37,193	50,487	29	408
25-49	13	461	8,721	75,818	121,593	44.9	207	333	8.7	4,095	31,391	97,047	128,438	57	981
50-99	11	735	15,352	157,237	228,078	58.6	431	626	10.2	8,055	51,147	109,972	161,119	76	2,779
100-199	8	1,055	33,978	214,397	303,693	55.6	587	833	6.3	28,563	110,332	286,843	397,175	93	5,827
200-299	3	797	34,981	182,314	248,841	62.7	500	682	5.2	27,106	78,648	238,792	317,440	61	5,208
300-399	0	0	0	0	0	00.0	0	0	0.0	0	0	0	0	0	0
400-499	0	0	0	0	0	00.0	0	0	0.0	0	0	0	0	0	0
500 or more	0	0	0	0	0	00.0	0	0	0.0	0	0	0	0	0	0
Nongovernment not-for-profit	11	1,242	47,060	257,721	370,237	57.0	708	1,015	5.5	36,631	122,142	405,801	527,943	97	6,934
Investor-owned (for-profit)	3	409	14,550	78,217	100,986	52.3	214	277	5.4	8,711	33,984	52,748	86,732	32	2,157
State and local government	29	1,549	35,011	314,720	465,365	55.6	861	1,276	9.0	24,463	128,686	311,298	439,984	187	6,112

*For information on community hospitals that excludes nursing-home-type data, refer to Hospital Units columns in tables 4A through 4D, pages 14 through 17.

CLASSIFICATION	FULL-TIME EQUIVALENT PERSONNEL					FULL-TIME EQUIVALENT TRAINEES			EXPENSES: LABOR				EXPENSES: TOTAL		
	Physicians and Dentists	Registered Nurses	Licensed Practical Nurses	Other Salaried Personnel	Total Personnel	Medical and Dental Residents	Other Trainees	Total Trainees	Payroll (in thousands)	Employee Benefits (in thousands)	Total (in thousands)	Percent of Total	Amount (in thousands)	Adjusted, per Admission	Adjusted, per Inpatient Day
IDAHO	65	2,667	764	8,134	11,630	2	34	36	$ 268,242	$ 52,128	$ 320,370	53.9	$ 594,861		
6-24 beds	22	106	29	511	668	0	0	0	16,475	3,166	19,641	70.9	27,694		
25-49	1	190	73	688	952	0	1	1	19,755	3,935	23,689	56.8	41,723		
50-99	4	357	104	1,217	1,682	0	0	0	34,600	7,137	41,737	55.4	75,332		
100-199	36	921	326	2,898	4,181	2	9	11	100,225	20,497	120,722	54.4	222,020		
200-299	2	1,093	232	2,820	4,147	0	24	24	97,188	17,392	114,580	50.2	228,092		
300-399	0	0	0	0	0	0	0	0	0	0	0	0.0	0		
400-499	0	0	0	0	0	0	0	0	0	0	0	0.0	0		
500 or more	0	0	0	0	0	0	0	0	0	0	0	0.0	0		
Psychiatric	7	66	67	913	1,053	0	12	12	21,918	5,845	27,763	72.4	38,328		
Hospitals	5	46	27	380	458	0	0	0	10,490	2,757	13,247	65.9	20,117		
Institutions for mentally retarded	2	20	40	533	595	0	12	12	11,428	3,087	14,515	79.7	18,211		
General	55	2,593	687	7,125	10,460	2	22	24	242,919	45,789	288,708	52.4	551,091		
Hospitals	55	2,593	687	7,125	10,460	2	22	24	242,919	45,789	288,708	52.4	551,091		
Hospital units of institutions	0	0	0	0	0	0	0	0	0	0	0	0.0	0		
TB and other respiratory diseases	0	0	0	0	0	0	0	0	0	0	0	0.0	0		
Obstetrics and gynecology	0	0	0	0	0	0	0	0	0	0	0	0.0	0		
Eye, ear, nose, and throat	0	0	0	0	0	0	0	0	0	0	0	0.0	0		
Rehabilitation	3	8	10	96	117	0	0	0	3,405	494	3,899	71.6	5,442		
Orthopedic	0	0	0	0	0	0	0	0	0	0	0	0.0	0		
Chronic disease	0	0	0	0	0	0	0	0	0	0	0	0.0	0		
All other	0	0	0	0	0	0	0	0	0	0	0	0.0	0		
Federal	54	145	17	699	915	2	9	11	26,950	5,117	32,067	72.5	44,254		
Psychiatric	0	0	0	0	0	0	0	0	0	0	0	0.0	0		
General and other special	54	145	17	699	915	2	9	11	26,950	5,117	32,067	72.5	44,254		
Nonfederal	11	2,522	747	7,435	10,715	0	25	25	241,293	47,010	288,303	52.4	550,607		
Psychiatric	7	66	67	913	1,053	0	12	12	21,918	5,845	27,763	72.4	38,328		
Hospitals	5	46	27	380	458	0	0	0	10,490	2,757	13,247	65.9	20,117		
Institutions for mentally retarded	2	20	40	533	595	0	12	12	11,428	3,087	14,515	79.7	18,211		
TB and other respiratory diseases	0	0	0	0	0	0	0	0	0	0	0	0.0	0		
Long-term general and other special	0	0	0	0	0	0	0	0	0	0	0	0.0	0		
Short-term general and other special	4	2,456	680	6,522	9,662	0	13	13	219,375	41,165	260,540	50.9	512,279		
Hospital units of institutions	0	0	0	0	0	0	0	0	0	0	0	0.0	0		
Community hospitals*	4	2,456	680	6,522	9,662	0	13	13	219,375	41,165	260,540	50.9	512,279	$3,700.85	$ 546.96
6-24 beds	0	65	22	252	339	0	0	0	7,063	1,511	8,574	54.4	15,755	2,599.01	458.23
25-49	1	181	70	666	918	0	1	1	19,052	3,745	22,797	56.8	40,143	2,755.19	330.14
50-99	3	339	101	1,111	1,554	0	0	0	30,976	6,369	37,345	55.4	67,370	3,011.09	295.38
100-199	0	798	295	2,206	3,299	0	0	0	76,524	15,236	91,760	51.2	179,130	3,761.73	589.84
200-299	0	1,073	192	2,287	3,552	0	12	12	85,760	14,305	100,065	47.7	209,881	4,391.09	843.43
300-399	0	0	0	0	0	0	0	0	0	0	0	0.0	0	0.00	0.00
400-499	0	0	0	0	0	0	0	0	0	0	0	0.0	0	0.00	0.00
500 or more	0	0	0	0	0	0	0	0	0	0	0	0.0	0	0.00	0.00
Nongovernment not-for-profit	3	1,363	230	3,169	4,765	0	12	12	116,186	19,870	136,056	51.9	261,958	3,866.42	707.54
Investor-owned (for-profit)	0	317	145	826	1,288	0	0	0	28,456	6,391	34,847	42.5	81,901	4,335.91	811.01
State and local government	1	776	305	2,527	3,609	0	1	1	74,733	14,904	89,637	53.2	168,421	3,252.56	361.91

*For information on community hospitals that excludes nursing-home-type data, refer to Hospital Units columns in tables 4A through 4D, pages 14 through 17.

(continued on next page)

Table

5C (Continued) Illinois

Utilization, Personnel, and Finances in States

Excludes AHA nonregistered hospitals (see Table 14, page 240).

CLASSIFICATION	HOSPITALS	BEDS	ADMISSIONS	INPATIENT DAYS	ADJUSTED PATIENT DAYS	OCCUPANCY, percent	AVERAGE DAILY CENSUS	ADJUSTED AVERAGE DAILY CENSUS	AVERAGE STAY, days	SURGICAL OPERATIONS	OUTPATIENT VISITS Emergency	OUTPATIENT VISITS Other	OUTPATIENT VISITS Total	NEWBORNS Bassinets	NEWBORNS Births
ILLINOIS	247	58,056	1,608,893	14,605,851		68.9	40,025			1,058,198	4,212,719	14,444,772	18,657,491	3,452	188,088
6-24 beds	4	89	1,798	7,244		22.5	20			910	31,977	169,423	201,400	0	0
25-49	13	531	14,794	79,003		40.9	217			6,187	63,921	133,366	197,287	32	476
50-99	53	3,861	101,579	747,004		52.9	2,043			46,654	298,736	1,237,658	1,536,394	236	5,202
100-199	70	9,942	273,419	2,202,721		60.7	6,038			178,538	840,655	2,243,646	3,084,301	678	31,170
200-299	42	10,565	334,315	2,650,852		68.8	7,265			225,992	857,046	2,617,779	3,474,825	798	39,327
300-399	28	9,665	297,684	2,456,396		69.7	6,733			209,054	808,678	2,299,976	3,108,654	644	39,435
400-499	15	6,854	199,768	1,734,801		69.4	4,754			141,170	495,483	1,729,117	2,224,600	396	24,275
500 or more	22	16,549	385,536	4,727,830		78.3	12,955			249,693	816,223	4,013,807	4,830,030	668	48,203
Psychiatric	24	5,986	37,634	1,928,496		88.3	5,284			2	5,842	50,822	56,664	0	0
Hospitals	23	5,478	37,604	1,752,315		87.6	4,801			0	5,546	49,973	55,519	0	0
Institutions for mentally retarded	1	508	30	176,181		95.1	483			2	296	849	1,145	0	0
General	217	50,610	1,563,224	12,220,592		66.2	33,491			1,056,085	4,203,476	14,238,450	18,441,926	3,452	188,088
Hospitals	215	50,570	1,563,106	12,220,090		66.2	33,490			1,055,988	4,188,814	14,203,274	18,392,088	3,452	188,088
Hospital units of institutions	2	40	118	502		02.5	1			97	14,662	35,176	49,838	0	0
TB and other respiratory diseases	0	0	0	0		00.0	0			0	0	0	0	0	0
Obstetrics and gynecology	0	0	0	0		00.0	0			0	0	0	0	0	0
Eye, ear, nose, and throat	0	0	0	0		00.0	0			0	0	0	0	0	0
Fehabilitation	3	347	3,948	109,306		86.2	299			0	0	85,554	85,554	0	0
Orthopedic	1	60	1,576	13,158		60.0	36			1,357	0	15,549	15,549	0	0
Chronic disease	1	988	1,159	316,613		87.8	867			754	371	40,208	40,579	0	0
All other	1	65	1,352	17,686		73.8	48			0	3,030	14,189	17,219	0	0
Federal	9	4,659	60,087	1,214,774		71.4	3,328			30,079	111,325	1,848,960	1,960,285	25	767
Psychiatric	0	0	0	0		00.0	0			0	0	0	0	0	0
General and other special	9	4,659	60,087	1,214,774		71.4	3,328			30,079	111,325	1,848,960	1,960,285	25	767
Nonfederal	238	53,397	1,548,806	13,391,077		68.7	36,697			1,028,119	4,101,394	12,595,812	16,697,206	3,427	187,321
Psychiatric	24	5,986	37,634	1,928,496		88.3	5,284			2	5,842	50,822	56,664	0	0
Hospitals	23	5,478	37,604	1,752,315		87.6	4,801			0	5,546	49,973	55,519	0	0
Institutions for mentally retarded	1	508	30	176,181		95.1	483			2	296	849	1,145	0	0
TB and other respiratory diseases	0	0	0	0		00.0	0			0	0	0	0	0	0
Long-term general and other special	2	1,306	11,619	409,078		85.8	1,120			6,347	23,075	143,233	166,308	22	2,046
Short-term general and other special	212	46,105	1,499,553	11,053,503		65.7	30,293			1,021,770	4,072,477	12,401,757	16,474,234	3,405	185,275
Hospital units of institutions	2	40	118	502		02.5	1			97	14,662	35,176	49,838	0	0
Community hospitals*	210	46,065	1,499,435	11,053,001	14,305,703	65.8	30,292	39,201	7.4	1,021,673	4,057,815	12,366,581	16,424,396	3,405	185,275
6-24 beds	1	18	563	3,258	6,093	50.0	9	17	5.8	239	2,788	25,091	27,879	0	0
25-49	12	489	14,181	71,043	105,009	39.9	195	288	5.0	6,187	63,921	133,366	197,287	32	476
50-99	48	3,432	88,877	637,762	899,101	50.8	1,744	2,460	7.2	44,299	279,570	752,370	1,031,940	236	5,202
100-199	61	8,658	258,688	1,825,308	2,506,878	57.8	5,004	6,876	7.1	174,917	812,364	1,947,848	2,760,212	653	30,403
200-299	38	9,638	324,565	2,351,014	3,081,924	66.9	6,444	8,441	7.2	224,471	819,384	2,581,880	3,401,264	798	39,327
300-399	22	7,677	272,606	1,848,287	2,403,581	66.0	5,066	6,586	6.8	200,918	781,271	2,014,348	2,795,619	622	37,389
400-499	13	5,875	189,867	1,454,975	1,841,742	67.9	3,988	5,048	7.7	136,942	491,754	1,469,462	1,961,216	396	24,275
500 or more	15	10,278	350,088	2,861,354	3,461,375	76.3	7,842	9,485	8.2	233,700	806,763	3,442,216	4,248,979	668	48,203
Nongovernment not-for-profit	163	40,704	1,349,604	9,940,774	12,824,181	66.9	27,237	35,132	7.4	947,677	3,517,731	10,977,309	14,495,040	3,011	167,309
Investor-owned (for-profit)	10	1,051	35,686	224,554	290,215	59.1	621	804	6.3	26,771	114,815	156,027	270,842	61	3,562
State and local government	37	4,310	114,145	887,673	1,191,307	56.5	2,434	3,265	7.8	47,225	425,269	1,233,245	1,658,514	333	14,404

*For information on community hospitals that excludes nursing-home-type data, refer to Hospital Units columns in tables 4A through 4D, pages 14 through 17.

CLASSIFICATION	FULL-TIME EQUIVALENT PERSONNEL: Physicians and Dentists	Registered Nurses	Licensed Practical Nurses	Other Salaried Personnel	Total Personnel	FULL-TIME EQUIVALENT TRAINEES: Medical and Dental Residents	Other Trainees	Total Trainees	EXPENSES: LABOR: Payroll (in thousands)	Employee Benefits (in thousands)	Total (in thousands)	Percent of Total	TOTAL: Amount (in thousands)	Adjusted, per Admission	Adjusted, per Inpatient Day
ILLINOIS	2,794	44,601	5,939	144,754	198,088	4,433	305	4,738	$ 5,319,513	$ 980,544	$ 6,300,056	55.1	$ 11,424,669		
6-24 beds	31	49	23	382	485	6	0	6	13,507	2,087	15,594	80.3	19,425		
25-49	1	251	89	1,085	1,426	1	0	1	26,849	4,403	31,252	54.4	57,424		
50-99	107	1,992	537	7,857	10,493	31	0	31	203,104	38,334	241,438	52.9	456,174		
100-199	242	6,874	1,141	21,009	29,266	118	24	142	688,064	131,971	820,035	53.3	1,539,525		
200-299	194	8,477	978	25,384	35,033	340	8	348	954,440	178,668	1,133,108	54.6	2,075,014		
300-399	412	8,004	1,135	25,690	35,241	451	52	503	943,739	157,768	1,101,507	56.9	1,934,739		
400-499	363	5,695	425	17,526	24,009	531	7	538	638,058	121,743	759,801	56.8	1,338,324		
500 or more	1,444	13,259	1,611	45,821	62,135	2,955	214	3,169	1,851,751	345,570	2,197,321	54.9	4,004,044		
Psychiatric	212	1,234	309	7,791	9,546	36	132	168	262,168	40,316	302,484	74.6	405,527		
Hospitals	209	1,207	288	6,904	8,608	36	132	168	242,002	35,463	277,465	74.1	374,517		
Institutions for mentally retarded	3	27	21	887	938	0	0	0	20,166	4,853	25,019	80.7	31,010		
General	2,472	42,740	5,459	133,660	184,331	4,343	173	4,516	4,955,140	915,530	5,870,671	54.3	10,817,647		
Hospitals	2,469	42,724	5,446	133,591	184,230	4,343	173	4,516	4,953,342	915,106	5,868,448	54.3	10,812,748		
Hospital units of institutions	3	16	13	69	101	0	0	0	1,798	424	2,222	45.4	4,899		
TB and other respiratory diseases	0	0	0	0	0	0	0	0	0	0	0	0.0	0		
Obstetrics and gynecology	0	0	0	0	0	0	0	0	0	0	0	0.0	0		
Eye, ear, nose, and throat	0	0	0	0	0	0	0	0	0	0	0	0.0	0		
Rehabilitation	12	345	75	1,243	1,675	20	0	20	42,651	7,609	50,261	57.0	88,169		
Orthopedic	14	78	0	160	252	5	0	5	3,364	664	4,028	53.7	7,502		
Chronic disease	84	163	84	1,631	1,962	29	0	29	47,253	14,935	62,188	70.4	88,319		
All other	0	41	12	269	322	0	0	0	8,936	1,489	10,425	59.6	17,505		
Federal	674	1,867	463	8,509	11,513	531	56	587	358,762	61,166	419,929	70.0	599,628		
Psychiatric	0	0	0	0	0	0	0	0	0	0	0	0.0	0		
General and other special	674	1,867	463	8,509	11,513	531	56	587	358,762	61,166	419,929	70.0	599,628		
Nonfederal	2,120	42,734	5,476	136,245	186,575	3,902	249	4,151	4,960,750	919,377	5,880,128	54.3	10,825,041		
Psychiatric	212	1,234	309	7,791	9,546	36	132	168	262,168	40,316	302,484	74.6	405,527		
Hospitals	209	1,207	288	6,904	8,608	36	132	168	242,002	35,463	277,465	74.1	374,517		
Institutions for mentally retarded	3	27	21	887	938	0	0	0	20,166	4,853	25,019	80.7	31,010		
TB and other respiratory diseases	0	0	0	0	0	0	0	0	0	0	0	0.0	0		
Long-term general and other special	108	488	98	2,723	3,417	76	10	86	81,248	21,398	102,646	64.0	160,502		
Short-term general and other special	1,800	41,012	5,069	125,731	173,612	3,790	107	3,897	4,617,334	857,664	5,474,998	53.4	10,259,012		
Hospital units of institutions	3	16	13	69	101	0	0	0	1,798	424	2,222	45.4	4,899		
Community hospitals*	1,797	40,996	5,056	125,662	173,511	3,790	107	3,897	4,615,536	857,240	5,472,776	53.4	10,254,113	$5,252.56	$ 716.79
6-24 beds	0	10	3	52	65	0	0	0	1,244	170	1,414	52.7	2,685	2,549.63	440.63
25-49	1	251	89	1,014	1,355	1	0	1	25,414	4,166	29,580	55.0	53,787	2,549.86	512.21
50-99	30	1,809	518	6,427	8,784	21	0	21	174,322	33,161	207,483	51.8	400,912	3,150.61	445.90
100-199	107	6,417	1,085	18,665	26,274	59	9	68	607,810	115,708	723,518	52.4	1,380,540	3,839.00	550.70
200-299	153	8,212	913	24,144	33,422	338	8	346	906,092	171,913	1,078,005	53.8	2,003,406	4,723.97	650.05
300-399	246	7,237	990	22,186	30,659	301	9	310	806,452	139,645	946,097	55.0	1,719,457	4,844.03	715.37
400-499	277	5,387	338	15,879	21,881	409	0	409	564,625	111,146	675,771	55.2	1,223,328	5,085.29	664.22
500 or more	983	11,673	1,120	37,295	51,071	2,661	81	2,742	1,529,577	281,330	1,810,908	52.2	3,470,000	8,191.90	1,002.49
Nongovernment not-for-profit	1,358	36,928	4,145	112,883	155,320	3,179	89	3,268	4,142,677	770,068	4,912,745	52.8	9,309,724	5,312.08	725.95
Investor-owned (for-profit)	7	812	194	2,502	3,515	20	0	20	77,828	14,624	92,452	45.3	203,936	4,408.00	702.71
State and local government	432	3,256	717	10,271	14,676	591	18	609	395,031	72,547	467,579	63.1	740,453	4,827.23	621.55

*For information on community hospitals that excludes nursing-home-type data, refer to Hospital Units columns in tables 4A through 4D, pages 14 through 17.

(continued on next page)

Table
5C (Continued) Indiana

Utilization, Personnel, and Finances in States
Excludes AHA nonregistered hospitals (see Table 14, page 240).

CLASSIFICATION	HOSPITALS	BEDS	ADMISSIONS	INPATIENT DAYS	ADJUSTED PATIENT DAYS	OCCUPANCY, percent	AVERAGE DAILY CENSUS	ADJUSTED AVERAGE DAILY CENSUS	AVERAGE STAY, days	SURGICAL OPERATIONS	OUTPATIENT VISITS Emergency	OUTPATIENT VISITS Other	OUTPATIENT VISITS Total	NEWBORNS Bassinets	NEWBORNS Births
INDIANA	135	26,501	753,940	6,147,509		63.6	16,843			587,363	2,062,479	7,231,963	9,294,442	1,832	83,915
6-24 beds	2	37	1,281	2,930		24.3	9			808	34,279	270,830	305,109	0	0
25-49	16	635	18,658	100,206		43.1	274			9,867	72,203	266,124	338,327	65	1,373
50-99	39	2,701	71,087	479,037		48.6	1,312			48,593	259,501	812,387	1,071,888	297	7,229
100-199	33	4,327	117,577	846,288		53.6	2,318			92,570	416,363	1,308,122	1,724,485	452	15,635
200-299	15	3,885	134,275	873,942		61.7	2,396			109,166	357,985	1,099,864	1,457,849	306	14,075
300-399	9	3,241	89,802	702,938		59.4	1,926			79,311	214,534	807,885	1,022,419	178	8,926
400-499	10	4,416	103,694	1,264,248		78.4	3,463			67,963	260,621	1,114,325	1,374,946	150	13,124
500 or more	11	7,259	217,566	1,877,920		70.9	5,145			179,085	446,993	1,552,426	1,999,419	384	23,553
Psychiatric	17	3,834	14,063	1,102,981		78.8	3,022			281	963	146,590	147,553	0	0
Hospitals	17	3,834	14,063	1,102,981		78.8	3,022			281	963	146,590	147,553	0	0
Institutions for mentally retarded	0	0	0	0		00.0	0			0	0	0	0	0	0
General	114	22,244	733,514	4,951,237		61.0	13,565			577,585	2,061,516	7,058,450	9,119,966	1,778	81,721
Hospitals	113	22,227	733,424	4,951,048		61.0	13,564			577,585	2,054,496	6,876,692	8,931,188	1,778	81,721
Hospital units of institutions	1	17	90	189		05.9	1			0	7,020	181,758	188,778	0	0
TB and other respiratory diseases	0	0	0	0		00.0	0			0	0	0	0	0	0
Obstetrics and gynecology	1	144	4,163	21,488		41.0	59			4,661	0	10,597	10,597	54	2,194
Eye, ear, nose, and throat	0	0	0	0		00.0	0			0	0	0	0	0	0
Rehabilitation	1	60	382	11,193		51.7	31			0	0	6,224	6,224	0	0
Orthopedic	0	0	0	0		00.0	0			0	0	0	0	0	0
Chronic disease	1	159	153	52,657		90.6	144			0	0	220	220	0	0
All other	1	60	1,665	7,953		36.7	22			4,836	0	9,882	9,882	0	0
Federal	4	1,205	14,647	313,703		71.4	860			8,121	36,126	312,202	348,328	0	0
Psychiatric	1	580	2,254	154,710		73.1	424			281	0	50,168	50,168	0	0
General and other special	3	625	12,393	158,993		69.8	436			7,840	36,126	262,034	298,160	0	0
Nonfederal	131	25,296	739,293	5,833,806		63.2	15,983			579,242	2,026,353	6,919,761	8,946,114	1,832	83,915
Psychiatric	16	3,254	11,809	948,271		79.8	2,598			0	963	96,422	97,385	0	0
Hospitals	16	3,254	11,809	948,271		79.8	2,598			0	963	96,422	97,385	0	0
Institutions for mentally retarded	0	0	0	0		00.0	0			0	0	0	0	0	0
TB and other respiratory diseases	0	0	0	0		00.0	0			0	0	0	0	0	0
Long-term general and other special	1	159	153	52,657		90.6	144			0	0	220	220	0	0
Short-term general and other special	114	21,883	727,331	4,832,878		60.5	13,241			579,242	2,025,390	6,823,119	8,848,509	1,832	83,915
Hospital units of institutions	1	17	90	189		05.9	1			0	7,020	181,758	188,778	0	0
Community hospitals*	113	21,866	727,241	4,832,689	6,585,205	60.6	13,240	18,044	6.6	579,242	2,018,370	6,641,361	8,659,731	1,832	83,915
6-24 beds	0	0	0	0	0	00.0	0	0	0.0	0	0	0	0	0	0
25-49	14	552	16,732	78,591	124,350	38.9	215	339	4.7	9,867	72,203	222,100	294,303	65	1,373
50-99	32	2,155	64,877	333,839	534,567	42.4	914	1,464	5.1	48,593	259,501	775,698	1,035,199	297	7,229
100-199	29	3,707	112,305	684,384	1,026,994	50.6	1,875	2,816	6.1	91,719	406,533	1,270,774	1,677,307	452	15,635
200-299	15	3,885	134,275	873,942	1,210,293	61.7	2,396	3,318	6.5	109,166	357,985	1,099,864	1,457,849	306	14,075
300-399	8	2,851	81,899	597,430	825,559	57.4	1,637	2,262	7.3	73,130	214,534	656,342	870,876	178	8,926
400-499	6	2,577	102,183	722,201	930,470	76.8	1,978	2,549	7.1	67,963	260,621	1,114,325	1,374,946	150	13,124
500 or more	9	6,139	214,970	1,542,302	1,932,972	68.8	4,225	5,296	7.2	178,804	446,993	1,502,258	1,949,251	384	23,553
Nongovernment not-for-profit	56	14,944	513,314	3,487,980	4,620,062	64.0	9,558	12,660	6.8	423,703	1,302,330	4,559,847	5,862,177	1,042	59,349
Investor-owned (for-profit)	7	960	23,081	169,754	222,598	48.5	466	610	7.4	18,800	49,355	133,279	182,634	96	3,442
State and local government	50	5,962	190,846	1,174,955	1,742,545	53.9	3,216	4,774	6.2	136,739	666,685	1,948,235	2,614,920	694	21,124

*For information on community hospitals that excludes nursing-home-type data, refer to Hospital Units columns in tables 4A through 4D, pages 14 through 17.

Table 5C (Continued) Indiana

CLASSIFICATION	FULL-TIME EQUIVALENT PERSONNEL					FULL-TIME EQUIVALENT TRAINEES			EXPENSES						
									LABOR				TOTAL		
	Physicians and Dentists	Registered Nurses	Licensed Practical Nurses	Other Salaried Personnel	Total Personnel	Medical and Dental Residents	Other Trainees	Total Trainees	Payroll (in thousands)	Employee Benefits (in thousands)	Total (in thousands)	Percent of Total	Amount (in thousands)	Adjusted, per Admission	Adjusted, per Inpatient Day
INDIANA	436	20,807	3,451	67,744	92,438	730	208	938	$ 2,163,023	$ 423,213	$ 2,586,236	54.3	$ 4,766,853		
6-24 beds	31	50	24	275	380	0	0	0	4,132	919	5,051	53.1	9,510		
25-49	15	383	136	1,547	2,081	0	5	5	40,020	7,601	47,621	54.7	87,025		
50-99	17	1,454	391	5,490	7,352	0	5	5	155,061	31,275	186,336	52.7	353,405		
100-199	55	2,701	468	9,694	12,918	13	0	13	288,776	56,630	345,406	54.5	633,663		
200-299	23	3,394	778	10,493	14,688	25	31	56	322,035	60,214	382,249	52.6	727,258		
300-399	83	2,782	349	7,614	10,828	103	34	137	268,791	50,876	319,666	54.0	592,001		
400-499	51	3,048	367	10,941	14,407	44	8	52	365,409	70,235	435,644	57.4	758,990		
500 or more	161	6,995	938	21,690	29,784	545	125	670	718,800	145,462	864,263	53.8	1,605,001		
Psychiatric	115	621	128	5,166	6,030	1	14	15	145,317	33,298	178,616	74.0	241,381		
Hospitals	115	621	128	5,166	6,030	1	14	15	145,317	33,298	178,616	74.0	241,381		
Institutions for mentally retarded	0	0	0	0	0	0	0	0	0	0	0	0.0	0		
General	320	19,949	3,292	61,855	85,416	729	194	923	1,999,512	385,975	2,385,487	53.3	4,477,309		
Hospitals	311	19,930	3,274	61,802	85,317	729	194	923	1,998,881	385,794	2,384,675	53.3	4,475,090		
Hospital units of institutions	9	19	18	53	99	0	0	0	631	181	812	36.6	2,219		
TB and other respiratory diseases	0	0	0	0	0	0	0	0	0	0	0	0.0	0		
Obstetrics and gynecology	0	136	1	244	381	0	0	0	7,420	1,672	9,092	43.0	21,123		
Eye, ear, nose, and throat	0	0	0	0	0	0	0	0	0	0	0	0.0	0		
Rehabilitation	0	29	9	127	165	0	0	0	3,584	623	4,208	56.9	7,399		
Orthopedic	0	0	0	0	0	0	0	0	0	0	0	0.0	0		
Chronic disease	0	10	14	220	244	0	0	0	3,329	779	4,108	55.0	7,471		
All other	1	62	7	132	202	0	0	0	3,861	864	4,725	38.8	12,170		
Federal	145	528	116	2,463	3,252	84	26	110	93,848	16,050	109,898	65.1	168,769		
Psychiatric	30	140	30	857	1,057	0	3	3	29,547	5,685	35,232	75.7	46,550		
General and other special	115	388	86	1,606	2,195	84	23	107	64,301	10,365	74,666	61.1	122,219		
Nonfederal	291	20,279	3,335	65,281	89,186	646	182	828	2,069,175	407,163	2,476,338	53.9	4,598,084		
Psychiatric	85	481	98	4,309	4,973	1	11	12	115,770	27,613	143,384	73.6	194,831		
Hospitals	85	481	98	4,309	4,973	1	11	12	115,770	27,613	143,384	73.6	194,831		
Institutions for mentally retarded	0	0	0	0	0	0	0	0	0	0	0	0.0	0		
TB and other respiratory diseases	0	0	0	0	0	0	0	0	0	0	0	0.0	0		
Long-term general and other special	0	10	14	220	244	0	0	0	3,329	779	4,108	55.0	7,471		
Short-term general and other special	206	19,788	3,223	60,752	83,969	645	171	816	1,950,076	378,770	2,328,846	53.0	4,395,782		
Hospital units of institutions	9	19	18	53	99	0	0	0	631	181	812	36.6	2,219		
Community hospitals*	197	19,769	3,205	60,699	83,870	645	171	816	1,949,445	378,589	2,328,034	53.0	4,393,563	$4,389.62	$ 667.19
6-24 beds	0	0	0	0	0	0	0	0	0	0	0	0.0	0	0.00	0.00
25-49	7	358	128	1,363	1,856	0	5	5	34,172	6,499	40,670	53.4	76,130	2,860.85	612.22
50-99	5	1,309	372	4,669	6,355	0	0	0	128,006	25,452	153,458	51.5	297,971	2,852.79	557.41
100-199	29	2,567	430	8,735	11,761	12	0	12	258,473	50,187	308,660	53.4	578,435	3,438.38	563.23
200-299	23	3,394	778	10,493	14,688	25	31	56	322,035	60,214	382,249	52.6	727,258	3,882.52	600.89
300-399	6	2,489	286	6,499	9,280	19	11	30	218,989	43,439	262,428	52.8	497,204	4,411.24	602.26
400-499	7	2,846	308	8,825	11,986	44	2	46	313,880	57,676	371,556	54.4	682,862	5,168.93	733.89
500 or more	120	6,806	903	20,115	27,944	545	122	667	673,890	135,123	809,013	52.7	1,533,703	5,691.53	793.44
Nongovernment not-for-profit	166	14,011	2,085	42,853	59,121	426	131	557	1,389,616	271,298	1,660,914	53.0	3,133,010	4,582.53	678.13
Investor-owned (for-profit)	0	661	149	1,593	2,406	0	2	2	55,604	11,063	66,666	44.5	149,932	4,847.47	673.56
State and local government	31	5,097	971	16,244	22,343	219	38	257	504,225	96,229	600,454	54.1	1,110,621	3,879.46	637.36

*For information on community hospitals that excludes nursing-home-type data, refer to Hospital Units columns in tables 4A through 4D, pages 14 through 17.

(continued on next page)

Table
5C (Continued) Iowa

Utilization, Personnel, and Finances in States
Excludes AHA nonregistered hospitals (see Table 14, page 240).

CLASSIFICATION	HOSPITALS	BEDS	ADMISSIONS	INPATIENT DAYS	ADJUSTED PATIENT DAYS	OCCUPANCY, percent	AVERAGE DAILY CENSUS	ADJUSTED AVERAGE DAILY CENSUS	AVERAGE STAY, days	SURGICAL OPERATIONS	OUTPATIENT VISITS Emergency	OUTPATIENT VISITS Other	OUTPATIENT VISITS Total	NEWBORNS Bassinets	NEWBORNS Births
IOWA	134	17,251	404,175	4,121,001		65.4	11,290			327,565	943,867	3,361,853	4,305,720	1,101	39,016
6-24 beds	5	103	2,282	13,557		35.9	37			934	4,402	46,483	50,885	20	263
25-49	47	1,789	36,301	288,373		44.3	792			19,943	104,373	368,720	473,093	226	3,608
50-99	37	2,504	51,623	528,520		57.8	1,448			33,030	167,616	471,552	639,168	244	5,216
100-199	16	2,165	37,902	517,356		65.5	1,417			33,087	128,665	396,576	525,241	133	3,649
200-299	15	3,730	101,274	864,460		63.5	2,368			66,516	230,831	758,121	988,952	184	9,930
300-399	4	1,454	41,268	349,029		65.7	956			27,791	76,843	310,663	387,506	96	5,241
400-499	5	2,181	50,503	561,965		70.6	1,539			40,857	131,248	253,589	384,837	106	4,874
500 or more	5	3,325	83,022	997,741		82.2	2,733			105,407	99,889	756,149	856,038	92	6,235
Psychiatric	8	2,461	7,688	812,223		90.3	2,223			0	0	42,774	42,774	0	0
Hospitals	6	1,460	7,626	456,497		85.5	1,249			0	0	42,774	42,774	0	0
Institutions for mentally retarded	2	1,001	62	355,726		97.3	974			0	0	0	0	0	0
General	126	14,790	396,487	3,308,778		61.3	9,067			327,565	943,867	3,319,079	4,262,946	1,101	39,016
Hospitals	126	14,790	396,487	3,308,778		61.3	9,067			327,565	943,867	3,319,079	4,262,946	1,101	39,016
Hospital units of institutions	0	0	0	0		00.0	0			0	0	0	0	0	0
TB and other respiratory diseases	0	0	0	0		00.0	0			0	0	0	0	0	0
Obstetrics and gynecology	0	0	0	0		00.0	0			0	0	0	0	0	0
Eye, ear, nose, and throat	0	0	0	0		00.0	0			0	0	0	0	0	0
Rehabilitation	0	0	0	0		00.0	0			0	0	0	0	0	0
Orthopedic	0	0	0	0		00.0	0			0	0	0	0	0	0
Chronic disease	0	0	0	0		00.0	0			0	0	0	0	0	0
All other	0	0	0	0		00.0	0			0	0	0	0	0	0
Federal	3	1,187	14,318	298,129		68.7	816			7,010	15,991	174,412	190,403	0	0
Psychiatric	1	636	2,969	195,761		84.3	536			0	0	39,737	39,737	0	0
General and other special	2	551	11,349	102,368		50.8	280			7,010	15,991	134,675	150,666	0	0
Nonfederal	131	16,064	389,857	3,822,872		65.2	10,474			320,555	927,876	3,187,441	4,115,317	1,101	39,016
Psychiatric	7	1,825	4,719	616,462		92.4	1,687			0	0	3,037	3,037	0	0
Hospitals	5	824	4,657	260,736		86.5	713			0	0	3,037	3,037	0	0
Institutions for mentally retarded	2	1,001	62	355,726		97.3	974			0	0	0	0	0	0
TB and other respiratory diseases	0	0	0	0		00.0	0			0	0	0	0	0	0
Long-term general and other special	0	0	0	0		00.0	0			0	0	0	0	0	0
Short-term general and other special	124	14,239	385,138	3,206,410		61.7	8,787			320,555	927,876	3,184,404	4,112,280	1,101	39,016
Hospital units of institutions	0	0	0	0		00.0	0			0	0	0	0	0	0
Community hospitals*	124	14,239	385,138	3,206,410	4,390,469	61.7	8,787	12,028	8.3	320,555	927,876	3,184,404	4,112,280	1,101	39,016
6-24 beds	5	103	2,282	13,557	23,133	35.9	37	63	5.9	934	4,402	46,483	50,885	20	263
25-49	46	1,743	36,067	271,938	418,072	42.9	747	1,147	7.5	19,943	104,373	368,720	473,093	226	3,608
50-99	37	2,504	51,623	528,520	788,493	57.8	1,448	2,159	10.2	33,030	167,616	471,552	639,168	244	5,216
100-199	14	1,880	36,445	423,228	591,354	61.7	1,160	1,619	11.6	33,087	128,665	395,498	524,163	133	3,649
200-299	11	2,686	86,959	611,919	812,418	62.4	1,677	2,227	7.0	59,506	214,840	621,487	836,327	184	9,930
300-399	4	1,454	41,268	349,029	471,489	65.7	956	1,292	8.5	27,791	76,843	310,663	387,506	96	5,241
400-499	4	1,755	50,473	412,925	539,015	64.4	1,131	1,476	8.2	40,857	131,248	253,589	384,837	106	4,874
500 or more	3	2,114	80,021	595,294	746,495	77.2	1,631	2,045	7.4	105,407	99,889	716,412	816,301	92	6,235
Nongovernment not-for-profit	57	9,429	269,991	2,216,043	2,957,401	64.4	6,072	8,101	8.2	198,633	624,912	1,916,714	2,541,626	689	28,648
Investor-owned (for-profit)	2	216	3,750	22,566	30,914	28.7	62	85	6.0	3,975	19,637	19,640	39,277	11	347
State and local government	65	4,594	111,397	967,801	1,402,154	57.7	2,653	3,842	8.7	117,947	283,327	1,248,050	1,531,377	401	10,021

*For information on community hospitals that excludes nursing-home-type data, refer to Hospital Units columns in tables 4A through 4D, pages 14 through 17.

CLASSIFICATION	FULL-TIME EQUIVALENT PERSONNEL					FULL-TIME EQUIVALENT TRAINEES			EXPENSES: LABOR				EXPENSES: TOTAL		
	Physicians and Dentists	Registered Nurses	Licensed Practical Nurses	Other Salaried Personnel	Total Personnel	Medical and Dental Residents	Other Trainees	Total Trainees	Payroll (in thousands)	Employee Benefits (in thousands)	Total (in thousands)	Percent of Total	Amount (in thousands)	Adjusted, per Admission	Adjusted, per Inpatient Day
IOWA	220	11,591	1,638	35,976	49,425	713	93	806	$ 1,125,147	$ 218,164	$ 1,343,311	55.4	$ 2,424,198		
6-24 beds	0	59	10	179	248	0	0	0	3,942	784	4,726	56.6	8,352		
25-49	3	894	235	2,613	3,745	0	0	0	68,629	12,389	81,018	55.3	146,460		
50-99	0	1,352	266	4,247	5,865	1	0	1	110,064	21,515	131,579	56.3	233,711		
100-199	10	964	205	3,338	4,517	37	0	37	101,545	19,928	121,473	55.6	218,658		
200-299	156	2,710	415	8,003	11,284	173	37	210	278,046	47,427	325,473	55.4	586,974		
300-399	1	1,139	187	3,166	4,493	20	0	20	104,726	21,407	126,134	55.0	229,229		
400-499	11	1,835	94	4,817	6,757	24	28	52	149,036	30,469	179,505	57.8	310,778		
500 or more	39	2,638	226	9,613	12,516	458	28	486	309,158	64,246	373,403	54.1	690,037		
Psychiatric	72	341	110	3,708	4,231	10	6	16	108,288	20,866	129,154	83.0	155,592		
Hospitals	55	273	97	1,707	2,132	10	6	16	58,681	9,633	68,314	78.8	86,740		
Institutions for mentally retarded	17	68	13	2,001	2,099	0	0	0	49,608	11,233	60,840	88.4	68,852		
General	148	11,250	1,528	32,268	45,194	703	87	790	1,016,859	197,298	1,214,157	53.5	2,268,606		
Hospitals	148	11,250	1,528	32,268	45,194	703	87	790	1,016,859	197,298	1,214,157	53.5	2,268,606		
Hospital units of institutions	0	0	0	0	0	0	0	0	0	0	0	0.0	0		
TB and other respiratory diseases	0	0	0	0	0	0	0	0	0	0	0	0.0	0		
Obstetrics and gynecology	0	0	0	0	0	0	0	0	0	0	0	0.0	0		
Eye, ear, nose, and throat	0	0	0	0	0	0	0	0	0	0	0	0.0	0		
Rehabilitation	0	0	0	0	0	0	0	0	0	0	0	0.0	0		
Orthopedic	0	0	0	0	0	0	0	0	0	0	0	0.0	0		
Chronic disease	0	0	0	0	0	0	0	0	0	0	0	0.0	0		
All other	0	0	0	0	0	0	0	0	0	0	0	0.0	0		
Federal	105	388	74	1,846	2,413	122	41	163	70,675	12,115	82,790	62.8	131,738		
Psychiatric	18	105	23	719	865	0	6	6	25,615	3,166	28,781	76.6	37,576		
General and other special	87	283	51	1,127	1,548	122	35	157	45,061	8,949	54,010	57.4	94,162		
Nonfederal	115	11,203	1,564	34,130	47,012	591	52	643	1,054,471	206,050	1,260,521	55.0	2,292,460		
Psychiatric	54	236	87	2,989	3,366	10	0	10	82,673	17,700	100,374	85.1	118,016		
Hospitals	37	168	74	988	1,267	10	0	10	33,066	6,467	39,533	80.4	49,165		
Institutions for mentally retarded	17	68	13	2,001	2,099	0	0	0	49,608	11,233	60,840	88.4	68,852		
TB and other respiratory diseases	0	0	0	0	0	0	0	0	0	0	0	0.0	0		
Long-term general and other special	0	0	0	0	0	0	0	0	0	0	0	0.0	0		
Short-term general and other special	61	10,967	1,477	31,141	43,646	581	52	633	971,798	188,349	1,160,147	53.4	2,174,443		
Hospital units of institutions	0	0	0	0	0	0	0	0	0	0	0	0.0	0		
Community hospitals*	61	10,967	1,477	31,141	43,646	581	52	633	971,798	188,349	1,160,147	53.4	2,174,443	$4,135.35	$ 495.26
6-24 beds	0	59	10	179	248	0	0	0	3,942	784	4,726	56.6	8,352	2,173.74	361.02
25-49	0	887	235	2,584	3,706	0	0	0	66,160	11,794	77,954	55.3	141,012	2,579.38	337.29
50-99	0	1,352	266	4,247	5,865	1	0	1	110,064	21,515	131,579	56.3	233,711	2,953.32	296.40
100-199	2	901	183	3,037	4,123	37	0	37	91,306	18,303	109,609	53.9	203,538	3,905.63	344.19
200-299	43	2,329	312	6,218	8,902	41	2	43	212,628	34,229	246,858	53.2	464,214	4,040.54	571.40
300-399	1	1,139	187	3,166	4,493	20	0	20	104,726	21,407	126,134	55.0	229,229	4,138.98	486.18
400-499	3	1,805	82	3,923	5,813	24	28	52	126,695	25,428	152,123	54.4	279,879	4,276.62	519.24
500 or more	12	2,495	202	7,787	10,496	458	22	480	256,277	54,888	311,164	50.6	614,508	6,124.07	823.19
Nongovernment not-for-profit	36	7,522	1,025	21,387	29,970	122	40	162	670,964	119,756	790,720	52.9	1,493,546	4,151.11	505.02
Investor-owned (for-profit)	0	89	10	266	365	7	0	7	10,677	2,350	13,028	43.8	29,774	5,844.85	963.11
State and local government	25	3,356	442	9,488	13,311	452	12	464	290,157	66,243	356,399	54.7	651,124	4,045.98	464.37

*For information on community hospitals that excludes nursing-home-type data, refer to Hospital Units columns in tables 4A through 4D, pages 14 through 17.

(continued on next page)

Table

5C (Continued) Kansas

Utilization, Personnel, and Finances in States

Excludes AHA nonregistered hospitals (see Table 14, page 240).

CLASSIFICATION	HOSPITALS	BEDS	ADMISSIONS	INPATIENT DAYS	ADJUSTED PATIENT DAYS	OCCUPANCY, percent	AVERAGE DAILY CENSUS	ADJUSTED AVERAGE DAILY CENSUS	AVERAGE STAY, days	SURGICAL OPERATIONS	OUTPATIENT VISITS Emergency	OUTPATIENT VISITS Other	OUTPATIENT VISITS Total	NEWBORNS Bassinets	NEWBORNS Births
KANSAS	160	16,139	335,204	3,607,924		61.3	9,892			215,820	792,239	3,272,567	4,064,806	1,080	37,906
6-24 beds	23	437	9,522	60,803		38.0	166			4,471	49,459	254,132	303,591	73	548
25-49	55	2,006	31,517	322,942		44.3	888			12,282	92,652	486,868	579,520	228	2,404
50-99	41	2,822	53,233	553,322		53.8	1,519			35,427	142,821	451,563	594,384	265	6,343
100-199	23	3,148	79,632	693,305		60.4	1,901			55,446	195,303	899,307	1,094,610	233	8,330
200-299	2	506	11,478	109,209		59.3	300			6,958	38,296	80,586	118,882	16	1,033
300-399	8	2,795	53,364	757,372		74.2	2,074			39,945	111,024	275,544	386,568	110	6,693
400-499	4	1,803	25,831	467,162		71.0	1,280			20,650	48,138	409,375	457,513	56	3,844
500 or more	4	2,622	70,627	643,809		67.3	1,764			40,641	114,546	415,192	529,738	99	8,711
Psychiatric	13	2,630	7,992	806,456		84.0	2,210			0	2,047	71,091	73,138	0	0
Hospitals	11	1,831	7,951	565,066		84.5	1,548			0	2,047	71,091	73,138	0	0
Institutions for mentally retarded	2	799	41	241,390		82.9	662			0	0	0	0	0	0
General	145	13,383	326,634	2,776,107		56.9	7,612			215,820	790,192	3,197,573	3,987,765	1,080	37,906
Hospitals	143	13,345	325,384	2,767,146		56.9	7,587			214,989	776,327	3,115,553	3,891,880	1,080	37,906
Hospital units of institutions	2	38	1,250	8,961		65.8	25			831	13,865	82,020	95,885	0	0
TB and other respiratory diseases	0	0	0	0		00.0	0			0	0	0	0	0	0
Obstetrics and gynecology	0	0	0	0		00.0	0			0	0	0	0	0	0
Eye, ear, nose, and throat	0	0	0	0		00.0	0			0	0	0	0	0	0
Rehabilitation	2	126	578	25,361		55.6	70			0	0	3,903	3,903	0	0
Orthopedic	0	0	0	0		00.0	0			0	0	0	0	0	0
Chronic disease	0	0	0	0		00.0	0			0	0	0	0	0	0
All other	0	0	0	0		00.0	0			0	0	0	0	0	0
Federal	7	1,649	22,540	388,791		64.7	1,067			10,363	96,694	1,010,685	1,107,379	25	1,160
Psychiatric	0	0	0	0		00.0	0			0	0	0	0	0	0
General and other special	7	1,649	22,540	388,791		64.7	1,067			10,363	96,694	1,010,685	1,107,379	25	1,160
Nonfederal	153	14,490	312,664	3,219,133		60.9	8,825			205,457	695,545	2,261,882	2,957,427	1,055	36,746
Psychiatric	13	2,630	7,992	806,456		84.0	2,210			0	2,047	71,091	73,138	0	0
Hospitals	11	1,831	7,951	565,066		84.5	1,548			0	2,047	71,091	73,138	0	0
Institutions for mentally retarded	2	799	41	241,390		82.9	662			0	0	0	0	0	0
TB and other respiratory diseases	0	0	0	0		00.0	0			0	0	0	0	0	0
Long-term general and other special	1	46	54	13,420		80.4	37			0	0	0	0	0	0
Short-term general and other special	139	11,814	304,618	2,399,257		55.7	6,578			205,457	693,498	2,190,791	2,884,289	1,055	36,746
Hospital units of institutions	1	18	67	5,448		83.3	15			0	0	0	0	0	0
Community hospitals*	138	11,796	304,551	2,393,809	3,213,322	55.6	6,563	8,806	7.9	205,457	693,498	2,190,791	2,884,289	1,055	36,746
6-24 beds	20	393	7,754	50,463	81,016	34.9	137	225	6.5	3,228	22,081	104,245	126,326	73	548
25-49	50	1,831	29,243	276,538	393,101	41.6	761	1,076	9.5	11,269	75,366	255,428	330,794	228	2,404
50-99	39	2,673	52,204	513,681	734,056	52.7	1,410	2,010	9.8	35,427	142,238	444,065	586,303	265	6,343
100-199	19	2,632	70,564	563,939	764,371	58.7	1,546	2,095	8.0	52,911	159,794	516,039	675,833	208	7,170
200-299	1	284	7,711	53,504	66,935	51.8	147	183	6.9	5,045	20,311	21,437	41,748	16	1,033
300-399	4	1,381	46,784	329,884	412,228	65.4	903	1,130	7.1	37,996	111,024	155,926	266,950	110	6,693
400-499	2	864	24,443	157,096	199,007	49.8	430	546	6.4	20,650	48,138	409,375	457,513	56	3,844
500 or more	3	1,738	65,848	448,704	562,608	70.7	1,229	1,541	6.8	38,931	114,546	284,276	398,822	99	8,711
Nongovernment not-for-profit	62	6,863	191,328	1,481,342	1,960,651	59.2	4,060	5,376	7.7	133,802	441,001	1,064,793	1,505,794	578	20,496
Investor-owned (for-profit)	8	1,301	39,988	240,966	302,608	50.7	660	829	6.0	25,674	68,809	193,113	261,922	100	8,343
State and local government	68	3,632	73,235	671,501	950,063	50.7	1,843	2,601	9.2	45,981	183,688	932,885	1,116,573	377	7,907

*For information on community hospitals that excludes nursing-home-type data, refer to Hospital Units columns in tables 4A through 4D, pages 14 through 17.

CLASSIFICATION	Physicians and Dentists	Registered Nurses	Licensed Practical Nurses	Other Salaried Personnel	Total Personnel	Medical and Dental Residents	Other Trainees	Total Trainees	Payroll (in thousands)	Employee Benefits (in thousands)	Total (in thousands)	Percent of Total	Amount (in thousands)	Adjusted, per Admission	Adjusted, per Inpatient Day
	FULL-TIME EQUIVALENT PERSONNEL					FULL-TIME EQUIVALENT TRAINEES			EXPENSES: LABOR				EXPENSES: TOTAL		
KANSAS	726	9,209	1,876	32,794	44,605	361	180	541	$ 1,004,420	$ 174,478	$ 1,178,898	56.1	$ 2,100,511		
6-24 beds	43	223	71	1,066	1,403	0	6	6	21,167	3,568	24,735	59.2	41,801		
25-49	50	670	219	3,010	3,949	0	0	0	72,298	13,541	85,838	56.5	151,858		
50-99	11	1,389	285	4,513	6,198	8	1	9	125,267	22,292	147,558	55.6	265,620		
100-199	83	1,840	384	6,099	8,406	12	3	15	180,644	32,799	213,442	53.5	398,686		
200-299	24	329	61	1,020	1,434	6	9	15	38,687	7,622	46,309	55.2	83,943		
300-399	78	1,793	266	6,172	8,309	35	8	43	220,731	39,197	259,929	60.0	433,103		
400-499	329	908	213	4,294	5,744	283	108	391	119,708	23,758	143,466	62.3	230,203		
500 or more	108	2,057	377	6,620	9,162	17	45	62	225,919	31,702	257,620	52.0	495,296		
Psychiatric	115	545	85	4,474	5,219	13	108	121	123,686	25,286	148,972	71.3	208,919		
Hospitals	104	498	34	2,929	3,565	13	0	13	88,296	17,313	105,608	68.8	153,481		
Institutions for mentally retarded	11	47	51	1,545	1,654	0	108	108	35,390	7,973	43,363	78.2	55,438		
General	609	8,608	1,772	28,090	39,079	348	72	420	873,106	147,846	1,020,951	54.5	1,874,446		
Hospitals	590	8,576	1,763	27,861	38,790	348	72	420	869,146	146,880	1,016,026	54.4	1,867,591		
Hospital units of institutions	19	32	9	229	289	0	0	0	3,960	966	4,925	71.8	6,856		
TB and other respiratory diseases	0	0	0	0	0	0	0	0	0	0	0	0.0	0		
Obstetrics and gynecology	0	0	0	0	0	0	0	0	0	0	0	0.0	0		
Eye, ear, nose, and throat	0	0	0	0	0	0	0	0	0	0	0	0.0	0		
Rehabilitation	2	56	19	230	307	0	0	0	7,629	1,347	8,975	52.3	17,145		
Orthopedic	0	0	0	0	0	0	0	0	0	0	0	0.0	0		
Chronic disease	0	0	0	0	0	0	0	0	0	0	0	0.0	0		
All other	0	0	0	0	0	0	0	0	0	0	0	0.0	0		
Federal	217	567	225	3,256	4,265	41	23	64	99,533	19,186	118,720	68.5	173,195		
Psychiatric	0	0	0	0	0	0	0	0	0	0	0	0.0	0		
General and other special	217	567	225	3,256	4,265	41	23	64	99,533	19,186	118,720	68.5	173,195		
Nonfederal	509	8,642	1,651	29,538	40,340	320	157	477	904,887	155,292	1,060,179	55.0	1,927,316		
Psychiatric	115	545	85	4,474	5,219	13	108	121	123,686	25,286	148,972	71.3	208,919		
Hospitals	104	498	34	2,929	3,565	13	0	13	88,296	17,313	105,608	68.8	153,481		
Institutions for mentally retarded	11	47	51	1,545	1,654	0	108	108	35,390	7,973	43,363	78.2	55,438		
TB and other respiratory diseases	0	0	0	0	0	0	0	0	0	0	0	0.0	0		
Long-term general and other special	2	13	7	110	132	0	0	0	3,903	847	4,750	63.6	7,474		
Short-term general and other special	392	8,084	1,559	24,954	34,989	307	49	356	777,298	129,159	906,457	53.0	1,710,922		
Hospital units of institutions	0	6	4	33	43	0	0	0	550	206	756	83.4	907		
Community hospitals*	392	8,078	1,555	24,921	34,946	307	49	356	776,748	128,953	905,701	53.0	1,710,015	$4,160.57	$ 532.16
6-24 beds	6	176	60	656	898	0	6	6	16,184	2,375	18,559	56.0	33,161	2,604.15	409.32
25-49	7	584	197	2,432	3,220	0	0	0	57,562	10,249	67,812	54.8	123,766	2,859.98	314.84
50-99	0	1,340	281	4,225	5,846	1	1	2	115,420	20,371	135,791	55.3	245,680	3,181.51	334.69
100-199	16	1,612	292	4,932	6,852	10	3	13	147,827	26,555	174,383	53.0	329,281	3,439.11	430.79
200-299	0	242	36	636	914	0	0	0	21,678	4,099	25,777	50.6	50,981	5,284.66	761.65
300-399	7	1,499	192	3,837	5,535	13	0	13	147,545	24,700	172,246	54.6	315,606	5,381.37	765.61
400-499	296	758	175	2,443	3,672	283	0	283	79,305	15,585	94,890	55.8	170,011	5,449.59	854.30
500 or more	60	1,867	322	5,760	8,009	0	39	39	191,226	25,018	216,243	49.0	441,529	5,349.47	784.79
Nongovernment not-for-profit	90	5,251	875	15,084	21,300	24	42	66	519,610	80,287	599,897	53.4	1,124,376	4,419.67	573.47
Investor-owned (for-profit)	0	1,070	194	3,245	4,509	0	0	0	78,351	16,000	94,351	45.3	208,506	4,125.41	689.03
State and local government	302	1,757	486	6,592	9,137	283	7	290	178,787	32,666	211,453	56.1	377,132	3,555.84	396.96

*For information on community hospitals that excludes nursing-home-type data, refer to Hospital Units columns in tables 4A through 4D, pages 14 through 17.

(continued on next page)

Table
5C (Continued) Kentucky

Utilization, Personnel, and Finances in States

Excludes AHA nonregistered hospitals (see Table 14, page 240).

CLASSIFICATION	HOSPITALS	BEDS	ADMISSIONS	INPATIENT DAYS	ADJUSTED PATIENT DAYS	OCCUPANCY, percent	AVERAGE DAILY CENSUS	ADJUSTED AVERAGE DAILY CENSUS	AVERAGE STAY, days	SURGICAL OPERATIONS	OUTPATIENT VISITS: Emergency	OUTPATIENT VISITS: Other	OUTPATIENT VISITS: Total	NEWBORNS: Bassinets	NEWBORNS: Births
KENTUCKY	123	18,845	580,166	4,466,765		65.0	12,242			401,478	1,649,666	4,165,943	5,815,609	1,149	54,735
6-24 beds	1	24	108	2,497		29.2	7			122	245	694	939	0	0
25-49	20	731	24,370	145,496		54.4	398			9,130	115,013	159,470	274,483	53	1,405
50-99	42	2,973	75,410	605,150		55.9	1,661			34,764	263,924	552,924	816,848	202	4,803
100-199	28	3,965	127,033	907,557		62.7	2,487			89,884	448,008	1,687,966	2,135,974	327	12,603
200-299	11	2,661	86,571	614,121		63.2	1,683			54,894	195,674	447,626	643,300	154	7,491
300-399	12	3,978	121,553	1,014,323		69.9	2,779			101,058	297,906	505,144	803,050	223	13,331
400-499	6	2,619	90,844	638,066		66.7	1,748			66,116	190,647	509,896	700,543	130	7,654
500 or more	3	1,894	54,277	539,555		78.1	1,479			45,510	138,249	302,223	440,472	60	7,448
Psychiatric	11	1,682	13,170	467,915		76.2	1,282			0	0	22,545	22,545	0	0
Hospitals	11	1,682	13,170	467,915		76.2	1,282			0	0	22,545	22,545	0	0
Institutions for mentally retarded	0	0	0	0		00.0	0			0	0	0	0	0	0
General	108	16,926	563,341	3,928,496		63.6	10,766			400,441	1,649,666	4,078,956	5,728,622	1,149	54,735
Hospitals	108	16,926	563,341	3,928,496		63.6	10,766			400,441	1,649,666	4,078,956	5,728,622	1,149	54,735
Hospital units of institutions	0	0	0	0		00.0	0			0	0	0	0	0	0
TB and other respiratory diseases	0	0	0	0		00.0	0			0	0	0	0	0	0
Obstetrics and gynecology	0	0	0	0		00.0	0			0	0	0	0	0	0
Eye, ear, nose, and throat	0	0	0	0		00.0	0			0	0	0	0	0	0
Rehabilitation	3	187	2,510	58,073		85.6	160			0	0	50,506	50,506	0	0
Orthopedic	1	50	1,145	12,281		68.0	34			1,037	0	13,936	13,936	0	0
Chronic disease	0	0	0	0		00.0	0			0	0	0	0	0	0
All other	0	0	0	0		00.0	0			0	0	0	0	0	0
Federal	4	1,419	35,023	411,107		79.4	1,126			24,947	136,522	1,256,384	1,392,906	43	2,401
Psychiatric	0	0	0	0		00.0	0			0	0	0	0	0	0
General and other special	4	1,419	35,023	411,107		79.4	1,126			24,947	136,522	1,256,384	1,392,906	43	2,401
Nonfederal	119	17,426	545,143	4,055,658		63.8	11,116			376,531	1,513,144	2,909,559	4,422,703	1,106	52,334
Psychiatric	11	1,682	13,170	467,915		76.2	1,282			0	0	22,545	22,545	0	0
Hospitals	11	1,682	13,170	467,915		76.2	1,282			0	0	22,545	22,545	0	0
Institutions for mentally retarded	0	0	0	0		00.0	0			0	0	0	0	0	0
TB and other respiratory diseases	0	0	0	0		00.0	0			0	0	0	0	0	0
Long-term general and other special	1	26	156	6,927		73.1	19			0	316	2,662	2,978	0	0
Short-term general and other special	107	15,718	531,817	3,580,816		62.4	9,815			376,531	1,512,828	2,884,352	4,397,180	1,106	52,334
Hospital units of institutions	0	0	0	0		00.0	0			0	0	0	0	0	0
Community hospitals*	107	15,718	531,817	3,580,816	4,693,845	62.4	9,815	12,861	6.7	376,531	1,512,828	2,884,352	4,397,180	1,106	52,334
6-24 beds	1	24	108	2,497	4,102	29.2	7	11	23.1	122	245	694	939	0	0
25-49	19	705	24,214	138,569	219,494	53.8	379	603	5.7	9,130	114,697	156,808	271,505	53	1,405
50-99	36	2,543	71,256	496,258	704,794	53.6	1,363	1,931	7.0	34,764	263,924	540,313	804,237	202	4,803
100-199	24	3,377	107,732	746,056	1,029,820	60.6	2,045	2,822	6.9	82,578	355,422	652,978	1,008,400	284	10,202
200-299	9	2,051	74,202	468,844	610,770	62.7	1,285	1,672	6.3	54,894	175,514	330,938	506,452	154	7,491
300-399	10	3,300	118,009	799,021	1,002,968	66.3	2,189	2,748	6.8	101,058	297,906	502,474	800,380	223	13,331
400-499	6	2,619	90,844	638,066	764,073	66.7	1,748	2,094	7.0	66,116	190,647	509,896	700,543	130	7,654
500 or more	2	1,099	45,452	291,505	357,824	72.7	799	980	6.4	27,869	114,473	190,251	304,724	60	7,448
Nongovernment not-for-profit	68	10,420	360,314	2,450,524	3,227,670	64.4	6,715	8,843	6.8	248,091	1,014,983	1,946,068	2,961,051	692	33,776
Investor-owned (for-profit)	21	3,223	106,346	643,688	822,508	54.8	1,765	2,255	6.1	86,834	311,200	508,501	819,701	280	12,530
State and local government	18	2,075	65,157	486,604	643,667	64.3	1,335	1,763	7.5	41,606	186,645	429,783	616,428	134	6,028

*For information on community hospitals that excludes nursing home type data, refer to Hospital Units columns in tables 4A through 4D, pages 14 through 17.

CLASSIFICATION	FULL-TIME EQUIVALENT PERSONNEL					FULL-TIME EQUIVALENT TRAINEES			EXPENSES						
									LABOR				TOTAL		
	Physicians and Dentists	Registered Nurses	Licensed Practical Nurses	Other Salaried Personnel	Total Personnel	Medical and Dental Residents	Other Trainees	Total Trainees	Payroll (in thousands)	Employee Benefits (in thousands)	Total (in thousands)	Percent of Total	Amount (in thousands)	Adjusted, per Admission	Adjusted, per Inpatient Day
KENTUCKY	511	13,065	3,613	41,230	58,419	227	102	329	$ 1,336,019	$ 256,175	$ 1,592,194	52.1	$ 3,054,213		
6-24 beds	0	10	6	42	58	0	0	0	510	96	607	55.1	1,102		
25-49	6	341	202	1,543	2,092	0	0	0	38,192	8,170	46,363	51.9	89,307		
50-99	24	1,444	481	5,282	7,231	14	18	32	144,567	28,829	173,396	52.4	330,755		
100-199	273	2,177	1,028	8,728	12,206	23	0	23	251,957	48,110	300,067	51.6	581,607		
200-299	86	1,908	582	5,818	8,394	45	12	57	189,791	36,398	226,189	52.9	427,749		
300-399	43	3,027	621	8,127	11,818	35	59	94	282,864	58,556	341,420	52.1	655,850		
400-499	3	2,639	397	7,425	10,464	2	3	5	241,451	40,260	281,711	48.0	587,326		
500 or more	76	1,519	296	4,265	6,156	108	10	118	186,687	35,755	222,442	58.5	380,518		
Psychiatric	49	431	157	2,192	2,829	8	4	12	74,250	15,726	89,976	62.5	143,960		
Hospitals	49	431	157	2,192	2,829	8	4	12	74,250	15,726	89,976	62.5	143,960		
Institutions for mentally retarded	0	0	0	0	0	0	0	0	0	0	0	0.0	0		
General	461	12,486	3,407	38,314	54,668	205	98	303	1,240,914	236,708	1,477,622	51.5	2,870,419		
Hospitals	461	12,486	3,407	38,314	54,668	205	98	303	1,240,914	236,708	1,477,622	51.5	2,870,419		
Hospital units of institutions	0	0	0	0	0	0	0	0	0	0	0	0.0	0		
TB and other respiratory diseases	0	0	0	0	0	0	0	0	0	0	0	0.0	0		
Obstetrics and gynecology	0	0	0	0	0	0	0	0	0	0	0	0.0	0		
Eye, ear, nose, and throat	0	0	0	0	0	0	0	0	0	0	0	0.0	0		
Rehabilitation	0	114	48	584	746	10	0	10	17,508	3,082	20,590	63.6	32,371		
Orthopedic	1	34	1	140	176	4	0	4	3,347	660	4,006	53.7	7,463		
Chronic disease	0	0	0	0	0	0	0	0	0	0	0	0.0	0		
All other	0	0	0	0	0	0	0	0	0	0	0	0.0	0		
Federal	355	737	371	3,615	5,078	157	22	179	147,615	24,620	172,235	65.2	264,071		
Psychiatric	0	0	0	0	0	0	0	0	0	0	0	0.0	0		
General and other special	355	737	371	3,615	5,078	157	22	179	147,615	24,620	172,235	65.2	264,071		
Nonfederal	156	12,328	3,242	37,615	53,341	70	80	150	1,188,404	231,555	1,419,959	50.9	2,790,142		
Psychiatric	49	431	157	2,192	2,829	8	4	12	74,250	15,726	89,976	62.5	143,960		
Hospitals	49	431	157	2,192	2,829	8	4	12	74,250	15,726	89,976	62.5	143,960		
Institutions for mentally retarded	0	0	0	0	0	0	0	0	0	0	0	0.0	0		
TB and other respiratory diseases	0	0	0	0	0	0	0	0	0	0	0	0.0	0		
Long-term general and other special	3	6	6	32	47	0	0	0	2,206	479	2,685	63.6	4,225		
Short-term general and other special	104	11,891	3,079	35,391	50,465	62	76	138	1,111,948	215,350	1,327,298	50.2	2,641,957		
Hospital units of institutions	0	0	0	0	0	0	0	0	0	0	0	0.0	0		
Community hospitals*	104	11,891	3,079	35,391	50,465	62	76	138	1,111,948	215,350	1,327,298	50.2	2,641,957	$3,761.81	$ 562.86
6-24 beds	0	10	6	42	58	0	0	0	510	96	607	55.1	1,102	6,225.16	268.61
25-49	3	335	196	1,511	2,045	0	0	0	35,986	7,692	43,678	51.3	85,082	2,230.90	387.63
50-99	17	1,322	457	4,640	6,436	14	18	32	124,479	24,495	148,974	52.0	286,257	2,721.49	406.16
100-199	41	1,831	843	6,463	9,178	0	0	0	188,489	37,379	225,868	49.3	458,409	3,072.14	445.14
200-299	16	1,611	511	4,759	6,897	0	0	0	143,954	27,635	171,589	50.7	338,648	3,504.69	554.46
300-399	18	2,917	557	7,348	10,840	27	55	82	253,416	51,867	305,283	50.4	605,732	4,090.24	603.94
400-499	3	2,639	397	7,425	10,464	2	3	5	241,451	40,260	281,711	48.0	587,326	5,382.88	768.68
500 or more	6	1,226	112	3,203	4,547	19	0	19	123,663	25,927	149,589	53.5	279,401	5,010.14	780.83
Nongovernment not-for-profit	97	7,971	2,136	24,397	34,601	60	76	136	778,077	151,001	929,078	51.7	1,795,851	3,742.15	556.39
Investor-owned (for-profit)	7	2,319	571	5,923	8,820	2	0	2	185,507	40,630	226,138	43.4	521,561	3,847.34	634.11
State and local government	0	1,601	372	5,071	7,044	0	0	0	148,364	23,719	172,083	53.0	324,545	3,736.94	504.21

*For information on community hospitals that excludes nursing-home-type data, refer to Hospital Units columns in tables 4A through 4D, pages 14 through 17.

(continued on next page)

Table
5C (Continued) Louisiana

Utilization, Personnel, and Finances in States

Excludes AHA nonregistered hospitals (see Table 14, page 240).

CLASSIFICATION	HOSPITALS	BEDS	ADMISSIONS	INPATIENT DAYS	ADJUSTED PATIENT DAYS	OCCUPANCY, percent	AVERAGE DAILY CENSUS	ADJUSTED AVERAGE DAILY CENSUS	AVERAGE STAY, days	SURGICAL OPERATIONS	OUTPATIENT VISITS: Emergency	OUTPATIENT VISITS: Other	OUTPATIENT VISITS: Total	NEWBORNS: Bassinets	NEWBORNS: Births
LOUISIANA	173	23,890	658,189	5,246,257		60.2	14,376			397,451	1,817,352	4,656,059	6,473,411	1,526	71,253
6-24 beds	4	68	2,250	8,953		36.8	25			1,390	26,184	101,066	127,250	0	23
25-49	41	1,556	41,286	267,851		47.1	733			15,229	149,200	374,682	523,882	96	1,882
50-99	48	3,487	83,118	641,950		50.6	1,763			41,053	205,764	322,601	528,365	252	8,218
100-199	46	6,602	189,333	1,287,556		53.4	3,527			121,819	564,630	1,133,424	1,698,054	605	29,715
200-299	16	4,093	123,525	969,043		64.8	2,653			85,361	256,082	715,548	971,630	232	11,463
300-399	7	2,625	78,111	673,271		70.3	1,845			48,452	171,306	769,213	940,519	167	9,846
400-499	6	2,648	56,557	684,932		70.9	1,878			31,146	165,500	382,838	548,338	74	2,632
500 or more	5	2,811	84,009	712,701		69.4	1,952			53,001	278,686	856,687	1,135,373	100	7,474
Psychiatric	26	3,060	17,087	755,514		67.6	2,070			0	3,721	45,431	49,152	0	0
Hospitals	26	3,060	17,087	755,514		67.6	2,070			0	3,721	45,431	49,152	0	0
Institutions for mentally retarded	0	0	0	0		00.0	0			0	0	0	0	0	0
General	137	19,536	617,492	4,220,492		59.2	11,565			383,465	1,796,359	4,433,351	6,229,710	1,392	64,360
Hospitals	137	19,536	617,492	4,220,492		59.2	11,565			383,465	1,796,359	4,433,351	6,229,710	1,392	64,360
Hospital units of institutions	0	0	0	0		00.0	0			0	0	0	0	0	0
TB and other respiratory diseases	0	0	0	0		00.0	0			0	0	0	0	0	0
Obstetrics and gynecology	1	177	10,408	38,265		59.3	105			5,340	2,726	42,783	45,509	70	5,327
Eye, ear, nose, and throat	1	39	744	1,962		12.8	5			2,520	0	25,952	25,952	0	0
Rehabilitation	4	414	3,521	57,178		37.9	157			0	0	34,624	34,624	0	0
Orthopedic	1	45	796	9,125		55.6	25			577	0	9,144	9,144	0	0
Chronic disease	1	418	205	113,429		74.4	311			0	0	0	0	0	0
All other	2	201	7,936	50,292		68.7	138			5,549	14,546	64,774	79,320	64	1,566
Federal	6	1,327	34,034	378,622		78.1	1,037			13,368	110,363	919,373	1,029,736	40	1,230
Psychiatric	0	0	0	0		00.0	0			0	0	0	0	0	0
General and other special	6	1,327	34,034	378,622		78.1	1,037			13,368	110,363	919,373	1,029,736	40	1,230
Nonfederal	167	22,563	624,155	4,867,635		59.1	13,339			384,083	1,706,989	3,736,686	5,443,675	1,486	70,023
Psychiatric	26	3,060	17,087	755,514		67.6	2,070			0	3,721	45,431	49,152	0	0
Hospitals	26	3,060	17,087	755,514		67.6	2,070			0	3,721	45,431	49,152	0	0
Institutions for mentally retarded	0	0	0	0		00.0	0			0	0	0	0	0	0
TB and other respiratory diseases	0	0	0	0		00.0	0			0	0	0	0	0	0
Long-term general and other special	1	418	205	113,429		74.4	311			0	0	0	0	0	0
Short-term general and other special	140	19,085	606,863	3,998,692		57.4	10,958			384,083	1,703,268	3,691,255	5,394,523	1,486	70,023
Hospital units of institutions	0	0	0	0		00.0	0			0	0	0	0	0	0
Community hospitals*	140	19,085	606,863	3,998,692	5,102,977	57.4	10,958	13,982	6.6	384,083	1,703,268	3,691,255	5,394,523	1,486	70,023
6-24 beds	3	53	1,220	5,791	10,136	30.2	16	28	4.7	503	8,089	27,294	35,383	0	23
25-49	34	1,273	35,464	199,524	295,831	43.0	547	814	5.6	13,662	119,913	200,066	319,979	78	1,482
50-99	37	2,660	76,450	467,500	615,265	48.3	1,284	1,684	6.1	41,053	204,030	303,612	507,642	252	8,218
100-199	39	5,554	177,367	1,079,079	1,439,949	53.2	2,956	3,945	6.1	117,481	531,878	827,790	1,359,668	583	28,885
200-299	14	3,533	113,369	799,155	973,801	61.9	2,188	2,668	7.0	83,361	255,713	596,268	851,981	232	11,463
300-399	5	1,917	68,942	456,543	587,806	65.3	1,251	1,610	6.6	46,123	160,292	563,160	723,452	167	9,846
400-499	4	1,778	55,718	428,100	522,667	66.0	1,174	1,432	7.7	31,146	165,305	379,767	545,072	74	2,632
500 or more	4	2,317	78,333	563,000	657,522	66.6	1,542	1,801	7.2	50,754	258,048	793,298	1,051,346	100	7,474
Nongovernment not-for-profit	34	7,917	261,494	1,832,497	2,293,600	63.4	5,021	6,284	7.0	173,401	533,363	1,645,134	2,178,497	458	22,401
Investor-owned (for-profit)	43	4,667	124,881	768,207	990,847	45.1	2,104	2,714	6.2	79,902	302,981	371,398	674,379	408	14,711
State and local government	63	6,501	220,488	1,397,988	1,818,530	59.0	3,833	4,984	6.3	130,780	866,924	1,674,723	2,541,647	620	32,911

*For information on community hospitals that excludes nursing home type data, refer to Hospital Units columns in tables 4A through 4D, pages 14 through 17.

CLASSIFICATION	FULL-TIME EQUIVALENT PERSONNEL					FULL-TIME EQUIVALENT TRAINEES			EXPENSES						
									LABOR				TOTAL		
	Physicians and Dentists	Registered Nurses	Licensed Practical Nurses	Other Salaried Personnel	Total Personnel	Medical and Dental Residents	Other Trainees	Total Trainees	Payroll (in thousands)	Employee Benefits (in thousands)	Total (in thousands)	Percent of Total	Amount (in thousands)	Adjusted, per Admission	Adjusted, per Inpatient Day
LOUISIANA	560	14,249	5,505	53,002	73,316	1,455	30	1,485	$ 1,725,427	$ 326,649	$ 2,052,076	49.7	$ 4,127,353		
6-24 beds	23	43	17	329	412	0	0	0	11,970	2,080	14,051	78.3	17,952		
25-49	51	648	383	3,075	4,157	6	0	6	81,300	15,989	97,288	52.0	187,232		
50-99	25	1,437	880	5,631	7,973	1	0	1	172,178	34,278	206,457	47.4	435,501		
100-199	106	3,996	1,484	13,102	18,688	119	0	119	426,304	88,394	514,698	48.0	1,072,143		
200-299	83	2,763	989	9,902	13,737	192	15	207	328,517	57,939	386,456	46.4	832,884		
300-399	146	1,859	622	7,399	10,026	325	11	336	269,200	51,002	320,201	55.1	580,621		
400-499	36	1,340	538	5,280	7,194	25	1	26	168,554	32,182	200,736	53.3	376,323		
500 or more	90	2,163	592	8,284	11,129	787	3	790	267,404	44,785	312,189	50.0	624,697		
Psychiatric	67	663	200	3,781	4,711	5	1	6	129,088	28,522	157,610	58.4	269,687		
Hospitals	67	663	200	3,781	4,711	5	1	6	129,088	28,522	157,610	58.4	269,687		
Institutions for mentally retarded	0	0	0	0	0	0	0	0	0	0	0	0.0	0		
General	479	12,943	5,146	46,761	65,329	1,435	29	1,464	1,527,650	284,593	1,812,243	49.0	3,696,948		
Hospitals	479	12,943	5,146	46,761	65,329	1,435	29	1,464	1,527,650	284,593	1,812,243	49.0	3,696,948		
Hospital units of institutions	0	0	0	0	0	0	0	0	0	0	0	0.0	0		
TB and other respiratory diseases	0	0	0	0	0	0	0	0	0	0	0	0.0	0		
Obstetrics and gynecology	0	282	17	539	838	0	0	0	19,798	3,593	23,391	54.1	43,199		
Eye, ear, nose, and throat	1	41	15	141	198	6	0	6	4,396	938	5,335	49.5	10,780		
Rehabilitation	1	82	66	598	747	0	0	0	16,354	3,630	19,984	44.8	44,648		
Orthopedic	2	17	7	96	122	0	0	0	3,401	643	4,044	52.5	7,704		
Chronic disease	4	11	19	371	405	0	0	0	6,913	1,048	7,961	69.7	11,416		
All other	6	210	35	715	966	9	0	9	17,827	3,682	21,508	50.1	42,971		
Federal	336	672	280	4,003	5,291	171	14	185	141,326	30,420	171,746	63.3	271,245		
Psychiatric	0	0	0	0	0	0	0	0	0	0	0	0.0	0		
General and other special	336	672	280	4,003	5,291	171	14	185	141,326	30,420	171,746	63.3	271,245		
Nonfederal	224	13,577	5,225	48,999	68,025	1,284	16	1,300	1,584,101	296,229	1,880,330	48.8	3,856,108		
Psychiatric	67	663	200	3,781	4,711	5	1	6	129,088	28,522	157,610	58.4	269,687		
Hospitals	67	663	200	3,781	4,711	5	1	6	129,088	28,522	157,610	58.4	269,687		
Institutions for mentally retarded	0	0	0	0	0	0	0	0	0	0	0	0.0	0		
TB and other respiratory diseases	0	0	0	0	0	0	0	0	0	0	0	0.0	0		
Long-term general and other special	4	11	19	371	405	0	0	0	6,913	1,048	7,961	69.7	11,416		
Short-term general and other special	153	12,903	5,006	44,847	62,909	1,279	15	1,294	1,448,100	266,659	1,714,759	48.0	3,575,006		
Hospital units of institutions	0	0	0	0	0	0	0	0	0	0	0	0.0	0		
Community hospitals*	153	12,903	5,006	44,847	62,909	1,279	15	1,294	1,448,100	266,659	1,714,759	48.0	3,575,006	$4,574.56	$ 700.57
6-24 beds	0	21	14	122	157	0	0	0	3,342	594	3,936	51.1	7,698	3,588.96	759.50
25-49	6	514	356	2,336	3,212	6	0	6	63,793	12,000	75,793	49.9	151,819	2,856.43	513.20
50-99	13	1,211	821	4,652	6,697	0	0	0	134,618	26,946	161,565	45.9	352,207	3,484.03	572.45
100-199	20	3,677	1,409	11,418	16,524	105	0	105	363,751	75,092	438,843	46.7	939,002	3,951.30	652.11
200-299	15	2,563	908	8,690	12,176	132	15	147	288,841	50,372	339,213	45.3	748,778	5,414.94	768.92
300-399	38	1,590	491	5,770	7,889	235	0	235	209,764	40,341	250,105	53.2	469,815	5,262.55	799.27
400-499	13	1,261	485	4,348	6,107	24	0	24	141,225	25,290	166,515	50.0	333,297	4,896.09	637.68
500 or more	48	2,066	522	7,511	10,147	777	0	777	242,764	36,024	278,789	48.7	572,389	6,232.66	870.52
Nongovernment not-for-profit	72	6,148	1,818	21,120	29,158	499	12	511	697,583	124,775	822,358	49.5	1,661,997	5,054.55	724.62
Investor-owned (for-profit)	6	2,689	954	7,395	11,044	0	0	0	253,939	60,784	314,722	41.2	763,716	4,697.74	770.77
State and local government	75	4,066	2,234	16,332	22,707	780	3	783	496,578	81,101	577,679	50.3	1,149,293	3,961.52	631.99

*For information on community hospitals that excludes nursing-home-type data, refer to Hospital Units columns in tables 4A through 4D, pages 14 through 17.

(continued on next page)

Table

5C (Continued) Maine

Utilization, Personnel, and Finances in States

Excludes AHA nonregistered hospitals (see Table 14, page 240).

CLASSIFICATION	HOSPITALS	BEDS	ADMISSIONS	INPATIENT DAYS	ADJUSTED PATIENT DAYS	OCCUPANCY, percent	AVERAGE DAILY CENSUS	ADJUSTED AVERAGE DAILY CENSUS	AVERAGE STAY, days	SURGICAL OPERATIONS	OUTPATIENT VISITS Emergency	OUTPATIENT VISITS Other	OUTPATIENT VISITS Total	NEWBORNS Bassinets	NEWBORNS Births
MAINE	44	5,636	155,909	1,518,325		73.8	4,160			110,978	621,369	1,489,082	2,110,451	408	16,692
6-24 beds	2	44	2,043	8,441		52.3	23			1,075	15,433	81,926	97,359	10	315
25-49	7	274	9,659	55,806		55.8	153			5,426	55,621	132,857	188,478	39	1,041
50-99	18	1,149	38,868	259,166		61.7	709			29,776	227,719	429,246	656,965	132	4,167
100-199	7	969	26,491	271,026		76.7	743			27,052	115,491	230,853	346,344	75	2,664
200-299	5	1,178	25,522	323,667		75.3	887			17,479	97,478	211,166	308,644	72	2,459
300-399	3	1,018	15,886	291,068		78.4	798			9,199	25,504	152,874	178,378	22	1,088
400-499	1	414	14,724	119,644		79.2	328			9,271	42,256	201,799	244,055	26	1,985
500 or more	1	590	22,716	189,507		88.0	519			11,700	41,867	48,361	90,228	32	2,973
Psychiatric	3	771	4,776	234,530		83.4	643			0	0	2,420	2,420	0	0
Hospitals	3	771	4,776	234,530		83.4	643			0	0	2,420	2,420	0	0
Institutions for mentally retarded	0	0	0	0		00.0	0			0	0	0	0	0	0
General	40	4,515	146,811	1,176,983		71.4	3,224			108,546	621,369	1,388,409	2,009,778	408	16,692
Hospitals	40	4,515	146,811	1,176,983		71.4	3,224			108,546	621,369	1,388,409	2,009,778	408	16,692
Hospital units of institutions	0	0	0	0		00.0	0			0	0	0	0	0	0
TB and other respiratory diseases	0	0	0	0		00.0	0			0	0	0	0	0	0
Obstetrics and gynecology	0	0	0	0		00.0	0			0	0	0	0	0	0
Eye, ear, nose, and throat	0	0	0	0		00.0	0			0	0	0	0	0	0
Rehabilitation	0	0	0	0		00.0	0			0	0	0	0	0	0
Orthopedic	0	0	0	0		00.0	0			0	0	0	0	0	0
Chronic disease	0	0	0	0		00.0	0			0	0	0	0	0	0
All other	1	350	4,322	106,812		83.7	293			2,432	0	98,253	98,253	0	0
Federal	2	370	5,564	110,453		81.9	303			2,873	10,897	162,715	173,612	10	315
Psychiatric	0	0	0	0		00.0	0			0	0	0	0	0	0
General and other special	2	370	5,564	110,453		81.9	303			2,873	10,897	162,715	173,612	10	315
Nonfederal	42	5,266	150,345	1,407,872		73.2	3,857			108,105	610,472	1,326,367	1,936,839	398	16,377
Psychiatric	3	771	4,776	234,530		83.4	643			0	0	2,420	2,420	0	0
Hospitals	3	771	4,776	234,530		83.4	643			0	0	2,420	2,420	0	0
Institutions for mentally retarded	0	0	0	0		00.0	0			0	0	0	0	0	0
TB and other respiratory diseases	0	0	0	0		00.0	0			0	0	0	0	0	0
Long-term general and other special	0	0	0	0		00.0	0			0	0	0	0	0	0
Short-term general and other special	39	4,495	145,569	1,173,342		71.5	3,214			108,105	610,472	1,323,947	1,934,419	398	16,377
Hospital units of institutions	0	0	0	0		00.0	0			0	0	0	0	0	0
Community hospitals*	39	4,495	145,569	1,173,342	1,600,755	71.5	3,214	4,386	8.1	108,105	610,472	1,323,947	1,934,419	398	16,377
6-24 beds	1	24	801	4,800	8,549	54.2	13	23	6.0	634	4,536	17,464	22,000	0	0
25-49	7	274	9,659	55,806	82,230	55.8	153	225	5.8	5,426	55,621	132,857	188,478	39	1,041
50-99	18	1,149	38,868	259,166	384,308	61.7	709	1,053	6.7	29,776	227,719	429,246	656,965	132	4,167
100-199	6	863	25,150	235,585	331,216	74.9	646	908	9.4	27,052	115,491	228,433	343,924	75	2,664
200-299	4	880	25,199	224,821	302,229	70.0	616	828	8.9	17,479	97,478	211,166	308,644	72	2,459
300-399	1	301	8,452	84,013	120,820	76.4	230	331	9.9	6,767	25,504	54,621	80,125	22	1,088
400-499	1	414	14,724	119,644	151,828	79.2	328	416	8.1	9,271	42,256	201,799	244,055	26	1,985
500 or more	1	590	22,716	189,507	219,575	88.0	519	602	8.3	11,700	41,867	48,361	90,228	32	2,973
Nongovernment not-for-profit	35	4,182	134,747	1,093,022	1,485,156	71.6	2,994	4,069	8.1	96,921	535,452	1,202,074	1,737,526	360	15,225
Investor-owned (for-profit)	0	0	0	0	0	00.0	0	0	0.0	0	0	0	0	0	0
State and local government	4	313	10,822	80,320	115,599	70.3	220	317	7.4	11,184	75,020	121,873	196,893	38	1,152

CLASSIFICATION	FULL-TIME EQUIVALENT PERSONNEL					FULL-TIME EQUIVALENT TRAINEES			EXPENSES						
									LABOR				TOTAL		
	Physicians and Dentists	Registered Nurses	Licensed Practical Nurses	Other Salaried Personnel	Total Personnel	Medical and Dental Residents	Other Trainees	Total Trainees	Payroll (in thousands)	Employee Benefits (in thousands)	Total (in thousands)	Percent of Total	Amount (in thousands)	Adjusted, per Admission	Adjusted, per Inpatient Day
MAINE	287	4,539	1,099	14,549	20,474	210	10	220	$ 519,161	$ 97,851	$ 617,012	59.4	$ 1,038,651		
6-24 beds	20	39	11	254	334	0	0	0	5,550	1,188	6,738	63.2	10,667		
25-49	3	241	69	730	1,043	0	0	0	24,316	4,445	28,761	59.6	48,253		
50-99	43	1,067	342	3,124	4,576	0	0	0	103,597	18,428	122,025	57.4	212,680		
100-199	17	731	141	2,239	3,188	19	0	19	81,993	15,099	97,092	59.1	164,399		
200-299	32	796	222	2,524	3,574	15	0	15	90,464	18,082	108,547	60.2	180,176		
300-399	83	475	111	2,046	2,715	9	10	19	77,751	15,394	93,145	69.1	134,884		
400-499	20	522	83	1,238	1,913	25	0	25	54,217	9,553	63,770	57.5	110,977		
500 or more	69	668	120	2,274	3,131	142	0	142	81,273	15,661	96,934	54.9	176,617		
Psychiatric	31	217	55	1,253	1,556	11	0	11	43,051	9,914	52,965	68.2	77,621		
Hospitals	31	217	55	1,253	1,556	11	0	11	43,051	9,914	52,965	68.2	77,621		
Institutions for mentally retarded	0	0	0	0	0	0	0	0	0	0	0	0.0	0		
General	212	4,180	1,022	12,537	17,951	196	0	196	450,290	82,696	532,986	57.7	924,148		
Hospitals	212	4,180	1,022	12,537	17,951	196	0	196	450,290	82,696	532,986	57.7	924,148		
Hospital units of institutions	0	0	0	0	0	0	0	0	0	0	0	0.0	0		
TB and other respiratory diseases	0	0	0	0	0	0	0	0	0	0	0	0.0	0		
Obstetrics and gynecology	0	0	0	0	0	0	0	0	0	0	0	0.0	0		
Eye, ear, nose, and throat	0	0	0	0	0	0	0	0	0	0	0	0.0	0		
Rehabilitation	0	0	0	0	0	0	0	0	0	0	0	0.0	0		
Orthopedic	0	0	0	0	0	0	0	0	0	0	0	0.0	0		
Chronic disease	0	0	0	0	0	0	0	0	0	0	0	0.0	0		
All other	44	142	22	759	967	3	10	13	25,820	5,241	31,061	84.2	36,883		
Federal	63	168	27	955	1,213	3	10	13	29,230	6,000	35,230	82.3	42,831		
Psychiatric	0	0	0	0	0	0	0	0	0	0	0	0.0	0		
General and other special	63	168	27	955	1,213	3	10	13	29,230	6,000	35,230	82.3	42,831		
Nonfederal	224	4,371	1,072	13,594	19,261	207	0	207	489,931	91,851	581,782	58.4	995,820		
Psychiatric	31	217	55	1,253	1,556	11	0	11	43,051	9,914	52,965	68.2	77,621		
Hospitals	31	217	55	1,253	1,556	11	0	11	43,051	9,914	52,965	68.2	77,621		
Institutions for mentally retarded	0	0	0	0	0	0	0	0	0	0	0	0.0	0		
TB and other respiratory diseases	0	0	0	0	0	0	0	0	0	0	0	0.0	0		
Long-term general and other special	0	0	0	0	0	0	0	0	0	0	0	0.0	0		
Short-term general and other special	193	4,154	1,017	12,341	17,705	196	0	196	446,880	81,937	528,817	57.6	918,199		
Hospital units of institutions	0	0	0	0	0	0	0	0	0	0	0	0.0	0		
Community hospitals*	193	4,154	1,017	12,341	17,705	196	0	196	446,880	81,937	528,817	57.6	918,199	$4,603.63	$ 573.60
6-24 beds	1	13	6	68	88	0	0	0	2,140	428	2,568	54.4	4,719	3,306.64	551.94
25-49	3	241	69	730	1,043	0	0	0	24,316	4,445	28,761	59.6	48,253	3,400.23	586.80
50-99	43	1,067	342	3,124	4,576	0	0	0	103,597	18,428	122,025	57.4	212,680	3,668.85	553.41
100-199	17	673	139	2,113	2,942	19	0	19	76,236	13,848	90,084	59.0	152,790	4,359.45	461.30
200-299	20	722	192	2,032	2,966	10	0	10	74,327	14,320	88,647	57.7	153,699	4,566.77	508.55
300-399	20	248	66	712	1,046	0	0	0	30,774	5,253	36,027	61.6	58,466	4,810.01	483.91
400-499	20	522	83	1,288	1,913	25	0	25	54,217	9,553	63,770	57.5	110,977	5,939.34	730.94
500 or more	69	668	120	2,274	3,131	142	0	142	81,273	15,661	96,934	54.9	176,617	6,710.36	804.36
Nongovernment not-for-profit	185	3,889	895	11,454	16,423	196	0	196	415,869	76,253	492,122	57.5	855,644	4,655.45	576.13
Investor-owned (for-profit)	0	0	0	0	0	0	0	0	0	0	0	0.0	0	0.00	0.00
State and local government	8	265	122	887	1,282	0	0	0	31,011	5,684	36,695	58.7	62,555	3,995.33	541.14

*For information on community hospitals that excludes nursing-home-type data, refer to Hospital Units columns in tables 4A through 4D, pages 14 through 17.

(continued on next page)

Table

5C (Continued) Maryland

Utilization, Personnel, and Finances in States

Excludes AHA nonregistered hospitals (see Table 14, page 240).

CLASSIFICATION	HOSPITALS	BEDS	ADMISSIONS	INPATIENT DAYS	ADJUSTED PATIENT DAYS	OCCUPANCY, percent	AVERAGE DAILY CENSUS	ADJUSTED AVERAGE DAILY CENSUS	AVERAGE STAY, days	SURGICAL OPERATIONS	OUTPATIENT VISITS Emergency	OUTPATIENT VISITS Other	OUTPATIENT VISITS Total	NEWBORNS Bassinets	NEWBORNS Births
MARYLAND	82	20,636	630,293	5,655,579		75.1	15,492			516,127	1,569,730	4,981,300	6,551,030	914	71,884
6-24 beds	2	44	979	10,818		68.2	30			2,294	15,454	84,996	100,450	8	326
25-49	4	176	2,958	46,251		72.2	127			850	10,885	35,751	46,636	0	0
50-99	11	856	19,921	212,444		68.0	582			14,469	58,046	328,905	386,951	16	603
100-199	17	2,262	57,603	638,414		77.2	1,747			42,145	195,519	429,787	625,306	78	3,218
200-299	22	5,261	185,250	1,474,788		76.8	4,039			157,544	517,799	1,407,824	1,925,623	290	20,111
300-399	13	4,405	156,599	1,269,194		78.9	3,477			146,947	337,968	1,418,662	1,756,630	220	17,623
400-499	7	3,067	126,836	841,025		75.2	2,305			107,928	275,165	632,639	907,804	222	23,096
500 or more	6	4,565	80,147	1,162,645		69.8	3,185			43,950	158,894	642,736	801,630	80	6,907
Psychiatric	16	3,985	15,452	969,159		66.7	2,657			287	743	141,322	142,065	0	0
Hospitals	16	3,985	15,452	969,159		66.7	2,657			287	743	141,322	142,065	0	0
Institutions for mentally retarded	0	0	0	0		00.0	0			0	0	0	0	0	0
General	55	14,559	597,353	4,147,704		78.0	11,360			506,143	1,565,603	4,580,530	6,146,133	914	71,884
Hospitals	55	14,559	597,353	4,147,704		78.0	11,360			506,143	1,565,603	4,580,530	6,146,133	914	71,884
Hospital units of institutions	0	0	0	0		00.0	0			0	0	0	0	0	0
TB and other respiratory diseases	0	0	0	0		00.0	0			0	0	0	0	0	0
Obstetrics and gynecology	0	0	0	0		00.0	0			0	0	0	0	0	0
Eye, ear, nose, and throat	0	0	0	0		00.0	0			0	0	0	0	0	0
Rehabilitation	1	135	877	40,185		81.5	110			0	0	1,919	1,919	0	0
Orthopedic	2	137	3,598	31,075		62.0	85			7,547	0	48,337	48,337	0	0
Chronic disease	3	658	2,122	199,180		82.8	545			104	3,384	29,773	33,157	0	0
All other	5	1,162	10,891	268,276		63.3	735			2,046	0	179,419	179,419	0	0
Federal	8	2,500	51,489	643,708		70.5	1,763			35,387	127,543	1,748,724	1,876,267	55	2,464
Psychiatric	1	759	3,085	220,174		79.4	603			287	5	63,462	63,467	0	0
General and other special	7	1,741	48,404	423,534		66.6	1,160			35,100	127,538	1,685,262	1,812,800	55	2,464
Nonfederal	74	18,136	578,804	5,011,871		75.7	13,729			480,740	1,442,187	3,232,576	4,674,763	859	69,420
Psychiatric	15	3,226	12,367	748,985		63.7	2,054			0	738	77,860	78,598	0	0
Hospitals	15	3,226	12,367	748,985		63.7	2,054			0	738	77,860	78,598	0	0
Institutions for mentally retarded	0	0	0	0		00.0	0			0	0	0	0	0	0
TB and other respiratory diseases	0	0	0	0		00.0	0			0	0	0	0	0	0
Long-term general and other special	7	1,438	4,157	398,904		75.9	1,092			104	3,384	31,692	35,076	0	0
Short-term general and other special	52	13,472	562,280	3,863,982		78.6	10,583			480,636	1,438,065	3,123,024	4,561,089	859	69,420
Hospital units of institutions	0	0	0	0		00.0	0			0	0	0	0	0	0
Community hospitals*	52	13,472	562,280	3,863,982	4,938,583	78.6	10,583	13,531	6.9	480,636	1,438,065	3,123,024	4,561,089	859	69,420
6-24 beds	0	0	0	0	0	00.0	0	0	0.0	0	0	0	0	0	0
25-49	3	134	2,782	34,266	46,220	70.1	94	127	12.3	850	10,526	33,972	44,498	0	0
50-99	4	277	10,281	66,108	88,750	65.3	181	243	6.4	12,128	29,135	95,183	124,318	16	603
100-199	9	1,106	47,677	296,388	393,574	73.2	810	1,078	6.2	38,334	156,555	253,647	410,202	78	3,218
200-299	18	4,177	174,153	1,207,884	1,550,156	79.2	3,308	4,248	6.9	154,056	469,827	963,101	1,432,928	255	19,128
300-399	9	2,970	136,139	847,026	1,083,041	78.1	2,320	2,966	6.2	125,723	337,968	716,142	1,054,110	208	16,468
400-499	6	2,596	117,519	742,749	967,331	78.4	2,036	2,650	6.3	105,882	275,165	481,705	756,870	222	23,096
500 or more	3	2,212	73,729	669,561	809,511	82.9	1,834	2,219	9.1	43,663	158,889	579,274	738,163	80	6,907
Nongovernment not-for-profit	50	12,914	540,955	3,713,249	4,754,135	78.8	10,170	13,025	6.9	455,015	1,380,800	3,098,651	4,479,451	843	67,946
Investor-owned (for-profit)	2	558	21,325	150,733	184,448	74.0	413	506	7.1	25,621	57,265	24,373	81,638	16	1,474
State and local government	0	0	0	0	0	00.0	0	0	0.0	0	0	0	0	0	0

CLASSIFICATION	FULL-TIME EQUIVALENT PERSONNEL					FULL-TIME EQUIVALENT TRAINEES			EXPENSES						
									LABOR				TOTAL		
	Physicians and Dentists	Registered Nurses	Licensed Practical Nurses	Other Salaried Personnel	Total Personnel	Medical and Dental Residents	Other Trainees	Total Trainees	Payroll (in thousands)	Employee Benefits (in thousands)	Total (in thousands)	Percent of Total	Amount (in thousands)	Adjusted, per Admission	Adjusted, per Inpatient Day
MARYLAND	1,371	17,797	2,103	55,934	77,205	1,517	136	1,653	$ 2,067,744	$ 413,273	$ 2,481,017	57.6	$ 4,310,555		
6-24 beds	11	28	5	230	274	0	0	0	3,387	1,868	5,256	61.2	8,585		
25-49	19	92	20	870	1,001	10	34	44	23,004	5,633	28,637	62.3	45,952		
50-99	73	448	75	1,878	2,474	1	13	14	65,019	12,871	77,891	58.5	133,194		
100-199	127	1,517	393	5,539	7,576	80	15	95	201,796	41,709	243,504	59.4	410,117		
200-299	341	4,594	619	14,318	19,872	231	8	239	519,581	99,412	618,993	56.4	1,098,188		
300-399	317	3,679	385	13,285	17,666	446	5	451	433,004	84,970	517,974	59.6	869,755		
400-499	293	3,581	184	9,532	13,590	337	61	398	407,577	77,601	485,178	56.9	852,408		
500 or more	190	3,858	422	10,282	14,752	412	0	412	414,375	89,210	503,585	56.4	892,356		
Psychiatric	225	1,016	392	5,525	7,158	49	9	58	219,486	53,104	272,590	66.0	412,759		
Hospitals	225	1,016	392	5,525	7,158	49	9	58	219,486	53,104	272,590	66.0	412,759		
Institutions for mentally retarded	0	0	0	0	0	0	0	0	0	0	0	0.0	0		
General	998	15,586	1,499	46,146	64,229	1,455	91	1,546	1,674,668	320,369	1,995,038	56.7	3,518,517		
Hospitals	998	15,586	1,499	46,146	64,229	1,455	91	1,546	1,674,668	320,369	1,995,038	56.7	3,518,517		
Hospital units of institutions	0	0	0	0	0	0	0	0	0	0	0	0.0	0		
TB and other respiratory diseases	0	0	0	0	0	0	0	0	0	0	0	0.0	0		
Obstetrics and gynecology	0	0	0	0	0	0	0	0	0	0	0	0.0	0		
Eye, ear, nose, and throat	0	0	0	0	0	0	0	0	0	0	0	0.0	0		
Rehabilitation	19	91	30	329	469	2	0	2	12,267	3,221	15,488	78.7	19,682		
Orthopedic	2	124	8	363	497	0	0	0	12,990	2,368	15,358	49.5	31,009		
Chronic disease	11	130	80	972	1,193	1	0	1	30,982	7,464	38,445	62.1	61,938		
All other	116	850	94	2,599	3,659	10	36	46	117,352	26,747	144,099	54.0	266,650		
Federal	520	1,863	165	7,260	9,808	455	5	460	232,106	51,237	283,343	57.7	491,409		
Psychiatric	42	164	63	931	1,200	8	0	8	34,432	6,400	40,832	55.8	73,192		
General and other special	478	1,699	102	6,329	8,608	447	5	452	197,674	44,836	242,511	58.0	418,217		
Nonfederal	851	15,934	1,938	48,674	67,397	1,062	131	1,193	1,835,638	362,037	2,197,675	57.5	3,819,146		
Psychiatric	183	852	329	4,594	5,958	41	9	50	185,054	46,704	231,758	68.3	339,567		
Hospitals	183	852	329	4,594	5,958	41	9	50	185,054	46,704	231,758	68.3	339,567		
Institutions for mentally retarded	0	0	0	0	0	0	0	0	0	0	0	0.0	0		
TB and other respiratory diseases	0	0	0	0	0	0	0	0	0	0	0	0.0	0		
Long-term general and other special	49	322	201	2,125	2,697	3	2	5	72,370	17,497	89,866	67.6	132,874		
Short-term general and other special	619	14,760	1,408	41,955	58,742	1,018	120	1,138	1,578,214	297,836	1,876,050	56.1	3,346,704		
Hospital units of institutions	0	0	0	0	0	0	0	0	0	0	0	0.0	0		
Community hospitals*	619	14,760	1,408	41,955	58,742	1,018	120	1,138	1,578,214	297,836	1,876,050	56.1	3,346,704	$4,640.37	$ 677.66
6-24 beds	0	0	0	0	0	0	0	0	0	0	0	0.0	0	0.00	0.00
25-49	17	83	19	796	915	10	34	44	20,750	5,090	25,840	63.1	40,979	11,214.75	886.60
50-99	6	247	36	723	1,012	0	3	3	25,003	5,236	30,239	54.2	55,750	4,022.07	628.17
100-199	11	958	194	3,100	4,263	2	11	13	104,538	19,864	124,401	54.5	228,236	3,585.80	579.91
200-299	191	4,245	518	12,194	17,148	147	6	153	456,188	88,860	545,048	55.2	988,118	4,408.23	637.43
300-399	115	3,039	325	9,243	12,725	130	5	135	344,751	58,276	403,027	57.4	702,571	4,019.28	648.70
400-499	213	2,863	182	8,275	11,533	337	61	398	334,037	61,602	395,639	59.5	664,722	4,372.22	687.17
500 or more	66	3,325	134	7,621	11,146	392	0	392	292,948	58,909	351,857	52.8	666,328	7,481.45	823.12
Nongovernment not-for-profit	602	14,405	1,315	40,783	57,110	1,018	120	1,138	1,529,124	289,616	1,818,740	56.4	3,227,327	4,642.83	678.85
Investor-owned (for-profit)	17	355	93	1,167	1,632	0	0	0	49,090	8,220	57,310	48.0	119,377	4,574.72	647.21
State and local government	0	0	0	0	0	0	0	0	0	0	0	0.0	0	0.00	0.00

*For information on community hospitals that excludes nursing-home-type data, refer to Hospital Units columns in tables 4A through 4D, pages 14 through 17.

(continued on next page)

Table

5C (Continued) Massachusetts

Utilization, Personnel, and Finances in States

Excludes AHA nonregistered hospitals (see Table 14, page 240).

CLASSIFICATION	HOSPITALS	BEDS	ADMISSIONS	INPATIENT DAYS	ADJUSTED PATIENT DAYS	OCCUPANCY, percent	AVERAGE DAILY CENSUS	ADJUSTED AVERAGE DAILY CENSUS	AVERAGE STAY, days	SURGICAL OPERATIONS	OUTPATIENT VISITS: Emergency	OUTPATIENT VISITS: Other	OUTPATIENT VISITS: Total	NEWBORNS: Bassinets	NEWBORNS: Births
MASSACHUSETTS	157	33,904	872,318	9,568,289		77.3	26,216			624,164	2,804,197	8,507,326	11,311,523	1,550	93,578
6-24 beds	4	93	1,340	13,480		40.9	38			512	6,226	45,224	51,450	4	98
25-49	9	329	5,641	81,177		67.5	222			2,925	32,722	62,401	95,123	10	154
50-99	30	2,134	45,487	559,317		71.8	1,532			23,284	176,890	691,678	868,568	24	768
100-199	48	7,269	193,689	1,922,289		72.4	5,264			144,382	746,931	1,912,055	2,658,986	389	20,715
200-299	29	7,188	207,709	1,945,190		74.1	5,329			164,879	796,400	1,877,896	2,674,296	373	21,130
300-399	22	7,437	199,988	2,237,288		82.5	6,132			147,559	575,854	1,526,640	2,102,494	327	18,751
400-499	6	2,835	75,184	851,265		82.3	2,334			53,194	192,276	699,335	891,611	136	9,430
500 or more	9	6,619	143,280	1,958,283		81.1	5,365			87,429	276,898	1,692,097	1,968,995	287	22,532
Psychiatric	24	5,224	26,624	1,611,315		84.5	4,416			0	7,576	326,015	333,591	0	0
Hospitals	24	5,224	26,624	1,611,315		84.5	4,416			0	7,576	326,015	333,591	0	0
Institutions for mentally retarded	0	0	0	0		00.0	0			0	0	0	0	0	0
General	101	23,217	808,771	6,250,118		73.8	17,129			603,616	2,743,451	7,722,876	10,466,327	1,501	90,482
Hospitals	97	23,124	807,180	6,235,095		73.9	17,087			603,379	2,739,607	7,691,601	10,431,208	1,501	90,482
Hospital units of institutions	4	93	1,591	15,023		45.2	42			237	3,844	31,275	35,119	0	0
TB and other respiratory diseases	0	0	0	0		00.0	0			0	0	0	0	0	0
Obstetrics and gynecology	1	114	4,818	27,505		65.8	75			840	0	17,239	17,239	49	3,096
Eye, ear, nose, and throat	1	109	8,766	23,192		58.7	64			15,150	38,463	81,777	120,240	0	0
Rehabilitation	9	1,290	11,752	387,400		82.2	1,060			356	0	225,718	225,718	0	0
Orthopedic	1	60	690	10,767		48.3	29			573	0	8,481	8,481	0	0
Chronic disease	13	2,820	2,737	936,276		90.9	2,563			42	0	19,878	19,878	0	0
All other	7	1,070	8,160	321,716		82.2	880			3,587	14,707	105,342	120,049	0	0
Federal	5	3,035	24,306	804,570		72.6	2,204			7,668	28,748	953,222	981,970	0	0
Psychiatric	2	1,395	5,659	397,748		78.1	1,090			0	0	215,532	215,532	0	0
General and other special	3	1,640	18,647	406,822		67.9	1,114			7,668	28,748	737,690	766,438	0	0
Nonfederal	152	30,869	848,012	8,763,719		77.8	24,012			616,496	2,775,449	7,554,104	10,329,553	1,550	93,578
Psychiatric	22	3,829	20,965	1,213,567		86.9	3,326			0	7,576	110,483	118,059	0	0
Hospitals	22	3,829	20,965	1,213,567		86.9	3,326			0	7,576	110,483	118,059	0	0
Institutions for mentally retarded	0	0	0	0		00.0	0			0	0	0	0	0	0
TB and other respiratory diseases	0	0	0	0		00.0	0			0	0	0	0	0	0
Long-term general and other special	25	5,072	14,465	1,613,751		87.1	4,419			1,525	0	275,481	275,481	0	0
Short-term general and other special	105	21,968	812,582	5,936,401		74.0	16,267			614,971	2,767,873	7,168,140	9,936,013	1,550	93,578
Hospital units of institutions	4	93	1,591	15,023		45.2	42			237	3,844	31,275	35,119	0	0
Community hospitals*	101	21,875	810,991	5,921,378	8,300,125	74.2	16,225	22,744	7.3	614,734	2,764,029	7,136,865	9,900,894	1,550	93,578
6-24 beds	1	34	613	3,127	11,102	26.5	9	30	5.1	372	4,301	16,559	20,860	4	98
25-49	3	113	3,811	26,468	43,999	63.7	72	121	6.9	2,646	26,181	31,360	57,541	10	154
50-99	17	1,143	35,210	287,034	448,584	68.8	786	1,230	8.2	22,222	157,464	475,493	632,957	24	768
100-199	35	5,228	182,707	1,350,556	2,050,583	70.8	3,699	5,617	7.4	144,208	746,931	1,737,823	2,484,754	389	20,715
200-299	22	5,499	200,560	1,414,289	2,008,318	70.5	3,875	5,503	7.1	163,752	796,400	1,803,347	2,599,747	373	21,130
300-399	15	5,063	192,476	1,432,545	1,906,241	77.5	3,926	5,224	7.4	147,559	573,578	1,460,304	2,033,882	327	18,751
400-499	4	1,899	71,448	530,132	729,465	76.6	1,454	2,000	7.4	53,194	192,276	586,488	778,764	136	9,430
500 or more	4	2,896	124,166	877,227	1,101,833	83.0	2,404	3,019	7.1	80,781	266,898	1,025,491	1,292,389	287	22,532
Nongovernment not-for-profit	89	19,755	743,211	5,330,026	7,493,594	73.9	14,605	20,534	7.2	571,932	2,517,911	6,380,237	8,898,148	1,467	89,405
Investor-owned (for-profit)	2	276	5,607	90,614	109,764	89.9	248	301	16.2	251	613	26,393	27,006	0	0
State and local government	10	1,844	62,173	500,738	696,767	74.4	1,372	1,909	8.1	42,551	245,505	730,235	975,740	83	4,173

*For information on community hospitals that excludes nursing home type data, refer to Hospital Units columns in tables 4A through 4D, pages 14 through 17.

CLASSIFICATION	FULL-TIME EQUIVALENT PERSONNEL: Physicians and Dentists	Registered Nurses	Licensed Practical Nurses	Other Salaried Personnel	Total Personnel	FULL-TIME EQUIVALENT TRAINEES: Medical and Dental Residents	Other Trainees	Total Trainees	EXPENSES: LABOR: Payroll (in thousands)	Employee Benefits (in thousands)	Total (in thousands)	Percent of Total	TOTAL: Amount (in thousands)	Adjusted, per Admission	Adjusted, per Inpatient Day
MINNESOTA	462	15,256	3,344	45,824	64,886	381	66	447	$ 1,893,220	$ 365,816	$ 2,259,036	58.8	$ 3,839,201		
6-24 beds	18	131	65	485	699	0	0	0	15,653	2,912	18,565	62.1	29,901		
25-49	6	664	228	2,035	2,933	0	0	0	70,173	12,341	82,513	55.1	149,631		
50-99	36	1,180	391	5,001	6,608	0	0	0	149,487	26,494	175,981	58.9	298,820		
100-199	50	2,697	701	8,424	11,872	3	0	3	298,418	54,981	353,399	57.1	619,395		
200-299	5	563	221	2,387	3,176	0	0	0	82,673	13,398	96,071	56.9	168,711		
300-399	58	2,882	527	8,602	12,069	52	10	62	380,385	73,534	453,919	60.7	747,869		
400-499	13	753	115	2,415	3,296	201	30	231	128,210	23,534	151,744	67.3	225,506		
500 or more	276	6,386	1,096	16,475	24,233	125	26	151	768,223	158,622	926,845	58.0	1,599,368		
Psychiatric	79	553	518	5,061	6,211	0	3	3	182,753	40,402	223,155	81.3	274,562		
Hospitals	73	528	461	4,205	5,267	0	3	3	156,813	32,882	189,695	80.2	236,519		
Institutions for mentally retarded	6	25	57	856	944	0	0	0	25,940	7,520	33,460	88.0	38,043		
General	375	14,568	2,801	40,247	57,991	381	63	444	1,692,709	322,382	2,015,091	57.2	3,525,089		
Hospitals	375	14,568	2,801	40,247	57,991	381	63	444	1,692,709	322,382	2,015,091	57.2	3,525,089		
Hospital units of institutions	0	0	0	0	0	0	0	0	0	0	0	0.0	0		
TB and other respiratory diseases	0	0	0	0	0	0	0	0	0	0	0	0.0	0		
Obstetrics and gynecology	0	0	0	0	0	0	0	0	0	0	0	0.0	0		
Eye, ear, nose, and throat	0	0	0	0	0	0	0	0	0	0	0	0.0	0		
Rehabilitation	0	0	0	0	0	0	0	0	0	0	0	0.0	0		
Orthopedic	3	30	2	89	124	0	0	0	3,234	610	3,843	52.5	7,325		
Chronic disease	0	0	0	0	0	0	0	0	0	0	0	0.0	0		
All other	5	105	23	427	560	0	0	0	14,524	2,423	16,947	52.6	32,224		
Federal	221	771	201	2,637	3,830	86	26	112	120,881	19,843	140,724	66.7	211,133		
Psychiatric	24	147	73	727	971	0	3	3	30,699	2,391	33,091	83.6	39,560		
General and other special	197	624	128	1,910	2,859	86	23	109	90,181	17,452	107,633	62.7	171,573		
Nonfederal	241	14,485	3,143	43,187	61,056	295	40	335	1,772,339	345,973	2,118,312	58.4	3,628,068		
Psychiatric	55	406	445	4,334	5,240	0	0	0	152,053	38,011	190,064	80.9	235,002		
Hospitals	49	381	388	3,478	4,296	0	0	0	126,113	30,491	156,604	79.5	196,959		
Institutions for mentally retarded	6	25	57	856	944	0	0	0	25,940	7,520	33,460	88.0	38,043		
TB and other respiratory diseases	0	0	0	0	0	0	0	0	0	0	0	0.0	0		
Long-term general and other special	3	34	21	205	263	0	0	0	7,411	1,311	8,721	50.4	17,306		
Short-term general and other special	183	14,045	2,677	38,648	55,553	295	40	335	1,612,875	306,651	1,919,526	56.9	3,375,761		
Hospital units of institutions	0	0	0	0	0	0	0	0	0	0	0	0.0	0		
Community hospitals*	183	14,045	2,677	38,648	55,553	295	40	335	1,612,875	306,651	1,919,526	56.9	3,375,761	$4,781.88	$ 536.47
6-24 beds	0	92	60	369	521	0	0	0	10,917	1,816	12,733	55.8	22,816	2,175.64	480.82
25-49	6	664	228	2,035	2,933	0	0	0	70,173	12,341	82,513	55.1	149,631	3,008.93	640.77
50-99	32	1,155	382	4,699	6,268	0	0	0	138,677	24,430	163,107	58.8	277,404	3,489.80	237.19
100-199	47	2,663	680	3,219	11,609	3	0	3	291,007	53,670	344,677	57.2	602,089	4,064.87	311.39
200-299	5	545	173	1,847	2,570	0	0	0	68,771	10,352	79,123	56.8	139,282	4,031.90	361.73
300-399	49	2,767	426	7,915	11,157	52	10	62	352,071	65,130	417,201	59.2	705,131	4,803.77	851.81
400-499	1	672	10	1,605	2,288	201	30	231	95,037	16,818	111,855	62.1	180,259	7,146.33	1,212.89
500 or more	43	5,487	718	11,959	18,207	39	0	39	586,223	122,094	708,317	54.5	1,299,148	6,140.63	839.80
Nongovernment not-for-profit	179	10,725	1,990	28,495	41,389	94	10	104	1,219,299	227,435	1,446,734	56.7	2,550,788	4,606.86	577.57
Investor-owned (for-profit)	0	0	0	0	0	0	0	0	0	0	0	0.0	0	0.00	0.00
State and local government	4	3,320	687	10,153	14,164	201	30	231	393,576	79,216	472,792	57.3	824,972	5,418.36	439.72

*For information on community hospitals that excludes nursing-home-type data, refer to Hospital Units columns in tables 4A through 4D, pages 14 through 17.

(continued on next page)

Table

5C (Continued) Mississippi

Utilization, Personnel, and Finances in States

Excludes AHA nonregistered hospitals (see Table 14, page 240).

CLASSIFICATION	HOSPITALS	BEDS	ADMISSIONS	INPATIENT DAYS	ADJUSTED PATIENT DAYS	OCCUPANCY, percent	AVERAGE DAILY CENSUS	ADJUSTED AVERAGE DAILY CENSUS	AVERAGE STAY, days	SURGICAL OPERATIONS	OUTPATIENT VISITS Emergency	OUTPATIENT VISITS Other	OUTPATIENT VISITS Total	NEWBORNS Bassinets	NEWBORNS Births
MISSISSIPPI	115	17,151	434,185	4,043,985		64.6	11,081			224,412	1,030,334	2,005,141	3,035,475	843	42,041
6-24 beds	4	71	2,591	12,251		47.9	34			440	10,535	60,918	71,453	0	0
25-49	23	924	22,051	166,378		49.7	459			3,315	75,477	159,593	235,070	27	663
50-99	41	3,104	75,847	643,318		56.7	1,761			26,480	225,395	277,969	503,364	171	7,066
100-199	25	3,406	88,447	712,417		57.3	1,952			60,531	204,531	320,258	524,789	248	10,189
200-299	9	2,196	72,493	436,784		54.5	1,197			40,272	163,913	184,313	348,226	133	6,959
300-399	4	1,281	48,930	308,439		66.0	845			26,598	131,224	455,797	587,021	106	5,228
400-499	2	836	33,084	225,747		73.9	618			19,052	68,303	75,204	143,507	40	2,871
500 or more	7	5,333	90,742	1,538,651		79.0	4,215			47,724	150,956	471,089	622,045	118	9,065
Psychiatric	6	2,504	6,726	801,627		87.7	2,197			0	3,516	3,343	6,859	0	0
Hospitals	6	2,504	6,726	801,627		87.7	2,197			0	3,516	3,343	6,859	0	0
Institutions for mentally retarded	0	0	0	0		00.0	0			0	0	0	0	0	0
General	106	14,397	422,609	3,191,709		60.7	8,745			220,202	1,026,400	1,994,437	3,020,837	803	40,195
Hospitals	106	14,397	422,609	3,191,709		60.7	8,745			220,202	1,026,400	1,994,437	3,020,837	803	40,195
Hospital units of institutions	0	0	0	0		00.0	0			0	0	0	0	0	0
TB and other respiratory diseases	0	0	0	0		00.0	0			0	0	0	0	0	0
Obstetrics and gynecology	1	111	3,342	13,040		32.4	36			2,808	418	618	1,036	40	1,846
Eye, ear, nose, and throat	0	0	0	0		00.0	0			0	0	0	0	0	0
Rehabilitation	1	104	1,323	27,502		72.1	75			1,382	0	6,743	6,743	0	0
Orthopedic	0	0	0	0		00.0	0			0	0	0	0	0	0
Chronic disease	1	35	185	10,107		80.0	28			20	0	0	0	0	0
All other	0	0	0	0		00.0	0			0	0	0	0	0	0
Federal	5	1,705	31,470	432,679		69.6	1,186			18,688	57,048	816,620	873,668	24	1,263
Psychiatric	0	0	0	0		00.0	0			0	0	0	0	0	0
General and other special	5	1,705	31,470	432,679		69.6	1,186			18,688	57,048	816,620	873,668	24	1,263
Nonfederal	110	15,446	402,715	3,611,306		64.1	9,895			205,724	973,286	1,188,521	2,161,807	819	40,778
Psychiatric	6	2,504	6,726	801,627		87.7	2,197			0	3,516	3,343	6,859	0	0
Hospitals	6	2,504	6,726	801,627		87.7	2,197			0	3,516	3,343	6,859	0	0
Institutions for mentally retarded	0	0	0	0		00.0	0			0	0	0	0	0	0
TB and other respiratory diseases	0	0	0	0		00.0	0			0	0	0	0	0	0
Long-term general and other special	1	35	185	10,107		80.0	28			20	0	0	0	0	0
Short-term general and other special	103	12,907	395,804	2,799,572		59.4	7,670			205,704	969,770	1,185,178	2,154,948	819	40,778
Hospital units of institutions	0	0	0	0		00.0	0			0	0	0	0	0	0
Community hospitals*	103	12,907	395,804	2,799,572	3,633,316	59.4	7,670	9,957	7.1	205,704	969,770	1,185,178	2,154,948	819	40,778
6-24 beds	3	64	1,874	9,995	13,418	43.8	28	37	5.3	1	4,830	4,346	9,176	0	0
25-49	21	857	20,198	150,583	207,471	48.4	415	571	7.5	2,342	59,136	69,421	128,557	21	423
50-99	38	2,918	74,031	606,368	829,781	56.9	1,659	2,274	8.2	26,480	221,879	276,879	498,758	171	7,066
100-199	24	3,295	86,972	680,759	907,563	56.6	1,865	2,486	7.8	60,531	204,531	318,005	522,536	248	10,189
200-299	9	2,196	72,493	436,784	574,280	54.5	1,197	1,574	6.0	40,272	163,913	184,313	348,226	133	6,959
300-399	3	972	37,156	225,591	285,124	63.6	618	781	6.1	21,393	96,222	92,626	188,848	88	4,205
400-499	2	836	33,084	225,747	266,580	73.9	618	730	6.8	19,052	68,303	75,204	143,507	40	2,871
500 or more	3	1,769	69,996	463,745	549,099	71.8	1,270	1,504	6.6	35,633	150,956	164,384	315,340	118	9,065
Nongovernment not-for-profit	32	4,734	163,415	1,095,186	1,379,755	63.4	2,999	3,779	6.7	90,952	330,177	401,172	731,349	250	13,791
Investor-owned (for-profit)	14	1,610	38,365	264,456	350,971	45.1	726	962	6.9	26,714	76,576	145,676	222,252	114	3,471
State and local government	57	6,563	194,024	1,439,930	1,902,590	60.1	3,945	5,216	7.4	88,038	563,017	638,330	1,201,347	455	23,516

*For information on community hospitals that excludes nursing home type data, refer to Hospital Units columns in tables 4A through 4D, pages 14 through 17.

CLASSIFICATION	FULL-TIME EQUIVALENT PERSONNEL					FULL-TIME EQUIVALENT TRAINEES			EXPENSES: LABOR				EXPENSES: TOTAL		
	Physicians and Dentists	Registered Nurses	Licensed Practical Nurses	Other Salaried Personnel	Total Personnel	Medical and Dental Residents	Other Trainees	Total Trainees	Payroll (in thousands)	Employee Benefits (in thousands)	Total (in thousands)	Percent of Total	Amount (in thousands)	Adjusted, per Admission	Adjusted, per Inpatient Day
MISSISSIPPI	394	7,940	3,564	30,413	42,311	541	122	663	$ 891,521	$ 164,035	$ 1,055,557	54.4	$ 1,939,029		
6-24 beds	16	47	15	255	333	0	0	0	3,104	564	3,668	57.8	6,347		
25-49	32	284	214	1,416	1,946	1	3	4	35,880	6,861	42,741	56.5	75,624		
50-99	8	1,153	748	4,414	6,323	0	1	1	115,167	21,925	137,092	52.9	259,230		
100-199	9	1,682	701	5,135	7,527	0	3	3	155,211	30,497	185,708	49.3	376,760		
200-299	6	1,318	702	3,916	5,942	0	0	0	124,777	20,955	145,732	49.7	293,350		
300-399	105	1,055	259	3,118	4,537	137	96	233	113,172	18,750	131,922	56.5	233,655		
400-499	3	748	185	2,206	3,142	0	0	0	65,275	9,576	74,851	50.9	146,997		
500 or more	215	1,653	740	9,953	12,561	403	19	422	278,935	54,908	333,843	61.0	547,066		
Psychiatric	37	191	166	2,910	3,304	5	2	7	53,240	13,487	66,728	68.6	97,305		
Hospitals	37	191	166	2,910	3,304	5	2	7	53,240	13,487	66,728	68.6	97,305		
Institutions for mentally retarded	0	0	0	0	0	0	0	0	0	0	0	0.0	0		
General	356	7,558	3,359	26,988	38,261	536	120	656	819,942	147,422	967,363	53.7	1,800,445		
Hospitals	356	7,558	3,359	26,988	38,261	536	120	656	819,942	147,422	967,363	53.7	1,800,445		
Hospital units of institutions	0	0	0	0	0	0	0	0	0	0	0	0.0	0		
TB and other respiratory diseases	0	0	0	0	0	0	0	0	0	0	0	0.0	0		
Obstetrics and gynecology	0	93	6	108	207	0	0	0	4,521	685	5,206	39.8	13,090		
Eye, ear, nose, and throat	0	0	0	0	0	0	0	0	0	0	0	0.0	0		
Rehabilitation	0	86	28	319	433	0	0	0	10,849	1,797	12,645	56.2	22,503		
Orthopedic	0	0	0	0	0	0	0	0	0	0	0	0.0	0		
Chronic disease	1	12	5	88	106	0	0	0	2,970	644	3,614	63.6	5,687		
All other	0	0	0	0	0	0	0	0	0	0	0	0.0	0		
Federal	279	686	287	3,544	4,796	217	109	326	138,257	23,445	161,702	67.0	241,434		
Psychiatric	0	0	0	0	0	0	0	0	0	0	0	0.0	0		
General and other special	279	686	287	3,544	4,796	217	109	326	138,257	23,445	161,702	67.0	241,434		
Nonfederal	115	7,254	3,277	26,869	37,515	324	13	337	753,265	140,590	893,855	52.7	1,697,595		
Psychiatric	37	191	166	2,910	3,304	5	2	7	53,240	13,487	66,728	68.6	97,305		
Hospitals	37	191	166	2,910	3,304	5	2	7	53,240	13,487	66,728	68.6	97,305		
Institutions for mentally retarded	0	0	0	0	0	0	0	0	0	0	0	0.0	0		
TB and other respiratory diseases	0	0	0	0	0	0	0	0	0	0	0	0.0	0		
Long-term general and other special	1	12	5	88	106	0	0	0	2,970	644	3,614	63.6	5,687		
Short-term general and other special	77	7,051	3,106	23,871	34,105	319	11	330	697,055	126,458	823,513	51.6	1,594,603		
Hospital units of institutions	0	0	0	0	0	0	0	0	0	0	0	0.0	0		
Community hospitals*	77	7,051	3,106	23,871	34,105	319	11	330	697,055	126,458	823,513	51.6	1,594,603	$3,115.80	$ 438.88
6-24 beds	1	27	15	89	132	0	0	0	1,910	299	2,209	51.8	4,265	1,725.50	317.89
25-49	9	239	201	1,123	1,572	1	3	4	27,514	5,071	32,586	53.3	61,120	2,227.81	294.60
50-99	8	1,090	735	4,195	6,028	0	0	0	106,377	20,279	126,656	52.6	240,781	2,337.50	290.17
100-199	9	1,639	692	4,990	7,330	0	3	3	149,848	29,359	179,207	49.1	364,976	3,174.04	402.15
200-299	6	1,318	702	3,916	5,942	0	0	0	124,777	20,955	145,732	49.7	293,350	3,086.27	510.81
300-399	0	865	191	2,064	3,120	0	0	0	78,584	15,192	93,776	52.7	177,863	3,780.55	623.81
400-499	3	748	185	2,206	3,142	0	0	0	65,275	9,576	74,851	50.9	146,997	3,760.56	551.42
500 or more	41	1,125	385	5,288	6,839	318	5	323	142,769	25,727	168,496	55.2	305,251	3,691.51	555.91
Nongovernment not-for-profit	20	2,742	1,248	10,059	14,069	0	5	5	290,179	50,757	340,936	51.7	659,442	3,222.12	477.94
Investor-owned (for-profit)	0	868	330	2,020	3,218	0	0	0	68,113	14,575	82,688	43.7	189,315	3,729.25	539.40
State and local government	57	3,441	1,528	11,792	16,818	319	6	325	338,763	61,126	399,889	53.6	745,846	2,909.45	392.02

*For information on community hospitals that excludes nursing-home-type data, refer to Hospital Units columns in tables 4A through 4D, pages 14 through 17.

(continued on next page)

Table

5C (Continued) Missouri

Utilization, Personnel, and Finances in States

Excludes AHA nonregistered hospitals (see Table 14, page 240).

CLASSIFICATION	HOSPITALS	BEDS	ADMISSIONS	INPATIENT DAYS	ADJUSTED PATIENT DAYS	OCCUPANCY, percent	AVERAGE DAILY CENSUS	ADJUSTED AVERAGE DAILY CENSUS	AVERAGE STAY, days	SURGICAL OPERATIONS	OUTPATIENT VISITS: Emergency	OUTPATIENT VISITS: Other	OUTPATIENT VISITS: Total	NEWBORNS: Bassinets	NEWBORNS: Births
MISSOURI	160	29,575	794,165	6,991,353		64.8	19,152			594,340	1,905,011	5,747,637	7,652,648	1,590	80,157
6-24 beds	6	118	4,529	20,854		49.2	58			1,419	15,832	124,165	139,997	11	354
25-49	25	949	23,525	156,132		45.1	428			11,332	98,030	190,506	288,536	96	1,136
50-99	46	3,149	79,444	592,378		51.6	1,625			49,105	249,959	711,174	961,133	222	5,734
100-199	32	4,531	121,985	930,644		56.2	2,547			84,240	395,127	732,579	1,127,706	275	11,809
200-299	17	4,129	109,119	1,055,647		70.0	2,891			76,773	304,789	1,026,635	1,331,424	203	11,481
300-399	16	5,240	139,232	1,229,057		64.2	3,366			136,845	255,410	1,175,274	1,430,684	230	13,409
400-499	4	1,776	56,238	425,218		65.6	1,165			50,265	74,027	410,428	484,455	117	7,871
500 or more	14	9,683	260,093	2,581,423		73.0	7,072			184,361	511,837	1,376,876	1,888,713	436	28,363
Psychiatric	15	2,542	12,903	744,343		80.2	2,038			0	12,274	204,915	217,189	0	0
Hospitals	15	2,542	12,903	744,343		80.2	2,038			0	12,274	204,915	217,189	0	0
Institutions for mentally retarded	0	0	0	0		00.0	0			0	0	0	0	0	0
General	140	26,729	776,811	6,176,729		63.3	16,921			592,470	1,886,860	5,492,902	7,379,762	1,590	80,157
Hospitals	139	26,014	775,148	5,953,164		62.7	16,308			592,019	1,885,429	5,463,626	7,349,055	1,590	80,157
Hospital units of institutions	1	715	1,663	223,565		85.7	613			451	1,431	29,276	30,707	0	0
TB and other respiratory diseases	0	0	0	0		00.0	0			0	0	0	0	0	0
Obstetrics and gynecology	0	0	0	0		00.0	0			0	0	0	0	0	0
Eye, ear, nose, and throat	0	0	0	0		00.0	0			0	0	0	0	0	0
Rehabilitation	3	182	1,673	49,884		75.3	137			0	1,740	26,316	28,056	0	0
Orthopedic	1	56	1,758	12,159		58.9	33			1,082	4,137	8,414	12,551	0	0
Chronic disease	0	0	0	0		00.0	0			0	0	0	0	0	0
All other	1	66	1,020	8,238		34.8	23			788	0	15,090	15,090	0	0
Federal	7	2,496	42,370	707,372		77.7	1,939			44,739	56,290	891,159	947,449	21	853
Psychiatric	0	0	0	0		00.0	0			0	0	0	0	0	0
General and other special	7	2,496	42,370	707,372		77.7	1,939			44,739	56,290	891,159	947,449	21	853
Nonfederal	153	27,079	751,795	6,283,981		63.6	17,213			549,601	1,848,721	4,856,478	6,705,199	1,569	79,304
Psychiatric	15	2,542	12,903	744,343		80.2	2,038			0	12,274	204,915	217,189	0	0
Hospitals	15	2,542	12,903	744,343		80.2	2,038			0	12,274	204,915	217,189	0	0
Institutions for mentally retarded	0	0	0	0		00.0	0			0	0	0	0	0	0
TB and other respiratory diseases	0	0	0	0		00.0	0			0	0	0	0	0	0
Long-term general and other special	3	182	1,673	49,884		75.3	137			0	1,740	26,316	28,056	0	0
Short-term general and other special	135	24,355	737,219	5,489,754		61.7	15,038			549,601	1,834,707	4,625,247	6,459,954	1,569	79,304
Hospital units of institutions	0	0	0	0		00.0	0			0	0	0	0	0	0
Community hospitals*	135	24,355	737,219	5,489,754	7,237,715	61.7	15,038	19,842	7.4	549,601	1,834,707	4,625,247	6,459,954	1,569	79,304
6-24 beds	4	86	2,566	13,837	20,929	44.2	38	58	5.4	517	7,665	25,352	33,017	2	45
25-49	25	949	23,525	156,132	245,784	45.1	428	675	6.6	11,332	98,030	190,506	288,536	96	1,136
50-99	39	2,640	74,555	458,530	680,933	47.7	1,259	1,877	6.2	49,105	248,219	644,681	892,900	222	5,734
100-199	27	3,942	117,322	805,617	1,100,564	55.9	2,205	3,015	6.9	84,240	389,445	727,659	1,117,104	275	11,809
200-299	12	3,014	92,993	735,700	957,847	66.8	2,014	2,623	7.9	65,180	259,693	571,191	830,884	191	10,937
300-399	13	4,245	124,566	952,413	1,208,192	61.5	2,609	3,311	7.6	108,895	255,410	949,502	1,204,912	230	13,409
400-499	4	1,776	56,238	425,218	526,466	65.6	1,165	1,443	7.6	50,265	74,027	410,428	484,455	117	7,871
500 or more	11	7,703	245,454	1,942,307	2,497,000	69.1	5,320	6,840	7.9	180,067	502,218	1,105,928	1,608,146	436	28,363
Nongovernment not-for-profit	84	19,332	600,520	4,439,016	5,800,048	62.9	12,161	15,900	7.4	454,498	1,479,636	3,613,035	5,092,671	1,183	67,515
Investor-owned (for-profit)	11	1,687	44,759	329,070	441,588	53.3	899	1,209	7.4	39,111	96,357	319,124	415,481	119	3,623
State and local government	40	3,336	91,940	721,668	996,079	59.3	1,978	2,733	7.8	55,992	258,714	693,088	951,802	267	8,166

*For information on community hospitals that excludes nursing-home-type data, refer to Hospital Units columns in tables 4A through 4D, pages 14 through 17.

CLASSIFICATION	FULL-TIME EQUIVALENT PERSONNEL					FULL-TIME EQUIVALENT TRAINEES			EXPENSES						
									LABOR				TOTAL		
	Physicians and Dentists	Registered Nurses	Licensed Practical Nurses	Other Salaried Personnel	Total Personnel	Medical and Dental Residents	Other Trainees	Total Trainees	Payroll (in thousands)	Employee Benefits (in thousands)	Total (in thousands)	Percent of Total	Amount (in thousands)	Adjusted, per Admission	Adjusted, per Inpatient Day
MISSOURI	1,308	22,195	5,001	74,127	102,631	1,836	166	2,002	$ 2,527,647	$ 455,796	$ 2,983,443	53.8	$ 5,550,266		
6-24 beds	26	80	45	542	693	0	0	0	10,061	2,177	12,238	62.2	19,672		
25-49	3	480	266	1,821	2,570	0	2	2	47,049	7,840	54,889	50.9	107,737		
50-99	67	1,925	840	3,838	9,670	14	15	29	196,886	34,361	231,247	51.8	446,142		
100-199	171	2,946	1,022	10,282	14,421	112	12	124	316,210	61,761	377,971	52.6	718,014		
200-299	189	2,880	643	10,414	14,126	174	8	182	351,938	61,655	413,593	55.2	748,920		
300-399	298	4,286	813	13,177	18,574	176	20	196	499,589	85,940	585,528	54.1	1,082,981		
400-499	10	1,709	368	6,652	8,739	201	7	208	212,649	38,756	251,406	54.6	460,508		
500 or more	544	7,889	1,004	24,401	33,838	1,159	102	1,261	893,266	163,306	1,056,572	53.7	1,966,292		
Psychiatric	122	729	247	4,869	5,967	62	24	86	132,292	32,411	164,703	73.4	224,381		
Hospitals	122	729	247	4,869	5,967	62	24	86	132,292	32,411	164,703	73.4	224,381		
Institutions for mentally retarded	0	0	0	0	0	0	0	0	0	0	0	0.0	0		
General	1,166	21,286	4,650	68,373	95,475	1,774	141	1,915	2,365,789	418,607	2,784,395	52.9	5,266,896		
Hospitals	1,148	21,222	4,604	67,789	94,763	1,774	141	1,915	2,344,849	413,700	2,758,549	52.8	5,228,446		
Hospital units of institutions	18	64	46	584	712	0	0	0	20,940	4,907	25,847	67.2	38,450		
TB and other respiratory diseases	0	0	0	0	0	0	0	0	0	0	0	0.0	0		
Obstetrics and gynecology	0	0	0	0	0	0	0	0	0	0	0	0.0	0		
Eye, ear, nose, and throat	0	0	0	0	0	0	0	0	0	0	0	0.0	0		
Rehabilitation	11	101	77	592	781	0	0	0	18,254	2,333	20,586	60.3	34,146		
Orthopedic	1	43	13	149	206	0	1	1	5,428	1,066	6,494	53.7	12,104		
Chronic disease	0	0	0	0	0	0	0	0	0	0	0	0.0	0		
All other	8	36	14	144	202	0	0	0	5,884	1,379	7,263	57.0	12,739		
Federal	347	998	384	4,906	6,635	302	80	382	209,513	33,985	243,498	64.9	375,231		
Psychiatric	0	0	0	0	0	0	0	0	0	0	0	0.0	0		
General and other special	347	998	384	4,906	6,635	302	80	382	209,513	33,985	243,498	64.9	375,231		
Nonfederal	961	21,197	4,617	69,221	95,996	1,534	86	1,620	2,318,134	421,811	2,739,944	52.9	5,175,035		
Psychiatric	122	729	247	4,869	5,967	62	24	86	132,292	32,411	164,703	73.4	224,381		
Hospitals	122	729	247	4,869	5,967	62	24	86	132,292	32,411	164,703	73.4	224,381		
Institutions for mentally retarded	0	0	0	0	0	0	0	0	0	0	0	0.0	0		
TB and other respiratory diseases	0	0	0	0	0	0	0	0	0	0	0	0.0	0		
Long-term general and other special	11	101	77	592	781	0	0	0	18,254	2,333	20,586	60.3	34,146		
Short-term general and other special	828	20,367	4,293	63,760	89,248	1,472	62	1,534	2,167,588	387,067	2,554,655	52.0	4,916,508		
Hospital units of institutions	0	0	0	0	0	0	0	0	0	0	0	0.0	0		
Community hospitals*	828	20,367	4,293	63,760	89,248	1,472	62	1,534	2,167,588	387,067	2,554,655	52.0	4,916,508	$5,021.87	$679.29
6-24 beds	2	46	38	228	314	0	0	0	4,192	721	4,914	50.3	9,766	2,431.88	466.65
25-49	3	480	266	1,821	2,570	0	2	2	47,049	7,840	54,889	50.9	107,737	2,899.36	438.34
50-99	46	1,700	733	5,844	8,323	3	9	12	160,622	28,507	189,129	50.6	373,761	3,341.21	548.90
100-199	154	2,771	980	9,517	13,422	94	4	98	291,309	56,308	347,617	51.8	671,255	4,161.68	609.92
200-299	55	2,436	458	7,620	10,569	141	1	142	261,322	46,179	307,501	50.8	605,023	5,007.27	631.65
300-399	149	3,833	638	10,833	15,453	89	16	105	410,071	69,940	480,011	51.7	928,705	5,857.64	768.67
400-499	10	1,709	368	6,652	8,739	201	7	208	212,649	38,756	251,406	54.6	460,508	6,611.07	874.71
500 or more	409	7,392	812	21,245	29,858	944	23	967	780,373	138,816	919,189	52.2	1,759,753	5,574.92	704.75
Nongovernment not-for-profit	749	17,073	2,970	52,216	73,008	1,247	33	1,280	1,840,443	318,097	2,158,539	52.0	4,151,477	5,258.29	715.77
Investor-owned (for-profit)	36	876	371	3,258	4,541	24	11	35	90,588	23,110	113,697	44.1	257,820	4,194.86	583.85
State and local government	43	2,418	952	8,286	11,699	201	18	219	236,557	45,861	282,418	55.7	507,211	3,961.10	509.21

*For information on community hospitals that excludes nursing-home-type data, refer to Hospital Units columns in tables 4A through 4D, pages 14 through 17.

(continued on next page)

Table 5C (Continued) Montana

Utilization, Personnel, and Finances in States

Excludes AHA nonregistered hospitals (see Table 14, page 240).

CLASSIFICATION	HOSPITALS	BEDS	ADMISSIONS	INPATIENT DAYS	ADJUSTED PATIENT DAYS	OCCUPANCY, percent	AVERAGE DAILY CENSUS	ADJUSTED AVERAGE DAILY CENSUS	AVERAGE STAY, days	SURGICAL OPERATIONS	OUTPATIENT VISITS			NEWBORNS	
											Emergency	Other	Total	Bassinets	Births
MONTANA	62	4,984	114,026	1,114,149		61.2	3,052			62,881	255,859	770,046	1,025,905	317	11,006
6-24 beds	8	142	1,496	26,621		51.4	73			86	5,855	36,662	42,517	13	60
25-49	20	753	13,823	144,218		52.5	395			5,365	54,766	195,355	250,121	81	1,563
50-99	18	1,210	21,018	305,864		69.3	839			10,748	46,425	112,017	158,442	82	2,576
100-199	11	1,410	33,415	322,563		62.6	883			18,138	55,073	278,653	333,726	86	3,175
200-299	4	1,043	34,736	214,022		56.2	586			22,999	72,875	112,737	185,612	37	2,575
300-399	0	0	0	0		00.0	0			0	0	0	0	0	0
400-499	1	426	9,538	100,861		64.8	276			5,545	20,865	34,622	55,487	18	1,057
500 or more	0	0	0	0		00.0	0			0	0	0	0	0	0
Psychiatric	1	21	73	6,505		85.7	18			0	0	3,330	3,330	0	0
Hospitals	1	21	73	6,505		85.7	18			0	0	3,330	3,330	0	0
Institutions for mentally retarded	0	0	0	0		00.0	0			0	0	0	0	0	0
General	61	4,963	113,953	1,107,644		61.1	3,034			62,881	255,859	766,716	1,022,575	317	11,006
Hospitals	61	4,963	113,953	1,107,644		61.1	3,034			62,881	255,859	766,716	1,022,575	317	11,006
Hospital units of institutions	0	0	0	0		00.0	0			0	0	0	0	0	0
TB and other respiratory diseases	0	0	0	0		00.0	0			0	0	0	0	0	0
Obstetrics and gynecology	0	0	0	0		00.0	0			0	0	0	0	0	0
Eye, ear, nose, and throat	0	0	0	0		00.0	0			0	0	0	0	0	0
Rehabilitation	0	0	0	0		00.0	0			0	0	0	0	0	0
Orthopedic	0	0	0	0		00.0	0			0	0	0	0	0	0
Chronic disease	0	0	0	0		00.0	0			0	0	0	0	0	0
All other	0	0	0	0		00.0	0			0	0	0	0	0	0
Federal	5	307	8,492	65,073		58.0	178			3,185	18,919	159,019	177,938	10	427
Psychiatric	0	0	0	0		00.0	0			0	0	0	0	0	0
General and other special	5	307	8,492	65,073		58.0	178			3,185	18,919	159,019	177,938	10	427
Nonfederal	57	4,677	105,534	1,049,076		61.4	2,874			59,696	236,940	611,027	847,967	307	10,579
Psychiatric	1	21	73	6,505		85.7	18			0	0	3,330	3,330	0	0
Hospitals	1	21	73	6,505		85.7	18			0	0	3,330	3,330	0	0
Institutions for mentally retarded	0	0	0	0		00.0	0			0	0	0	0	0	0
TB and other respiratory diseases	0	0	0	0		00.0	0			0	0	0	0	0	0
Long-term general and other special	1	23	56	7,406		87.0	20			0	398	772	1,170	0	0
Short-term general and other special	55	4,633	105,405	1,035,165		61.2	2,836			59,696	236,542	606,925	843,467	307	10,579
Hospital units of institutions	0	0	0	0		00.0	0			0	0	0	0	0	0
Community hospitals*	55	4,633	105,405	1,035,165	1,364,420	61.2	2,836	3,741	9.8	59,696	236,542	606,925	843,467	307	10,579
6-24 beds	5	82	943	11,181	15,844	37.8	31	44	11.9	86	2,110	12,754	14,864	13	60
25-49	18	692	11,039	134,783	200,132	53.3	369	550	12.2	4,517	39,194	109,423	148,617	71	1,136
50-99	18	1,210	21,018	305,864	413,407	69.3	839	1,133	14.6	10,748	46,425	112,017	158,442	82	2,576
100-199	9	1,180	28,131	268,454	353,302	62.3	735	968	9.5	15,801	55,073	225,372	280,445	86	3,175
200-299	4	1,043	34,736	214,022	258,786	56.2	586	709	6.2	22,999	72,875	112,737	185,612	37	2,575
300-399	0	0	0	0	0	00.0	0	0	0.0	0	0	0	0	0	0
400-499	1	426	9,538	100,861	122,949	64.8	276	337	10.6	5,545	20,865	34,622	55,487	18	1,057
500 or more	0	0	0	0	0	00.0	0	0	0.0	0	0	0	0	0	0
Nongovernment not-for-profit	42	3,914	98,961	861,721	1,140,626	60.3	2,361	3,128	8.7	58,202	219,256	570,432	789,688	276	10,164
Investor-owned (for-profit)	1	44	655	12,843	16,685	79.5	35	46	19.6	345	1,358	2,862	4,220	0	0
State and local government	12	675	5,789	160,601	207,109	65.2	440	567	27.7	1,149	15,928	33,631	49,559	31	415

*For information on community hospitals that excludes nursing-home-type data, refer to Hospital Units columns in tables 4A through 4D, pages 14 through 17.

CLASSIFICATION	FULL-TIME EQUIVALENT PERSONNEL: Physicians and Dentists	Registered Nurses	Licensed Practical Nurses	Other Salaried Personnel	Total Personnel	FULL-TIME EQUIVALENT TRAINEES: Medical and Dental Residents	Other Trainees	Total Trainees	EXPENSES — LABOR: Payroll (in thousands)	Employee Benefits (in thousands)	Total (in thousands)	Percent of Total	TOTAL: Amount (in thousands)	Adjusted, per Admission	Adjusted, per Inpatient Day
MONTANA	78	2,700	648	8,909	12,335	0	14	14	$ 278,190	$ 51,870	$ 330,059	54.9	$ 601,648		
6-24 beds	12	54	17	220	303	0	0	0	6,385	1,139	7,524	66.2	11,367		
25-49	33	309	76	1,268	1,686	0	4	4	30,541	5,710	36,251	58.3	62,210		
50-99	3	392	92	1,775	2,262	0	5	5	42,697	7,523	50,219	55.3	90,886		
100-199	29	745	215	2,586	3,575	0	3	3	79,908	14,935	94,843	57.9	163,933		
200-299	1	945	201	2,328	3,475	0	2	2	89,247	17,107	106,354	49.0	217,238		
300-399	0	0	0	0	0	0	0	0	0	0	0	0.0	0		
400-499	0	255	47	732	1,034	0	0	0	29,412	5,456	34,868	62.2	56,014		
500 or more	0	0	0	0	0	0	0	0	0	0	0	0.0	0		
Psychiatric	4	9	5	74	92	0	0	0	2,501	429	2,930	64.8	4,519		
Hospitals	4	9	5	74	92	0	0	0	2,501	429	2,930	64.8	4,519		
Institutions for mentally retarded	0	0	0	0	0	0	0	0	0	0	0	0.0	0		
General	74	2,691	643	8,835	12,243	0	14	14	275,689	51,441	327,130	54.8	597,128		
Hospitals	74	2,691	643	8,835	12,243	0	14	14	275,689	51,441	327,130	54.8	597,128		
Hospital units of institutions	0	0	0	0	0	0	0	0	0	0	0	0.0	0		
TB and other respiratory diseases	0	0	0	0	0	0	0	0	0	0	0	0.0	0		
Obstetrics and gynecology	0	0	0	0	0	0	0	0	0	0	0	0.0	0		
Eye, ear, nose, and throat	0	0	0	0	0	0	0	0	0	0	0	0.0	0		
Rehabilitation	0	0	0	0	0	0	0	0	0	0	0	0.0	0		
Orthopedic	0	0	0	0	0	0	0	0	0	0	0	0.0	0		
Chronic disease	0	0	0	0	0	0	0	0	0	0	0	0.0	0		
All other	0	0	0	0	0	0	0	0	0	0	0	0.0	0		
Federal	66	183	64	662	975	0	0	0	25,759	4,989	30,747	71.0	43,331		
Psychiatric	0	0	0	0	0	0	0	0	0	0	0	0.0	0		
General and other special	66	183	64	662	975	0	0	0	25,759	4,989	30,747	71.0	43,331		
Nonfederal	12	2,517	584	8,247	11,360	0	14	14	252,431	46,881	299,312	53.6	558,317		
Psychiatric	4	9	5	74	92	0	0	0	2,501	429	2,930	64.8	4,519		
Hospitals	4	9	5	74	92	0	0	0	2,501	429	2,930	64.8	4,519		
Institutions for mentally retarded	0	0	0	0	0	0	0	0	0	0	0	0.0	0		
TB and other respiratory diseases	0	0	0	0	0	0	0	0	0	0	0	0.0	0		
Long-term general and other special	0	3	1	13	17	0	0	0	431	45	475	57.6	825		
Short-term general and other special	8	2,505	578	8,160	11,251	0	14	14	249,500	46,407	295,907	53.5	552,973		
Hospital units of institutions	0	0	0	0	0	0	0	0	0	0	0	0.0	0		
Community hospitals*	8	2,505	578	8,160	11,251	0	14	14	249,500	46,407	295,907	53.5	552,973	$3,972.79	$ 405.28
6-24 beds	0	26	6	92	124	0	0	0	2,148	300	2,448	59.5	4,116	2,548.80	259.80
25-49	2	232	61	1,034	1,329	0	4	4	23,861	3,736	27,596	54.6	50,551	2,839.30	252.59
50-99	3	392	92	1,775	2,262	0	5	5	42,697	7,523	50,219	55.3	90,886	3,150.30	219.85
100-199	2	655	171	2,199	3,027	0	3	3	62,136	12,286	74,422	55.5	134,168	3,609.57	379.75
200-299	1	945	201	2,328	3,475	0	2	2	89,247	17,107	106,354	49.0	217,238	5,157.10	839.45
300-399	0	0	0	0	0	0	0	0	0	0	0	0.0	0	0.00	0.00
400-499	0	255	47	732	1,034	0	0	0	29,412	5,456	34,868	62.2	56,014	4,817.56	455.59
500 or more	0	0	0	0	0	0	0	0	0	0	0	0.0	0	0.00	0.00
Nongovernment not-for-profit	7	2,408	548	7,339	10,302	0	10	10	235,096	43,576	278,672	53.4	521,622	3,990.41	457.31
Investor-owned (for-profit)	0	13	0	69	82	0	0	0	1,377	265	1,642	54.5	3,012	3,539.38	180.52
State and local government	1	84	30	752	867	0	4	4	13,027	2,566	15,593	55.0	28,338	3,718.93	136.83

*For information on community hospitals that excludes nursing-home-type data, refer to Hospital Units columns in tables 4A through 4D, pages 14 through 17.

(continued on next page)

Table

5C (Continued) Nebraska

Utilization, Personnel, and Finances in States

Excludes AHA nonregistered hospitals (see Table 14, page 240).

CLASSIFICATION	HOSPI-TALS	BEDS	ADMISSIONS	INPATIENT DAYS	ADJUSTED PATIENT DAYS	OCCU-PANCY, percent	AVERAGE DAILY CENSUS	ADJUSTED AVERAGE DAILY CENSUS	AVERAGE STAY, days	SURGICAL OPERATIONS	OUTPATIENT VISITS Emergency	OUTPATIENT VISITS Other	OUTPATIENT VISITS Total	NEWBORNS Bassinets	NEWBORNS Births
NEBRASKA	102	10,561	212,324	2,360,956		61.2	6,468			177,784	398,580	1,746,405	2,144,985	779	24,283
6-24 beds	18	345	5,698	39,791		31.9	110			2,340	10,735	43,726	54,461	72	391
25-49	35	1,314	24,722	165,541		34.4	452			12,128	44,679	215,580	260,259	219	2,919
50-99	17	1,203	16,039	278,165		63.5	764			11,298	33,187	110,216	143,403	117	2,343
100-199	15	2,242	43,127	487,736		59.6	1,336			34,275	99,868	591,961	691,829	118	4,891
200-299	10	2,472	52,833	676,222		74.9	1,852			44,982	80,324	421,343	501,667	105	4,604
300-399	4	1,433	35,998	314,842		60.2	862			37,819	57,120	122,890	180,010	76	4,735
400-499	1	407	10,831	80,034		53.8	219			11,750	28,136	45,402	73,538	16	939
500 or more	2	1,145	23,076	318,625		76.2	873			23,192	44,531	195,287	239,818	56	3,461
Psychiatric	4	720	4,830	205,962		78.3	564			0	857	19,665	20,522	0	0
Hospitals	4	720	4,830	205,962		78.3	564			0	857	19,665	20,522	0	0
Institutions for mentally retarded	0	0	0	0		00.0	0			0	0	0	0	0	0
General	95	9,028	204,648	1,913,188		58.1	5,241			176,322	392,873	1,709,839	2,102,712	779	24,283
Hospitals	95	9,028	204,648	1,913,188		58.1	5,241			176,322	392,873	1,709,839	2,102,712	779	24,283
Hospital units of institutions	0	0	0	0		00.0	0			0	0	0	0	0	0
TB and other respiratory diseases	0	0	0	0		00.0	0			0	0	0	0	0	0
Obstetrics and gynecology	0	0	0	0		00.0	0			0	0	0	0	0	0
Eye, ear, nose, and throat	0	0	0	0		00.0	0			0	0	0	0	0	0
Rehabilitation	1	252	1,217	86,510		94.0	237			0	1,373	6,093	7,466	0	0
Orthopedic	0	0	0	0		00.0	0			0	0	0	0	0	0
Chronic disease	0	0	0	0		00.0	0			0	0	0	0	0	0
All other	2	561	1,629	155,296		75.9	426			1,462	3,477	10,808	14,285	0	0
Federal	5	726	17,527	177,706		67.1	487			8,977	29,559	475,595	505,154	22	830
Psychiatric	0	0	0	0		00.0	0			0	0	0	0	0	0
General and other special	5	726	17,527	177,706		67.1	487			8,977	29,559	475,595	505,154	22	830
Nonfederal	97	9,835	194,797	2,183,250		60.8	5,981			168,807	369,021	1,270,810	1,639,831	757	23,453
Psychiatric	4	720	4,830	205,962		78.3	564			0	857	19,665	20,522	0	0
Hospitals	4	720	4,830	205,962		78.3	564			0	857	19,665	20,522	0	0
Institutions for mentally retarded	0	0	0	0		00.0	0			0	0	0	0	0	0
TB and other respiratory diseases	0	0	0	0		00.0	0			0	0	0	0	0	0
Long-term general and other special	3	504	1,990	166,681		90.7	457			223	3,152	12,131	15,283	0	0
Short-term general and other special	90	8,611	187,977	1,810,607		57.6	4,960			168,584	365,012	1,239,014	1,604,026	757	23,453
Hospital units of institutions	0	0	0	0		00.0	0			0	0	0	0	0	0
Community hospitals*	90	8,611	187,977	1,810,607	2,431,589	57.6	4,960	6,663	9.6	168,584	365,012	1,239,014	1,604,026	757	23,453
6-24 beds	17	325	5,546	33,950	53,434	28.9	94	147	6.1	2,266	10,220	43,298	53,518	72	391
25-49	34	1,284	24,096	159,870	250,314	34.0	436	686	6.6	11,916	44,079	184,219	228,298	219	2,919
50-99	17	1,203	16,039	278,165	394,353	63.5	764	1,081	17.3	11,298	33,187	110,216	143,403	117	2,343
100-199	9	1,284	28,204	269,735	382,721	57.6	739	1,048	9.6	27,877	70,052	230,624	300,676	96	4,061
200-299	6	1,530	44,187	355,386	467,600	63.6	973	1,282	8.0	42,466	77,687	307,078	384,765	105	4,604
300-399	4	1,433	35,998	314,842	386,351	60.2	862	1,059	8.7	37,819	57,120	122,890	180,010	76	4,735
400-499	1	407	10,831	80,034	97,925	53.8	219	268	7.4	11,750	28,136	45,402	73,538	16	939
500 or more	2	1,145	23,076	318,625	398,891	76.2	873	1,092	13.8	23,192	44,531	195,287	239,818	56	3,461
Nongovernment not-for-profit	46	5,559	133,841	1,170,802	1,568,697	57.7	3,205	4,295	8.7	129,590	248,003	923,652	1,171,655	479	18,439
Investor-owned (for-profit)	1	407	10,831	80,034	97,925	53.8	219	268	7.4	11,750	28,136	45,402	73,538	16	939
State and local government	43	2,645	43,305	559,771	764,967	58.1	1,536	2,100	12.9	27,244	88,873	269,960	358,833	262	4,075

*For information on community hospitals that excludes nursing-home-type data, refer to Hospital Units columns in tables 4A through 4D, pages 14 through 17.

CLASSIFICATION	FULL-TIME EQUIVALENT PERSONNEL: Physicians and Dentists	Registered Nurses	Licensed Practical Nurses	Other Salaried Personnel	Total Personnel	FULL-TIME EQUIVALENT TRAINEES: Medical and Dental Residents	Other Trainees	Total Trainees	EXPENSES, LABOR: Payroll (in thousands)	Employee Benefits (in thousands)	Total (in thousands)	Percent of Total	EXPENSES, TOTAL: Amount (in thousands)	Adjusted, per Admission	Adjusted, per Inpatient Day
NEBRASKA	234	5,940	1,682	21,261	29,117	449	15	464	$ 621,479	$ 116,675	$ 738,154	52.4	$ 1,407,628		
6-24 beds	1	99	51	450	601	0	0	0	11,230	1,986	13,216	56.5	23,387		
25-49	8	495	235	1,690	2,428	0	0	0	42,350	6,468	48,819	55.8	87,437		
50-99	3	338	199	1,418	1,958	0	1	1	34,226	4,679	38,905	55.7	69,862		
100-199	119	1,259	273	4,527	6,178	19	0	19	123,501	23,386	146,886	53.3	275,726		
200-299	76	1,561	539	5,480	7,656	79	14	93	174,157	31,281	205,439	55.8	368,010		
300-399	20	1,318	224	4,076	5,638	351	0	351	128,279	25,750	154,029	48.8	315,860		
400-499	2	303	74	1,171	1,550	0	0	0	35,904	8,488	44,392	39.4	112,619		
500 or more	5	567	87	2,449	3,108	0	0	0	71,831	14,637	86,469	55.9	154,727		
Psychiatric	22	187	41	1,226	1,476	5	0	5	33,659	7,314	40,973	63.0	65,022		
Hospitals	22	187	41	1,226	1,476	5	0	5	33,659	7,314	40,973	63.0	65,022		
Institutions for mentally retarded	0	0	0	0	0	0	0	0	0	0	0	0.0	0		
General	189	5,582	1,584	18,661	26,016	421	15	436	557,190	102,723	659,913	51.2	1,287,673		
Hospitals	189	5,582	1,584	18,661	26,016	421	15	436	557,190	102,723	659,913	51.2	1,287,673		
Hospital units of institutions	0	0	0	0	0	0	0	0	0	0	0	0.0	0		
TB and other respiratory diseases	0	0	0	0	0	0	0	0	0	0	0	0.0	0		
Obstetrics and gynecology	0	0	0	0	0	0	0	0	0	0	0	0.0	0		
Eye, ear, nose, and throat	0	0	0	0	0	0	0	0	0	0	0	0.0	0		
Rehabilitation	3	21	12	596	632	1	0	1	9,998	1,613	11,611	73.9	15,715		
Orthopedic	0	0	0	0	0	0	0	0	0	0	0	0.0	0		
Chronic disease	0	0	0	0	0	0	0	0	0	0	0	0.0	0		
All other	20	150	45	778	993	22	0	22	20,633	5,024	25,657	65.4	39,218		
Federal	150	431	126	1,890	2,597	89	0	89	54,465	12,485	66,950	59.4	112,668		
Psychiatric	0	0	0	0	0	0	0	0	0	0	0	0.0	0		
General and other special	150	431	126	1,890	2,597	89	0	89	54,465	12,485	66,950	59.4	112,668		
Nonfederal	84	5,509	1,556	19,371	26,520	360	15	375	567,014	104,190	671,204	51.8	1,294,960		
Psychiatric	22	187	41	1,226	1,476	5	0	5	33,659	7,314	40,973	63.0	65,022		
Hospitals	22	187	41	1,226	1,476	5	0	5	33,659	7,314	40,973	63.0	65,022		
Institutions for mentally retarded	0	0	0	0	0	0	0	0	0	0	0	0.0	0		
TB and other respiratory diseases	0	0	0	0	0	0	0	0	0	0	0	0.0	0		
Long-term general and other special	11	67	39	1,001	1,118	3	0	3	23,482	5,133	28,615	73.6	38,868		
Short-term general and other special	51	5,255	1,476	17,144	23,926	352	15	367	509,873	91,743	601,616	50.5	1,191,070		
Hospital units of institutions	0	0	0	0	0	0	0	0	0	0	0	0.0	0		
Community hospitals*	51	5,255	1,476	17,144	23,926	352	15	367	509,873	91,743	601,616	50.5	1,191,070	$4,675.43	$ 489.83
6-24 beds	1	93	48	398	540	0	0	0	9,533	1,618	11,151	55.4	20,137	2,297.69	376.86
25-49	2	476	229	1,634	2,341	0	0	0	39,718	5,951	45,669	54.7	83,559	2,149.71	333.82
50-99	3	338	199	1,418	1,958	0	1	1	34,226	4,679	38,905	55.7	69,862	2,925.77	177.16
100-199	16	893	168	2,515	3,592	1	0	1	74,650	11,368	86,018	51.3	167,746	4,185.79	438.30
200-299	2	1,267	447	3,483	5,199	0	14	14	115,732	19,253	134,984	50.6	266,560	4,632.60	570.06
300-399	20	1,318	224	4,076	5,638	351	0	351	128,279	25,750	154,029	48.8	315,860	7,282.08	817.55
400-499	2	303	74	1,171	1,550	0	0	0	35,904	8,488	44,392	39.4	112,619	8,498.26	1,150.05
500 or more	5	567	87	2,449	3,108	0	0	0	71,831	14,637	86,469	55.9	154,727	5,335.98	387.89
Nongovernment not-for-profit	34	3,737	1,068	11,352	16,191	13	15	28	352,447	62,832	415,279	51.6	804,850	4,455.40	513.07
Investor-owned (for-profit)	2	303	74	1,171	1,550	0	0	0	35,904	8,488	44,392	39.4	112,619	8,498.26	1,150.05
State and local government	15	1,215	334	4,621	6,185	339	0	339	121,522	20,424	141,946	51.9	273,602	4,496.11	357.66

*For information on community hospitals that excludes nursing-home-type data, refer to Hospital Units columns in tables 4A through 4D, pages 14 through 17.

(continued on next page)

Table
5C (Continued) Nevada

Utilization, Personnel, and Finances in States

Excludes AHA nonregistered hospitals (see Table 14, page 240).

CLASSIFICATION	HOSPITALS	BEDS	ADMISSIONS	INPATIENT DAYS	ADJUSTED PATIENT DAYS	OCCUPANCY, percent	AVERAGE DAILY CENSUS	ADJUSTED AVERAGE DAILY CENSUS	AVERAGE STAY, days	SURGICAL OPERATIONS	OUTPATIENT VISITS			NEWBORNS	
											Emergency	Other	Total	Bassinets	Births
NEVADA	31	4,118	129,596	917,080		61.0	2,512			92,617	415,192	1,149,147	1,564,339	263	20,146
6-24 beds	3	43	1,878	7,154		46.5	20			1,205	22,447	124,034	146,481	0	0
25-49	8	318	7,875	59,647		51.6	164			3,982	53,565	250,314	303,879	55	1,379
50-99	10	695	14,185	145,747		57.3	398			7,864	32,752	100,815	133,567	44	4,410
100-199	3	385	9,872	54,335		38.4	148			6,398	65,305	40,878	106,183	18	573
200-299	2	426	12,743	111,451		71.6	305			9,302	28,932	140,797	169,729	0	0
300-399	2	677	25,986	150,002		60.7	411			22,823	48,352	151,406	199,758	63	3,576
400-499	2	886	35,103	227,947		70.5	625			18,851	112,567	292,885	405,452	43	6,859
500 or more	1	688	21,954	160,797		64.1	441			22,192	51,272	48,018	99,290	40	3,349
Psychiatric	6	465	4,848	109,154		63.9	297			0	1,287	36,924	38,211	0	0
Hospitals	6	465	4,848	109,154		63.9	297			0	1,287	36,924	38,211	0	0
Institutions for mentally retarded	0	0	0	0		00.0	0			0	0	0	0	0	0
General	24	3,586	121,284	798,569		61.0	2,189			89,874	413,905	1,102,143	1,516,048	243	17,371
Hospitals	24	3,586	121,284	798,569		61.0	2,189			89,874	413,905	1,102,143	1,516,048	243	17,371
Hospital units of institutions	0	0	0	0		00.0	0			0	0	0	0	0	0
TB and other respiratory diseases	0	0	0	0		00.0	0			0	0	0	0	0	0
Obstetrics and gynecology	1	67	3,464	9,357		38.8	26			2,743	0	10,080	10,080	20	2,775
Eye, ear, nose, and throat	0	0	0	0		00.0	0			0	0	0	0	0	0
Rehabilitation	0	0	0	0		00.0	0			0	0	0	0	0	0
Orthopedic	0	0	0	0		00.0	0			0	0	0	0	0	0
Chronic disease	0	0	0	0		00.0	0			0	0	0	0	0	0
All other	0	0	0	0		00.0	0			0	0	0	0	0	0
Federal	4	280	8,753	66,221		65.0	182			4,770	45,090	394,787	439,877	20	629
Psychiatric	0	0	0	0		00.0	0			0	0	0	0	0	0
General and other special	4	280	8,753	66,221		65.0	182			4,770	45,090	394,787	439,877	20	629
Nonfederal	27	3,838	120,843	850,859		60.7	2,330			87,847	370,102	754,360	1,124,462	243	19,517
Psychiatric	6	465	4,848	109,154		63.9	297			0	1,287	36,924	38,211	0	0
Hospitals	6	465	4,848	109,154		63.9	297			0	1,287	36,924	38,211	0	0
Institutions for mentally retarded	0	0	0	0		00.0	0			0	0	0	0	0	0
TB and other respiratory diseases	0	0	0	0		00.0	0			0	0	0	0	0	0
Long-term general and other special	0	0	0	0		00.0	0			0	0	0	0	0	0
Short-term general and other special	21	3,373	115,995	741,705		60.3	2,033			87,847	368,815	717,436	1,086,251	243	19,517
Hospital units of institutions	0	0	0	0		00.0	0			0	0	0	0	0	0
Community hospitals*	21	3,373	115,995	741,705	925,916	60.3	2,033	2,535	6.4	87,847	368,815	717,436	1,086,251	243	19,517
6-24 beds	1	14	163	2,061	3,385	42.9	6	9	12.6	0	2,344	5,104	7,448	0	0
25-49	7	283	4,697	52,137	88,568	50.5	143	243	11.1	2,847	28,578	60,206	88,784	35	750
50-99	4	230	9,337	36,593	52,604	43.9	101	143	3.9	7,864	31,465	63,891	95,356	44	4,410
100-199	3	385	9,872	54,335	73,105	38.4	148	200	5.5	6,398	65,305	40,878	106,183	18	573
200-299	1	210	8,883	57,833	70,761	75.2	158	194	6.5	6,872	28,932	55,048	83,980	0	0
300-399	2	677	25,986	150,002	174,670	60.7	411	478	5.8	22,823	48,352	151,406	199,758	63	3,576
400-499	2	886	35,103	227,947	266,081	70.5	625	729	6.5	18,851	112,567	292,885	405,452	43	6,859
500 or more	1	688	21,954	160,797	196,742	64.1	441	539	7.3	22,192	51,272	48,018	99,290	40	3,349
Nongovernment not-for-profit	6	996	37,590	229,421	287,946	63.2	629	789	6.1	24,659	118,920	258,146	377,066	84	6,688
Investor-owned (for-profit)	5	1,415	50,114	324,671	390,168	62.8	889	1,068	6.5	46,782	111,765	150,120	261,885	75	7,449
State and local government	10	962	28,291	187,613	247,802	53.5	515	678	6.6	16,406	138,130	309,170	447,300	84	5,380

*For information on community hospitals that excludes nursing-home-type data, refer to Hospital Units columns in tables 4A through 4D, pages 14 through 17.

Table 5C (Continued) Nevada

CLASSIFICATION	FULL-TIME EQUIVALENT PERSONNEL: Physicians and Dentists	Registered Nurses	Licensed Practical Nurses	Other Salaried Personnel	Total Personnel	FULL-TIME EQUIVALENT TRAINEES: Medical and Dental Residents	Other Trainees	Total Trainees	EXPENSES — LABOR: Payroll (in thousands)	Employee Benefits (in thousands)	Total (in thousands)	Percent of Total	EXPENSES — TOTAL: Amount (in thousands)	Adjusted, per Admission	Adjusted, per Inpatient Day
NEVADA	150	3,630	646	9,578	14,004	25	15	40	$ 379,900	$ 83,231	$ 463,131	51.3	$ 903,072		
6-24 beds	27	45	13	317	402	0	0	0	6,039	1,310	7,349	66.9	10,989		
25-49	60	174	60	1,005	1,299	0	4	4	19,019	4,491	23,511	58.7	40,026		
50-99	13	250	78	1,245	1,586	1	1	2	45,009	9,981	54,990	53.5	102,709		
100-199	0	257	41	637	935	0	0	0	31,339	5,387	36,726	51.4	71,439		
200-299	32	274	59	965	1,330	13	10	23	48,962	7,305	56,267	57.8	97,265		
300-399	0	708	108	1,542	2,358	0	0	0	69,625	14,033	83,657	50.4	165,915		
400-499	18	1,065	132	2,644	3,859	11	0	11	103,530	28,546	132,075	51.3	257,641		
500 or more	0	857	155	1,223	2,235	0	0	0	56,377	12,178	68,555	43.6	157,087		
Psychiatric	12	110	28	766	916	1	1	2	26,216	5,551	31,766	59.0	53,826		
Hospitals	12	110	28	766	916	1	1	2	26,216	5,551	31,766	59.0	53,826		
Institutions for mentally retarded	0	0	0	0	0	0	0	0	0	0	0	0.0	0		
General	137	3,479	600	8,677	12,893	24	14	38	348,048	76,418	424,466	50.9	833,672		
Hospitals	137	3,479	600	8,677	12,893	24	14	38	348,048	76,418	424,466	50.9	833,672		
Hospital units of institutions	0	0	0	0	0	0	0	0	0	0	0	0.0	0		
TB and other respiratory diseases	0	0	0	0	0	0	0	0	0	0	0	0.0	0		
Obstetrics and gynecology	1	41	18	135	195	0	0	0	5,636	1,263	6,898	44.3	15,574		
Eye, ear, nose, and throat	0	0	0	0	0	0	0	0	0	0	0	0.0	0		
Rehabilitation	0	0	0	0	0	0	0	0	0	0	0	0.0	0		
Orthopedic	0	0	0	0	0	0	0	0	0	0	0	0.0	0		
Chronic disease	0	0	0	0	0	0	0	0	0	0	0	0.0	0		
All other	0	0	0	0	0	0	0	0	0	0	0	0.0	0		
Federal	115	242	51	1,274	1,682	13	10	23	34,946	5,988	40,934	69.7	58,748		
Psychiatric	0	0	0	0	0	0	0	0	0	0	0	0.0	0		
General and other special	115	242	51	1,274	1,682	13	10	23	34,946	5,988	40,934	69.7	58,748		
Nonfederal	35	3,388	595	8,304	12,322	12	5	17	344,954	77,243	422,196	50.0	844,324		
Psychiatric	12	110	28	766	916	1	1	2	26,216	5,551	31,766	59.0	53,826		
Hospitals	12	110	28	766	916	1	1	2	26,216	5,551	31,766	59.0	53,826		
Institutions for mentally retarded	0	0	0	0	0	0	0	0	0	0	0	0.0	0		
TB and other respiratory diseases	0	0	0	0	0	0	0	0	0	0	0	0.0	0		
Long-term general and other special	0	0	0	0	0	0	0	0	0	0	0	0.0	0		
Short-term general and other special	23	3,278	567	7,538	11,406	11	4	15	318,738	71,692	390,430	49.4	790,498		
Hospital units of institutions	0	0	0	0	0	0	0	0	0	0	0	0.0	0		
Community hospitals*	23	3,278	567	7,538	11,406	11	4	15	318,738	71,692	390,430	49.4	790,498	$5,510.96	$ 853.75
6-24 beds	0	7	5	33	45	0	0	0	1,095	209	1,304	55.1	2,364	8,821.20	698.40
25-49	4	89	38	505	636	0	4	4	13,118	3,239	16,357	53.8	30,382	4,019.86	343.04
50-99	1	140	50	479	670	0	0	0	18,793	4,431	23,224	47.5	48,883	3,680.66	929.26
100-199	0	257	41	637	935	0	0	0	31,339	5,387	36,726	51.4	71,439	5,324.14	977.22
200-299	0	155	38	475	668	0	0	0	24,861	3,671	28,532	50.2	56,786	5,224.59	802.51
300-399	0	708	108	1,542	2,358	0	0	0	69,625	14,033	83,657	50.4	165,915	5,490.60	949.88
400-499	18	1,065	132	2,644	3,859	11	0	11	103,530	28,546	132,075	51.3	257,641	6,289.00	968.28
500 or more	0	857	155	1,223	2,235	0	0	0	56,377	12,178	68,555	43.6	157,087	5,847.94	798.44
Nongovernment not-for-profit	1	993	118	2,976	4,088	0	0	0	115,471	27,876	143,346	51.4	279,112	5,998.80	969.32
Investor-owned (for-profit)	1	1,399	295	2,421	4,116	0	0	0	119,400	21,624	141,024	45.0	313,206	5,203.27	802.75
State and local government	21	886	154	2,141	3,202	11	4	15	83,868	22,192	106,060	53.5	198,180	5,397.20	799.75

*For information on community hospitals that excludes nursing-home-type data, refer to Hospital Units columns in tables 4A through 4D, pages 14 through 17.

(continued on next page)

Table

5C (Continued) New Hampshire

Utilization, Personnel, and Finances in States

Excludes AHA nonregistered hospitals (see Table 14, page 240).

CLASSIFICATION	HOSPITALS	BEDS	ADMISSIONS	INPATIENT DAYS	ADJUSTED PATIENT DAYS	OCCUPANCY, percent	AVERAGE DAILY CENSUS	ADJUSTED AVERAGE DAILY CENSUS	AVERAGE STAY, days	SURGICAL OPERATIONS	OUTPATIENT VISITS			NEWBORNS	
											Emergency	Other	Total	Bassinets	Births
NEW HAMPSHIRE	40	4,953	138,302	1,249,054		69.1	3,424			86,285	488,654	1,247,996	1,736,650	350	16,807
6-24 beds	1	10	362	1,140		30.0	3			56	0	17,231	17,231	0	0
25-49	5	216	4,811	37,323		47.2	102			2,364	29,663	45,954	75,617	30	403
50-99	17	1,282	25,461	292,802		62.7	804			15,607	108,652	299,497	408,149	80	2,776
100-199	9	1,256	42,551	303,202		66.2	831			25,436	122,689	326,460	449,149	110	5,964
200-299	5	1,179	37,567	321,121		74.6	880			26,626	119,546	331,714	451,260	92	4,588
300-399	3	1,010	27,550	293,466		79.6	804			16,196	108,104	227,140	335,244	38	3,076
400-499	0	0	0	0		00.0	0			0	0	0	0	0	0
500 or more	0	0	0	0		00.0	0			0	0	0	0	0	0
Psychiatric	10	1,171	10,633	313,532		73.4	859			0	2,705	24,296	27,001	0	0
Hospitals	10	1,171	10,633	313,532		73.4	859			0	2,705	24,296	27,001	0	0
Institutions for mentally retarded	0	0	0	0		00.0	0			0	0	0	0	0	0
General	28	3,618	126,615	884,504		67.0	2,425			86,285	485,949	1,188,165	1,674,114	350	16,807
Hospitals	27	3,608	126,253	883,364		67.1	2,422			86,229	485,949	1,170,934	1,656,883	350	16,807
Hospital units of institutions	1	10	362	1,140		30.0	3			56	0	17,231	17,231	0	0
TB and other respiratory diseases	0	0	0	0		00.0	0			0	0	0	0	0	0
Obstetrics and gynecology	0	0	0	0		00.0	0			0	0	0	0	0	0
Eye, ear, nose, and throat	0	0	0	0		00.0	0			0	0	0	0	0	0
Rehabilitation	2	164	1,054	51,018		85.4	140			0	0	35,535	35,535	0	0
Orthopedic	0	0	0	0		00.0	0			0	0	0	0	0	0
Chronic disease	0	0	0	0		00.0	0			0	0	0	0	0	0
All other	0	0	0	0		00.0	0			0	0	0	0	0	0
Federal	1	240	2,751	65,603		75.0	180			2,503	0	79,114	79,114	0	0
Psychiatric	0	0	0	0		00.0	0			0	0	0	0	0	0
General and other special	1	240	2,751	65,603		75.0	180			2,503	0	79,114	79,114	0	0
Nonfederal	39	4,713	135,551	1,183,451		68.8	3,244			83,782	488,654	1,168,882	1,657,536	350	16,807
Psychiatric	10	1,171	10,633	313,532		73.4	859			0	2,705	24,296	27,001	0	0
Hospitals	10	1,171	10,633	313,532		73.4	859			0	2,705	24,296	27,001	0	0
Institutions for mentally retarded	0	0	0	0		00.0	0			0	0	0	0	0	0
TB and other respiratory diseases	0	0	0	0		00.0	0			0	0	0	0	0	0
Long-term general and other special	1	62	24	22,630		100.0	62			0	0	0	0	0	0
Short-term general and other special	28	3,480	124,894	847,289		66.8	2,323			83,782	485,949	1,144,586	1,630,535	350	16,807
Hospital units of institutions	1	10	362	1,140		30.0	3			56	0	17,231	17,231	0	0
Community hospitals*	27	3,470	124,532	846,149	1,200,534	66.9	2,320	3,289	6.8	83,726	485,949	1,127,355	1,613,304	350	16,807
6-24 beds	0	0	0	0	0	00.0	0	0	0.0	0	0	0	0	0	0
25-49	4	175	4,639	25,623	42,188	40.0	70	116	5.5	2,364	29,313	44,217	73,530	30	403
50-99	10	705	19,593	149,246	240,528	58.2	410	659	7.6	15,607	107,340	286,925	394,265	80	2,776
100-199	7	973	38,842	231,135	324,529	65.2	634	888	6.0	25,436	121,646	316,473	438,119	110	5,964
200-299	4	939	34,816	255,518	351,603	74.5	700	963	7.3	24,123	119,546	252,600	372,146	92	4,588
300-399	2	678	26,642	184,627	241,686	74.6	506	663	6.9	16,196	108,104	227,140	335,244	38	3,076
400-499	0	0	0	0	0	00.0	0	0	0.0	0	0	0	0	0	0
500 or more	0	0	0	0	0	00.0	0	0	0.0	0	0	0	0	0	0
Nongovernment not-for-profit	24	3,171	113,633	772,504	1,093,800	66.8	2,118	2,998	6.8	76,192	438,663	1,010,048	1,448,711	320	15,174
Investor-owned (for-profit)	3	299	10,899	73,645	106,734	67.6	202	291	6.8	7,534	47,286	117,307	164,593	30	1,633
State and local government	0	0	0	0	0	00.0	0	0	0.0	0	0	0	0	0	0

*For information on community hospitals that excludes nursing-home-type data, refer to Hospital Units columns in tables 4A through 4D, pages 14 through 17.

CLASSIFICATION	Physicians and Dentists	Registered Nurses	Licensed Practical Nurses	Other Salaried Personnel	Total Personnel	Medical and Dental Residents	Other Trainees	Total Trainees	Payroll (in thousands)	Employee Benefits (in thousands)	Total (in thousands)	Percent of Total	Amount (in thousands)	Adjusted, per Admission	Adjusted, per Inpatient Day
	FULL-TIME EQUIVALENT PERSONNEL					FULL-TIME EQUIVALENT TRAINEES			EXPENSES: LABOR				EXPENSES: TOTAL		
NEW HAMPSHIRE	112	4,083	564	12,120	16,879	246	6	252	$ 461,518	$ 94,053	$ 555,570	57.2	$ 970,898		
6-24 beds	1	8	1	14	24	0	0	0	805	202	1,007	61.3	1,643		
25-49	4	131	35	434	604	0	0	0	14,100	2,443	16,543	56.7	29,162		
50-99	31	764	132	2,514	3,441	0	0	0	89,696	16,519	106,215	57.4	185,199		
100-199	17	1,176	183	3,142	4,518	1	0	1	121,147	23,698	144,845	55.4	261,566		
200-299	36	1,012	139	2,962	4,149	8	6	14	120,374	22,454	142,828	54.3	262,977		
300-399	23	992	74	3,054	4,143	237	0	237	115,395	28,737	144,132	62.6	230,352		
400-499	0	0	0	0	0	0	0	0	0	0	0	0.0	0		
500 or more	0	0	0	0	0	0	0	0	0	0	0	0.0	0		
Psychiatric	41	315	48	1,903	2,307	1	0	1	62,155	14,289	76,445	65.5	116,658		
Hospitals	41	315	48	1,903	2,307	1	0	1	62,155	14,289	76,445	65.5	116,658		
Institutions for mentally retarded	0	0	0	0	0	0	0	0	0	0	0	0.0	0		
General	71	3,708	488	9,553	13,820	245	6	251	383,338	76,926	460,264	56.2	819,348		
Hospitals	70	3,700	487	9,539	13,796	245	6	251	382,533	76,724	459,256	56.2	817,705		
Hospital units of institutions	1	8	1	14	24	0	0	0	805	202	1,007	61.3	1,643		
TB and other respiratory diseases	0	0	0	0	0	0	0	0	0	0	0	0.0	0		
Obstetrics and gynecology	0	0	0	0	0	0	0	0	0	0	0	0.0	0		
Eye, ear, nose, and throat	0	0	0	0	0	0	0	0	0	0	0	0.0	0		
Rehabilitation	0	60	28	664	752	0	0	0	16,025	2,837	18,862	54.1	34,892		
Orthopedic	0	0	0	0	0	0	0	0	0	0	0	0.0	0		
Chronic disease	0	0	0	0	0	0	0	0	0	0	0	0.0	0		
All other	0	0	0	0	0	0	0	0	0	0	0	0.0	0		
Federal	32	92	14	442	580	8	0	8	18,519	3,547	22,067	62.4	35,382		
Psychiatric	0	0	0	0	0	0	0	0	0	0	0	0.0	0		
General and other special	32	92	14	442	580	8	0	8	18,519	3,547	22,067	62.4	35,382		
Nonfederal	80	3,991	550	11,678	16,299	238	6	244	442,998	90,505	533,504	57.0	935,516		
Psychiatric	41	315	48	1,903	2,307	1	0	1	62,155	14,289	76,445	65.5	116,658		
Hospitals	41	315	48	1,903	2,307	1	0	1	62,155	14,289	76,445	65.5	116,658		
Institutions for mentally retarded	0	0	0	0	0	0	0	0	0	0	0	0.0	0		
TB and other respiratory diseases	0	0	0	0	0	0	0	0	0	0	0	0.0	0		
Long-term general and other special	0	14	4	405	423	0	0	0	7,721	615	8,336	69.4	12,008		
Short-term general and other special	39	3,662	498	9,370	13,569	237	6	243	373,122	75,601	448,722	55.6	806,850		
Hospital units of institutions	1	8	1	14	24	0	0	0	805	202	1,007	61.3	1,643		
Community hospitals*	38	3,654	497	9,356	13,545	237	6	243	372,317	75,398	447,715	55.6	805,208	$4,543.65	$ 670.71
6-24 beds	0	0	0	0	0	0	0	0	0	0	0	0.0	0	0.00	0.00
25-49	1	122	34	362	519	0	0	0	11,899	1,913	13,812	56.8	24,307	3,160.43	576.16
50-99	10	563	107	1,498	2,178	0	0	0	54,061	10,609	64,670	54.7	118,123	3,746.83	491.10
100-199	15	1,122	175	2,766	4,078	0	0	0	109,806	21,308	131,114	55.2	237,443	4,285.04	731.65
200-299	4	920	125	2,520	3,569	0	6	6	101,855	18,906	120,761	53.1	227,595	4,791.98	647.31
300-399	8	927	56	2,210	3,201	237	0	237	94,696	22,662	117,358	59.3	197,740	5,634.91	818.17
400-499	0	0	0	0	0	0	0	0	0	0	0	0.0	0	0.00	0.00
500 or more	0	0	0	0	0	0	0	0	0	0	0	0.0	0	0.00	0.00
Nongovernment not-for-profit	38	3,326	441	8,602	12,407	237	6	243	341,937	68,139	410,076	56.9	720,809	4,494.88	658.99
Investor-owned (for-profit)	0	328	56	754	1,138	0	0	0	30,379	7,260	37,639	44.6	84,399	5,007.66	790.74
State and local government	0	0	0	0	0	0	0	0	0	0	0	0.0	0	0.00	0.00

*For information on community hospitals that excludes nursing-home-type data, refer to Hospital Units columns in tables 4A through 4D, pages 14 through 17.

(continued on next page)

Table
5C (Continued) New Jersey

Utilization, Personnel, and Finances in States

Excludes AHA nonregistered hospitals (see Table 14, page 240).

CLASSIFICATION	HOSPITALS	BEDS	ADMISSIONS	INPATIENT DAYS	ADJUSTED PATIENT DAYS	OCCUPANCY, percent	AVERAGE DAILY CENSUS	ADJUSTED AVERAGE DAILY CENSUS	AVERAGE STAY, days	SURGICAL OPERATIONS	OUTPATIENT VISITS Emergency	OUTPATIENT VISITS Other	OUTPATIENT VISITS Total	NEWBORNS Bassinets	NEWBORNS Births
NEW JERSEY	119	38,143	1,173,615	11,294,417		81.1	30,948			683,356	2,471,373	8,360,980	10,832,353	1,995	114,045
6-24 beds	1	21	463	1,787		23.8	5			60	1,185	1,612	2,797	0	0
25-49	2	76	1,898	6,624		25.0	19			513	15,750	142,743	158,493	0	0
50-99	9	725	12,178	217,492		82.2	596			6,397	34,708	350,403	385,111	0	0
100-199	21	2,860	86,828	737,521		70.7	2,021			53,884	218,727	843,909	1,062,636	97	3,984
200-299	28	6,706	269,597	1,937,512		79.2	5,310			158,188	597,618	2,074,378	2,671,996	438	26,063
300-399	22	7,783	246,095	2,274,905		80.1	6,233			158,165	523,807	1,317,217	1,841,024	490	22,986
400-499	19	8,408	324,551	2,583,133		84.2	7,076			179,908	706,943	1,852,787	2,559,730	626	38,202
500 or more	17	11,564	232,005	3,535,443		83.8	9,688			126,241	372,635	1,777,931	2,150,566	344	22,810
Psychiatric	11	4,382	10,125	1,422,171		88.9	3,896			0	2,150	169,153	171,303	0	0
Hospitals	11	4,382	10,125	1,422,171		88.9	3,896			0	2,150	169,153	171,303	0	0
Institutions for mentally retarded	0	0	0	0		00.0	0			0	0	0	0	0	0
General	96	31,180	1,144,400	9,086,922		79.9	24,900			680,566	2,465,734	7,820,543	10,286,277	1,995	114,045
Hospitals	93	30,934	1,143,315	9,029,001		80.0	24,742			680,159	2,463,144	7,813,762	10,276,906	1,995	114,045
Hospital units of institutions	3	246	1,085	57,921		64.2	158			407	2,590	6,781	9,371	0	0
TB and other respiratory diseases	0	0	0	0		00.0	0			0	0	0	0	0	0
Obstetrics and gynecology	0	0	0	0		00.0	0			0	0	0	0	0	0
Eye, ear, nose, and throat	0	0	0	0		00.0	0			0	0	0	0	0	0
Rehabilitation	7	827	10,003	246,425		81.5	674			48	0	319,972	319,972	0	0
Orthopedic	0	0	0	0		00.0	0			0	0	0	0	0	0
Chronic disease	1	558	996	181,666		89.2	498			0	0	9,157	9,157	0	0
All other	4	1,196	8,091	357,233		81.9	980			2,742	3,489	42,155	45,644	0	0
Federal	4	2,189	20,260	582,861		73.0	1,598			4,932	46,856	652,916	699,772	0	0
Psychiatric	0	0	0	0		00.0	0			0	0	0	0	0	0
General and other special	4	2,189	20,260	582,861		73.0	1,598			4,932	46,856	652,916	699,772	0	0
Nonfederal	115	35,954	1,153,355	10,711,556		81.6	29,350			678,424	2,424,517	7,708,064	10,132,581	1,995	114,045
Psychiatric	11	4,382	10,125	1,422,171		88.9	3,896			0	2,150	169,153	171,303	0	0
Hospitals	11	4,382	10,125	1,422,171		88.9	3,896			0	2,150	169,153	171,303	0	0
Institutions for mentally retarded	0	0	0	0		00.0	0			0	0	0	0	0	0
TB and other respiratory diseases	0	0	0	0		00.0	0			0	0	0	0	0	0
Long-term general and other special	7	2,580	11,188	809,458		86.0	2,218			1,630	14,052	209,856	223,908	0	0
Short-term general and other special	97	28,992	1,132,042	8,479,927		80.1	23,236			676,794	2,408,315	7,329,055	9,737,370	1,995	114,045
Hospital units of institutions	2	146	533	41,011		76.7	112			78	1,266	1,911	3,177	0	0
Community hospitals*	95	28,846	1,131,509	8,438,916	10,619,506	80.2	23,124	29,094	7.5	676,716	2,407,049	7,327,144	9,734,193	1,995	114,045
6-24 beds	0	0	0	0	0	00.0	0	0	0.0	0	0	0	0	0	0
25-49	1	27	360	1,326	1,326	14.8	4	4	3.7	0	0	38,702	38,702	0	0
50-99	5	424	10,297	116,926	159,077	75.5	320	435	11.4	6,349	33,452	79,854	113,306	0	0
100-199	16	2,291	80,093	587,206	755,323	70.3	1,610	2,070	7.3	52,349	188,576	528,966	717,542	97	3,984
200-299	27	6,419	267,040	1,857,996	2,363,528	79.3	5,092	6,474	7.0	158,188	597,618	2,055,291	2,652,909	438	26,063
300-399	19	6,696	244,582	1,899,841	2,363,273	77.7	5,206	6,474	7.8	158,165	523,753	1,315,878	1,839,631	490	22,986
400-499	18	8,008	324,513	2,465,157	3,089,250	84.3	6,753	8,465	7.6	179,908	706,943	1,841,285	2,548,228	626	38,202
500 or more	9	4,981	204,624	1,510,464	1,887,729	83.1	4,139	5,172	7.4	121,757	356,707	1,467,168	1,823,875	344	22,810
Nongovernment not-for-profit	91	27,874	1,111,343	8,160,577	10,260,252	80.2	22,361	28,109	7.3	670,555	2,350,264	7,123,292	9,473,556	1,970	111,139
Investor-owned (for-profit)	1	151	3,425	47,232	62,422	85.4	129	171	13.8	0	0	29,982	29,982	0	0
State and local government	3	821	16,741	231,107	296,832	77.2	634	814	13.8	6,161	56,785	173,870	230,655	25	2,906

*For information on community hospitals that excludes nursing-home-type data, refer to Hospital Units columns in tables 4A through 4D, pages 14 through 17.

CLASSIFICATION	Physicians and Dentists	Registered Nurses	Licensed Practical Nurses	Other Salaried Personnel	Total Personnel	Medical and Dental Residents	Other Trainees	Total Trainees	Payroll (in thousands)	Employee Benefits (in thousands)	Labor Total (in thousands)	Percent of Total	Total Amount (in thousands)	Adjusted, per Admission	Adjusted, per Inpatient Day
	FULL-TIME EQUIVALENT PERSONNEL					FULL-TIME EQUIVALENT TRAINEES			EXPENSES: LABOR				EXPENSES: TOTAL		
NEW JERSEY	2,139	26,887	6,122	91,661	126,809	1,992	63	2,055	$ 3,707,414	$ 710,849	$ 4,418,263	59.7	$ 7,395,640		
6-24 beds	0	5	3	37	45	0	0	0	1,191	221	1,412	60.9	2,318		
25-49	38	54	15	334	441	0	0	0	9,520	1,197	10,717	86.2	12,430		
50-99	55	473	135	2,259	2,922	15	5	20	79,869	18,399	98,268	63.6	154,418		
100-199	202	1,801	486	6,830	9,319	74	6	80	279,910	53,732	333,642	59.9	556,754		
200-299	96	5,245	1,290	16,279	22,910	70	0	70	658,269	124,493	782,762	58.3	1,343,796		
300-399	243	5,352	1,412	18,385	25,392	308	6	314	736,184	146,361	882,545	58.3	1,513,529		
400-499	833	7,469	1,430	23,768	33,500	675	3	678	997,907	196,147	1,194,054	58.9	2,028,860		
500 or more	672	6,488	1,351	23,769	32,280	850	43	893	944,563	170,299	1,114,862	62.5	1,783,536		
Psychiatric	215	897	535	7,020	8,667	22	4	26	243,958	52,188	296,146	77.4	382,675		
Hospitals	215	897	535	7,020	8,667	22	4	26	243,958	52,188	296,146	77.4	382,675		
Institutions for mentally retarded	0	0	0	0	0	0	0	0	0	0	0	0.0	0		
General	1,778	25,160	5,364	79,757	112,059	1,900	58	1,958	3,277,294	615,921	3,893,216	58.4	6,666,673		
Hospitals	1,758	25,108	5,322	79,340	111,528	1,900	52	1,952	3,265,504	613,150	3,878,654	58.3	6,648,057		
Hospital units of institutions	20	52	42	417	531	0	6	6	11,790	2,772	14,562	78.2	18,616		
TB and other respiratory diseases	0	0	0	0	0	0	0	0	0	0	0	0.0	0		
Obstetrics and gynecology	0	0	0	0	0	0	0	0	0	0	0	0.0	0		
Eye, ear, nose, and throat	0	0	0	0	0	0	0	0	0	0	0	0.0	0		
Rehabilitation	52	345	111	2,060	2,568	9	0	9	72,540	15,844	88,385	64.4	137,204		
Orthopedic	0	0	0	0	0	0	0	0	0	0	0	0.0	0		
Chronic disease	7	11	11	664	693	0	0	0	21,143	5,478	26,621	73.0	36,482		
All other	87	474	101	2,160	2,822	61	1	62	92,479	21,417	113,896	66.0	172,606		
Federal	287	667	142	3,861	4,957	149	11	160	163,468	18,628	182,096	73.2	248,646		
Psychiatric	0	0	0	0	0	0	0	0	0	0	0	0.0	0		
General and other special	287	667	142	3,861	4,957	149	11	160	163,468	18,628	182,096	73.2	248,646		
Nonfederal	1,852	26,220	5,980	87,800	121,852	1,843	52	1,895	3,543,946	692,221	4,236,167	59.3	7,146,994		
Psychiatric	215	897	535	7,020	8,667	22	4	26	243,958	52,188	296,146	77.4	382,675		
Hospitals	215	897	535	7,020	8,667	22	4	26	243,958	52,188	296,146	77.4	382,675		
Institutions for mentally retarded	0	0	0	0	0	0	0	0	0	0	0	0.0	0		
TB and other respiratory diseases	0	0	0	0	0	0	0	0	0	0	0	0.0	0		
Long-term general and other special	128	578	246	4,124	5,076	62	1	63	142,480	36,545	179,025	72.2	248,053		
Short-term general and other special	1,509	24,745	5,199	76,656	108,109	1,759	47	1,806	3,157,508	603,488	3,760,996	57.7	6,516,266		
Hospital units of institutions	2	14	13	290	319	0	6	6	7,079	1,638	8,718	76.7	11,372		
Community hospitals*	1,507	24,731	5,186	76,366	107,790	1,759	41	1,800	3,150,429	601,849	3,752,279	57.7	6,504,894	$4,572.56	$ 612.54
6-24 beds	0	0	0	0	0	0	0	0	0	0	0	0.0	0	0.00	0.00
25-49	6	24	0	20	50	0	0	0	1,246	48	1,294	83.5	1,549	4,302.63	1,168.13
50-99	14	309	89	819	1,231	0	1	1	35,306	7,347	42,653	56.9	75,025	5,326.23	471.63
100-199	123	1,600	406	5,441	7,570	63	0	63	228,047	46,129	274,176	59.1	463,822	4,446.75	614.07
200-299	96	5,113	1,283	15,606	22,098	70	0	70	639,861	119,813	759,674	57.9	1,311,702	3,847.25	554.98
300-399	213	5,200	1,331	16,789	23,533	294	6	300	676,286	129,960	806,246	57.0	1,415,281	4,676.30	598.86
400-499	802	7,384	1,348	23,147	32,681	675	3	678	970,588	188,667	1,159,255	58.2	1,990,796	4,920.19	644.43
500 or more	253	5,101	729	14,544	20,627	657	31	688	599,096	109,886	708,982	56.9	1,246,718	4,877.08	660.43
Nongovernment not-for-profit	1,163	23,920	5,065	74,223	104,371	1,729	41	1,770	3,038,404	574,159	3,612,564	57.7	6,260,133	4,482.43	610.13
Investor-owned (for-profit)	0	61	18	221	300	0	0	0	5,950	1,350	7,300	43.1	16,939	3,741.82	271.37
State and local government	344	750	103	1,922	3,119	30	0	30	106,074	26,341	132,415	58.1	227,821	10,610.64	767.51

*For information on community hospitals that excludes nursing-home-type data, refer to Hospital Units columns in tables 4A through 4D, pages 14 through 17.

(continued on next page)

Table
5C (Continued) New Mexico

Utilization, Personnel, and Finances in States

Excludes AHA nonregistered hospitals (see Table 14, page 240).

CLASSIFICATION	HOSPITALS	BEDS	ADMISSIONS	INPATIENT DAYS	ADJUSTED PATIENT DAYS	OCCUPANCY, percent	AVERAGE DAILY CENSUS	ADJUSTED AVERAGE DAILY CENSUS	AVERAGE STAY, days	SURGICAL OPERATIONS	OUTPATIENT VISITS			NEWBORNS	
											Emergency	Other	Total	Bassinets	Births
NEW MEXICO	60	6,597	190,546	1,521,279		63.2	4,167			132,804	508,164	2,593,944	3,102,108	472	26,523
6-24 beds	3	57	2,801	10,072		49.1	28			1,131	14,978	117,221	132,199	16	341
25-49	19	627	20,135	88,974		38.9	244			7,208	79,840	589,237	669,077	73	2,380
50-99	16	1,089	31,835	246,434		62.0	675			13,831	86,332	447,093	533,425	76	4,869
100-199	11	1,495	43,974	321,179		58.9	880			33,709	125,377	882,344	1,007,721	129	5,969
200-299	6	1,432	43,713	315,436		60.3	864			36,576	112,196	177,531	289,727	94	5,890
300-399	3	1,045	17,189	328,675		86.1	900			8,535	42,922	164,914	207,836	36	3,752
400-499	2	852	30,899	210,509		67.6	576			31,814	46,519	215,604	262,123	48	3,322
500 or more	0	0	0	0		00.0	0			0	0	0	0	0	0
Psychiatric	11	1,555	6,691	450,201		79.3	1,233			0	6,434	83,062	89,496	0	0
Hospitals	10	1,198	6,686	324,161		74.1	888			0	6,434	83,062	89,496	0	0
Institutions for mentally retarded	1	357	5	126,040		96.6	345			0	0	0	0	0	0
General	46	4,943	182,545	1,045,259		57.9	2,864			132,057	501,730	2,468,135	2,969,865	472	26,523
Hospitals	46	4,943	182,545	1,045,259		57.9	2,864			132,057	501,730	2,468,135	2,969,865	472	26,523
Hospital units of institutions	0	0	0	0		00.0	0			0	0	0	0	0	0
TB and other respiratory diseases	0	0	0	0		00.0	0			0	0	0	0	0	0
Obstetrics and gynecology	0	0	0	0		00.0	0			0	0	0	0	0	0
Eye, ear, nose, and throat	0	0	0	0		00.0	0			0	0	0	0	0	0
Rehabilitation	2	75	857	22,912		82.7	62			0	0	32,055	32,055	0	0
Orthopedic	1	24	453	2,907		33.3	8			747	0	10,692	10,692	0	0
Chronic disease	0	0	0	0		00.0	0			0	0	0	0	0	0
All other	0	0	0	0		00.0	0			0	0	0	0	0	0
Federal	12	850	30,536	191,226		61.6	524			20,152	107,380	1,067,859	1,175,239	65	3,740
Psychiatric	0	0	0	0		00.0	0			0	0	0	0	0	0
General and other special	12	850	30,536	191,226		61.6	524			20,152	107,380	1,067,859	1,175,239	65	3,740
Nonfederal	48	5,747	160,010	1,330,053		63.4	3,643			112,652	400,784	1,526,085	1,926,869	407	22,783
Psychiatric	11	1,555	6,691	450,201		79.3	1,233			0	6,434	83,062	89,496	0	0
Hospitals	10	1,198	6,686	324,161		74.1	888			0	6,434	83,062	89,496	0	0
Institutions for mentally retarded	1	357	5	126,040		96.6	345			0	0	0	0	0	0
TB and other respiratory diseases	0	0	0	0		00.0	0			0	0	0	0	0	0
Long-term general and other special	0	0	0	0		00.0	0			0	0	0	0	0	0
Short-term general and other special	37	4,192	153,319	879,852		57.5	2,410			112,652	394,350	1,443,023	1,837,373	407	22,783
Hospital units of institutions	0	0	0	0		00.0	0			0	0	0	0	0	0
Community hospitals*	37	4,192	153,319	879,852	1,222,121	57.5	2,410	3,347	5.7	112,652	394,350	1,443,023	1,837,373	407	22,783
6-24 beds	1	24	453	2,907	4,499	33.3	8	12	6.4	747	0	10,692	10,692	0	0
25-49	11	359	9,782	42,609	64,375	32.6	117	177	4.4	3,990	35,441	68,165	103,606	46	1,252
50-99	8	514	18,775	104,968	148,634	55.8	287	407	5.6	9,640	52,965	125,284	178,249	54	2,598
100-199	10	1,380	43,400	307,725	463,778	61.1	843	1,270	7.1	33,709	125,377	882,344	1,007,721	129	5,969
200-299	5	1,201	43,408	237,208	304,619	54.1	650	834	5.5	36,576	112,196	177,531	289,727	94	5,890
300-399	1	295	16,523	84,311	110,752	78.3	231	303	5.1	8,535	42,922	164,914	207,836	36	3,752
400-499	1	419	20,978	100,124	125,464	65.4	274	344	4.8	19,455	25,449	14,093	39,542	48	3,322
500 or more	0	0	0	0	0	00.0	0	0	0.0	0	0	0	0	0	0
Nongovernment not-for-profit	23	2,368	86,160	473,891	640,361	54.8	1,298	1,754	5.5	72,352	214,325	259,168	473,493	203	10,496
Investor-owned (for-profit)	4	688	23,516	151,361	250,293	60.3	415	685	6.4	16,056	61,210	829,191	890,401	79	3,860
State and local government	10	1,136	43,643	254,600	331,467	61.4	697	908	5.8	24,244	118,815	354,664	473,479	125	8,427

*For information on community hospitals that excludes nursing-home-type data, refer to Hospital Units columns in tables 4A through 4D, pages 14 through 17.

CLASSIFICATION	FULL-TIME EQUIVALENT PERSONNEL: Physicians and Dentists	Registered Nurses	Licensed Practical Nurses	Other Salaried Personnel	Total Personnel	FULL-TIME EQUIVALENT TRAINEES: Medical and Dental Residents	Other Trainees	Total Trainees	EXPENSES — LABOR: Payroll (in thousands)	Employee Benefits (in thousands)	Total (in thousands)	Percent of Total	EXPENSES — TOTAL: Amount (in thousands)	Adjusted, per Admission	Adjusted, per Inpatient Day
NEW MEXICO	395	4,387	994	16,351	22,127	49	35	84	$ 539,373	$ 113,906	$ 653,279	53.7	$ 1,216,644		
6-24 beds	28	50	10	297	385	4	0	4	12,293	781	13,075	93.2	14,030		
25-49	142	417	105	1,806	2,470	1	0	1	58,866	12,084	70,950	65.9	107,647		
50-99	102	806	187	2,619	3,714	37	7	44	88,349	16,020	104,369	58.3	179,084		
100-199	5	965	285	3,587	4,842	0	1	1	113,194	28,711	141,905	40.7	348,471		
200-299	13	881	175	2,720	3,789	7	25	32	88,115	18,323	106,438	49.9	213,142		
300-399	24	542	85	3,038	3,689	0	0	0	76,366	17,786	94,152	63.6	148,007		
400-499	81	726	147	2,284	3,238	0	2	2	102,190	20,201	122,390	59.3	206,264		
500 or more	0	0	0	0	0	0	0	0	0	0	0	0.0	0		
Psychiatric	38	288	74	2,937	3,337	26	5	31	64,830	18,158	82,988	67.9	122,218		
Hospitals	33	259	52	2,126	2,470	26	5	31	50,944	13,724	64,668	65.5	98,781		
Institutions for mentally retarded	5	29	22	811	867	0	0	0	13,886	4,434	18,320	78.2	23,437		
General	353	4,050	898	13,139	18,440	19	30	49	465,228	93,826	559,054	52.0	1,075,052		
Hospitals	353	4,050	898	13,139	18,440	19	30	49	465,228	93,826	559,054	52.0	1,075,052		
Hospital units of institutions	0	0	0	0	0	0	0	0	0	0	0	0.0	0		
TB and other respiratory diseases	0	0	0	0	0	0	0	0	0	0	0	0.0	0		
Obstetrics and gynecology	0	0	0	0	0	0	0	0	0	0	0	0.0	0		
Eye, ear, nose, and throat	0	0	0	0	0	0	0	0	0	0	0	0.0	0		
Rehabilitation	1	38	15	193	247	0	0	0	6,759	1,378	8,137	59.1	13,756		
Orthopedic	3	11	7	82	103	4	0	4	2,557	544	3,100	55.2	5,618		
Chronic disease	0	0	0	0	0	0	0	0	0	0	0	0.0	0		
All other	0	0	0	0	0	0	0	0	0	0	0	0.0	0		
Federal	333	813	160	3,103	4,409	13	2	15	122,480	22,799	145,279	73.6	197,353		
Psychiatric	0	0	0	0	0	0	0	0	0	0	0	0.0	0		
General and other special	333	813	160	3,103	4,409	13	2	15	122,480	22,799	145,279	73.6	197,353		
Nonfederal	62	3,574	834	13,248	17,718	36	33	69	416,893	91,107	508,000	49.8	1,019,291		
Psychiatric	38	288	74	2,937	3,337	26	5	31	64,830	18,158	82,988	67.9	122,218		
Hospitals	33	259	52	2,126	2,470	26	5	31	50,944	13,724	64,668	65.5	98,781		
Institutions for mentally retarded	5	29	22	811	867	0	0	0	13,886	4,434	18,320	78.2	23,437		
TB and other respiratory diseases	0	0	0	0	0	0	0	0	0	0	0	0.0	0		
Long-term general and other special	0	0	0	0	0	0	0	0	0	0	0	0.0	0		
Short-term general and other special	24	3,286	760	10,311	14,381	10	28	38	352,063	72,949	425,012	47.4	897,073		
Hospital units of institutions	0	0	0	0	0	0	0	0	0	0	0	0.0	0		
Community hospitals*	24	3,286	760	10,311	14,381	10	28	38	352,063	72,949	425,012	47.4	897,073	$4,172.47	$ 734.03
6-24 beds	3	11	7	82	103	4	0	4	2,557	544	3,100	55.2	5,618	8,014.46	1,248.75
25-49	2	165	61	607	835	0	0	0	17,561	4,075	21,636	53.1	40,708	2,674.98	632.36
50-99	3	393	129	1,121	1,646	0	0	0	37,805	5,127	42,932	47.5	90,389	3,319.46	608.13
100-199	5	953	283	3,487	4,728	0	1	1	110,370	28,017	138,387	40.5	341,473	5,022.48	736.29
200-299	10	864	171	2,441	3,486	6	25	31	83,397	16,585	99,982	48.8	204,721	3,664.37	672.06
300-399	1	478	32	1,400	1,911	0	0	0	46,044	7,956	53,999	55.7	96,885	4,463.70	874.79
400-499	0	422	77	1,173	1,672	0	2	2	54,330	10,645	64,975	55.4	117,279	4,461.48	934.76
500 or more	0	0	0	0	0	0	0	0	0	0	0	0.0	0	0.00	0.00
Nongovernment not-for-profit	18	1,772	385	4,876	7,051	10	3	13	194,188	35,372	229,560	50.7	452,347	3,863.11	706.39
Investor-owned (for-profit)	0	517	218	2,441	3,176	0	0	0	64,231	20,255	84,487	35.5	237,886	5,829.82	950.43
State and local government	6	997	157	2,994	4,154	0	25	25	93,644	17,322	110,966	53.6	206,840	3,622.48	624.01

*For information on community hospitals that excludes nursing-home-type data, refer to Hospital Units columns in tables 4A through 4D, pages 14 through 17.

(continued on next page)

Table

5C (Continued) New York

Utilization, Personnel, and Finances in States

Excludes AHA nonregistered hospitals (see Table 14, page 240).

CLASSIFICATION	HOSPITALS	BEDS	ADMISSIONS	INPATIENT DAYS	ADJUSTED PATIENT DAYS	OCCUPANCY, percent	AVERAGE DAILY CENSUS	ADJUSTED AVERAGE DAILY CENSUS	AVERAGE STAY, days	SURGICAL OPERATIONS	OUTPATIENT VISITS Emergency	OUTPATIENT VISITS Other	OUTPATIENT VISITS Total	NEWBORNS Bassinets	NEWBORNS Births
NEW YORK	305	104,935	2,449,532	33,041,861		86.3	90,529			1,646,357	6,991,334	26,557,436	33,548,770	4,702	294,356
6-24 beds	4	63	2,420	8,751		38.1	24			8,681	29,660	185,241	214,901	10	379
25-49	16	597	13,679	149,099		68.7	410			8,256	74,188	213,177	287,365	31	1,135
50-99	39	2,820	79,465	767,328		74.5	2,102			56,141	291,197	1,175,606	1,466,803	213	8,180
100-199	62	9,517	239,432	2,761,307		79.5	7,563			194,743	760,912	2,696,335	3,457,247	483	17,380
200-299	60	14,172	413,431	4,294,563		83.0	11,769			320,212	1,240,245	3,123,585	4,363,830	832	40,554
300-399	32	10,721	310,773	3,330,813		85.1	9,127			209,129	895,651	2,825,626	3,721,277	746	40,461
400-499	22	10,128	281,995	3,244,450		87.8	8,890			172,577	821,248	3,204,923	4,026,171	602	41,069
500 or more	70	56,917	1,108,337	18,485,550		89.0	50,644			676,618	2,878,233	13,132,943	16,011,176	1,785	145,198
Psychiatric	47	21,093	51,082	6,826,533		88.7	18,703			699	99,247	1,929,508	2,028,755	0	0
Hospitals	46	20,382	51,040	6,579,948		88.4	18,027			696	98,832	1,928,320	2,027,152	0	0
Institutions for mentally retarded	1	711	42	246,585		95.1	676			3	415	1,188	1,603	0	0
General	236	77,397	2,304,899	24,119,937		85.4	66,085			1,550,159	6,798,444	23,761,204	30,559,648	4,607	287,961
Hospitals	235	77,372	2,304,622	24,114,468		85.4	66,070			1,550,058	6,797,411	23,743,913	30,541,324	4,607	287,961
Hospital units of institutions	1	25	277	5,469		60.0	15			101	1,033	17,291	18,324	0	0
TB and other respiratory diseases	0	0	0	0		00.0	0			0	0	0	0	0	0
Obstetrics and gynecology	1	52	3,871	12,568		65.4	34			3,139	11,052	13,803	24,855	28	2,232
Eye, ear, nose, and throat	3	238	15,789	39,441		45.4	108			36,271	26,740	202,353	229,093	0	0
Rehabilitation	5	557	4,349	172,932		84.9	473			396	1	43,517	43,518	0	0
Orthopedic	2	392	12,314	119,408		83.4	327			15,515	0	180,810	180,810	0	0
Chronic disease	3	2,356	3,970	820,807		95.5	2,249			0	0	0	0	0	0
All other	8	2,850	53,258	930,235		89.5	2,550			40,178	55,850	426,241	482,091	67	4,163
Federal	15	7,226	70,974	2,068,657		78.4	5,667			95,157	196,733	1,974,294	2,171,027	19	562
Psychiatric	1	897	3,262	261,527		79.9	717			0	0	76,067	76,067	0	0
General and other special	14	6,329	67,712	1,807,130		78.2	4,950			95,157	196,733	1,898,227	2,094,960	19	562
Nonfederal	290	97,709	2,378,558	30,973,204		86.9	84,862			1,551,200	6,794,601	24,583,142	31,377,743	4,683	293,794
Psychiatric	46	20,196	47,820	6,565,006		89.1	17,986			699	99,247	1,853,441	1,952,688	0	0
Hospitals	45	19,485	47,778	6,318,421		88.8	17,310			696	98,832	1,852,253	1,951,085	0	0
Institutions for mentally retarded	1	711	42	246,585		95.1	676			3	415	1,188	1,603	0	0
TB and other respiratory diseases	0	0	0	0		00.0	0			0	0	0	0	0	0
Long-term general and other special	8	3,012	8,952	1,030,430		93.7	2,823			403	0	62,287	62,287	0	0
Short-term general and other special	236	74,501	2,321,786	23,377,768		86.0	64,053			1,550,098	6,695,354	22,667,414	29,362,768	4,683	293,794
Hospital units of institutions	1	25	277	5,469		60.0	15			101	1,033	17,291	18,324	0	0
Community hospitals*	235	74,476	2,321,509	23,372,299	30,239,515	86.0	64,038	82,852	10.1	1,549,997	6,694,321	22,650,123	29,344,444	4,683	293,794
6-24 beds	2	40	707	3,289	9,773	22.5	9	27	4.7	7,470	1,899	16,737	18,636	0	0
25-49	11	418	12,816	99,601	153,593	65.6	274	420	7.8	8,155	72,908	194,657	267,565	31	1,135
50-99	26	1,854	65,489	504,377	750,068	74.5	1,382	2,054	7.7	53,248	271,653	804,734	1,076,387	204	7,997
100-199	51	7,782	226,480	2,244,855	3,157,470	79.0	6,149	8,652	9.9	194,077	742,414	2,411,745	3,154,159	483	17,380
200-299	54	12,858	397,872	3,871,878	5,182,911	82.5	10,610	14,203	9.7	318,497	1,209,117	2,878,741	4,087,858	832	40,554
300-399	28	9,276	301,629	2,860,638	3,659,023	84.5	7,840	10,026	9.5	206,372	847,297	2,497,114	3,344,411	746	40,461
400-499	18	8,173	272,419	2,621,492	3,411,128	87.9	7,183	9,346	9.6	168,987	794,693	2,985,273	3,779,966	602	41,069
500 or more	45	34,075	1,044,097	11,166,169	13,915,549	89.8	30,591	38,124	10.7	593,191	2,754,340	10,861,122	13,615,462	1,785	145,198
Nongovernment not-for-profit	194	59,669	1,903,142	18,648,883	24,323,727	85.6	51,096	66,644	9.8	1,339,581	5,068,143	17,100,914	22,169,057	3,898	239,569
Investor-owned (for-profit)	13	2,592	87,537	775,463	949,214	81.9	2,123	2,601	8.9	74,472	206,939	155,361	362,300	111	5,937
State and local government	28	12,215	330,830	3,947,953	4,966,574	88.6	10,819	13,607	11.9	135,944	1,419,239	5,393,848	6,813,087	674	48,288

*For information on community hospitals that excludes nursing-home-type data, refer to Hospital Units columns in tables 4A through 4D, pages 14 through 17.

CLASSIFICATION	FULL-TIME EQUIVALENT PERSONNEL					FULL-TIME EQUIVALENT TRAINEES			EXPENSES: LABOR				EXPENSES: TOTAL		
	Physicians and Dentists	Registered Nurses	Licensed Practical Nurses	Other Salaried Personnel	Total Personnel	Medical and Dental Residents	Other Trainees	Total Trainees	Payroll (in thousands)	Employee Benefits (in thousands)	Total (in thousands)	Percent of Total	Amount (in thousands)	Adjusted, per Admission	Adjusted, per Inpatient Day
NEW YORK	11,825	75,637	13,150	269,670	370,282	14,330	399	14,729	$11,452,512	$ 2,261,389	$13,713,902	61.8	$ 22,175,079		
6-24 beds	40	91	32	572	735	0	0	0	8,547	1,768	10,316	61.3	16,817		
25-49	17	325	151	1,343	1,836	0	0	0	40,763	7,768	48,531	54.6	88,827		
50-99	249	1,757	546	7,515	10,067	38	17	55	232,441	44,954	277,395	60.9	455,633		
100-199	483	6,374	1,630	23,274	31,761	211	5	216	811,161	156,968	968,129	58.3	1,661,126		
200-299	908	11,431	2,265	34,547	49,151	484	8	492	1,377,732	249,511	1,627,243	59.4	2,738,783		
300-399	943	8,947	1,480	27,057	38,427	803	3	806	1,129,266	232,149	1,361,415	61.3	2,221,923		
400-499	1,074	8,359	1,303	29,391	40,127	1,580	15	1,595	1,247,739	257,166	1,504,905	63.8	2,358,952		
500 or more	8,111	38,353	5,743	145,971	198,178	11,214	351	11,565	6,604,863	1,311,105	7,915,968	62.7	12,633,017		
Psychiatric	1,317	4,084	1,353	31,160	37,914	135	54	189	1,082,914	204,407	1,287,320	81.6	1,577,832		
Hospitals	1,311	4,047	1,324	29,919	36,601	135	54	189	1,054,689	197,615	1,252,304	81.6	1,534,430		
Institutions for mentally retarded	6	37	29	1,241	1,313	0	0	0	28,224	6,792	35,016	80.7	43,401		
General	9,711	68,032	11,368	222,483	311,594	13,756	342	14,098	9,692,402	1,910,955	11,603,358	60.2	19,262,680		
Hospitals	9,708	68,023	11,359	222,455	311,545	13,756	342	14,098	9,691,475	1,910,689	11,602,164	60.2	19,259,416		
Hospital units of institutions	3	9	9	28	49	0	0	0	928	266	1,194	36.6	3,264		
TB and other respiratory diseases	0	0	0	0	0	0	0	0	0	0	0	0.0	0		
Obstetrics and gynecology	1	75	6	178	260	0	0	0	7,329	1,140	8,468	62.1	13,637		
Eye, ear, nose, and throat	6	201	22	1,277	1,506	64	0	64	38,941	12,311	51,252	56.5	90,736		
Rehabilitation	42	271	74	1,454	1,841	3	0	3	56,192	12,640	68,832	63.8	107,833		
Orthopedic	145	346	69	1,580	2,140	68	0	68	76,295	16,029	92,323	57.3	161,070		
Chronic disease	106	283	102	4,031	4,522	15	0	15	142,988	36,911	179,899	79.6	226,063		
All other	497	2,345	156	7,507	10,505	289	3	292	355,451	66,997	422,448	57.5	735,229		
Federal	1,010	2,709	809	13,213	17,741	661	77	738	579,922	91,058	670,980	72.3	927,938		
Psychiatric	52	182	67	1,366	1,667	7	7	14	41,224	7,531	48,755	70.4	69,285		
General and other special	958	2,527	742	11,847	16,074	654	70	724	538,697	83,528	622,225	72.5	858,654		
Nonfederal	10,815	72,928	12,341	256,457	352,541	13,669	322	13,991	10,872,590	2,170,331	13,042,921	61.4	21,247,140		
Psychiatric	1,265	3,902	1,286	29,794	36,247	128	47	175	1,041,689	196,876	1,238,565	82.1	1,508,547		
Hospitals	1,259	3,865	1,257	28,553	34,934	128	47	175	1,013,465	190,084	1,203,549	82.1	1,465,146		
Institutions for mentally retarded	6	37	29	1,241	1,313	0	0	0	28,224	6,792	35,016	80.7	43,401		
TB and other respiratory diseases	0	0	0	0	0	0	0	0	0	0	0	0.0	0		
Long-term general and other special	159	597	155	5,765	6,676	18	0	18	213,750	53,521	267,271	74.2	360,190		
Short-term general and other special	9,391	68,429	10,900	220,898	309,618	13,523	275	13,798	9,617,151	1,919,934	11,537,085	59.5	19,378,404		
Hospital units of institutions	3	9	9	28	49	0	0	0	928	266	1,194	36.6	3,264		
Community hospitals*	9,388	68,420	10,891	220,870	309,569	13,523	275	13,798	9,616,223	1,919,668	11,535,891	59.5	19,375,140	$6,396.57	$ 640.72
6-24 beds	2	37	21	183	243	0	0	0	4,626	895	5,521	55.3	9,976	2,890.69	1,020.75
25-49	6	283	138	1,077	1,504	0	0	0	32,084	5,575	37,659	55.6	67,675	3,444.91	440.61
50-99	30	1,357	465	5,091	6,943	31	3	34	153,160	29,737	182,897	57.3	319,368	3,104.79	425.79
100-199	349	5,729	1,503	19,479	27,060	192	4	196	683,791	130,152	813,943	57.3	1,421,136	4,403.44	450.09
200-299	789	10,901	2,095	31,798	45,583	409	4	413	1,269,779	226,791	1,496,570	58.8	2,544,278	4,777.66	490.90
300-399	809	8,446	1,383	24,399	35,037	793	2	795	1,024,183	213,983	1,238,166	59.9	2,068,597	5,371.75	565.34
400-499	918	7,789	1,087	26,308	36,102	1,504	2	1,506	1,105,225	231,211	1,336,436	62.2	2,147,072	6,031.08	629.43
500 or more	6,485	33,878	4,199	112,535	157,097	10,594	260	10,854	5,343,374	1,081,324	6,424,699	59.5	10,797,039	8,263.01	775.90
Nongovernment not-for-profit	6,234	55,412	8,113	171,022	240,781	9,426	223	9,649	7,338,666	1,455,800	8,794,467	58.4	15,062,670	6,026.00	619.26
Investor-owned (for-profit)	77	2,075	438	5,079	7,669	0	0	0	217,598	45,541	263,139	52.2	503,935	4,647.30	530.90
State and local government	3,077	10,933	2,340	44,769	31,119	4,097	52	4,149	2,059,958	418,327	2,478,285	65.1	3,808,536	9,047.71	766.83

*For information on community hospitals that excludes nursing-home-type data, refer to Hospital Units columns in tables 4A through 4D, pages 14 through 17.

(continued on next page)

Table
5C (Continued) North Carolina

Utilization, Personnel, and Finances in States

Excludes AHA nonregistered hospitals (see Table 14, page 240).

CLASSIFICATION	HOSPITALS	BEDS	ADMISSIONS	INPATIENT DAYS	ADJUSTED PATIENT DAYS	OCCUPANCY, percent	AVERAGE DAILY CENSUS	ADJUSTED AVERAGE DAILY CENSUS	AVERAGE STAY, days	SURGICAL OPERATIONS	OUTPATIENT VISITS Emergency	OUTPATIENT VISITS Other	OUTPATIENT VISITS Total	NEWBORNS Bassinets	NEWBORNS Births
NORTH CAROLINA	155	30,122	867,970	8,229,917		74.9	22,550			599,526	2,574,069	5,456,592	8,030,661	1,880	104,091
6-24 beds	2	44	269	6,043		38.6	17			2,210	710	46,758	47,468	0	0
25-49	18	753	21,845	153,484		55.9	421			6,696	124,742	354,149	478,891	72	1,556
50-99	47	3,482	90,851	817,111		64.2	2,237			57,838	386,729	480,177	866,906	224	6,914
100-199	45	5,951	184,778	1,478,025		68.1	4,053			143,328	715,100	1,040,529	1,755,629	570	22,527
200-299	14	3,527	131,251	898,039		69.8	2,462			74,906	434,843	1,305,640	1,740,483	402	17,292
300-399	11	3,858	143,518	1,067,027		75.8	2,924			106,056	346,852	576,573	923,425	219	16,725
400-499	3	1,364	39,341	377,263		75.7	1,033			31,747	103,425	212,210	315,635	74	7,161
500 or more	15	11,143	256,117	3,432,925		84.4	9,403			176,745	461,668	1,440,556	1,902,224	319	31,916
Psychiatric	21	6,060	30,060	1,850,637		83.7	5,070			2,361	7,307	115,675	122,982	0	0
Hospitals	20	5,154	29,941	1,546,819		82.2	4,238			2,361	7,117	113,912	121,029	0	0
Institutions for mentally retarded	1	906	119	303,818		91.8	832			0	190	1,763	1,953	0	0
General	129	23,700	833,684	6,297,905		72.8	17,257			588,983	2,564,781	5,242,435	7,807,216	1,880	104,091
Hospitals	127	23,528	830,846	6,263,017		72.9	17,161			588,154	2,553,401	5,183,007	7,736,408	1,880	104,091
Hospital units of institutions	2	172	2,838	34,888		55.8	96			829	11,380	59,428	70,808	0	0
TB and other respiratory diseases	0	0	0	0		00.0	0			0	0	0	0	0	0
Obstetrics and gynecology	0	0	0	0		00.0	0			0	0	0	0	0	0
Eye, ear, nose, and throat	1	24	164	268		04.2	1			2,199	324	44,673	44,997	0	0
Rehabilitation	3	222	1,412	66,438		82.0	182			128	0	25,792	25,792	0	0
Orthopedic	1	116	2,650	14,669		34.5	40			5,855	1,657	28,017	29,674	0	0
Chronic disease	0	0	0	0		00.0	0			0	0	0	0	0	0
All other	0	0	0	0		00.0	0			0	0	0	0	0	0
Federal	9	2,557	55,192	696,475		74.6	1,908			31,321	147,723	1,624,450	1,772,173	99	4,137
Psychiatric	1	843	6,051	280,639		91.2	769			1,514	0	83,239	83,239	0	0
General and other special	8	1,714	49,141	415,836		66.5	1,139			29,807	147,723	1,541,211	1,688,934	99	4,137
Nonfederal	146	27,565	812,778	7,533,442		74.9	20,642			568,205	2,426,346	3,832,142	6,258,488	1,781	99,954
Psychiatric	20	5,217	24,009	1,569,998		82.4	4,301			847	7,307	32,436	39,743	0	0
Hospitals	19	4,311	23,890	1,266,180		80.5	3,469			847	7,117	30,673	37,790	0	0
Institutions for mentally retarded	1	906	119	303,818		91.8	832			0	190	1,763	1,953	0	0
TB and other respiratory diseases	0	0	0	0		00.0	0			0	0	0	0	0	0
Long-term general and other special	4	242	1,517	72,213		81.8	198			139	386	27,877	28,263	0	0
Short-term general and other special	122	22,106	787,252	5,891,231		73.0	16,143			567,219	2,418,653	3,771,829	6,190,482	1,781	99,954
Hospital units of institutions	2	172	2,838	34,888		55.8	96			829	11,380	59,428	70,808	0	0
Community hospitals*	120	21,934	784,414	5,856,343	7,647,972	73.2	16,047	20,958	7.5	566,390	2,407,273	3,712,401	6,119,674	1,781	99,954
6-24 beds	1	24	164	268	7,348	04.2	1	20	1.6	2,199	324	44,673	44,997	0	0
25-49	12	528	15,400	105,697	155,136	54.9	290	425	6.9	5,803	72,404	70,081	142,485	36	535
50-99	35	2,557	79,638	580,383	858,668	62.1	1,588	2,353	7.3	57,009	373,820	386,067	759,887	224	6,914
100-199	39	5,222	172,509	1,295,193	1,807,778	68.0	3,552	4,955	7.5	139,271	678,995	808,629	1,487,624	538	21,632
200-299	13	3,255	115,392	832,369	1,102,002	70.1	2,282	3,019	7.2	74,906	375,911	532,716	908,627	371	15,071
300-399	9	3,110	129,966	882,360	1,125,282	77.7	2,418	3,084	6.8	89,733	346,852	384,801	731,653	219	16,725
400-499	2	908	32,908	256,671	319,940	77.4	703	877	7.8	23,085	97,489	133,368	230,857	74	7,161
500 or more	9	6,330	238,437	1,903,402	2,271,818	82.4	5,213	6,225	8.0	174,384	461,478	1,352,066	1,813,544	319	31,916
Nongovernment not-for-profit	72	13,527	487,946	3,682,813	4,799,046	74.6	10,091	13,150	7.5	353,452	1,440,891	2,072,612	3,513,503	1,095	59,592
Investor-owned (for-profit)	13	1,445	45,007	296,008	406,501	56.1	810	1,114	6.6	47,093	149,807	236,553	386,360	80	3,860
State and local government	35	6,962	251,461	1,877,522	2,442,425	73.9	5,146	6,694	7.5	165,845	816,575	1,403,236	2,219,811	606	36,502

*For information on community hospitals that excludes nursing home type data, refer to Hospital Units columns in tables 4A through 4D, pages 14 through 17.

CLASSIFICATION	FULL-TIME EQUIVALENT PERSONNEL: Physicians and Dentists	Registered Nurses	Licensed Practical Nurses	Other Salaried Personnel	Total Personnel	FULL-TIME EQUIVALENT TRAINEES: Medical and Dental Residents	Other Trainees	Total Trainees	EXPENSES — LABOR: Payroll (in thousands)	Employee Benefits (in thousands)	Total (in thousands)	Percent of Total	TOTAL: Amount (in thousands)	Adjusted, per Admission	Adjusted, per Inpatient Day
NORTH CAROLINA	1,257	24,901	5,486	74,823	106,467	1,679	135	1,814	$ 2,562,800	$ 472,624	$ 3,035,424	56.6	$ 5,363,024		
6-24 beds	3	23	14	137	177	0	0	0	6,097	1,030	7,127	62.3	11,435		
25-49	68	441	161	2,009	2,679	0	1	1	52,544	9,963	62,507	61.9	101,031		
50-99	92	2,030	624	6,813	9,559	11	1	12	208,630	36,423	245,053	52.9	463,242		
100-199	95	4,453	1,317	13,338	19,203	0	9	9	400,503	72,490	472,992	53.5	884,915		
200-299	153	3,205	759	9,026	13,143	45	12	57	313,874	50,943	364,817	55.6	656,017		
300-399	104	3,880	641	10,347	14,972	117	11	128	402,833	64,585	467,418	56.8	823,199		
400-499	56	1,187	291	3,290	4,824	54	0	54	125,724	23,683	149,406	61.4	243,345		
500 or more	686	9,682	1,679	29,863	41,910	1,452	101	1,553	1,052,596	213,507	1,266,103	58.1	2,179,840		
Psychiatric	192	1,168	475	8,866	10,701	1	3	4	244,264	59,800	304,064	72.0	422,293		
Hospitals	186	1,121	407	7,135	8,849	1	3	4	208,681	50,390	259,071	69.7	371,748		
Institutions for mentally retarded	6	47	68	1,731	1,852	0	0	0	35,583	9,410	44,993	89.0	50,545		
General	1,055	23,512	4,964	65,172	94,703	1,678	131	1,809	2,289,774	407,941	2,697,715	55.3	4,879,073		
Hospitals	1,027	23,454	4,922	65,002	94,405	1,678	131	1,809	2,283,392	406,109	2,689,501	55.4	4,856,620		
Hospital units of institutions	28	58	42	170	298	0	0	0	6,383	1,832	8,214	36.6	22,453		
TB and other respiratory diseases	0	0	0	0	0	0	0	0	0	0	0	0.0	0		
Obstetrics and gynecology	0	0	0	0	0	0	0	0	0	0	0	0.0	0		
Eye, ear, nose, and throat	3	17	11	86	117	0	0	0	4,400	662	5,062	61.8	8,185		
Rehabilitation	7	86	35	504	632	0	1	1	15,762	2,201	17,963	63.4	28,316		
Orthopedic	0	118	1	195	314	0	0	0	8,600	2,020	10,620	42.2	25,158		
Chronic disease	0	0	0	0	0	0	0	0	0	0	0	0.0	0		
All other	0	0	0	0	0	0	0	0	0	0	0	0.0	0		
Federal	493	1,212	391	6,098	8,194	184	23	207	228,768	35,563	264,331	65.8	401,893		
Psychiatric	47	192	86	1,054	1,379	0	2	2	37,571	7,463	45,034	65.6	68,691		
General and other special	446	1,020	305	5,044	6,815	184	21	205	191,197	28,100	219,297	65.8	333,202		
Nonfederal	764	23,689	5,095	68,725	98,273	1,495	112	1,607	2,334,032	437,061	2,771,092	55.9	4,961,131		
Psychiatric	145	976	389	7,812	9,322	1	1	2	206,693	52,337	259,030	73.3	353,601		
Hospitals	139	929	321	6,081	7,470	1	1	2	171,110	42,927	214,037	70.6	303,056		
Institutions for mentally retarded	6	47	68	1,731	1,852	0	0	0	35,583	9,410	44,993	89.0	50,545		
TB and other respiratory diseases	0	0	0	0	0	0	0	0	0	0	0	0.0	0		
Long-term general and other special	7	92	38	555	692	0	1	1	17,459	2,570	20,028	63.4	31,566		
Short-term general and other special	612	22,621	4,668	60,358	88,259	1,494	110	1,604	2,109,880	382,155	2,492,035	54.5	4,575,964		
Hospital units of institutions	28	58	42	170	298	0	0	0	6,383	1,832	8,214	36.6	22,453		
Community hospitals*	584	22,563	4,626	60,188	87,961	1,494	110	1,604	2,103,497	380,323	2,483,820	54.5	4,553,511	$4,408.28	$ 595.39
6-24 beds	3	17	11	86	117	0	0	0	4,400	662	5,062	61.8	8,185	1,820.14	1,113.93
25-49	1	298	125	1,140	1,564	0	0	0	29,306	5,274	34,580	56.4	61,283	2,697.67	395.03
50-99	45	1,796	532	5,538	7,911	11	1	12	167,079	27,661	194,740	52.8	369,009	3,123.17	429.75
100-199	19	4,109	1,240	11,271	16,639	0	8	8	350,354	64,114	414,468	53.2	779,447	3,204.44	431.16
200-299	1	2,986	652	7,994	11,633	0	2	2	261,911	47,872	309,783	54.5	568,580	3,710.00	515.95
300-399	0	3,512	550	8,883	12,945	0	0	0	333,939	52,562	386,502	55.0	702,507	4,243.04	624.29
400-499	2	1,004	245	2,573	3,824	32	0	32	95,410	17,907	113,317	59.2	191,287	4,659.85	597.88
500 or more	513	8,841	1,271	22,703	33,328	1,451	99	1,550	861,098	164,271	1,025,369	54.7	1,873,213	6,585.02	824.54
Nongovernment not-for-profit	63	14,012	2,817	36,473	53,365	856	71	927	1,293,500	222,528	1,516,028	54.8	2,768,994	4,339.74	576.99
Investor-owned (for-profit)	11	1,323	258	2,861	4,453	0	0	0	96,549	22,783	119,332	44.4	268,634	4,118.32	660.84
State and local government	510	7,228	1,551	20,854	30,143	638	39	677	713,448	135,012	848,460	56.0	1,515,883	4,598.32	620.65

*For information on community hospitals that excludes nursing-home-type data, refer to Hospital Units columns in tables 4A through 4D, pages 14 through 17.

(continued on next page)

Table

5C (Continued) North Dakota

Utilization, Personnel, and Finances in States

Excludes AHA nonregistered hospitals (see Table 14, page 240).

CLASSIFICATION	HOSPITALS	BEDS	ADMISSIONS	INPATIENT DAYS	ADJUSTED PATIENT DAYS	OCCUPANCY, percent	AVERAGE DAILY CENSUS	ADJUSTED AVERAGE DAILY CENSUS	AVERAGE STAY, days	SURGICAL OPERATIONS	OUTPATIENT VISITS: Emergency	OUTPATIENT VISITS: Other	OUTPATIENT VISITS: Total	NEWBORNS: Bassinets	NEWBORNS: Births
NORTH DAKOTA	57	5,298	109,302	1,239,706		64.1	3,398			72,426	207,896	704,781	912,677	379	10,665
6-24 beds	7	145	2,935	19,566		37.2	54			433	5,981	53,612	59,593	29	154
25-49	23	772	16,652	124,512		44.3	342			8,733	53,232	364,832	418,064	98	1,404
50-99	14	953	20,100	231,546		66.6	635			14,565	39,618	104,516	144,134	136	2,390
100-199	6	928	17,792	238,439		70.4	653			11,012	33,633	64,893	98,526	39	1,171
200-299	4	1,020	29,523	255,146		68.5	699			26,530	44,278	88,963	133,241	49	3,245
300-399	1	384	14,629	101,444		72.4	278			7,099	25,584	11,931	37,515	16	1,610
400-499	1	545	2,304	126,628		63.7	347			0	0	0	0	0	0
500 or more	1	551	5,367	142,425		70.8	390			4,054	5,570	16,034	21,604	12	691
Psychiatric	2	583	3,019	134,065		63.0	367			0	0	3,971	3,971	0	0
Hospitals	2	583	3,019	134,065		63.0	367			0	0	3,971	3,971	0	0
Institutions for mentally retarded	0	0	0	0		00.0	0			0	0	0	0	0	0
General	54	4,663	105,464	1,093,196		64.3	2,997			72,426	207,896	659,165	867,061	379	10,665
Hospitals	54	4,663	105,464	1,093,196		64.3	2,997			72,426	207,896	659,165	867,061	379	10,665
Hospital units of institutions	0	0	0	0		00.0	0			0	0	0	0	0	0
TB and other respiratory diseases	0	0	0	0		00.0	0			0	0	0	0	0	0
Obstetrics and gynecology	0	0	0	0		00.0	0			0	0	0	0	0	0
Eye, ear, nose, and throat	0	0	0	0		00.0	0			0	0	0	0	0	0
Rehabilitation	1	52	819	12,445		65.4	34			0	0	41,645	41,645	0	0
Orthopedic	0	0	0	0		00.0	0			0	0	0	0	0	0
Chronic disease	0	0	0	0		00.0	0			0	0	0	0	0	0
All other	0	0	0	0		00.0	0			0	0	0	0	0	0
Federal	5	303	10,300	72,021		64.7	196			7,096	42,771	325,722	368,493	39	862
Psychiatric	0	0	0	0		00.0	0			0	0	0	0	0	0
General and other special	5	303	10,300	72,021		64.7	196			7,096	42,771	325,722	368,493	39	862
Nonfederal	52	4,995	99,002	1,167,685		64.1	3,202			65,330	165,125	379,059	544,184	340	9,803
Psychiatric	2	583	3,019	134,065		63.0	367			0	0	3,971	3,971	0	0
Hospitals	2	583	3,019	134,065		63.0	367			0	0	3,971	3,971	0	0
Institutions for mentally retarded	0	0	0	0		00.0	0			0	0	0	0	0	0
TB and other respiratory diseases	0	0	0	0		00.0	0			0	0	0	0	0	0
Long-term general and other special	0	0	0	0		00.0	0			0	0	0	0	0	0
Short-term general and other special	50	4,412	95,983	1,033,620		64.3	2,835			65,330	165,125	375,088	540,213	340	9,803
Hospital units of institutions	0	0	0	0		00.0	0			0	0	0	0	0	0
Community hospitals*	50	4,412	95,983	1,033,620	1,323,463	64.3	2,835	3,626	10.8	65,330	165,125	375,088	540,213	340	9,803
6-24 beds	6	129	2,377	17,937	27,792	38.8	50	74	7.5	433	4,996	25,132	30,128	22	128
25-49	19	629	10,579	101,098	150,120	44.4	279	413	9.6	3,122	17,633	105,782	123,415	66	568
50-99	14	953	20,100	231,546	320,217	66.6	635	877	11.5	14,565	39,618	104,516	144,134	136	2,390
100-199	5	746	13,408	184,024	220,346	67.6	504	604	13.7	9,527	27,446	22,730	50,176	39	1,171
200-299	4	1,020	29,523	255,146	314,533	68.5	699	862	8.6	26,530	44,278	88,963	133,241	49	3,245
300-399	1	384	14,629	101,444	114,841	72.4	278	315	6.9	7,099	25,584	11,931	37,515	16	1,610
400-499	0	0	0	0	0	00.0	0	0	0.0	0	0	0	0	0	0
500 or more	1	551	5,367	142,425	175,614	70.8	390	481	26.5	4,054	5,570	16,034	21,604	12	691
Nongovernment not-for-profit	49	4,360	95,164	1,021,175	1,302,268	64.2	2,801	3,568	10.7	65,330	165,125	333,443	498,568	340	9,803
Investor-owned (for-profit)	0	0	0	0	0	00.0	0	0	0.0	0	0	0	0	0	0
State and local government	1	52	819	12,445	21,195	65.4	34	58	15.2	0	0	41,645	41,645	0	0

CLASSIFICATION	FULL-TIME EQUIVALENT PERSONNEL					FULL-TIME EQUIVALENT TRAINEES			EXPENSES						
									LABOR				TOTAL		
	Physicians and Dentists	Registered Nurses	Licensed Practical Nurses	Other Salaried Personnel	Total Personnel	Medical and Dental Residents	Other Trainees	Total Trainees	Payroll (in thousands)	Employee Benefits (in thousands)	Total (in thousands)	Percent of Total	Amount (in thousands)	Adjusted, per Admission	Adjusted, per Inpatient Day
NORTH DAKOTA	144	2,920	745	9,052	12,861	21	44	65	$ 300,788	$ 55,184	$ 355,972	54.9	$ 648,238		
6-24 beds	8	47	14	210	279	0	0	0	6,860	1,346	8,205	58.6	13,997		
25-49	83	301	100	1,545	2,029	2	0	2	42,115	7,593	49,708	65.9	75,484		
50-99	3	401	178	1,479	2,061	0	0	0	44,576	7,416	51,993	55.3	94,103		
100-199	23	535	129	1,584	2,271	19	23	42	53,174	9,670	62,844	56.1	112,043		
200-299	12	898	160	2,124	3,194	0	18	18	78,218	13,429	91,647	48.3	189,785		
300-399	0	566	73	926	1,565	0	0	0	42,996	7,810	50,806	51.4	98,921		
400-499	15	51	45	512	623	0	0	0	14,793	4,538	19,331	78.4	24,669		
500 or more	0	121	46	672	839	0	3	3	18,056	3,382	21,438	54.6	39,237		
Psychiatric	15	57	48	533	653	0	0	0	15,644	4,692	20,336	76.7	26,529		
Hospitals	15	57	48	533	653	0	0	0	15,644	4,692	20,336	76.7	26,529		
Institutions for mentally retarded	0	0	0	0	0	0	0	0	0	0	0	0.0	0		
General	125	2,846	679	8,320	11,970	21	44	65	279,217	48,854	328,072	53.7	610,660		
Hospitals	125	2,846	679	8,320	11,970	21	44	65	279,217	48,854	328,072	53.7	610,660		
Hospital units of institutions	0	0	0	0	0	0	0	0	0	0	0	0.0	0		
TB and other respiratory diseases	0	0	0	0	0	0	0	0	0	0	0	0.0	0		
Obstetrics and gynecology	0	0	0	0	0	0	0	0	0	0	0	0.0	0		
Eye, ear, nose, and throat	0	0	0	0	0	0	0	0	0	0	0	0.0	0		
Rehabilitation	4	17	18	199	238	0	0	0	5,926	1,638	7,564	68.5	11,050		
Orthopedic	0	0	0	0	0	0	0	0	0	0	0	0.0	0		
Chronic disease	0	0	0	0	0	0	0	0	0	0	0	0.0	0		
All other	0	0	0	0	0	0	0	0	0	0	0	0.0	0		
Federal	103	183	42	1,005	1,333	21	23	44	36,851	6,984	43,835	76.7	57,144		
Psychiatric	0	0	0	0	0	0	0	0	0	0	0	0.0	0		
General and other special	103	183	42	1,005	1,333	21	23	44	36,851	6,984	43,835	76.7	57,144		
Nonfederal	41	2,737	703	8,047	11,528	0	21	21	263,936	48,200	312,137	52.8	591,094		
Psychiatric	15	57	48	533	653	0	0	0	15,644	4,692	20,336	76.7	26,529		
Hospitals	15	57	48	533	653	0	0	0	15,644	4,692	20,336	76.7	26,529		
Institutions for mentally retarded	0	0	0	0	0	0	0	0	0	0	0	0.0	0		
TB and other respiratory diseases	0	0	0	0	0	0	0	0	0	0	0	0.0	0		
Long-term general and other special	0	0	0	0	0	0	0	0	0	0	0	0.0	0		
Short-term general and other special	26	2,680	655	7,514	10,875	0	21	21	248,293	43,509	291,801	51.7	564,565		
Hospital units of institutions	0	0	0	0	0	0	0	0	0	0	0	0.0	0		
Community hospitals*	26	2,680	655	7,514	10,875	0	21	21	248,293	43,509	291,801	51.7	564,565	$4,468.16	$ 426.58
6-24 beds	1	42	13	159	215	0	0	0	4,132	738	4,870	52.7	9,238	2,524.67	332.39
25-49	10	211	91	940	1,252	0	0	0	23,108	4,069	27,177	58.0	46,897	2,946.89	312.40
50-99	3	401	178	1,479	2,061	0	0	0	44,576	7,416	51,993	55.3	94,103	3,192.86	293.87
100-199	0	441	94	1,214	1,749	0	0	0	37,208	6,664	43,872	50.8	86,385	5,189.20	392.04
200-299	12	898	160	2,124	3,194	0	18	18	78,218	13,429	91,647	48.3	189,785	5,063.51	603.39
300-399	0	566	73	926	1,565	0	0	0	42,996	7,810	50,806	51.4	98,921	5,973.10	861.37
400-499	0	0	0	0	0	0	0	0	0	0	0	0.0	0	0.00	0.00
500 or more	0	121	46	672	839	0	3	3	18,056	3,382	21,438	54.6	39,237	5,928.79	223.43
Nongovernment not-for-profit	22	2,663	637	7,315	10,637	0	21	21	242,366	41,871	284,237	51.4	553,515	4,429.61	425.04
Investor-owned (for-profit)	0	0	0	0	0	0	0	0	0	0	0	0.0	0	0.00	0.00
State and local government	4	17	18	199	238	0	0	0	5,926	1,638	7,564	68.5	11,050	7,920.90	521.33

*For information on community hospitals that excludes nursing-home-type data, refer to Hospital Units columns in tables 4A through 4D, pages 14 through 17.

(continued on next page)

Table
5C (Continued) Ohio

Utilization, Personnel, and Finances in States

Excludes AHA nonregistered hospitals (see Table 14, page 240).

CLASSIFICATION	HOSPITALS	BEDS	ADMISSIONS	INPATIENT DAYS	ADJUSTED PATIENT DAYS	OCCUPANCY, percent	AVERAGE DAILY CENSUS	ADJUSTED AVERAGE DAILY CENSUS	AVERAGE STAY, days	SURGICAL OPERATIONS	OUTPATIENT VISITS: Emergency	OUTPATIENT VISITS: Other	OUTPATIENT VISITS: Total	NEWBORNS: Bassinets	NEWBORNS: Births
OHIO	224	52,205	1,580,337	12,813,756		67.2	35,104			1,118,600	4,690,029	13,744,458	18,434,487	3,119	165,836
6-24 beds	1	23	300	1,508		17.4	4			226	1,615	3,889	5,504	0	0
25-49	16	616	16,758	93,960		41.9	258			11,016	100,305	321,264	421,569	65	1,643
50-99	51	3,666	109,200	670,704		50.1	1,837			74,808	429,164	1,024,719	1,453,883	377	12,897
100-199	62	9,124	268,876	2,028,681		60.9	5,556			191,064	895,396	2,005,893	2,901,289	698	26,624
200-299	38	9,636	323,921	2,293,667		65.2	6,283			251,786	1,093,936	3,304,123	4,398,059	552	23,248
300-399	24	8,448	220,020	2,149,365		69.7	5,888			155,801	757,221	1,709,485	2,466,706	363	18,006
400-499	12	5,509	182,449	1,448,331		72.0	3,968			135,605	420,169	1,396,056	1,816,225	339	25,948
500 or more	20	15,183	458,813	4,127,540		74.5	11,310			298,294	992,223	3,979,029	4,971,252	725	57,470
Psychiatric	26	5,391	31,118	1,569,951		79.7	4,299			764	5,908	116,948	122,856	0	0
Hospitals	25	5,243	30,535	1,543,205		80.6	4,226			764	5,908	116,535	122,443	0	0
Institutions for mentally retarded	1	148	583	26,746		49.3	73			0	0	413	413	0	0
General	189	45,448	1,525,175	10,906,699		65.7	29,881			1,104,261	4,617,957	13,374,998	17,992,955	3,119	165,836
Hospitals	189	45,448	1,525,175	10,906,699		65.7	29,881			1,104,261	4,617,957	13,374,998	17,992,955	3,119	165,836
Hospital units of institutions	0	0	0	0		00.0	0			0	0	0	0	0	0
TB and other respiratory diseases	0	0	0	0		00.0	0			0	0	0	0	0	0
Obstetrics and gynecology	0	0	0	0		00.0	0			0	0	0	0	0	0
Eye, ear, nose, and throat	0	0	0	0		00.0	0			0	0	0	0	0	0
Rehabilitation	5	908	4,666	223,914		67.6	614			0	0	38,492	38,492	0	0
Orthopedic	0	0	0	0		00.0	0			0	0	0	0	0	0
Chronic disease	0	0	0	0		00.0	0			0	0	0	0	0	0
All other	4	458	19,378	113,192		67.7	310			13,575	66,164	214,020	280,184	0	0
Federal	5	3,520	41,129	1,049,599		81.7	2,876			16,443	59,379	1,183,753	1,243,132	30	973
Psychiatric	1	642	6,042	185,854		79.3	509			764	1,640	70,934	72,574	0	0
General and other special	4	2,878	35,087	863,745		82.2	2,367			15,679	57,739	1,112,819	1,170,558	30	973
Nonfederal	219	48,685	1,539,208	11,764,157		66.2	32,228			1,102,157	4,630,650	12,560,705	17,191,355	3,089	164,863
Psychiatric	25	4,749	25,076	1,384,097		79.8	3,790			0	4,268	46,014	50,282	0	0
Hospitals	24	4,601	24,493	1,357,351		80.8	3,717			0	4,268	45,601	49,869	0	0
Institutions for mentally retarded	1	148	583	26,746		49.3	73			0	0	413	413	0	0
TB and other respiratory diseases	0	0	0	0		00.0	0			0	0	0	0	0	0
Long-term general and other special	4	793	2,477	192,633		66.6	528			110	3,597	32,213	35,810	0	0
Short-term general and other special	190	43,143	1,511,655	10,187,427		64.7	27,910			1,102,047	4,622,785	12,482,478	17,105,263	3,089	164,863
Hospital units of institutions	0	0	0	0		00.0	0			0	0	0	0	0	0
Community hospitals*	190	43,143	1,511,655	10,187,427	13,649,109	64.7	27,910	37,399	6.7	1,102,047	4,622,785	12,482,478	17,105,263	3,089	164,863
6-24 beds	1	23	300	1,508	2,923	17.4	4	8	5.0	226	1,615	3,889	5,504	0	0
25-49	16	616	16,758	93,960	164,645	41.9	258	451	5.6	11,016	100,305	321,264	421,569	65	1,643
50-99	44	3,155	104,571	550,734	866,884	47.8	1,509	2,377	5.3	74,808	428,259	1,011,870	1,440,129	377	12,897
100-199	48	7,120	251,119	1,502,249	2,165,789	57.8	4,114	5,932	6.0	190,954	888,436	1,947,448	2,835,884	698	26,624
200-299	36	9,105	314,102	2,136,385	2,915,503	64.3	5,852	7,990	6.8	247,204	1,066,265	2,752,179	3,818,444	522	22,275
300-399	18	6,255	209,666	1,480,162	1,986,602	64.8	4,055	5,443	7.1	153,407	752,677	1,571,056	2,323,733	363	18,006
400-499	10	4,563	181,822	1,152,396	1,464,931	69.2	3,157	4,014	6.3	135,605	420,169	1,396,056	1,816,225	339	25,948
500 or more	17	12,306	433,317	3,270,033	4,081,832	72.8	8,961	11,184	7.5	288,827	965,059	3,478,716	4,443,775	725	57,470
Nongovernment not-for-profit	165	38,726	1,377,313	9,082,840	12,193,042	64.3	24,883	33,409	6.6	1,020,490	4,214,267	10,894,183	15,108,450	2,731	146,563
Investor-owned (for-profit)	1	43	966	6,581	9,188	41.9	18	25	6.8	773	2,426	3,984	6,410	0	0
State and local government	24	4,374	133,376	1,098,006	1,446,879	68.8	3,009	3,965	8.2	80,784	406,092	1,584,311	1,990,403	358	18,300

*For information on community hospitals that excludes nursing home-type data, refer to Hospital Units columns in tables 4A through 4D, pages 14 through 17.

CLASSIFICATION	FULL-TIME EQUIVALENT PERSONNEL					FULL-TIME EQUIVALENT TRAINEES			EXPENSES: LABOR				EXPENSES: TOTAL		
	Physicians and Dentists	Registered Nurses	Licensed Practical Nurses	Other Salaried Personnel	Total Personnel	Medical and Dental Residents	Other Trainees	Total Trainees	Payroll (in thousands)	Employee Benefits (in thousands)	Total (in thousands)	Percent of Total	Amount (in thousands)	Adjusted, per Admission	Adjusted, per Inpatient Day
OHIO	1,894	44,281	8,536	135,796	190,507	4,957	311	5,268	$ 4,986,563	$ 1,060,491	$ 6,047,054	56.2	$ 10,754,712		
6-24 beds	0	9	3	42	54	0	0	0	710	140	850	53.4	1,591		
25-49	5	415	118	1,510	2,048	1	2	3	41,550	8,827	50,377	53.5	94,167		
50-99	144	2,688	837	7,448	11,117	31	7	38	245,497	55,608	301,104	55.2	545,558		
100-199	149	6,466	1,842	21,319	29,776	202	0	202	737,918	155,746	893,664	55.5	1,609,876		
200-299	306	8,509	2,016	24,936	35,767	637	12	649	939,259	195,679	1,134,938	55.8	2,034,747		
300-399	277	6,346	1,337	21,576	29,536	438	9	447	753,929	160,663	914,593	57.0	1,604,094		
400-499	293	4,847	848	14,108	20,096	643	25	668	555,065	104,277	659,343	56.9	1,158,941		
500 or more	720	15,001	1,535	44,857	62,113	3,005	256	3,261	1,712,634	379,550	2,092,185	56.5	3,705,739		
Psychiatric	240	1,157	443	7,386	9,226	26	0	26	267,779	58,399	326,178	71.1	458,629		
Hospitals	240	1,147	417	7,131	8,935	26	0	26	262,870	56,614	319,483	71.2	448,873		
Institutions for mentally retarded	0	10	26	255	291	0	0	0	4,909	1,786	6,695	68.6	9,756		
General	1,618	42,212	7,929	124,837	176 596	4,856	302	5,158	4,601,664	976,613	5,578,277	55.4	10,064,284		
Hospitals	1,618	42,212	7,929	124,837	176 596	4,856	302	5,158	4,601,664	976,613	5,578,277	55.4	10,064,284		
Hospital units of institutions	0	0	0	0	0	0	0	0	0	0	0	0.0	0		
TB and other respiratory diseases	0	0	0	0	0	0	0	0	0	0	0	0.0	0		
Obstetrics and gynecology	0	0	0	0	0	0	0	0	0	0	0	0.0	0		
Eye, ear, nose, and throat	0	0	0	0	0	0	0	0	0	0	0	0.0	0		
Rehabilitation	18	246	112	1,619	1,995	1	0	1	49,708	14,947	64,655	66.7	96,990		
Orthopedic	0	0	0	0	0	0	0	0	0	0	0	0.0	0		
Chronic disease	0	0	0	0	0	0	0	0	0	0	0	0.0	0		
All other	18	666	52	1,954	2,690	74	9	83	67,412	10,531	77,943	57.8	134,809		
Federal	450	1,298	259	6,395	8,402	232	29	261	248,787	40,163	288,951	66.0	437,902		
Psychiatric	42	162	46	1,036	1,286	6	0	6	34,267	6,499	40,766	73.2	55,728		
General and other special	408	1,136	213	5,359	7,116	226	29	255	214,520	33,664	248,184	64.9	382,174		
Nonfederal	1,444	42,983	8,277	129,401	182,105	4,725	282	5,007	4,737,775	1,020,327	5,758,103	55.8	10,316,810		
Psychiatric	198	995	397	6,350	7,940	20	0	20	233,511	51,900	285,412	70.8	402,901		
Hospitals	198	985	371	6,095	7,649	20	0	20	228,602	50,115	278,717	70.9	393,145		
Institutions for mentally retarded	0	10	26	255	291	0	0	0	4,909	1,786	6,695	68.6	9,756		
TB and other respiratory diseases	0	0	0	0	0	0	0	0	0	0	0	0.0	0		
Long-term general and other special	22	199	110	1,518	1,849	2	0	2	49,029	11,771	60,801	65.7	92,524		
Short-term general and other special	1,224	41,789	7,770	121,533	172,316	4,703	282	4,985	4,455,235	956,656	5,411,891	55.1	9,821,385		
Hospital units of institutions	0	0	0	0	0	0	0	0	0	0	0	0.0	0		
Community hospitals*	1,224	41,789	7,770	121,533	172,316	4,703	282	4,985	4,455,235	956,656	5,411,891	55.1	9,821,385	$4,801.23	$ 719.56
6-24 beds	0	9	3	42	54	0	0	0	710	140	850	53.4	1,591	2,734.03	544.37
25-49	5	415	118	1,510	2,048	1	2	3	41,550	8,827	50,377	53.5	94,167	3,238.87	571.94
50-99	119	2,502	801	6,612	10,034	30	7	37	216,534	48,529	265,062	54.5	486,784	2,937.43	561.53
100-199	64	5,887	1,633	18,156	25,740	181	0	181	621,035	129,707	750,742	54.3	1,381,472	3,794.72	637.86
200-299	162	8,183	1,979	23,509	33,833	531	12	543	876,650	192,129	1,068,778	55.1	1,940,114	4,487.02	665.45
300-399	186	5,894	1,143	18,432	25,655	393	9	402	635,590	132,286	767,876	54.8	1,400,271	4,954.91	704.86
400-499	238	4,734	755	12,939	18,666	643	25	668	517,799	96,012	613,811	55.5	1,105,118	4,784.52	754.38
500 or more	450	14,165	1,338	40,333	56,286	2,924	227	3,151	1,545,367	349,028	1,894,395	55.5	3,411,869	6,315.83	835.87
Nongovernment not-for-profit	940	37,348	7,094	108,084	153,466	3,337	225	3,562	3,948,338	809,198	4,757,536	54.7	8,701,008	4,672.92	713.60
Investor-owned (for-profit)	0	14	9	64	87	0	0	0	2,359	483	2,841	46.5	6,112	4,530.53	665.18
State and local government	284	4,427	667	13,385	18,763	1,366	57	1,423	504,539	146,975	651,514	58.5	1,114,266	6,114.14	770.12

*For information on community hospitals that excludes nursing-home-type data, refer to Hospital Units columns in tables 4A through 4D, pages 14 through 17.

(continued on next page)

Table

5C (Continued) Oklahoma

Utilization, Personnel, and Finances in States

Excludes AHA nonregistered hospitals (see Table 14, page 240).

CLASSIFICATION	HOSPI-TALS	BEDS	ADMISSIONS	INPATIENT DAYS	ADJUSTED PATIENT DAYS	OCCU-PANCY, percent	AVERAGE DAILY CENSUS	ADJUSTED AVERAGE DAILY CENSUS	AVERAGE STAY, days	SURGICAL OPERATIONS	OUTPATIENT VISITS			NEWBORNS	
											Emergency	Other	Total	Bassinets	Births
OKLAHOMA	137	15,033	431,097	3,302,291		60.2	9,047			279,690	1,104,605	2,844,679	3,949,284	1,181	46,625
6-24 beds	11	224	5,253	22,645		26.8	60			2,036	28,805	193,958	222,763	33	367
25-49	48	1,806	42,110	261,407		39.6	716			15,983	133,206	413,204	546,410	204	3,281
50-99	32	2,115	53,835	358,018		46.4	981			29,091	227,851	385,479	613,330	234	7,595
100-199	27	3,522	103,946	723,595		56.3	1,984			63,829	298,837	893,886	1,192,723	294	10,142
200-299	5	1,252	38,741	327,393		71.6	897			23,221	88,435	68,680	157,115	117	4,557
300-399	8	2,580	64,662	691,460		73.4	1,894			60,561	111,151	333,355	444,506	112	6,454
400-499	2	1,012	30,382	248,968		67.4	682			20,316	43,581	80,066	123,647	44	3,625
500 or more	4	2,522	92,168	668,805		72.7	1,833			64,653	172,739	476,051	648,790	143	10,604
Psychiatric	13	1,600	10,875	467,006		79.9	1,278			357	7,530	63,048	70,578	0	0
Hospitals	13	1,600	10,875	467,006		79.9	1,278			357	7,530	63,048	70,578	0	0
Institutions for mentally retarded	0	0	0	0		00.0	0			0	0	0	0	0	0
General	121	13,259	417,201	2,805,934		58.0	7,688			276,225	1,094,473	2,776,817	3,871,290	1,181	46,625
Hospitals	119	13,187	417,010	2,805,599		58.3	7,687			276,005	1,087,413	2,654,486	3,741,899	1,181	46,625
Hospital units of institutions	2	72	191	335		01.4	1			220	7,060	122,331	129,391	0	0
TB and other respiratory diseases	0	0	0	0		00.0	0			0	0	0	0	0	0
Obstetrics and gynecology	0	0	0	0		00.0	0			0	0	0	0	0	0
Eye, ear, nose, and throat	0	0	0	0		00.0	0			0	0	0	0	0	0
Rehabilitation	2	72	453	10,739		41.7	30			0	254	3,903	4,157	0	0
Orthopedic	1	102	2,568	18,612		50.0	51			3,108	2,348	911	3,259	0	0
Chronic disease	0	0	0	0		00.0	0			0	0	0	0	0	0
All other	0	0	0	0		00.0	0			0	0	0	0	0	0
Federal	11	936	38,103	217,023		63.6	595			32,333	215,233	1,256,507	1,471,740	129	5,239
Psychiatric	0	0	0	0		00.0	0			0	0	0	0	0	0
General and other special	11	936	38,103	217,023		63.6	595			32,333	215,233	1,256,507	1,471,740	129	5,239
Nonfederal	126	14,097	392,994	3,085,268		60.0	8,452			247,357	889,372	1,588,172	2,477,544	1,052	41,386
Psychiatric	13	1,600	10,875	467,006		79.9	1,278			357	7,530	63,048	70,578	0	0
Hospitals	13	1,600	10,875	467,006		79.9	1,278			357	7,530	63,048	70,578	0	0
Institutions for mentally retarded	0	0	0	0		00.0	0			0	0	0	0	0	0
TB and other respiratory diseases	0	0	0	0		00.0	0			0	0	0	0	0	0
Long-term general and other special	0	0	0	0		00.0	0			0	0	0	0	0	0
Short-term general and other special	113	12,497	382,119	2,618,262		57.4	7,174			247,000	881,842	1,525,124	2,406,966	1,052	41,386
Hospital units of institutions	2	72	191	335		01.4	1			220	7,060	122,331	129,391	0	0
Community hospitals*	111	12,425	381,928	2,617,927	3,308,489	57.7	7,173	9,063	6.9	246,780	874,782	1,402,793	2,277,575	1,052	41,386
6-24 beds	8	175	3,148	16,585	25,832	25.1	44	71	5.3	722	9,093	17,112	26,205	23	96
25-49	41	1,549	35,770	201,583	287,514	35.6	552	785	5.6	13,589	101,262	158,332	259,594	169	2,365
50-99	25	1,703	43,034	290,208	404,892	46.7	795	1,110	6.7	24,907	141,060	155,300	296,360	172	4,424
100-199	22	2,887	87,987	565,098	734,681	53.7	1,550	2,014	6.4	58,900	218,764	309,166	527,930	272	9,261
200-299	4	998	36,149	237,908	299,553	65.3	652	819	6.6	22,864	88,435	64,195	152,630	117	4,557
300-399	5	1,579	53,290	388,772	481,370	67.4	1,065	1,319	7.3	40,829	99,848	142,571	242,419	112	6,454
400-499	2	1,012	30,382	248,968	300,325	67.4	682	823	8.2	20,316	43,581	80,066	123,647	44	3,625
500 or more	4	2,522	92,168	668,805	774,322	72.7	1,833	2,122	7.3	64,653	172,739	476,051	648,790	143	10,604
Nongovernment not-for-profit	39	6,687	220,818	1,571,165	1,932,148	64.4	4,305	5,294	7.1	154,307	443,854	699,529	1,143,383	485	24,097
Investor-owned (for-profit)	13	1,347	37,554	251,082	324,311	51.2	689	889	6.7	30,338	92,713	134,697	227,410	111	4,211
State and local government	59	4,391	123,556	795,680	1,052,030	49.6	2,179	2,880	6.4	62,135	338,215	568,567	906,782	456	13,078

CLASSIFICATION	FULL-TIME EQUIVALENT PERSONNEL: Physicians and Dentists	Registered Nurses	Licensed Practical Nurses	Other Salaried Personnel	Total Personnel	FULL-TIME EQUIVALENT TRAINEES: Medical and Dental Residents	Other Trainees	Total Trainees	EXPENSES — LABOR: Payroll (in thousands)	Employee Benefits (in thousands)	Total (in thousands)	Percent of Total	EXPENSES — TOTAL: Amount (in thousands)	Adjusted, per Admission	Adjusted, per Inpatient Day
OKLAHOMA	499	9,301	3,539	37,042	50,381	731	135	866	$ 1,092,778	$ 208,458	$ 1,301,236	52.5	$ 2,479,018		
6-24 beds	37	105	51	581	774	0	0	0	11,449	2,422	13,871	59.1	23,472		
25-49	77	612	429	3,264	4,382	5	6	11	76,244	13,223	89,467	56.0	159,904		
50-99	103	1,058	601	3,881	5,643	11	0	11	114,464	23,210	137,674	56.5	243,514		
100-199	108	1,920	925	7,840	10,793	24	0	24	226,091	46,518	272,609	49.8	546,933		
200-299	18	764	351	2,895	4,028	22	0	22	90,544	16,578	107,122	55.6	192,723		
300-399	137	1,534	552	6,737	8,960	203	89	292	210,695	41,391	252,086	52.9	476,317		
400-499	4	829	158	2,589	3,580	4	4	8	94,297	14,061	108,359	51.6	210,122		
500 or more	15	2,479	472	9,255	12,221	462	36	498	268,992	51,055	320,048	51.1	626,033		
Psychiatric	73	392	139	2,786	3,390	31	1	32	81,939	19,333	101,272	69.2	146,252		
Hospitals	73	392	139	2,786	3,390	31	1	32	81,939	19,333	101,272	69.2	146,252		
Institutions for mentally retarded	0	0	0	0	0	0	0	0	0	0	0	0.0	0		
General	425	8,831	3,316	33,345	46,517	700	134	834	999,870	187,202	1,187,071	51.5	2,304,365		
Hospitals	410	8,807	3,306	33,368	46,391	700	134	834	997,087	186,414	1,183,501	51.5	2,298,669		
Hospital units of institutions	15	24	10	77	126	0	0	0	2,783	788	3,571	62.7	5,696		
TB and other respiratory diseases	0	0	0	0	0	0	0	0	0	0	0	0.0	0		
Obstetrics and gynecology	0	0	0	0	0	0	0	0	0	0	0	0.0	0		
Eye, ear, nose, and throat	0	0	0	0	0	0	0	0	0	0	0	0.0	0		
Rehabilitation	1	24	16	37	178	0	0	0	3,456	702	4,157	49.0	8,487		
Orthopedic	0	54	68	74	296	0	0	0	7,514	1,222	8,735	43.9	19,914		
Chronic disease	0	0	0	0	0	0	0	0	0	0	0	0.0	0		
All other	0	0	0	0	0	0	0	0	0	0	0	0.0	0		
Federal	348	811	319	3,822	5,300	184	6	190	119,278	21,213	140,490	59.5	236,004		
Psychiatric	0	0	0	0	0	0	0	0	0	0	0	0.0	0		
General and other special	348	811	319	3,822	5,300	184	6	190	119,278	21,213	140,490	59.5	236,004		
Nonfederal	151	8,490	3,220	33,220	45,081	547	129	676	973,500	187,245	1,160,746	51.7	2,243,014		
Psychiatric	73	392	139	2,786	3,390	31	1	32	81,939	19,333	101,272	69.2	146,252		
Hospitals	73	392	139	2,786	3,390	31	1	32	81,939	19,333	101,272	69.2	146,252		
Institutions for mentally retarded	0	0	0	0	0	0	0	0	0	0	0	0.0	0		
TB and other respiratory diseases	0	0	0	0	0	0	0	0	0	0	0	0.0	0		
Long-term general and other special	0	0	0	0	0	0	0	0	0	0	0	0.0	0		
Short-term general and other special	78	8,098	3,081	30,434	41,691	516	128	644	891,561	167,913	1,059,474	50.5	2,096,762		
Hospital units of institutions	15	24	10	77	126	0	0	0	2,783	788	3,571	62.7	5,696		
Community hospitals*	63	8,074	3,071	30,357	41,565	516	128	644	888,778	167,124	1,055,903	50.5	2,091,066	$4,301.98	$ 632.03
6-24 beds	0	54	37	243	334	0	0	0	5,496	1,054	6,549	55.0	11,902	2,436.45	460.75
25-49	12	455	381	2,440	3,288	0	6	6	56,841	9,190	66,030	53.2	124,217	2,432.57	432.04
50-99	2	774	519	3,003	4,298	0	0	0	78,252	15,143	93,395	51.7	180,633	3,013.71	446.13
100-199	5	1,629	785	5,873	8,292	14	0	14	177,288	36,793	214,081	48.3	443,303	3,841.48	603.39
200-299	0	694	316	2,389	3,399	0	0	0	77,083	12,758	89,841	52.8	170,053	3,739.89	567.69
300-399	25	1,160	403	4,565	6,153	36	82	118	130,529	27,071	157,600	48.5	324,805	4,934.15	674.75
400-499	4	829	158	2,589	3,580	4	4	8	94,297	14,061	108,359	51.6	210,122	5,726.79	699.65
500 or more	15	2,479	472	9,255	12,221	462	36	498	268,992	51,055	320,048	51.1	626,033	5,861.89	808.49
Nongovernment not-for-profit	44	5,016	1,540	18,149	24,749	62	122	184	535,307	91,280	626,587	50.5	1,240,219	4,538.65	641.89
Investor-owned (for-profit)	2	658	263	2,874	3,797	0	0	0	90,823	22,297	113,120	43.2	261,772	5,376.08	807.16
State and local government	17	2,400	1,268	9,334	13,019	454	6	460	262,648	53,547	316,196	53.7	589,075	3,589.25	559.94

*For information on community hospitals that excludes nursing-home-type data, refer to Hospital Units columns in tables 4A through 4D, pages 14 through 17.

(continued on next page)

Table
5C (Continued) Oregon

Utilization, Personnel, and Finances in States
Excludes AHA nonregistered hospitals (see Table 14, page 240).

CLASSIFICATION	HOSPITALS	BEDS	ADMISSIONS	INPATIENT DAYS	ADJUSTED PATIENT DAYS	OCCUPANCY, percent	AVERAGE DAILY CENSUS	ADJUSTED AVERAGE DAILY CENSUS	AVERAGE STAY, days	SURGICAL OPERATIONS	OUTPATIENT VISITS: Emergency	OUTPATIENT VISITS: Other	OUTPATIENT VISITS: Total	NEWBORNS: Bassinets	NEWBORNS: Births
OREGON	77	10,322	321,756	2,367,544		62.9	6,490			255,765	965,701	2,736,381	3,702,082	715	42,796
6-24 beds	4	81	1,907	6,711		23.5	19			978	10,027	19,589	29,616	8	212
25-49	24	953	27,774	126,337		36.3	346			20,837	118,448	255,859	374,307	138	3,853
50-99	19	1,336	40,634	264,046		54.3	725			34,753	191,332	334,811	526,143	118	5,365
100-199	16	2,243	87,964	467,210		57.1	1,280			80,054	300,040	412,909	712,949	199	11,231
200-299	2	562	16,125	112,989		55.2	310			13,308	49,831	136,425	186,256	40	2,775
300-399	5	1,697	45,010	441,668		71.3	1,210			30,910	81,511	468,348	549,859	74	6,786
400-499	5	2,106	89,363	514,707		67.0	1,411			66,270	191,603	921,740	1,113,343	138	12,574
500 or more	2	1,344	12,979	433,876		88.5	1,189			8,655	22,909	186,700	209,609	0	0
Psychiatric	5	1,331	4,562	438,693		90.2	1,201			0	2,807	15,973	18,780	0	0
Hospitals	5	1,331	4,562	438,693		90.2	1,201			0	2,807	15,973	18,780	0	0
Institutions for mentally retarded	0	0	0	0		00.0	0			0	0	0	0	0	0
General	71	8,951	316,003	1,921,865		58.9	5,270			254,784	962,894	2,710,419	3,673,313	715	42,796
Hospitals	71	8,951	316,003	1,921,865		58.9	5,270			254,784	962,894	2,710,419	3,673,313	715	42,796
Hospital units of institutions	0	0	0	0		00.0	0			0	0	0	0	0	0
TB and other respiratory diseases	0	0	0	0		00.0	0			0	0	0	0	0	0
Obstetrics and gynecology	0	0	0	0		00.0	0			0	0	0	0	0	0
Eye, ear, nose, and throat	0	0	0	0		00.0	0			0	0	0	0	0	0
Rehabilitation	0	0	0	0		00.0	0			0	0	0	0	0	0
Orthopedic	1	40	1,191	6,986		47.5	19			981	0	9,989	9,989	0	0
Chronic disease	0	0	0	0		00.0	0			0	0	0	0	0	0
All other	0	0	0	0		00.0	0			0	0	0	0	0	0
Federal	2	918	15,291	257,288		76.8	705			10,007	24,425	245,582	270,007	0	0
Psychiatric	0	0	0	0		00.0	0			0	0	0	0	0	0
General and other special	2	918	15,291	257,288		76.8	705			10,007	24,425	245,582	270,007	0	0
Nonfederal	75	9,404	306,465	2,110,256		61.5	5,785			245,758	941,276	2,490,799	3,432,075	715	42,796
Psychiatric	5	1,331	4,562	438,693		90.2	1,201			0	2,807	15,973	18,780	0	0
Hospitals	5	1,331	4,562	438,693		90.2	1,201			0	2,807	15,973	18,780	0	0
Institutions for mentally retarded	0	0	0	0		00.0	0			0	0	0	0	0	0
TB and other respiratory diseases	0	0	0	0		00.0	0			0	0	0	0	0	0
Long-term general and other special	0	0	0	0		00.0	0			0	0	0	0	0	0
Short-term general and other special	70	8,073	301,903	1,671,563		56.8	4,584			245,758	938,469	2,474,826	3,413,295	715	42,796
Hospital units of institutions	0	0	0	0		00.0	0			0	0	0	0	0	0
Community hospitals*	70	8,073	301,903	1,671,563	2,392,458	56.8	4,584	6,553	5.5	245,758	938,469	2,474,826	3,413,295	715	42,796
6-24 beds	4	81	1,907	6,711	13,085	23.5	19	37	3.5	978	10,027	19,589	29,616	8	212
25-49	24	953	27,774	126,337	226,144	36.3	346	621	4.5	20,837	118,448	255,859	374,307	138	3,853
50-99	16	1,146	39,262	214,825	328,913	51.6	591	899	5.5	34,753	190,667	330,841	521,508	118	5,365
100-199	16	2,243	87,964	467,210	667,159	57.1	1,280	1,827	5.3	80,054	300,040	412,909	712,949	199	11,231
200-299	2	562	16,125	112,989	170,280	55.2	310	466	7.0	13,308	49,831	136,425	186,256	40	2,775
300-399	3	982	39,508	228,784	297,245	63.8	627	814	5.8	29,558	77,853	397,463	475,316	74	6,786
400-499	5	2,106	89,363	514,707	689,632	67.0	1,411	1,889	5.8	66,270	191,603	921,740	1,113,343	138	12,574
500 or more	0	0	0	0	0	00.0	0	0	0.0	0	0	0	0	0	0
Nongovernment not-for-profit	43	6,223	248,317	1,329,637	1,881,918	58.6	3,645	5,156	5.4	206,119	754,894	2,036,421	2,791,315	546	35,874
Investor-owned (for-profit)	8	585	17,246	85,678	125,148	40.3	236	342	5.0	15,946	88,918	108,030	196,948	52	1,797
State and local government	19	1,265	36,340	256,248	385,392	55.6	703	1,055	7.1	23,693	94,657	330,375	425,032	117	5,125

*For information on community hospitals that excludes nursing home type data, refer to Hospital Units columns in tables 4A through 4D, pages 14 through 17.

Table 5C (Continued) Oregon

CLASSIFICATION	FULL-TIME EQUIVALENT PERSONNEL					FULL-TIME EQUIVALENT TRAINEES			EXPENSES						
									LABOR				TOTAL		
	Physicians and Dentists	Registered Nurses	Licensed Practical Nurses	Other Salaried Personnel	Total Personnel	Medical and Dental Residents	Other Trainees	Total Trainees	Payroll (in thousands)	Employee Benefits (in thousands)	Total (in thousands)	Percent of Total	Amount (in thousands)	Adjusted, per Admission	Adjusted, per Inpatient Day
OREGON	775	10,256	1,075	25 631	37,737	452	34	486	$ 1,005,256	$ 219,086	$ 1,224,342	56.5	$ 2,167,448		
6-24 beds	1	49	6	156	212	0	0	0	4,536	954	5,490	55.1	9,964		
25-49	13	810	104	2,073	3,000	2	1	3	70,686	15,244	85,930	54.7	157,171		
50-99	24	1,106	194	3,156	4,480	11	0	11	103,338	22,819	126,157	54.1	232,982		
100-199	449	2,482	208	4,381	8,120	1	8	9	196,845	38,289	235,134	53.2	441,770		
200-299	17	538	35	1,422	2,012	0	0	0	49,644	9,849	59,492	55.7	106,831		
300-399	69	1,904	129	4,797	6,899	279	1	280	213,005	46,460	259,465	58.7	442,107		
400-499	47	2,835	288	6,304	9,974	97	0	97	277,817	61,340	339,157	55.7	609,188		
500 or more	155	532	111	2,242	3,040	62	24	86	89,385	24,132	113,517	67.8	167,434		
Psychiatric	48	218	58	1,679	2,003	3	1	4	53,551	17,698	71,250	75.5	94,361		
Hospitals	48	218	58	1,679	2,003	3	1	4	53,551	17,698	71,250	75.5	94,361		
Institutions for mentally retarded	0	0	0	0	0	0	0	0	0	0	0	0.0	0		
General	723	10,010	1,017	23,803	35,553	447	32	479	947,313	200,561	1,147,874	55.6	2,063,139		
Hospitals	723	10,010	1,017	23,803	35,553	447	32	479	947,313	200,561	1,147,874	55.6	2,063,139		
Hospital units of institutions	0	0	0	0	0	0	0	0	0	0	0	0.0	0		
TB and other respiratory diseases	0	0	0	0	0	0	0	0	0	0	0	0.0	0		
Obstetrics and gynecology	0	0	0	0	0	0	0	0	0	0	0	0.0	0		
Eye, ear, nose, and throat	0	0	0	0	0	0	0	0	0	0	0	0.0	0		
Rehabilitation	0	0	0	0	0	0	0	0	0	0	0	0.0	0		
Orthopedic	4	28	0	149	181	2	1	3	4,392	827	5,218	52.5	9,948		
Chronic disease	0	0	0	0	0	0	0	0	0	0	0	0.0	0		
All other	0	0	0	0	0	0	0	0	0	0	0	0.0	0		
Federal	157	545	129	1,896	2,727	62	24	86	85,394	17,508	102,902	64.2	160,285		
Psychiatric	0	0	0	0	0	0	0	0	0	0	0	0.0	0		
General and other special	157	545	129	1,896	2,727	62	24	86	85,394	17,508	102,902	64.2	160,285		
Nonfederal	618	9,711	946	23,735	35,010	390	10	400	919,862	201,578	1,121,440	55.9	2,007,163		
Psychiatric	48	218	58	1,673	2,003	3	1	4	53,551	17,698	71,250	75.5	94,361		
Hospitals	48	218	58	1,673	2,003	3	1	4	53,551	17,698	71,250	75.5	94,361		
Institutions for mentally retarded	0	0	0	0	0	0	0	0	0	0	0	0.0	0		
TB and other respiratory diseases	0	0	0	0	0	0	0	0	0	0	0	0.0	0		
Long-term general and other special	0	0	0	0	0	0	0	0	0	0	0	0.0	0		
Short-term general and other special	570	9,493	888	22,056	33,007	387	9	396	866,310	183,880	1,050,190	54.9	1,912,802		
Hospital units of institutions	0	0	0	0	0	0	0	0	0	0	0	0.0	0		
Community hospitals*	570	9,493	888	22,056	33,007	387	9	396	866,310	183,880	1,050,190	54.9	1,912,802	$4,431.64	$ 799.51
6-24 beds	1	49	6	156	212	0	0	0	4,536	954	5,490	55.1	9,964	2,683.66	761.51
25-49	13	810	104	2,073	3,000	2	1	3	70,686	15,244	85,930	54.7	157,171	3,323.00	695.00
50-99	17	1,058	188	2,887	4,150	11	0	11	92,270	20,478	112,748	53.5	210,780	3,490.08	640.84
100-199	449	2,482	208	4,981	8,120	1	8	9	196,845	38,289	235,134	53.2	441,770	3,547.67	662.17
200-299	17	538	35	1,422	2,012	0	0	0	49,644	9,849	59,492	55.7	106,831	4,231.42	627.38
300-399	26	1,721	59	3,733	5,539	276	0	276	174,513	37,727	212,240	56.3	377,097	7,346.24	1,268.64
400-499	47	2,835	288	6,804	9,974	97	0	97	277,817	61,340	339,157	55.7	609,188	5,114.24	883.35
500 or more	0	0	0	0	0	0	0	0	0	0	0	0.0	0	0.00	0.00
Nongovernment not-for-profit	551	7,621	672	17,467	26,311	144	6	150	701,841	137,935	839,776	55.0	1,526,027	4,328.04	810.89
Investor-owned (for-profit)	3	492	102	1,311	1,908	11	0	11	41,658	7,835	49,492	46.5	106,384	4,214.71	850.06
State and local government	16	1,380	114	3,278	4,788	232	3	235	122,811	38,110	160,922	57.4	280,392	5,212.52	727.55

*For information on community hospitals that excludes nursing-home-type data, refer to Hospital Units columns in tables 4A through 4D, pages 14 through 17.

(continued on next page)

Table

5C (Continued) Pennsylvania

Utilization, Personnel, and Finances in States

Excludes AHA nonregistered hospitals (see Table 14, page 240).

CLASSIFICATION	HOSPITALS	BEDS	ADMISSIONS	INPATIENT DAYS	ADJUSTED PATIENT DAYS	OCCUPANCY, percent	AVERAGE DAILY CENSUS	ADJUSTED AVERAGE DAILY CENSUS	AVERAGE STAY, days	SURGICAL OPERATIONS	OUTPATIENT VISITS: Emergency	OUTPATIENT VISITS: Other	OUTPATIENT VISITS: Total	NEWBORNS: Bassinets	NEWBORNS: Births
PENNSYLVANIA	302	68,354	1,886,477	18,786,058		75.3	51,466			1,420,281	5,169,721	17,597,937	22,767,658	3,167	169,833
6-24 beds	5	72	2,287	13,520		50.0	36			3,920	12,349	83,799	96,148	0	0
25-49	17	625	10,845	149,519		65.4	409			5,302	23,059	188,236	211,295	12	95
50-99	53	3,968	89,588	921,028		63.6	2,524			57,914	364,031	1,259,346	1,623,377	187	5,642
100-199	85	11,860	348,636	2,998,828		69.3	8,216			252,014	1,238,297	3,221,258	4,459,555	528	22,452
200-299	69	16,288	529,645	4,280,220		72.0	11,728			432,025	1,654,809	5,010,131	6,664,940	1,066	49,252
300-399	23	7,830	280,525	2,157,019		75.5	5,910			202,760	719,062	2,480,987	3,200,049	530	30,877
400-499	24	10,892	270,435	3,274,222		82.3	8,969			219,466	534,363	2,316,488	2,850,851	438	30,639
500 or more	26	16,819	354,516	4,991,702		81.3	13,674			246,880	623,751	3,037,692	3,661,443	406	30,876
Psychiatric	45	11,597	48,926	3,606,602		85.2	9,882			56	14,986	333,439	348,425	0	0
Hospitals	44	11,459	48,920	3,559,819		85.1	9,754			56	14,986	333,439	348,425	0	0
Institutions for mentally retarded	1	138	6	46,783		92.8	128			0	0	0	0	0	0
General	228	53,242	1,787,499	14,166,853		72.9	38,812			1,391,732	5,112,820	16,569,305	21,682,125	3,036	160,266
Hospitals	225	53,188	1,786,117	14,157,585		72.9	38,787			1,390,889	5,099,355	16,480,146	21,579,501	3,036	160,266
Hospital units of institutions	3	54	1,382	9,268		46.3	25			843	13,465	89,159	102,624	0	0
TB and other respiratory diseases	0	0	0	0		00.0	0			0	0	0	0	0	0
Obstetrics and gynecology	1	319	17,604	78,649		67.4	215			10,231	13,547	33,172	46,719	131	9,567
Eye, ear, nose, and throat	0	0	0	0		00.0	0			0	0	0	0	0	0
Rehabilitation	18	1,701	18,090	493,596		79.4	1,351			0	3,459	512,466	515,925	0	0
Orthopedic	2	110	1,369	17,921		45.5	50			896	0	18,681	18,681	0	0
Chronic disease	0	0	0	0		00.0	0			0	0	0	0	0	0
All other	8	1,385	12,989	422,437		83.5	1,156			17,366	24,909	130,874	155,783	0	0
Federal	11	4,628	43,348	1,323,916		78.4	3,627			15,301	69,699	1,076,425	1,146,124	0	0
Psychiatric	2	1,536	7,259	441,083		78.6	1,208			0	1,821	150,721	152,542	0	0
General and other special	9	3,092	36,089	882,833		78.2	2,419			15,301	67,878	925,704	993,582	0	0
Nonfederal	291	63,726	1,843,129	17,462,142		75.1	47,839			1,404,980	5,100,022	16,521,512	21,621,534	3,167	169,833
Psychiatric	43	10,061	41,667	3,165,519		86.2	8,674			56	13,165	182,718	195,883	0	0
Hospitals	42	9,923	41,661	3,118,736		86.1	8,546			56	13,165	182,718	195,883	0	0
Institutions for mentally retarded	1	138	6	46,783		92.8	128			0	0	0	0	0	0
TB and other respiratory diseases	0	0	0	0		00.0	0			0	0	0	0	0	0
Long-term general and other special	8	1,239	5,032	350,749		77.6	961			0	5,199	235,685	240,884	0	0
Short-term general and other special	240	52,426	1,796,430	13,945,874		72.9	38,204			1,404,924	5,081,658	16,103,109	21,184,767	3,167	169,833
Hospital units of institutions	2	37	376	6,282		45.9	17			137	1,680	19,442	21,122	0	0
Community hospitals*	238	52,389	1,796,054	13,939,592	18,582,523	72.9	38,187	50,902	7.8	1,404,787	5,079,978	16,083,667	21,163,645	3,167	169,833
6-24 beds	2	21	768	3,110	6,393	38.1	8	17	4.0	3,186	0	13,314	13,314	0	0
25-49	10	395	9,118	86,743	165,508	60.0	237	453	9.5	5,193	21,732	161,680	183,412	12	95
50-99	39	2,906	77,636	644,386	934,515	60.7	1,765	2,558	8.3	55,829	339,490	902,438	1,241,928	187	5,642
100-199	70	9,742	327,032	2,385,093	3,373,163	67.1	6,534	9,241	7.3	249,390	1,232,234	3,088,262	4,320,496	528	22,452
200-299	63	14,820	516,651	3,853,049	5,346,030	71.2	10,557	14,643	7.5	432,025	1,649,497	4,864,486	6,513,983	1,066	49,252
300-399	22	7,485	277,954	2,050,081	2,624,672	75.0	5,617	7,189	7.4	202,760	719,062	2,424,974	3,144,036	530	30,877
400-499	16	7,094	254,659	2,007,859	2,520,499	77.5	5,500	6,906	7.9	213,674	500,326	1,945,291	2,445,617	438	30,639
500 or more	16	9,926	332,236	2,909,271	3,611,743	80.3	7,969	9,895	8.8	242,730	617,637	2,683,222	3,300,859	406	30,876
Nongovernment not-for-profit	225	51,284	1,777,967	13,675,219	18,235,402	73.1	37,464	49,951	7.7	1,395,420	5,022,227	15,832,907	20,855,134	3,128	169,428
Investor-owned (for-profit)	7	553	7,236	153,372	195,574	75.8	419	536	21.2	714	3,258	131,996	135,254	8	57
State and local government	6	552	10,851	111,001	151,547	55.1	304	415	10.2	8,653	54,493	118,764	173,257	31	348

Table 5C (Continued) Pennsylvania

CLASSIFICATION	FULL-TIME EQUIVALENT PERSONNEL: Physicians and Dentists	Registered Nurses	Licensed Practical Nurses	Other Salaried Personnel	Total Personnel	FULL-TIME EQUIVALENT TRAINEES: Medical and Dental Residents	Other Trainees	Total Trainees	EXPENSES — LABOR: Payroll (in thousands)	Employee Benefits (in thousands)	Total (in thousands)	Percent of Total	EXPENSES — TOTAL: Amount (in thousands)	Adjusted, per Admission	Adjusted, per Inpatient Day
PENNSYLVANIA	3,771	56,404	10,725	170,926	241,826	5,471	324	5,795	$ 6,483,820	$ 1,342,573	$ 7,826,393	56.6	$ 13,821,348		
6-24 beds	21	71	12	329	433	0	0	0	7,793	1,581	9,375	60.2	15,567		
25-49	40	268	76	1,214	1,598	1	0	1	36,046	6,645	42,691	56.2	76,012		
50-99	118	2,492	896	8,725	12,231	15	12	27	289,510	55,993	345,503	56.2	614,987		
100-199	297	9,162	2,156	28,065	39,680	349	28	377	1,002,241	209,242	1,211,482	55.4	2,184,888		
200-299	693	14,182	2,920	43,112	60,907	599	22	621	1,567,945	322,869	1,890,814	57.3	3,302,404		
300-399	1,014	7,885	1,392	21,699	31,990	920	0	920	872,238	181,821	1,054,058	55.3	1,906,753		
400-499	620	9,245	1,398	26,913	38,176	960	118	1,078	1,070,942	218,981	1,289,923	57.6	2,239,623		
500 or more	968	13,099	1,875	40,869	56,811	2,627	144	2,771	1,637,106	345,442	1,982,548	57.0	3,481,113		
Psychiatric	609	2,726	725	15,886	19,946	115	62	177	547,332	156,223	703,555	73.8	953,533		
Hospitals	608	2,720	718	15,712	19,758	115	62	177	540,831	154,659	695,490	73.7	943,537		
Institutions for mentally retarded	1	6	7	174	188	0	0	0	6,501	1,564	8,065	80.7	9,996		
General	3,029	51,765	9,436	147,016	211,246	5,296	241	5,537	5,681,085	1,129,636	6,810,721	55.2	12,346,266		
Hospitals	3,009	51,731	9,421	146,801	210,962	5,296	241	5,537	5,676,618	1,128,597	6,805,215	55.2	12,336,581		
Hospital units of institutions	20	34	15	215	284	0	0	0	4,468	1,038	5,506	56.9	9,685		
TB and other respiratory diseases	0	0	0	0	0	0	0	0	0	0	0	0.0	0		
Obstetrics and gynecology	0	472	86	957	1,515	0	0	0	45,869	8,972	54,841	55.9	98,075		
Eye, ear, nose, and throat	0	0	0	0	0	0	0	0	0	0	0	0.0	0		
Rehabilitation	81	981	373	4,485	5,920	16	3	19	147,810	30,579	178,389	62.4	285,740		
Orthopedic	3	57	1	243	309	6	0	6	6,354	1,237	7,591	53.4	14,224		
Chronic disease	0	0	0	0	0	0	0	0	0	0	0	0.0	0		
All other	49	403	104	2,334	2,890	38	18	56	55,371	15,925	71,295	57.7	123,509		
Federal	467	1,462	438	7,277	9,644	220	105	325	301,674	53,137	354,811	66.5	533,430		
Psychiatric	84	326	118	1,910	2,438	2	13	15	72,296	12,946	85,241	73.1	116,536		
General and other special	383	1,136	320	5,367	7,206	218	92	310	229,378	40,191	269,569	64.7	416,893		
Nonfederal	3,304	54,942	10,287	163,649	232,182	5,251	219	5,470	6,182,147	1,289,436	7,471,582	56.2	13,287,918		
Psychiatric	525	2,400	607	13,976	17,508	113	49	162	475,036	143,278	618,313	73.9	836,997		
Hospitals	524	2,394	600	13,802	17,320	113	49	162	468,535	141,713	610,249	73.8	827,001		
Institutions for mentally retarded	1	6	7	174	188	0	0	0	6,501	1,564	8,065	80.7	9,996		
TB and other respiratory diseases	0	0	0	0	0	0	0	0	0	0	0	0.0	0		
Long-term general and other special	54	429	217	2,610	3,310	2	27	29	79,349	19,750	99,099	69.0	143,651		
Short-term general and other special	2,725	52,113	9,463	147,063	211,364	5,136	143	5,279	5,627,762	1,126,408	6,754,170	54.9	12,307,270		
Hospital units of institutions	4	12	11	48	75	0	0	0	1,569	393	1,962	42.4	4,628		
Community hospitals*	2,721	52,101	9,452	147,015	211,289	5,136	143	5,279	5,626,193	1,126,015	6,752,208	54.9	12,302,642	$5,120.14	$ 662.05
6-24 beds	4	33	6	97	140	0	0	0	3,052	578	3,630	56.4	6,439	2,625.88	1,007.14
25-49	22	173	58	882	1,135	1	0	1	23,104	3,880	26,984	57.5	46,924	3,466.62	283.52
50-99	51	2,044	805	6,156	9,056	15	0	15	210,879	40,964	251,843	54.3	463,761	3,909.70	496.26
100-199	198	8,521	2,045	24,501	35,265	334	28	362	875,809	179,957	1,055,765	54.3	1,944,941	4,127.18	576.59
200-299	533	13,604	2,772	39,428	56,337	512	20	532	1,434,538	293,138	1,727,676	56.3	3,070,190	4,283.94	574.29
300-399	996	7,798	1,357	21,238	31,389	920	0	920	854,865	178,766	1,033,632	55.1	1,877,551	5,272.51	715.35
400-499	315	8,338	1,008	21,932	31,593	831	16	847	881,997	168,909	1,050,905	54.5	1,929,321	6,019.74	765.45
500 or more	602	11,590	1,401	32,781	46,374	2,523	79	2,602	1,341,948	259,825	1,601,773	54.0	2,963,515	7,341.59	820.52
Nongovernment not-for-profit	2,718	51,451	9,203	145,071	208,443	5,135	143	5,278	5,561,601	1,109,081	6,670,681	54.9	12,149,090	5,107.93	666.24
Investor-owned (for-profit)	3	331	165	1,174	1,673	1	0	1	31,621	7,577	39,198	48.7	80,431	8,134.24	411.26
State and local government	0	319	84	770	1,173	0	0	0	32,971	9,357	42,329	57.9	73,121	5,067.62	482.50

*For information on community hospitals that excludes nursing-home-type data, refer to Hospital Units columns in tables 4A through 4D, pages 14 through 17.

(continued on next page)

Table

5C (Continued) Rhode Island

Utilization, Personnel, and Finances in States

Excludes AHA nonregistered hospitals (see Table 14, page 240).

CLASSIFICATION	HOSPITALS	BEDS	ADMISSIONS	INPATIENT DAYS	ADJUSTED PATIENT DAYS	OCCUPANCY, percent	AVERAGE DAILY CENSUS	ADJUSTED AVERAGE DAILY CENSUS	AVERAGE STAY, days	SURGICAL OPERATIONS	OUTPATIENT VISITS: Emergency	OUTPATIENT VISITS: Other	OUTPATIENT VISITS: Total	NEWBORNS: Bassinets	NEWBORNS: Births
RHODE ISLAND	19	4,464	137,597	1,341,763		82.3	3,675			118,830	515,246	943,347	1,458,593	195	15,896
6-24 beds	0	0	0	0		00.0	0			0	0	0	0	0	0
25-49	0	0	0	0		00.0	0			0	0	0	0	0	0
50-99	3	198	5,082	54,413		74.7	148			7,229	29,347	138,425	167,772	0	0
100-199	7	1,079	41,135	327,057		83.0	896			24,018	130,498	224,308	354,806	95	11,714
200-299	5	1,293	34,933	379,231		80.4	1,039			35,810	137,719	372,330	510,049	46	1,597
300-399	2	739	15,218	253,694		94.0	695			16,650	67,724	59,910	127,634	42	1,677
400-499	1	436	14,453	116,182		72.9	318			17,410	60,620	69,014	129,634	12	908
500 or more	1	719	26,776	211,186		80.5	579			17,713	89,338	79,360	168,698	0	0
Psychiatric	3	371	4,056	120,923		89.2	331			0	172	16,798	16,970	0	0
Hospitals	3	371	4,056	120,923		89.2	331			0	172	16,798	16,970	0	0
Institutions for mentally retarded	0	0	0	0		00.0	0			0	0	0	0	0	0
General	13	3,254	118,873	927,616		78.1	2,541			113,136	495,364	899,624	1,394,988	135	6,158
Hospitals	13	3,254	118,873	927,616		78.1	2,541			113,136	495,364	899,624	1,394,988	135	6,158
Hospital units of institutions	0	0	0	0		00.0	0			0	0	0	0	0	0
TB and other respiratory diseases	0	0	0	0		00.0	0			0	0	0	0	0	0
Obstetrics and gynecology	1	197	14,388	67,975		94.4	186			5,694	19,710	26,925	46,635	60	9,738
Eye, ear, nose, and throat	0	0	0	0		00.0	0			0	0	0	0	0	0
Rehabilitation	0	0	0	0		00.0	0			0	0	0	0	0	0
Orthopedic	0	0	0	0		00.0	0			0	0	0	0	0	0
Chronic disease	1	380	248	138,514		99.7	379			0	0	0	0	0	0
All other	1	262	32	86,735		90.8	238			0	0	0	0	0	0
Federal	2	271	6,531	74,296		74.9	203			17,563	42,075	245,861	287,936	0	0
Psychiatric	0	0	0	0		00.0	0			0	0	0	0	0	0
General and other special	2	271	6,531	74,296		74.9	203			17,563	42,075	245,861	287,936	0	0
Nonfederal	17	4,193	131,066	1,267,467		82.8	3,472			101,267	473,171	697,486	1,170,657	195	15,896
Psychiatric	3	371	4,056	120,923		89.2	331			0	172	16,798	16,970	0	0
Hospitals	3	371	4,056	120,923		89.2	331			0	172	16,798	16,970	0	0
Institutions for mentally retarded	0	0	0	0		00.0	0			0	0	0	0	0	0
TB and other respiratory diseases	0	0	0	0		00.0	0			0	0	0	0	0	0
Long-term general and other special	2	642	280	225,249		96.1	617			0	0	0	0	0	0
Short-term general and other special	12	3,180	126,730	921,295		79.4	2,524			101,267	472,999	680,688	1,153,687	195	15,896
Hospital units of institutions	0	0	0	0		00.0	0			0	0	0	0	0	0
Community hospitals*	12	3,180	126,730	921,295	1,273,481	79.4	2,524	3,491	7.3	101,267	472,999	680,688	1,153,687	195	15,896
6-24 beds	0	0	0	0	0	00.0	0	0	0.0	0	0	0	0	0	0
25-49	0	0	0	0	0	00.0	0	0	0.0	0	0	0	0	0	0
50-99	1	79	2,290	16,919	30,602	58.2	46	84	7.4	3,910	13,628	15,210	28,838	0	0
100-199	5	768	37,458	226,349	317,197	80.7	620	870	6.0	24,018	130,326	209,133	339,459	95	11,714
200-299	3	819	30,783	235,479	327,015	78.8	645	897	7.6	21,566	111,363	248,061	359,424	46	1,597
300-399	1	359	14,970	115,180	163,154	88.0	316	447	7.7	16,650	67,724	59,910	127,634	42	1,677
400-499	1	436	14,453	116,182	160,747	72.9	318	440	8.0	17,410	60,620	69,014	129,634	12	908
500 or more	1	719	26,776	211,186	274,766	80.5	579	753	7.9	17,713	89,338	79,360	168,698	0	0
Nongovernment not-for-profit	12	3,180	126,730	921,295	1,273,481	79.4	2,524	3,491	7.3	101,267	472,999	680,688	1,153,687	195	15,896
Investor-owned (for-profit)	0	0	0	0	0	00.0	0	0	0.0	0	0	0	0	0	0
State and local government	0	0	0	0	0	00.0	0	0	0.0	0	0	0	0	0	0

CLASSIFICATION	FULL-TIME EQUIVALENT PERSONNEL: Physicians and Dentists	Registered Nurses	Licensed Practical Nurses	Other Salaried Personnel	Total Personnel	FULL-TIME EQUIVALENT TRAINEES: Medical and Dental Residents	Other Trainees	Total Trainees	EXPENSES: LABOR: Payroll (in thousands)	Employee Benefits (in thousands)	Total (in thousands)	Percent of Total	TOTAL: Amount (in thousands)	Adjusted, per Admission	Adjusted, per Inpatient Day
RHODE ISLAND	482	3,809	850	13,300	18,441	571	23	594	$ 535,011	$ 121,302	$ 656,313	63.1	$ 1,040,695		
6-24 beds	0	0	0	0	0	0	0	0	0	0	0	0.0	0		
25-49	0	0	0	0	0	0	0	0	0	0	0	0.0	0		
50-99	53	140	18	927	1,138	27	19	46	25,577	4,540	30,118	67.1	44,851		
100-199	112	1,044	117	3,617	4,890	104	0	104	141,327	33,714	175,041	62.7	279,297		
200-299	125	933	166	3,378	4,602	123	4	127	138,647	30,756	169,403	61.9	273,551		
300-399	33	511	309	1,424	2,277	0	0	0	64,427	20,473	84,900	66.1	128,360		
400-499	20	360	173	1,159	1,712	0	0	0	50,461	11,717	62,178	69.0	90,143		
500 or more	139	821	67	2,795	3,822	317	0	317	114,571	20,102	134,673	60.0	224,493		
Psychiatric	28	198	7	981	1,214	49	19	68	36,810	10,809	47,618	71.7	66,451		
Hospitals	28	198	7	981	1,214	49	19	68	36,810	10,809	47,618	71.7	66,451		
Institutions for mentally retarded	0	0	0	0	0	0	0	0	0	0	0	0.0	0		
General	387	3,179	751	10,481	14,798	492	4	496	426,603	85,561	512,165	61.5	832,144		
Hospitals	387	3,179	751	10,481	14,798	492	4	496	426,603	85,561	512,165	61.5	832,144		
Hospital units of institutions	0	0	0	0	0	0	0	0	0	0	0	0.0	0		
TB and other respiratory diseases	0	0	0	0	0	0	0	0	0	0	0	0.0	0		
Obstetrics and gynecology	35	320	21	893	1,274	16	0	16	39,090	8,940	48,030	62.6	76,756		
Eye, ear, nose, and throat	0	0	0	0	0	0	0	0	0	0	0	0.0	0		
Rehabilitation	0	0	0	0	0	0	0	0	0	0	0	0.0	0		
Orthopedic	0	0	0	0	0	0	0	0	0	0	0	0.0	0		
Chronic disease	27	80	54	625	787	0	0	0	22,962	12,028	34,991	73.7	47,472		
All other	5	32	17	314	368	14	0	14	9,545	3,964	13,509	75.6	17,873		
Federal	96	204	33	1,040	1,373	39	4	43	38,466	6,610	45,076	70.1	64,304		
Psychiatric	0	0	0	0	0	0	0	0	0	0	0	0.0	0		
General and other special	96	204	33	1,040	1,373	39	4	43	38,466	6,610	45,076	70.1	64,304		
Nonfederal	386	3,605	817	12,260	17,068	532	19	551	496,545	114,692	611,237	62.6	976,392		
Psychiatric	28	198	7	981	1,214	49	19	68	36,810	10,809	47,618	71.7	66,451		
Hospitals	28	198	7	981	1,214	49	19	68	36,810	10,809	47,618	71.7	66,451		
Institutions for mentally retarded	0	0	0	0	0	0	0	0	0	0	0	0.0	0		
TB and other respiratory diseases	0	0	0	0	0	0	0	0	0	0	0	0.0	0		
Long-term general and other special	32	112	71	940	1,155	14	0	14	32,507	15,992	48,500	74.2	65,345		
Short-term general and other special	326	3,295	739	10,339	14,699	469	0	469	427,227	87,891	515,118	61.0	844,596		
Hospital units of institutions	0	0	0	0	0	0	0	0	0	0	0	0.0	0		
Community hospitals*	326	3,295	739	10,339	14,699	469	0	469	427,227	87,891	515,118	61.0	844,596	$4,838.68	$ 663.22
6-24 beds	0	0	0	0	0	0	0	0	0	0	0	0.0	0	0.00	0.00
25-49	0	0	0	0	0	0	0	0	0	0	0	0.0	0	0.00	0.00
50-99	0	47	9	172	228	12	0	12	6,885	953	7,838	53.1	14,751	3,561.38	482.04
100-199	97	892	110	2,939	4,038	70	0	70	116,307	25,005	141,312	61.1	231,156	4,469.71	728.74
200-299	64	744	125	2,476	3,409	70	0	70	97,538	21,669	119,207	58.7	203,165	4,763.09	621.27
300-399	6	431	255	798	1,490	0	0	0	41,465	8,445	49,910	61.7	80,888	3,814.56	495.78
400-499	20	360	173	1,159	1,712	0	0	0	50,461	11,717	62,178	69.0	90,143	4,507.84	560.78
500 or more	139	821	67	2,795	3,822	317	0	317	114,571	20,102	134,673	60.0	224,493	6,444.10	817.03
Nongovernment not-for-profit	326	3,295	739	10,339	14,699	469	0	469	427,227	87,891	515,118	61.0	844,596	4,838.68	663.22
Investor-owned (for-profit)	0	0	0	0	0	0	0	0	0	0	0	0.0	0	0.00	0.00
State and local government	0	0	0	0	0	0	0	0	0	0	0	0.0	0	0.00	0.00

*For information on community hospitals that excludes nursing-home-type data, refer to Hospital Units columns in tables 4A through 4D, pages 14 through 17.

(continued on next page)

Table
5C (Continued) South Carolina

Utilization, Personnel, and Finances in States
Excludes AHA nonregistered hospitals (see Table 14, page 240).

CLASSIFICATION	HOSPITALS	BEDS	ADMISSIONS	INPATIENT DAYS	ADJUSTED PATIENT DAYS	OCCUPANCY, percent	AVERAGE DAILY CENSUS	ADJUSTED AVERAGE DAILY CENSUS	AVERAGE STAY, days	SURGICAL OPERATIONS	OUTPATIENT VISITS: Emergency	OUTPATIENT VISITS: Other	OUTPATIENT VISITS: Total	NEWBORNS: Bassinets	NEWBORNS: Births
SOUTH CAROLINA	89	14,550	460,309	3,799,785		71.7	10,427			325,867	1,429,520	3,251,296	4,680,816	985	55,577
6-24 beds	2	30	1,068	4,039		36.7	11			623	10,398	61,516	71,914	0	0
25-49	14	554	13,707	110,710		54.5	302			6,307	85,736	203,033	288,769	28	499
50-99	24	1,729	49,129	355,797		56.4	975			29,346	173,496	371,567	545,063	175	5,571
100-199	26	3,561	113,677	866,474		67.0	2,387			86,651	494,035	1,019,820	1,513,855	287	11,548
200-299	10	2,447	85,366	653,383		73.3	1,793			64,176	247,922	322,223	570,145	155	9,152
300-399	3	980	41,826	262,853		73.6	721			25,674	106,533	160,626	267,159	74	6,613
400-499	3	1,251	52,565	352,735		77.2	966			38,604	116,165	278,110	394,275	94	6,976
500 or more	7	3,998	102,971	1,193,794		81.8	3,272			74,486	195,235	834,401	1,029,636	172	15,218
Psychiatric	10	1,969	9,446	567,619		79.0	1,556			0	102	17,175	17,277	0	0
Hospitals	10	1,969	9,446	567,619		79.0	1,556			0	102	17,175	17,277	0	0
Institutions for mentally retarded	0	0	0	0		00.0	0			0	0	0	0	0	0
General	76	12,382	449,319	3,204,909		71.0	8,797			323,540	1,429,418	3,155,256	4,584,674	985	55,577
Hospitals	73	12,243	446,994	3,193,052		71.6	8,764			323,512	1,425,785	3,150,318	4,576,103	979	55,499
Hospital units of institutions	3	139	2,325	11,857		23.7	33			28	3,633	4,938	8,571	6	78
TB and other respiratory diseases	0	0	0	0		00.0	0			0	0	0	0	0	0
Obstetrics and gynecology	0	0	0	0		00.0	0			0	0	0	0	0	0
Eye, ear, nose, and throat	0	0	0	0		00.0	0			0	0	0	0	0	0
Rehabilitation	2	139	660	16,135		31.7	44			0	0	69,330	69,330	0	0
Orthopedic	1	60	884	11,122		50.0	30			2,327	0	9,535	9,535	0	0
Chronic disease	0	0	0	0		00.0	0			0	0	0	0	0	0
All other	0	0	0	0		00.0	0			0	0	0	0	0	0
Federal	7	1,234	35,493	320,455		71.2	878			38,740	128,216	1,090,120	1,218,336	60	1,895
Psychiatric	0	0	0	0		00.0	0			0	0	0	0	0	0
General and other special	7	1,234	35,493	320,455		71.2	878			38,740	128,216	1,090,120	1,218,336	60	1,895
Nonfederal	82	13,316	424,816	3,479,330		71.7	9,549			287,127	1,301,304	2,161,176	3,462,480	925	53,682
Psychiatric	10	1,969	9,446	567,619		79.0	1,556			0	102	17,175	17,277	0	0
Hospitals	10	1,969	9,446	567,619		79.0	1,556			0	102	17,175	17,277	0	0
Institutions for mentally retarded	0	0	0	0		00.0	0			0	0	0	0	0	0
TB and other respiratory diseases	0	0	0	0		00.0	0			0	0	0	0	0	0
Long-term general and other special	0	0	0	0		00.0	0			0	0	0	0	0	0
Short-term general and other special	72	11,347	415,370	2,911,711		70.4	7,993			287,127	1,301,202	2,144,001	3,445,203	925	53,682
Hospital units of institutions	3	139	2,325	11,857		23.7	33			28	3,633	4,938	8,571	6	78
Community hospitals*	69	11,208	413,045	2,899,854	3,792,993	71.0	7,960	10,411	7.0	287,099	1,297,569	2,139,063	3,436,632	919	53,604
6-24 beds	1	15	181	1,405	1,632	26.7	4	4	7.8	0	0	0	0	0	0
25-49	10	408	10,543	81,709	124,809	54.7	223	342	7.8	5,116	65,309	90,319	155,628	23	199
50-99	17	1,212	40,304	253,005	361,445	57.1	692	990	6.3	28,159	155,242	283,214	438,456	146	5,170
100-199	23	3,146	95,793	778,152	1,065,462	68.2	2,145	2,937	8.1	71,001	420,880	429,067	849,947	255	10,276
200-299	8	1,937	78,347	517,437	673,255	73.3	1,420	1,844	6.6	61,287	238,205	234,647	472,852	155	9,152
300-399	3	980	41,826	262,853	329,933	73.6	721	904	6.3	25,674	106,533	160,626	267,159	74	6,613
400-499	3	1,251	52,565	352,735	444,679	77.2	966	1,220	6.7	38,604	116,165	278,110	394,275	94	6,976
500 or more	4	2,259	93,486	652,558	791,778	79.2	1,789	2,170	7.0	57,258	195,235	663,080	858,315	172	15,218
Nongovernment not-for-profit	29	5,666	216,692	1,539,990	2,030,774	74.5	4,219	5,566	7.1	154,072	591,959	1,220,529	1,812,488	433	27,168
Investor-owned (for-profit)	11	1,631	57,673	330,517	432,663	55.6	907	1,185	5.7	45,969	218,165	189,710	407,875	146	8,114
State and local government	29	3,911	138,680	1,029,347	1,329,556	72.5	2,834	3,660	7.4	87,058	487,445	728,824	1,216,269	340	18,322

Table 5C (Continued) South Carolina

CLASSIFICATION	FULL-TIME EQUIVALENT PERSONNEL					FULL-TIME EQUIVALENT TRAINEES			EXPENSES						
									LABOR				TOTAL		
	Physicians and Dentists	Registered Nurses	Licensed Practical Nurses	Other Salaried Personnel	Total Personnel	Medical and Dental Residents	Other Trainees	Total Trainees	Payroll (in thousands)	Employee Benefits (in thousands)	Total (in thousands)	Percent of Total	Amount (in thousands)	Adjusted, per Admission	Adjusted, per Inpatient Day
SOUTH CAROLINA	521	10,853	3,268	34,801	49,443	925	158	1,083	$ 1,189,122	$ 222,470	$ 1,411,592	53.3	$ 2,649,885		
6-24 beds	14	22	8	151	195	0	0	0	2,785	629	3,414	68.8	4,960		
25-49	28	264	127	1,244	1,663	0	0	0	30,677	6,293	36,970	58.0	63,688		
50-99	44	995	303	3,674	5,016	7	4	11	107,644	20,241	127,885	54.7	233,618		
100-199	168	2,333	968	7,538	11,007	24	25	49	259,992	41,984	301,976	53.5	564,888		
200-299	72	2,042	467	5,919	8,500	67	40	107	202,760	40,331	243,091	51.4	473,304		
300-399	15	913	290	2,802	4,020	35	24	59	98,118	19,393	117,511	51.3	229,029		
400-499	9	1,214	331	3,905	5,459	19	15	34	122,500	17,808	140,308	50.5	277,701		
500 or more	171	3,070	774	9,568	13,583	773	50	823	364,646	75,791	440,438	54.9	802,697		
Psychiatric	76	402	149	2,374	3,001	38	1	39	87,206	20,850	108,055	71.0	152,110		
Hospitals	76	402	149	2,374	3,001	38	1	39	87,206	20,850	108,055	71.0	152,110		
Institutions for mentally retarded	0	0	0	0	0	0	0	0	0	0	0	0.0	0		
General	431	10,341	3,103	32,001	45,876	880	157	1,037	1,088,721	199,234	1,287,955	52.0	2,474,769		
Hospitals	431	10,302	3,086	31,856	45,675	880	157	1,037	1,086,644	198,570	1,285,214	52.1	2,468,883		
Hospital units of institutions	0	39	17	145	201	0	0	0	2,077	665	2,741	46.6	5,887		
TB and other respiratory diseases	0	0	0	0	0	0	0	0	0	0	0	0.0	0		
Obstetrics and gynecology	0	0	0	0	0	0	0	0	0	0	0	0.0	0		
Eye, ear, nose, and throat	0	0	0	0	0	0	0	0	0	0	0	0.0	0		
Rehabilitation	3	58	16	262	339	0	0	0	8,244	1,410	9,654	80.7	11,964		
Orthopedic	11	52	0	164	227	7	0	7	4,951	976	5,927	53.7	11,041		
Chronic disease	0	0	0	0	0	0	0	0	0	0	0	0.0	0		
All other	0	0	0	0	0	0	0	0	0	0	0	0.0	0		
Federal	338	649	228	3,992	5,207	91	5	96	152,020	18,650	170,670	66.9	254,964		
Psychiatric	0	0	0	0	0	0	0	0	0	0	0	0.0	0		
General and other special	338	649	228	3,992	5,207	91	5	96	152,020	18,650	170,670	66.9	254,964		
Nonfederal	183	10,204	3,040	30,809	44,236	834	153	987	1,037,103	203,820	1,240,922	51.8	2,394,920		
Psychiatric	76	402	149	2,374	3,001	38	1	39	87,206	20,850	108,055	71.0	152,110		
Hospitals	76	402	149	2,374	3,001	38	1	39	87,206	20,850	108,055	71.0	152,110		
Institutions for mentally retarded	0	0	0	0	0	0	0	0	0	0	0	0.0	0		
TB and other respiratory diseases	0	0	0	0	0	0	0	0	0	0	0	0.0	0		
Long-term general and other special	0	0	0	0	0	0	0	0	0	0	0	0.0	0		
Short-term general and other special	107	9,802	2,891	28,435	41,235	796	152	948	949,897	182,970	1,132,867	50.5	2,242,810		
Hospital units of institutions	0	39	17	145	201	0	0	0	2,077	665	2,741	46.6	5,887		
Community hospitals*	107	9,763	2,874	28,290	41,034	796	152	948	947,820	182,305	1,130,126	50.5	2,236,923	$4,167.57	$ 589.75
6-24 beds	0	2	4	4	10	0	0	0	227	59	287	57.5	498	2,372.50	305.28
25-49	1	189	100	810	1,100	0	0	0	20,173	3,754	23,927	54.7	43,767	2,740.90	350.67
50-99	21	797	274	2,696	3,788	7	4	11	79,663	14,976	94,639	53.2	178,036	3,109.19	492.57
100-199	2	2,077	857	5,857	8,793	0	25	25	182,650	36,874	219,524	49.3	445,466	3,444.97	418.10
200-299	1	1,835	396	4,960	7,192	0	35	35	162,517	32,596	195,113	48.5	402,085	3,952.59	597.23
300-399	15	913	290	2,802	4,020	35	24	59	98,118	19,393	117,511	51.3	229,029	4,358.72	694.17
400-499	9	1,214	331	3,905	5,459	19	15	34	122,500	17,808	140,308	50.5	277,701	4,183.00	624.50
500 or more	58	2,736	622	7,256	10,672	735	49	784	281,972	56,845	338,817	51.3	660,341	5,826.35	834.00
Nongovernment not-for-profit	67	5,217	1,333	14,638	21,255	163	63	226	506,907	89,002	595,908	51.5	1,157,322	4,082.65	569.89
Investor-owned (for-profit)	3	1,308	397	3,322	5,030	0	0	0	102,554	24,820	127,374	44.1	288,650	3,816.40	667.15
State and local government	37	3,238	1,144	10,330	14,749	633	89	722	338,360	68,484	406,844	51.4	790,951	4,452.60	594.90

*For information on community hospitals that excludes nursing-home-type data, refer to Hospital Units columns in tables 4A through 4D, pages 14 through 17.

(continued on next page)

Table
5C (Continued) South Dakota

Utilization, Personnel, and Finances in States
Excludes AHA nonregistered hospitals (see Table 14, page 240).

CLASSIFICATION	HOSPITALS	BEDS	ADMISSIONS	INPATIENT DAYS	ADJUSTED PATIENT DAYS	OCCUPANCY, percent	AVERAGE DAILY CENSUS	ADJUSTED AVERAGE DAILY CENSUS	AVERAGE STAY, days	SURGICAL OPERATIONS	OUTPATIENT VISITS Emergency	OUTPATIENT VISITS Other	OUTPATIENT VISITS Total	NEWBORNS Bassinets	NEWBORNS Births
SOUTH DAKOTA	66	5,428	114,299	1,260,419		63.6	3,454			64,390	207,710	1,028,503	1,236,213	441	11,229
6-24 beds	12	219	4,040	22,744		28.8	63			592	8,497	69,432	77,929	49	202
25-49	22	759	18,796	95,587		34.4	261			6,463	60,885	388,341	449,226	121	2,179
50-99	18	1,333	16,884	326,278		67.1	895			8,241	35,825	123,049	158,874	104	1,560
100-199	7	875	11,556	242,835		76.0	665			8,976	22,484	147,898	170,382	47	1,194
200-299	4	1,030	29,085	259,640		69.0	711			17,917	47,340	150,434	197,774	64	3,220
300-399	1	349	3,610	95,460		75.1	262			2,814	0	42,353	42,353	0	0
400-499	2	863	30,328	217,875		69.2	597			19,387	32,679	106,996	139,675	56	2,874
500 or more	0	0	0	0		00.0	0			0	0	0	0	0	0
Psychiatric	1	60	620	14,431		66.7	40			0	0	5,854	5,854	0	0
Hospitals	1	60	620	14,431		66.7	40			0	0	5,854	5,854	0	0
Institutions for mentally retarded	0	0	0	0		00.0	0			0	0	0	0	0	0
General	63	5,221	113,170	1,206,495		63.3	3,306			64,390	207,710	1,009,354	1,217,064	441	11,229
Hospitals	63	5,221	113,170	1,206,495		63.3	3,306			64,390	207,710	1,009,354	1,217,064	441	11,229
Hospital units of institutions	0	0	0	0		00.0	0			0	0	0	0	0	0
TB and other respiratory diseases	0	0	0	0		00.0	0			0	0	0	0	0	0
Obstetrics and gynecology	0	0	0	0		00.0	0			0	0	0	0	0	0
Eye, ear, nose, and throat	0	0	0	0		00.0	0			0	0	0	0	0	0
Rehabilitation	2	147	509	39,493		73.5	108			0	0	13,295	13,295	0	0
Orthopedic	0	0	0	0		00.0	0			0	0	0	0	0	0
Chronic disease	0	0	0	0		00.0	0			0	0	0	0	0	0
All other	0	0	0	0		00.0	0			0	0	0	0	0	0
Federal	10	1,016	19,193	242,538		65.6	667			8,872	36,311	519,035	555,346	39	1,162
Psychiatric	0	0	0	0		00.0	0			0	0	0	0	0	0
General and other special	10	1,016	19,193	242,538		65.6	667			8,872	36,311	519,035	555,346	39	1,162
Nonfederal	56	4,412	95,106	1,017,881		63.2	2,787			55,518	171,399	509,468	680,867	402	10,067
Psychiatric	1	60	620	14,431		66.7	40			0	0	5,854	5,854	0	0
Hospitals	1	60	620	14,431		66.7	40			0	0	5,854	5,854	0	0
Institutions for mentally retarded	0	0	0	0		00.0	0			0	0	0	0	0	0
TB and other respiratory diseases	0	0	0	0		00.0	0			0	0	0	0	0	0
Long-term general and other special	2	152	65	50,936		92.1	140			0	416	2,346	2,762	0	0
Short-term general and other special	53	4,200	94,421	952,514		62.1	2,607			55,518	170,983	501,268	672,251	402	10,067
Hospital units of institutions	0	0	0	0		00.0	0			0	0	0	0	0	0
Community hospitals*	53	4,200	94,421	952,514	1,215,750	62.1	2,607	3,329	10.1	55,518	170,983	501,268	672,251	402	10,067
6-24 beds	10	178	3,363	19,902	28,142	29.8	53	76	5.9	592	7,853	22,875	30,728	44	197
25-49	17	583	11,187	70,739	99,108	33.1	193	270	6.3	4,952	25,218	86,823	112,041	87	1,022
50-99	15	1,121	16,199	260,911	338,915	63.8	715	930	16.1	8,241	35,409	114,849	150,258	104	1,560
100-199	6	706	8,793	201,609	263,744	78.2	552	722	22.9	6,003	22,484	72,141	94,625	47	1,194
200-299	3	749	24,551	181,478	238,623	66.4	497	654	7.4	16,343	47,340	97,584	144,924	64	3,220
300-399	0	0	0	0	0	00.0	0	0	0.0	0	0	0	0	0	0
400-499	2	863	30,328	217,875	247,218	69.2	597	677	7.2	19,387	32,679	106,996	139,675	56	2,874
500 or more	0	0	0	0	0	00.0	0	0	0.0	0	0	0	0	0	0
Nongovernment not-for-profit	45	3,851	89,782	883,597	1,124,275	62.8	2,417	3,079	9.8	53,475	158,197	460,878	619,075	362	9,703
Investor-owned (for-profit)	0	0	0	0	0	00.0	0	0	0.0	0	0	0	0	0	0
State and local government	8	349	4,639	68,917	91,475	54.4	190	250	14.9	2,043	12,786	40,390	53,176	40	364

*For information on community hospitals [illegible] refer to Hospital Unit columns in tables 4A through 4D, pages 14 through 17.

CLASSIFICATION	FULL-TIME EQUIVALENT PERSONNEL					FULL-TIME EQUIVALENT TRAINEES			EXPENSES						
									LABOR				TOTAL		
	Physicians and Dentists	Registered Nurses	Licensed Practical Nurses	Other Salaried Personnel	Total Personnel	Medical and Dental Residents	Other Trainees	Total Trainees	Payroll (in thousands)	Employee Benefits (in thousands)	Total (in thousands)	Percent of Total	Amount (in thousands)	Adjusted, per Admission	Adjusted, per Inpatient Day
SOUTH DAKOTA	161	3,509	521	9,687	13,878	63	25	88	$ 305,792	$ 57,325	$ 363,117	58.6	$ 619,635		
6-24 beds	13	98	27	311	449	0	0	0	9,942	2,121	12,063	61.5	19,627		
25-49	73	366	98	1,405	1,942	0	0	0	37,127	10,051	47,178	64.3	73,318		
50-99	1	425	93	1,657	2,176	0	2	2	39,834	7,095	46,930	56.1	83,661		
100-199	21	238	91	1,279	1,629	0	3	3	33,859	6,423	40,282	63.8	63,142		
200-299	27	760	111	2,066	2,964	33	0	33	75,738	12,601	88,339	56.8	155,451		
300-399	26	85	28	449	588	0	2	2	16,872	3,384	20,256	68.9	29,403		
400-499	0	1,537	73	2,520	4,130	30	18	48	92,419	15,650	108,069	55.4	195,033		
500 or more	0	0	0	0	0	0	0	0	0	0	0	0.0	0		
Psychiatric	0	26	0	85	111	0	0	0	2,423	482	2,905	50.2	5,783		
Hospitals	0	26	0	85	111	0	0	0	2,423	482	2,905	50.2	5,783		
Institutions for mentally retarded	0	0	0	0	0	0	0	0	0	0	0	0.0	0		
General	161	3,455	505	9,333	13,454	63	25	88	298,739	55,985	354,723	58.6	604,897		
Hospitals	161	3,455	505	9,333	13,454	63	25	88	298,739	55,985	354,723	58.6	604,897		
Hospital units of institutions	0	0	0	0	0	0	0	0	0	0	0	0.0	0		
TB and other respiratory diseases	0	0	0	0	0	0	0	0	0	0	0	0.0	0		
Obstetrics and gynecology	0	0	0	0	0	0	0	0	0	0	0	0.0	0		
Eye, ear, nose, and throat	0	0	0	0	0	0	0	0	0	0	0	0.0	0		
Rehabilitation	0	28	16	269	313	0	0	0	4,630	859	5,489	61.3	8,954		
Orthopedic	0	0	0	0	0	0	0	0	0	0	0	0.0	0		
Chronic disease	0	0	0	0	0	0	0	0	0	0	0	0.0	0		
All other	0	0	0	0	0	0	0	0	0	0	0	0.0	0		
Federal	155	435	135	1,968	2,693	33	5	38	73,837	18,343	92,180	69.4	132,807		
Psychiatric	0	0	0	0	0	0	0	0	0	0	0	0.0	0		
General and other special	155	435	135	1,968	2,693	33	5	38	73,837	18,343	92,180	69.4	132,807		
Nonfederal	6	3,074	386	7,719	11,185	30	20	50	231,955	38,982	270,938	55.7	486,828		
Psychiatric	0	26	0	85	111	0	0	0	2,423	482	2,905	50.2	5,783		
Hospitals	0	26	0	85	111	0	0	0	2,423	482	2,905	50.2	5,783		
Institutions for mentally retarded	0	0	0	0	0	0	0	0	0	0	0	0.0	0		
TB and other respiratory diseases	0	0	0	0	0	0	0	0	0	0	0	0.0	0		
Long-term general and other special	0	21	8	261	290	0	0	0	3,523	710	4,232	67.5	6,271		
Short-term general and other special	6	3,027	378	7,373	10,784	30	20	50	226,009	37,791	263,800	55.6	474,773		
Hospital units of institutions	0	0	0	0	0	0	0	0	0	0	0	0.0	0		
Community hospitals*	6	3,027	378	7,373	10,784	30	20	50	226,009	37,791	263,800	55.6	474,773	$3,904.51	$ 390.52
6-24 beds	4	71	24	229	328	0	0	0	5,248	754	6,003	53.0	11,328	2,240.00	402.52
25-49	1	210	63	745	1,019	0	0	0	17,055	2,944	19,998	58.0	34,462	2,162.24	347.72
50-99	1	378	85	1,311	1,775	0	2	2	33,888	5,904	39,792	55.6	71,606	3,290.72	211.28
100-199	0	181	65	906	1,152	0	0	0	19,594	3,620	23,214	58.4	39,727	3,340.61	150.63
200-299	0	650	68	1,662	2,380	0	0	0	57,805	8,919	66,724	54.4	122,618	3,772.51	513.86
300-399	0	0	0	0	0	0	0	0	0	0	0	0.0	0	0.00	0.00
400-499	0	1,537	73	2,520	4,130	30	18	48	92,419	15,650	108,069	55.4	195,033	5,661.99	788.91
500 or more	0	0	0	0	0	0	0	0	0	0	0	0.0	0	0.00	0.00
Nongovernment not-for-profit	5	2,936	353	6,987	10,281	30	20	50	217,199	36,276	253,475	55.4	457,830	3,973.04	407.22
Investor-owned (for-profit)	0	0	0	0	0	0	0	0	0	0	0	0.0	0	0.00	0.00
State and local government	1	91	25	386	503	0	0	0	8,811	1,514	10,325	60.9	16,943	2,663.23	185.22

*For information on community hospitals that excludes nursing-home-type data, refer to Hospital Units columns in tables 4A through 4D, pages 14 through 17.

(continued on next page)

Table
5C (Continued) Tennessee

Utilization, Personnel, and Finances in States
Excludes AHA nonregistered hospitals (see Table 14, page 240).

CLASSIFICATION	HOSPITALS	BEDS	ADMISSIONS	INPATIENT DAYS	ADJUSTED PATIENT DAYS	OCCUPANCY, percent	AVERAGE DAILY CENSUS	ADJUSTED AVERAGE DAILY CENSUS	AVERAGE STAY, days	SURGICAL OPERATIONS	OUTPATIENT VISITS Emergency	OUTPATIENT VISITS Other	OUTPATIENT VISITS Total	NEWBORNS Bassinets	NEWBORNS Births
TENNESSEE	156	29,480	850,816	7,265,984		67.6	19,917			549,897	2,266,720	3,775,447	6,042,167	1,551	75,717
6-24 beds	1	23	310	2,409		30.4	7			351	904	444	1,348	0	0
25-49	22	854	24,706	151,872		48.9	418			9,944	79,859	177,714	257,573	65	620
50-99	48	3,511	91,734	591,829		46.4	1,629			46,009	400,851	385,097	785,948	268	5,197
100-199	44	6,167	178,466	1,373,590		61.0	3,764			105,406	615,603	976,936	1,592,539	405	16,927
200-299	13	3,067	95,455	757,011		67.6	2,073			70,726	254,480	340,462	594,942	184	7,214
300-399	7	2,365	65,983	656,593		76.1	1,799			57,235	148,711	347,316	496,027	50	1,522
400-499	7	3,073	101,977	887,470		79.2	2,433			59,330	249,495	409,293	658,788	199	14,425
500 or more	14	10,420	292,185	2,845,210		74.8	7,794			200,896	516,817	1,138,185	1,655,002	380	29,812
Psychiatric	14	2,771	17,786	866,440		85.8	2,377			0	2,080	66,660	68,740	0	0
Hospitals	14	2,771	17,786	866,440		85.8	2,377			0	2,080	66,660	68,740	0	0
Institutions for mentally retarded	0	0	0	0		00.0	0			0	0	0	0	0	0
General	137	25,947	830,160	6,196,608		65.5	16,984			547,525	2,262,214	3,673,136	5,935,350	1,537	75,679
Hospitals	136	25,842	828,996	6,173,636		65.5	16,921			547,098	2,257,873	3,600,516	5,858,389	1,537	75,679
Hospital units of institutions	1	105	1,164	22,972		60.0	63			427	4,341	72,620	76,961	0	0
TB and other respiratory diseases	0	0	0	0		00.0	0			0	0	0	0	0	0
Obstetrics and gynecology	0	0	0	0		00.0	0			0	0	0	0	0	0
Eye, ear, nose, and throat	0	0	0	0		00.0	0			0	0	0	0	0	0
Rehabilitation	2	125	596	18,632		40.8	51			0	1,261	11,615	12,876	0	0
Orthopedic	0	0	0	0		00.0	0			0	0	0	0	0	0
Chronic disease	1	550	178	172,458		85.8	472			0	0	0	0	0	0
All other	2	87	2,096	11,846		37.9	33			2,372	1,165	24,036	25,201	14	38
Federal	5	2,492	33,290	671,749		73.9	1,841			17,963	76,529	613,527	690,056	24	492
Psychiatric	0	0	0	0		00.0	0			0	0	0	0	0	0
General and other special	5	2,492	33,290	671,749		73.9	1,841			17,963	76,529	613,527	690,056	24	492
Nonfederal	151	26,988	817,526	6,594,235		67.0	18,076			531,934	2,190,191	3,161,920	5,352,111	1,527	75,225
Psychiatric	14	2,771	17,786	866,440		85.8	2,377			0	2,080	66,660	68,740	0	0
Hospitals	14	2,771	17,786	866,440		85.8	2,377			0	2,080	66,660	68,740	0	0
Institutions for mentally retarded	0	0	0	0		00.0	0			0	0	0	0	0	0
TB and other respiratory diseases	0	0	0	0		00.0	0			0	0	0	0	0	0
Long-term general and other special	2	595	404	180,063		82.9	493			0	0	10,040	10,040	0	0
Short-term general and other special	135	23,622	799,336	5,547,732		64.4	15,206			531,934	2,188,111	3,085,220	5,273,331	1,527	75,225
Hospital units of institutions	1	105	1,164	22,972		60.0	63			427	4,341	72,620	76,961	0	0
Community hospitals*	134	23,517	798,172	5,524,760	7,036,047	64.4	15,143	19,285	6.9	531,507	2,183,770	3,012,600	5,196,370	1,527	75,225
6-24 beds	1	23	310	2,409	3,309	30.4	7	9	7.8	351	904	444	1,348	0	0
25-49	19	734	23,536	126,552	187,061	47.4	348	511	5.4	9,944	78,794	108,534	187,328	65	620
50-99	44	3,227	86,188	517,824	723,709	44.2	1,425	1,990	6.0	42,916	346,185	304,354	650,539	244	4,705
100-199	39	5,497	173,142	1,175,429	1,627,543	58.6	3,220	4,461	6.8	104,979	610,247	896,796	1,507,043	405	16,927
200-299	11	2,554	91,172	595,517	806,745	63.8	1,630	2,210	6.5	70,726	254,480	340,462	594,942	184	7,214
300-399	5	1,641	56,714	424,475	515,943	70.9	1,163	1,415	7.5	51,549	148,711	229,244	377,955	50	1,522
400-499	5	2,127	93,115	597,859	731,704	77.1	1,639	2,005	6.4	55,480	239,111	271,389	510,500	199	14,425
500 or more	10	7,714	273,995	2,084,695	2,440,033	74.0	5,711	6,684	7.6	195,562	505,338	861,377	1,366,715	380	29,812
Nongovernment not-for-profit	56	13,427	477,683	3,421,860	4,231,239	69.8	9,376	11,595	7.2	324,452	1,157,194	1,638,152	2,795,346	802	44,165
Investor-owned (for-profit)	46	4,705	140,841	853,163	1,134,898	49.6	2,336	3,107	6.1	90,031	446,860	495,269	942,129	288	10,407
State and local government	32	5,385	179,648	1,249,737	1,669,910	63.7	3,431	4,583	7.0	117,024	579,716	879,179	1,458,895	437	20,653

*For information on community hospitals that excludes nursing home type data, refer to Hospital Units columns in tables 4A through 4D, pages 14 through 17.

CLASSIFICATION	Full-Time Equivalent Personnel: Physicians and Dentists	Registered Nurses	Licensed Practical Nurses	Other Salaried Personnel	Total Personnel	Full-Time Equivalent Trainees: Medical and Dental Residents	Other Trainees	Total Trainees	Expenses: Labor: Payroll (in thousands)	Employee Benefits (in thousands)	Total (in thousands)	Percent of Total	Total: Amount (in thousands)	Adjusted, per Admission	Adjusted, per Inpatient Day
TENNESSEE	675	19,837	6,544	65,416	92,472	964	262	1,226	$ 2,160,091	$ 432,569	$ 2,592,661	51.7	$ 5,013,968		
6-24 beds	0	10	4	35	49	2	0	2	773	134	907	46.6	1,947		
25-49	8	562	298	2,552	3,420	1	26	27	45,253	9,266	54,519	50.8	107,325		
50-99	56	1,396	940	5,471	7,863	5	2	7	151,559	31,198	182,756	47.4	385,386		
100-199	52	3,238	1,699	10,982	15,971	4	17	21	341,726	74,963	416,689	49.5	841,770		
200-299	46	2,330	632	7,253	10,261	12	9	21	228,443	45,198	273,641	52.0	526,546		
300-399	94	1,570	407	5,701	7,772	109	5	114	190,656	38,815	229,470	52.4	438,234		
400-499	78	2,548	890	8,063	11,579	63	82	145	282,708	56,077	338,785	51.6	656,237		
500 or more	341	8,183	1,674	25,359	35,557	768	121	889	918,973	176,919	1,095,893	53.3	2,056,523		
Psychiatric	95	595	145	4,180	5,015	4	1	5	112,548	28,450	140,998	69.7	202,241		
Hospitals	95	595	145	4,180	5,015	4	1	5	112,548	28,450	140,998	69.7	202,241		
Institutions for mentally retarded	0	0	0	0	0	0	0	0	0	0	0	0.0	0		
General	572	18,931	6,262	59,449	85,214	959	235	1,194	2,023,214	396,694	2,419,908	50.8	4,759,407		
Hospitals	551	18,890	6,223	59,343	85,007	959	235	1,194	2,019,318	395,576	2,414,894	50.9	4,745,700		
Hospital units of institutions	21	41	39	106	207	0	0	0	3,897	1,118	5,015	36.6	13,707		
TB and other respiratory diseases	0	0	0	0	0	0	0	0	0	0	0	0.0	0		
Obstetrics and gynecology	0	0	0	0	0	0	0	0	0	0	0	0.0	0		
Eye, ear, nose, and throat	0	0	0	0	0	0	0	0	0	0	0	0.0	0		
Rehabilitation	0	41	15	229	285	0	0	0	4,937	1,040	5,978	44.1	13,547		
Orthopedic	0	0	0	0	0	0	0	0	0	0	0	0.0	0		
Chronic disease	3	9	23	532	567	0	0	0	11,883	4,931	16,813	79.2	21,234		
All other	5	261	99	1,026	1,391	1	26	27	7,509	1,454	8,963	51.1	17,539		
Federal	350	979	222	4,972	6,523	272	29	301	175,091	34,268	209,359	66.5	314,845		
Psychiatric	0	0	0	0	0	0	0	0	0	0	0	0.0	0		
General and other special	350	979	222	4,972	6,523	272	29	301	175,091	34,268	209,359	66.5	314,845		
Nonfederal	325	18,858	6,322	60,444	85,949	692	233	925	1,985,001	398,301	2,383,302	50.7	4,699,123		
Psychiatric	95	595	145	4,180	5,015	4	1	5	112,548	28,450	140,998	69.7	202,241		
Hospitals	95	595	145	4,180	5,015	4	1	5	112,548	28,450	140,998	69.7	202,241		
Institutions for mentally retarded	0	0	0	0	0	0	0	0	0	0	0	0.0	0		
TB and other respiratory diseases	0	0	0	0	0	0	0	0	0	0	0	0.0	0		
Long-term general and other special	3	25	27	677	732	0	0	0	13,990	5,338	19,328	71.7	26,962		
Short-term general and other special	227	18,238	6,150	55,587	80,202	688	232	920	1,858,462	364,513	2,222,975	49.7	4,469,920		
Hospital units of institutions	21	41	39	106	207	0	0	0	3,897	1,118	5,015	36.6	13,707		
Community hospitals*	206	18,197	6,111	55,431	79,995	688	232	920	1,854,566	363,395	2,217,961	49.8	4,456,213	$4,339.98	$ 633.34
6-24 beds	0	10	4	35	49	2	0	2	773	134	907	46.6	1,947	4,570.61	588.42
25-49	8	510	292	2,192	3,002	1	26	27	37,202	7,940	45,142	49.4	91,393	2,532.01	488.57
50-99	4	1,200	906	4,664	6,774	4	1	5	130,380	26,850	157,230	45.7	344,179	2,834.75	475.58
100-199	6	3,055	1,625	9,900	14,586	1	17	18	310,339	65,234	375,573	48.9	768,391	3,215.47	472.12
200-299	21	2,221	608	6,490	9,340	11	9	20	209,624	40,733	250,356	50.4	496,562	4,017.26	615.51
300-399	1	1,299	321	4,383	6,004	0	0	0	141,902	27,810	169,713	48.9	346,745	4,993.95	672.06
400-499	1	2,276	821	6,351	9,449	0	78	78	230,506	45,213	275,719	48.9	564,265	4,957.43	771.17
500 or more	165	7,626	1,534	21,466	30,791	669	101	770	793,840	149,482	943,322	51.2	1,842,732	5,704.72	755.21
Nongovernment not-for-profit	83	11,664	3,408	35,576	50,731	497	184	681	1,187,921	232,566	1,420,486	50.7	2,799,702	4,688.47	661.67
Investor-owned (for-profit)	4	2,627	1,148	7,769	11,548	3	1	4	266,224	58,221	324,446	42.3	766,759	4,051.63	675.62
State and local government	119	3,906	1,555	12,136	17,716	188	47	235	400,421	72,608	473,028	53.2	889,752	3,701.29	532.81

*For information on community hospitals that excludes nursing-home-type data, refer to Hospital Units columns in tables 4A through 4D, pages 14 through 17.

(continued on next page)

Table
5C (Continued) Texas

Utilization, Personnel, and Finances in States
Excludes AHA nonregistered hospitals (see Table 14, page 240).

CLASSIFICATION	HOSPITALS	BEDS	ADMISSIONS	INPATIENT DAYS	ADJUSTED PATIENT DAYS	OCCUPANCY, percent	AVERAGE DAILY CENSUS	ADJUSTED AVERAGE DAILY CENSUS	AVERAGE STAY, days	SURGICAL OPERATIONS	OUTPATIENT VISITS Emergency	OUTPATIENT VISITS Other	OUTPATIENT VISITS Total	NEWBORNS Bassinets	NEWBORNS Births
TEXAS	537	79,056	2,227,166	17,365,703		60.3	47,683			1,454,729	5,251,840	13,688,074	18,939,914	5,383	306,182
6-24 beds	42	799	18,064	82,743		28.4	227			9,334	86,832	279,189	366,021	107	1,536
25-49	129	4,871	112,959	630,932		35.6	1,735			43,290	388,614	694,869	1,083,483	449	10,949
50-99	131	9,534	213,773	1,732,065		50.3	4,798			144,282	583,740	857,897	1,441,637	519	23,792
100-199	120	16,942	465,957	3,455,586		56.2	9,517			328,476	1,284,992	2,142,949	3,427,941	1,221	59,917
200-299	48	11,501	371,586	2,483,956		59.2	6,806			287,012	959,629	1,871,022	2,830,651	1,078	47,492
300-399	26	8,928	302,053	2,144,854		65.8	5,875			205,208	632,423	988,782	1,621,205	658	53,362
400-499	12	5,320	176,085	1,259,241		64.8	3,449			118,509	312,370	1,129,117	1,441,487	363	27,293
500 or more	29	21,161	566,689	5,576,326		72.2	15,276			318,618	1,003,240	5,724,249	6,727,489	988	81,841
Psychiatric	75	11,247	72,375	2,748,091		67.2	7,553			1,125	21,469	364,640	386,109	5	177
Hospitals	75	11,247	72,375	2,748,091		67.2	7,553			1,125	21,469	364,640	386,109	5	177
Institutions for mentally retarded	0	0	0	0		00.0	0			0	0	0	0	0	0
General	433	65,107	2,101,466	14,016,372		59.0	38,443			1,425,527	5,176,353	12,616,822	17,793,175	5,260	296,655
Hospitals	431	65,081	2,101,013	14,013,736		59.1	38,436			1,425,463	5,176,064	12,608,284	17,784,348	5,235	296,350
Hospital units of institutions	2	26	453	2,636		26.9	7			64	289	8,538	8,827	25	305
TB and other respiratory diseases	1	115	1,211	29,224		69.6	80			1,806	0	15,790	15,790	0	0
Obstetrics and gynecology	2	311	14,024	52,989		46.6	145			10,593	9,839	42,723	52,562	103	8,050
Eye, ear, nose, and throat	0	0	0	0		00.0	0			0	0	0	0	0	0
Rehabilitation	18	1,226	10,378	268,303		63.1	774			799	9,975	78,435	88,410	0	0
Orthopedic	2	104	2,461	19,157		51.0	53			1,859	0	42,244	42,244	0	0
Chronic disease	0	0	0	0		00.0	0			0	0	0	0	0	0
All other	6	946	25,251	231,567		67.1	635			13,020	34,204	527,420	561,624	15	1,300
Federal	21	8,212	167,791	2,191,754		73.1	6,007			105,155	349,912	4,622,533	4,972,445	191	6,978
Psychiatric	1	799	4,325	250,599		86.0	687			0	0	78,741	78,741	0	0
General and other special	20	7,413	163,466	1,941,155		71.8	5,320			105,155	349,912	4,543,792	4,893,704	191	6,978
Nonfederal	516	70,844	2,059,375	15,173,949		58.8	41,676			1,349,574	4,901,928	9,065,541	13,967,469	5,192	299,204
Psychiatric	74	10,448	68,050	2,497,492		65.7	6,866			1,125	21,469	285,899	307,368	5	177
Hospitals	74	10,448	68,050	2,497,492		65.7	6,866			1,125	21,469	285,899	307,368	5	177
Institutions for mentally retarded	0	0	0	0		00.0	0			0	0	0	0	0	0
TB and other respiratory diseases	1	115	1,211	29,224		69.6	80			1,806	0	15,790	15,790	0	0
Long-term general and other special	11	910	3,402	246,417		75.7	689			760	1,696	27,927	29,623	0	0
Short-term general and other special	430	59,371	1,986,712	12,400,816		57.3	34,041			1,345,883	4,878,763	8,735,925	13,614,688	5,187	299,027
Hospital units of institutions	2	26	453	2,636		26.9	7			64	289	8,538	8,827	25	305
Community hospitals*	428	59,345	1,986,259	12,398,180	15,986,034	57.3	34,034	43,898	6.2	1,345,819	4,878,474	8,727,387	13,605,861	5,162	298,722
6-24 beds	35	695	15,269	66,969	114,958	26.5	184	317	4.4	7,828	55,201	104,721	159,922	75	1,141
25-49	120	4,514	108,301	568,447	812,708	34.6	1,563	2,239	5.2	41,474	356,781	516,930	873,711	430	10,687
50-99	86	6,177	182,647	1,058,734	1,467,098	47.3	2,919	4,045	5.8	141,628	566,789	710,149	1,276,938	514	23,615
100-199	95	13,378	431,533	2,615,583	3,470,817	53.9	7,211	9,567	6.1	320,692	1,235,164	1,549,164	2,784,328	1,189	58,776
200-299	43	10,433	339,511	2,192,513	2,779,930	57.6	6,007	7,617	6.5	243,474	871,221	1,067,388	1,938,609	1,040	45,022
300-399	23	7,899	296,033	1,830,149	2,279,124	63.5	5,013	6,245	6.2	203,337	628,721	930,994	1,559,715	658	53,362
400-499	9	4,033	154,178	903,180	1,089,768	61.3	2,473	2,986	5.9	107,645	251,283	507,934	759,217	338	25,824
500 or more	17	12,216	458,787	3,162,605	3,971,631	70.9	8,664	10,882	6.9	279,741	913,314	3,340,107	4,253,421	918	80,295
Nongovernment not-for-profit	132	26,952	988,368	6,223,209	7,818,676	63.2	17,047	21,418	6.3	697,891	2,166,581	3,600,509	5,767,090	2,045	128,546
Investor-owned (for-profit)	138	18,699	543,951	3,303,349	4,238,814	48.7	9,112	11,702	6.1	425,390	1,246,049	1,644,438	2,890,487	1,369	78,142
State and local government	158	13,694	453,940	2,871,622	3,928,544	57.5	7,875	10,778	6.3	222,538	1,465,844	3,482,440	4,948,284	1,748	92,034

*For information on community hospitals that excludes nursing-home-type data, refer to Hospital Units columns in tables 4A through 4D, pages 14 through 17.

CLASSIFICATION	FULL-TIME EQUIVALENT PERSONNEL					FULL-TIME EQUIVALENT TRAINEES			EXPENSES						
									LABOR				TOTAL		
	Physicians and Dentists	Registered Nurses	Licensed Practical Nurses	Other Salaried Personnel	Total Personnel	Medical and Dental Residents	Other Trainees	Total Trainees	Payroll (in thousands)	Employee Benefits (in thousands)	Total (in thousands)	Percent of Total	Amount (in thousands)	Adjusted, per Admission	Adjusted, per Inpatient Day
TEXAS	2,511	51,348	19,444	175,337	248,940	4,080	741	4,821	$ 6,174,668	$ 1,220,862	$ 7,395,530	51.4	$ 14,387,115		
6-24 beds	44	335	305	1,529	2,213	0	0	0	46,125	9,983	56,108	60.1	93,287		
25-49	78	1,795	1,628	7,797	11,298	2	12	14	213,363	40,762	254,125	52.4	484,714		
50-99	73	4,435	2,381	15,934	22,823	22	0	22	550,185	118,187	668,372	49.3	1,356,232		
100-199	263	10,417	4,078	32,516	47,274	188	45	233	1,167,457	248,815	1,416,272	48.0	2,953,334		
200-299	270	8,324	3,213	25,048	36,855	186	65	251	957,448	179,983	1,137,431	49.2	2,312,849		
300-399	67	6,744	2,404	21,100	30,315	291	28	319	709,266	143,754	853,020	49.6	1,720,731		
400-499	221	3,939	1,117	12,308	17,585	283	56	339	485,311	82,192	567,503	53.3	1,064,557		
500 or more	1,495	15,359	4,318	59,405	80,577	3,108	535	3,643	2,045,512	397,187	2,442,699	55.5	4,401,411		
Psychiatric	282	2,586	944	15,493	19,305	67	37	104	502,758	101,935	604,693	61.7	979,965		
Hospitals	282	2,586	944	15,493	19,305	67	37	104	502,758	101,935	604,693	61.7	979,965		
Institutions for mentally retarded	0	0	0	0	0	0	0	0	0	0	0	0.0	0		
General	1,836	46,802	17,867	150,789	217,294	3,838	376	4,214	5,367,870	1,040,815	6,408,685	50.3	12,728,817		
Hospitals	1,836	46,784	17,851	150,762	217,233	3,838	376	4,214	5,366,811	1,040,616	6,407,426	50.3	12,726,380		
Hospital units of institutions	0	18	16	27	61	0	0	0	1,060	200	1,259	51.7	2,437		
TB and other respiratory diseases	14	44	26	238	322	0	0	0	6,993	866	7,859	65.4	12,019		
Obstetrics and gynecology	0	310	60	430	830	0	0	0	25,569	5,763	31,332	43.0	72,788		
Eye, ear, nose, and throat	0	0	0	0	0	0	0	0	0	0	0	0.0	0		
Rehabilitation	20	461	312	2,636	3,459	0	0	0	86,407	17,457	103,864	51.3	202,449		
Orthopedic	11	85	14	477	587	8	0	8	12,014	2,343	14,358	53.4	26,889		
Chronic disease	0	0	0	0	0	0	0	0	0	0	0	0.0	0		
All other	348	1,060	221	5,514	7,143	167	328	495	173,057	51,682	224,739	61.7	364,188		
Federal	1,706	3,720	1,371	18,770	25,567	1,404	122	1,526	738,890	134,725	873,615	65.7	1,328,853		
Psychiatric	43	154	89	1,139	1,425	2	0	2	36,720	6,708	43,429	70.4	61,715		
General and other special	1,663	3,566	1,282	17,631	24,142	1,402	122	1,524	702,170	128,017	830,186	65.5	1,267,137		
Nonfederal	805	47,628	18,073	156,867	223,373	2,676	619	3,295	5,435,777	1,086,138	6,521,915	49.9	13,058,263		
Psychiatric	239	2,432	855	14,354	17,880	65	37	102	466,037	95,227	561,264	61.1	918,250		
Hospitals	239	2,432	855	14,354	17,880	65	37	102	466,037	95,227	561,264	61.1	918,250		
Institutions for mentally retarded	0	0	0	0	0	0	0	0	0	0	0	0.0	0		
TB and other respiratory diseases	14	44	26	238	322	0	0	0	6,993	866	7,859	65.4	12,019		
Long-term general and other special	8	217	148	1,511	1,884	0	0	0	52,942	10,381	63,322	58.4	108,359		
Short-term general and other special	544	44,935	17,044	140,764	203,287	2,611	582	3,193	4,909,805	979,664	5,889,469	49.0	12,019,635		
Hospital units of institutions	0	18	16	27	61	0	0	0	1,060	200	1,259	51.7	2,437		
Community hospitals*	544	44,917	17,028	140,737	203,226	2,611	582	3,193	4,908,745	979,464	5,888,210	49.0	12,017,198	$4,663.50	$ 751.73
6-24 beds	8	265	278	1,064	1,615	0	0	0	30,602	6,164	36,766	54.1	67,945	2,482.36	591.04
25-49	25	1,654	1,565	7,045	10,289	2	12	14	189,585	35,855	225,440	51.3	439,490	2,806.49	540.77
50-99	32	3,391	2,044	11,565	17,032	21	0	21	359,061	79,657	438,718	46.6	940,579	3,676.71	641.12
100-199	61	9,203	3,841	27,162	40,267	136	43	179	957,727	204,247	1,161,974	46.3	2,507,035	4,361.65	722.32
200-299	5	7,772	2,990	22,626	33,393	97	51	148	828,564	164,366	992,931	47.5	2,091,222	4,852.58	752.26
300-399	27	6,616	2,300	19,616	28,559	291	26	317	673,454	135,322	808,775	48.7	1,660,809	4,492.80	728.70
400-499	7	3,320	888	9,357	13,572	107	1	108	350,937	64,972	415,910	48.5	857,253	4,613.50	786.64
500 or more	379	12,696	3,122	42,302	58,499	1,957	449	2,406	1,518,815	288,881	1,807,696	52.4	3,452,866	5,996.04	869.38
Nongovernment not-for-profit	104	23,787	8,308	72,806	105,005	857	156	1,013	2,570,581	500,718	3,071,298	50.5	6,078,607	4,868.53	777.45
Investor-owned (for-profit)	18	11,482	4,418	31,044	46,962	16	33	49	1,144,597	258,704	1,403,301	43.0	3,263,069	4,624.23	769.81
State and local government	422	9,648	4,302	36,887	51,259	1,738	393	2,131	1,193,568	220,042	1,413,610	52.8	2,675,523	4,296.88	681.05

*For information on community hospitals that excludes nursing-home-type data, refer to Hospital Units columns in tables 4A through 4D, pages 14 through 17.

(continued on next page)

Table

5C (Continued) Utah

Utilization, Personnel, and Finances in States

Excludes AHA nonregistered hospitals (see Table 14, page 240).

CLASSIFICATION	HOSPITALS	BEDS	ADMISSIONS	INPATIENT DAYS	ADJUSTED PATIENT DAYS	OCCUPANCY, percent	AVERAGE DAILY CENSUS	ADJUSTED AVERAGE DAILY CENSUS	AVERAGE STAY, days	SURGICAL OPERATIONS	OUTPATIENT VISITS Emergency	OUTPATIENT VISITS Other	OUTPATIENT VISITS Total	NEWBORNS Bassinets	NEWBORNS Births
UTAH	52	5,585	190,235	1,235,849		60.6	3,386			146,341	577,111	2,112,877	2,689,988	645	35,783
6-24 beds	9	185	5,485	29,867		44.9	83			3,128	26,666	98,568	125,234	48	1,678
25-49	17	619	15,829	111,454		49.3	305			9,949	92,224	272,273	364,497	106	2,978
50-99	8	602	15,702	125,377		57.0	343			10,555	70,590	116,897	187,487	65	3,201
100-199	8	1,016	41,473	167,270		45.2	459			39,974	147,864	450,782	598,646	168	9,352
200-299	4	865	38,272	211,435		66.9	579			30,654	100,649	266,554	367,203	84	6,180
300-399	5	1,836	52,862	478,362		71.4	1,310			32,469	115,776	615,293	731,069	101	8,794
400-499	1	462	20,612	112,084		66.5	307			19,612	23,342	292,510	315,852	73	3,600
500 or more	0	0	0	0		00.0	0			0	0	0	0	0	0
Psychiatric	8	755	4,696	200,699		72.8	550			0	247	15,044	15,291	0	0
Hospitals	8	755	4,696	200,699		72.8	550			0	247	15,044	15,291	0	0
Institutions for mentally retarded	0	0	0	0		00.0	0			0	0	0	0	0	0
General	42	4,705	184,390	1,009,491		58.8	2,766			145,785	576,864	2,085,016	2,661,880	645	35,783
Hospitals	42	4,705	184,390	1,009,491		58.8	2,766			145,785	576,864	2,085,016	2,661,880	645	35,783
Hospital units of institutions	0	0	0	0		00.0	0			0	0	0	0	0	0
TB and other respiratory diseases	0	0	0	0		00.0	0			0	0	0	0	0	0
Obstetrics and gynecology	0	0	0	0		00.0	0			0	0	0	0	0	0
Eye, ear, nose, and throat	0	0	0	0		00.0	0			0	0	0	0	0	0
Rehabilitation	1	80	591	16,510		56.3	45			0	0	9,154	9,154	0	0
Orthopedic	1	45	558	9,149		55.6	25			556	0	3,663	3,663	0	0
Chronic disease	0	0	0	0		00.0	0			0	0	0	0	0	0
All other	0	0	0	0		00.0	0			0	0	0	0	0	0
Federal	2	422	10,067	90,641		58.8	248			4,944	51,156	253,012	304,168	13	404
Psychiatric	0	0	0	0		00.0	0			0	0	0	0	0	0
General and other special	2	422	10,067	90,641		58.8	248			4,944	51,156	253,012	304,168	13	404
Nonfederal	50	5,163	180,168	1,145,208		60.8	3,138			141,397	525,955	1,859,865	2,385,820	632	35,379
Psychiatric	8	755	4,696	200,699		72.8	550			0	247	15,044	15,291	0	0
Hospitals	8	755	4,696	200,699		72.8	550			0	247	15,044	15,291	0	0
Institutions for mentally retarded	0	0	0	0		00.0	0			0	0	0	0	0	0
TB and other respiratory diseases	0	0	0	0		00.0	0			0	0	0	0	0	0
Long-term general and other special	0	0	0	0		00.0	0			0	0	0	0	0	0
Short-term general and other special	42	4,408	175,472	944,509		58.7	2,588			141,397	525,708	1,844,821	2,370,529	632	35,379
Hospital units of institutions	0	0	0	0		00.0	0			0	0	0	0	0	0
Community hospitals*	42	4,408	175,472	944,509	1,312,716	58.7	2,588	3,597	5.4	141,397	525,708	1,844,821	2,370,529	632	35,379
6-24 beds	9	185	5,485	29,867	60,367	44.9	83	166	5.4	3,128	26,666	98,568	125,234	48	1,678
25-49	13	465	12,605	76,803	127,757	45.2	210	350	6.1	8,343	69,607	124,663	194,270	93	2,574
50-99	5	400	13,035	80,684	120,498	55.3	221	330	6.2	10,555	70,590	104,228	174,818	65	3,201
100-199	7	914	40,856	155,657	232,471	46.7	427	637	3.8	39,974	147,864	450,782	598,646	168	9,352
200-299	4	865	38,272	211,435	273,792	66.9	579	750	5.5	30,654	100,649	266,554	367,203	84	6,180
300-399	3	1,117	44,607	277,979	351,978	68.1	761	964	6.2	29,131	86,990	507,516	594,506	101	8,794
400-499	1	462	20,612	112,084	145,853	66.5	307	400	5.4	19,612	23,342	292,510	315,852	73	3,600
500 or more	0	0	0	0	0	00.0	0	0	0.0	0	0	0	0	0	0
Nongovernment not-for-profit	24	2,758	120,460	596,805	836,001	59.3	1,636	2,291	5.0	95,410	338,909	1,409,086	1,747,995	405	25,381
Investor-owned (for-profit)	9	961	34,795	159,751	224,802	45.6	438	616	4.6	35,170	142,238	220,108	362,346	153	6,851
State and local government	9	689	20,217	187,953	251,913	74.6	514	690	9.3	10,817	44,561	215,627	260,188	74	3,147

*For information on community hospitals that excludes nursing-home-type data, refer to Hospital Units columns in tables 4A through 4D, pages 14 through 17.

CLASSIFICATION	FULL-TIME EQUIVALENT PERSONNEL					FULL-TIME EQUIVALENT TRAINEES			EXPENSES						
									LABOR				TOTAL		
	Physicians and Dentists	Registered Nurses	Licensed Practical Nurses	Other Salaried Personnel	Total Personnel	Medical and Dental Residents	Other Trainees	Total Trainees	Payroll (in thousands)	Employee Benefits (in thousands)	Total (in thousands)	Percent of Total	Amount (in thousands)	Adjusted, per Admission	Adjusted, per Inpatient Day
UTAH	211	4,914	953	14,665	20,743	209	14	223	$ 521,603	$ 131,623	$ 653,225	52.1	$ 1,253,033		
6-24 beds	10	104	41	326	481	0	0	0	10,542	2,694	13,236	52.2	25,344		
25-49	42	343	95	1,327	1,807	3	0	3	38,204	9,243	47,446	52.5	90,298		
50-99	0	329	94	1,147	1,570	0	2	2	37,758	8,724	46,482	49.3	94,249		
100-199	1	812	180	2,089	3,082	0	0	0	80,388	19,553	99,941	51.0	195,883		
200-299	14	1,184	136	2,657	3,991	2	0	2	99,568	25,356	124,925	49.5	252,210		
300-399	114	1,552	321	5,470	7,457	189	12	201	187,558	49,344	236,902	55.4	427,619		
400-499	30	590	86	1,649	2,355	15	0	15	67,585	16,708	84,292	50.3	167,429		
500 or more	0	0	0	0	0	0	0	0	0	0	0	0.0	0		
Psychiatric	11	173	40	1,051	1,275	0	4	4	31,378	6,902	38,280	58.4	65,512		
Hospitals	11	173	40	1,051	1,275	0	4	4	31,378	6,902	38,280	58.4	65,512		
Institutions for mentally retarded	0	0	0	0	0	0	0	0	0	0	0	0.0	0		
General	194	4,669	897	13,345	19,105	206	10	216	482,315	123,067	605,382	51.9	1,167,281		
Hospitals	194	4,669	897	13,345	19,105	206	10	216	482,315	123,067	605,382	51.9	1,167,281		
Hospital units of institutions	0	0	0	0	0	0	0	0	0	0	0	0.0	0		
TB and other respiratory diseases	0	0	0	0	0	0	0	0	0	0	0	0.0	0		
Obstetrics and gynecology	0	0	0	0	0	0	0	0	0	0	0	0.0	0		
Eye, ear, nose, and throat	0	0	0	0	0	0	0	0	0	0	0	0.0	0		
Rehabilitation	0	50	13	202	265	0	0	0	4,661	1,040	5,702	44.3	12,881		
Orthopedic	6	22	3	67	98	3	0	3	3,249	614	3,862	52.5	7,359		
Chronic disease	0	0	0	0	0	0	0	0	0	0	0	0.0	0		
All other	0	0	0	0	0	0	0	0	0	0	0	0.0	0		
Federal	109	207	50	1,108	1,474	50	0	50	47,778	9,513	57,292	60.4	94,895		
Psychiatric	0	0	0	0	0	0	0	0	0	0	0	0.0	0		
General and other special	109	207	50	1,108	1,474	50	0	50	47,778	9,513	57,292	60.4	94,895		
Nonfederal	102	4,707	903	13,557	19,269	159	14	173	473,824	122,109	595,934	51.5	1,158,138		
Psychiatric	11	173	40	1,051	1,275	0	4	4	31,378	6,902	38,280	58.4	65,512		
Hospitals	11	173	40	1,051	1,275	0	4	4	31,378	6,902	38,280	58.4	65,512		
Institutions for mentally retarded	0	0	0	0	0	0	0	0	0	0	0	0.0	0		
TB and other respiratory diseases	0	0	0	0	0	0	0	0	0	0	0	0.0	0		
Long-term general and other special	0	0	0	0	0	0	0	0	0	0	0	0.0	0		
Short-term general and other special	91	4,534	863	12,506	17,994	159	10	169	442,447	115,207	557,654	51.0	1,092,626		
Hospital units of institutions	0	0	0	0	0	0	0	0	0	0	0	0.0	0		
Community hospitals*	91	4,534	863	12,506	17,994	159	10	169	442,447	115,207	557,654	51.0	1,092,626	$4,409.36	$ 832.34
6-24 beds	10	104	41	326	481	0	0	0	10,542	2,694	13,236	52.2	25,344	2,513.05	419.83
25-49	13	272	80	887	1,252	3	0	3	25,694	6,623	32,317	49.1	65,823	2,936.30	515.22
50-99	0	271	84	822	1,177	0	1	1	27,844	6,610	34,454	49.0	70,267	3,452.92	583.14
100-199	1	796	174	2,017	2,988	0	0	0	75,459	18,508	93,967	50.8	185,054	3,025.10	796.03
200-299	14	1,184	136	2,657	3,991	2	0	2	99,568	25,356	124,925	49.5	252,210	5,022.71	921.17
300-399	23	1,317	262	4,148	5,750	139	9	148	135,755	38,708	174,463	53.4	326,498	5,754.70	927.61
400-499	30	590	86	1,649	2,355	15	0	15	67,585	16,708	84,292	50.3	167,429	6,242.21	1,147.93
500 or more	0	0	0	0	0	0	0	0	0	0	0	0.0	0	0.00	0.00
Nongovernment not-for-profit	87	3,015	541	8,203	11,846	20	1	21	313,409	81,061	394,470	53.5	737,532	4,301.38	882.21
Investor-owned (for-profit)	0	839	190	1,916	2,945	0	0	0	65,108	14,416	79,525	43.7	182,124	3,676.16	810.15
State and local government	4	680	132	2,387	3,203	139	9	148	63,929	19,730	83,659	48.4	172,969	6,456.25	686.62

*For information on community hospitals that excludes nursing-home-type data, refer to Hospital Units columns in tables 4A through 4D, pages 14 through 17.

(continued on next page)

Table

5C (Continued) Vermont

Utilization, Personnel, and Finances in States

Excludes AHA nonregistered hospitals (see Table 14, page 240).

CLASSIFICATION	HOSPITALS	BEDS	ADMISSIONS	INPATIENT DAYS	ADJUSTED PATIENT DAYS	OCCUPANCY, percent	AVERAGE DAILY CENSUS	ADJUSTED AVERAGE DAILY CENSUS	AVERAGE STAY, days	SURGICAL OPERATIONS	OUTPATIENT VISITS Emergency	OUTPATIENT VISITS Other	OUTPATIENT VISITS Total	NEWBORNS Bassinets	NEWBORNS Births
VERMONT	18	2,270	62,770	577,490		69.7	1,582			39,888	196,133	604,867	801,000	187	7,797
6-24 beds	0	0	0	0		00.0	0			0	0	0	0	0	0
25-49	2	75	1,760	18,238		66.7	50			1,289	6,075	22,962	29,037	12	382
50-99	8	594	16,846	123,349		56.9	338			12,801	89,237	149,594	238,831	73	2,138
100-199	6	864	24,248	213,322		67.6	584			14,441	70,465	296,696	367,161	64	2,438
200-299	1	253	1,300	80,401		87.0	220			0	290	6,069	6,359	0	0
300-399	0	0	0	0		00.0	0			0	0	0	0	0	0
400-499	1	484	18,616	142,180		80.6	390			11,357	30,066	129,546	159,612	38	2,839
500 or more	0	0	0	0		00.0	0			0	0	0	0	0	0
Psychiatric	2	383	1,733	111,914		79.9	306			0	290	6,069	6,359	0	0
Hospitals	2	383	1,733	111,914		79.9	306			0	290	6,069	6,359	0	0
Institutions for mentally retarded	0	0	0	0		00.0	0			0	0	0	0	0	0
General	16	1,887	61,037	465,576		67.6	1,276			39,888	195,843	598,798	794,641	187	7,797
Hospitals	16	1,887	61,037	465,576		67.6	1,276			39,888	195,843	598,798	794,641	187	7,797
Hospital units of institutions	0	0	0	0		00.0	0			0	0	0	0	0	0
TB and other respiratory diseases	0	0	0	0		00.0	0			0	0	0	0	0	0
Obstetrics and gynecology	0	0	0	0		00.0	0			0	0	0	0	0	0
Eye, ear, nose, and throat	0	0	0	0		00.0	0			0	0	0	0	0	0
Rehabilitation	0	0	0	0		00.0	0			0	0	0	0	0	0
Orthopedic	0	0	0	0		00.0	0			0	0	0	0	0	0
Chronic disease	0	0	0	0		00.0	0			0	0	0	0	0	0
All other	0	0	0	0		00.0	0			0	0	0	0	0	0
Federal	1	171	3,332	44,282		70.8	121			0	0	69,409	69,409	0	0
Psychiatric	0	0	0	0		00.0	0			0	0	0	0	0	0
General and other special	1	171	3,332	44,282		70.8	121			0	0	69,409	69,409	0	0
Nonfederal	17	2,099	59,438	533,208		69.6	1,461			39,888	196,133	535,458	731,591	187	7,797
Psychiatric	2	383	1,733	111,914		79.9	306			0	290	6,069	6,359	0	0
Hospitals	2	383	1,733	111,914		79.9	306			0	290	6,069	6,359	0	0
Institutions for mentally retarded	0	0	0	0		00.0	0			0	0	0	0	0	0
TB and other respiratory diseases	0	0	0	0		00.0	0			0	0	0	0	0	0
Long-term general and other special	0	0	0	0		00.0	0			0	0	0	0	0	0
Short-term general and other special	15	1,716	57,705	421,294		67.3	1,155			39,888	195,843	529,389	725,232	187	7,797
Hospital units of institutions	0	0	0	0		00.0	0			0	0	0	0	0	0
Community hospitals*	15	1,716	57,705	421,294	596,952	67.3	1,155	1,636	7.3	39,888	195,843	529,389	725,232	187	7,797
6-24 beds	0	0	0	0	0	00.0	0	0	0.0	0	0	0	0	0	0
25-49	2	75	1,760	18,238	33,125	66.7	50	91	10.4	1,289	6,075	22,962	29,037	12	382
50-99	8	594	16,846	123,349	195,853	56.9	338	536	7.3	12,801	89,237	149,594	238,831	73	2,138
100-199	4	563	20,483	137,527	193,270	67.0	377	530	6.7	14,441	70,465	227,287	297,752	64	2,438
200-299	0	0	0	0	0	00.0	0	0	0.0	0	0	0	0	0	0
300-399	0	0	0	0	0	00.0	0	0	0.0	0	0	0	0	0	0
400-499	1	484	18,616	142,180	174,704	80.6	390	479	7.6	11,357	30,066	129,546	159,612	38	2,839
500 or more	0	0	0	0	0	00.0	0	0	0.0	0	0	0	0	0	0
Nongovernment not-for-profit	15	1,716	57,705	421,294	596,952	67.3	1,155	1,636	7.3	39,888	195,843	529,389	725,232	187	7,797
Investor-owned (for-profit)	0	0	0	0	0	00.0	0	0	0.0	0	0	0	0	0	0
State and local government	0	0	0	0	0	00.0	0	0	0.0	0	0	0	0	0	0

*For information on community hospitals that excludes nursing-home-type data, refer to Hospital Units columns in tables 4A through 4D, pages 14 through 17.

CLASSIFICATION	FULL-TIME EQUIVALENT PERSONNEL					FULL-TIME EQUIVALENT TRAINEES			EXPENSES: LABOR				EXPENSES: TOTAL		
	Physicians and Dentists	Registered Nurses	Licensed Practical Nurses	Other Salaried Personnel	Total Personnel	Medical and Dental Residents	Other Trainees	Total Trainees	Payroll (in thousands)	Employee Benefits (in thousands)	Total (in thousands)	Percent of Total	Amount (in thousands)	Adjusted, per Admission	Adjusted, per Inpatient Day
VERMONT	125	1,796	468	5,511	7,900	241	17	258	$ 208,081	$ 38,773	$ 246,854	57.1	$ 432,003		
6-24 beds	0	0	0	0	0	0	0	0	0	0	0	0.0	0		
25-49	5	49	12	161	227	0	0	0	5,698	981	6,679	63.7	10,493		
50-99	22	469	166	1,342	1,999	0	0	0	48,372	9,920	58,292	58.2	100,136		
100-199	82	669	196	2,058	3,005	45	1	46	80,342	14,763	95,105	59.5	159,956		
200-299	15	69	3	489	576	0	0	0	9,980	1,532	11,512	48.3	23,822		
300-399	0	0	0	0	0	0	0	0	0	0	0	0.0	0		
400-499	1	540	91	1,461	2,093	196	16	212	63,689	11,577	75,265	54.7	137,595		
500 or more	0	0	0	0	0	0	0	0	0	0	0	0.0	0		
Psychiatric	21	89	9	726	845	0	0	0	16,353	3,235	19,588	56.5	34,649		
Hospitals	21	89	9	726	845	0	0	0	16,353	3,235	19,588	56.5	34,649		
Institutions for mentally retarded	0	0	0	0	0	0	0	0	0	0	0	0.0	0		
General	104	1,707	459	4,785	7,055	241	17	258	191,728	35,537	227,265	57.2	397,353		
Hospitals	104	1,707	459	4,785	7,055	241	17	258	191,728	35,537	227,265	57.2	397,353		
Hospital units of institutions	0	0	0	0	0	0	0	0	0	0	0	0.0	0		
TB and other respiratory diseases	0	0	0	0	0	0	0	0	0	0	0	0.0	0		
Obstetrics and gynecology	0	0	0	0	0	0	0	0	0	0	0	0.0	0		
Eye, ear, nose, and throat	0	0	0	0	0	0	0	0	0	0	0	0.0	0		
Rehabilitation	0	0	0	0	0	0	0	0	0	0	0	0.0	0		
Orthopedic	0	0	0	0	0	0	0	0	0	0	0	0.0	0		
Chronic disease	0	0	0	0	0	0	0	0	0	0	0	0.0	0		
All other	0	0	0	0	0	0	0	0	0	0	0	0.0	0		
Federal	47	114	28	449	638	45	1	46	19,809	3,598	23,407	57.6	40,615		
Psychiatric	0	0	0	0	0	0	0	0	0	0	0	0.0	0		
General and other special	47	114	28	449	638	45	1	46	19,809	3,598	23,407	57.6	40,615		
Nonfederal	78	1,682	440	5,062	7,262	196	16	212	188,272	35,174	223,446	57.1	391,387		
Psychiatric	21	89	9	726	845	0	0	0	16,353	3,235	19,588	56.5	34,649		
Hospitals	21	89	9	726	845	0	0	0	16,353	3,235	19,588	56.5	34,649		
Institutions for mentally retarded	0	0	0	0	0	0	0	0	0	0	0	0.0	0		
TB and other respiratory diseases	0	0	0	0	0	0	0	0	0	0	0	0.0	0		
Long-term general and other special	0	0	0	0	0	0	0	0	0	0	0	0.0	0		
Short-term general and other special	57	1,593	431	4,336	6,417	196	16	212	171,919	31,939	203,858	57.1	356,738		
Hospital units of institutions	0	0	0	0	0	0	0	0	0	0	0	0.0	0		
Community hospitals*	57	1,593	431	4,336	6,417	196	16	212	171,919	31,939	203,858	57.1	356,738	$4,343.47	$ 597.60
6-24 beds	0	0	0	0	0	0	0	0	0	0	0	0.0	0	0.00	0.00
25-49	5	49	12	161	227	0	0	0	5,698	981	6,679	63.7	10,493	2,949.16	316.77
50-99	22	469	166	1,342	1,999	0	0	0	48,372	9,920	58,292	58.2	100,136	3,732.53	511.28
100-199	29	535	162	1,372	2,098	0	0	0	54,160	9,461	63,621	58.6	108,514	3,758.57	561.46
200-299	0	0	0	0	0	0	0	0	0	0	0	0.0	0	0.00	0.00
300-399	0	0	0	0	0	0	0	0	0	0	0	0.0	0	0.00	0.00
400-499	1	540	91	1,461	2,093	196	16	212	63,689	11,577	75,265	54.7	137,595	6,015.09	787.59
500 or more	0	0	0	0	0	0	0	0	0	0	0	0.0	0	0.00	0.00
Nongovernment not-for-profit	57	1,593	431	4,336	6,417	196	16	212	171,919	31,939	203,858	57.1	356,738	4,343.47	597.60
Investor-owned (for-profit)	0	0	0	0	0	0	0	0	0	0	0	0.0	0	0.00	0.00
State and local government	0	0	0	0	0	0	0	0	0	0	0	0.0	0	0.00	0.00

*For information on community hospitals that excludes nursing-home-type data, refer to Hospital Units columns in tables 4A through 4D, pages 14 through 17.

(continued on next page)

Table
5C (Continued) Virginia

Utilization, Personnel, and Finances in States
Excludes AHA nonregistered hospitals (see Table 14, page 240).

CLASSIFICATION	HOSPITALS	BEDS	ADMISSIONS	INPATIENT DAYS	ADJUSTED PATIENT DAYS	OCCUPANCY, percent	AVERAGE DAILY CENSUS	ADJUSTED AVERAGE DAILY CENSUS	AVERAGE STAY, days	SURGICAL OPERATIONS	OUTPATIENT VISITS Emergency	OUTPATIENT VISITS Other	OUTPATIENT VISITS Total	NEWBORNS Bassinets	NEWBORNS Births
VIRGINIA	135	29,298	798,164	7,726,947		72.3	21,173			522,145	2,295,431	6,449,291	8,744,722	1,564	94,924
6-24 beds	2	25	1,282	2,625		28.0	7			2,136	0	2,049	2,049	0	0
25-49	10	368	11,225	82,462		61.7	227			5,606	67,286	415,939	483,225	11	227
50-99	30	2,115	60,495	472,857		61.2	1,294			27,966	229,244	1,315,193	1,544,437	94	3,777
100-199	42	6,161	180,901	1,373,493		61.1	3,766			134,119	624,850	1,083,605	1,708,455	452	19,246
200-299	21	4,872	132,456	1,248,470		70.2	3,420			97,869	421,512	580,450	1,001,962	279	14,485
300-399	16	5,562	201,514	1,483,924		73.1	4,067			136,461	515,819	1,582,938	2,098,757	415	28,973
400-499	1	470	15,920	109,429		63.8	300			13,328	40,425	104,585	145,010	35	2,346
500 or more	13	9,725	194,371	2,953,687		83.2	8,092			104,660	396,295	1,364,532	1,760,827	278	25,870
Psychiatric	24	5,976	27,640	1,877,099		86.0	5,142			25	4,131	37,785	41,916	0	0
Hospitals	23	4,623	27,597	1,383,485		82.0	3,790			0	1,977	31,631	33,608	0	0
Institutions for mentally retarded	1	1,353	43	493,614		99.9	1,352			25	2,154	6,154	8,308	0	0
General	101	22,367	762,191	5,600,751		68.6	15,348			512,769	2,277,648	6,285,277	8,562,925	1,564	94,924
Hospitals	100	22,327	761,748	5,592,000		68.6	15,324			512,607	2,275,995	6,257,612	8,533,607	1,564	94,924
Hospital units of institutions	1	40	443	8,751		60.0	24			162	1,653	27,665	29,318	0	0
TB and other respiratory diseases	0	0	0	0		00.0	0			0	0	0	0	0	0
Obstetrics and gynecology	0	0	0	0		00.0	0			0	0	0	0	0	0
Eye, ear, nose, and throat	2	71	1,773	3,405		12.7	9			5,980	0	5,033	5,033	0	0
Rehabilitation	3	164	1,235	50,197		83.5	137			49	0	42,903	42,903	0	0
Orthopedic	2	164	3,803	29,612		50.0	82			3,322	13,652	78,293	91,945	0	0
Chronic disease	1	332	518	96,717		79.8	265			0	0	0	0	0	0
All other	2	224	1,004	69,166		84.8	190			0	0	0	0	0	0
Federal	8	2,571	61,980	708,403		75.5	1,942			26,046	211,462	2,570,014	2,781,476	66	3,340
Psychiatric	0	0	0	0		00.0	0			0	0	0	0	0	0
General and other special	8	2,571	61,980	708,403		75.5	1,942			26,046	211,462	2,570,014	2,781,476	66	3,340
Nonfederal	127	26,727	736,184	7,018,544		72.0	19,231			496,099	2,083,969	3,879,277	5,963,246	1,498	91,584
Psychiatric	24	5,976	27,640	1,877,099		86.0	5,142			25	4,131	37,785	41,916	0	0
Hospitals	23	4,623	27,597	1,383,485		82.0	3,790			0	1,977	31,631	33,608	0	0
Institutions for mentally retarded	1	1,353	43	493,614		99.9	1,352			25	2,154	6,154	8,308	0	0
TB and other respiratory diseases	0	0	0	0		00.0	0			0	0	0	0	0	0
Long-term general and other special	5	706	1,861	213,935		83.0	586			49	0	42,903	42,903	0	0
Short-term general and other special	98	20,045	706,683	4,927,510		67.4	13,503			496,025	2,079,838	3,798,589	5,878,427	1,498	91,584
Hospital units of institutions	1	40	443	8,751		60.0	24			162	1,653	27,665	29,318	0	0
Community hospitals*	97	20,005	706,240	4,918,759	6,430,948	67.4	13,479	17,624	7.0	495,863	2,078,185	3,770,924	5,849,109	1,498	91,584
6-24 beds	2	25	1,282	2,625	6,271	28.0	7	17	2.0	2,136	0	2,049	2,049	0	0
25-49	5	177	5,694	29,780	45,601	46.3	82	124	5.2	3,057	27,963	72,629	100,592	11	227
50-99	16	1,137	36,471	213,753	303,583	51.5	585	834	5.9	23,393	131,859	211,644	343,503	65	1,708
100-199	35	5,099	168,162	1,105,027	1,553,864	59.4	3,030	4,258	6.6	134,119	623,500	1,066,417	1,689,917	452	19,246
200-299	18	4,179	130,419	1,024,530	1,377,612	67.1	2,806	3,777	7.9	97,869	421,512	580,450	1,001,962	279	14,485
300-399	14	4,841	184,331	1,286,694	1,625,346	72.9	3,527	4,453	7.0	124,908	474,381	849,723	1,324,104	378	27,702
400-499	1	470	15,920	109,429	133,891	63.8	300	367	6.9	13,328	40,425	104,585	145,010	35	2,346
500 or more	6	4,077	163,961	1,146,921	1,384,780	77.1	3,142	3,794	7.0	97,053	358,545	883,427	1,241,972	278	25,870
Nongovernment not-for-profit	77	14,811	519,277	3,608,253	4,797,057	66.8	9,890	13,147	6.9	380,945	1,568,895	2,656,351	4,225,246	1,187	70,267
Investor-owned (for-profit)	15	3,006	100,716	680,607	851,650	62.0	1,864	2,334	6.8	74,091	266,428	532,204	798,632	158	9,979
State and local government	5	2,188	86,247	629,899	782,241	78.8	1,725	2,143	7.3	40,827	242,862	582,369	825,231	153	11,338

*For information on community hospitals that excludes nursing-home-type data, refer to Hospital Units columns in tables 4A through 4D, pages 14 through 17.

CLASSIFICATION	FULL-TIME EQUIVALENT PERSONNEL: Physicians and Dentists	Registered Nurses	Licensed Practical Nurses	Other Salaried Personnel	Total Personnel	FULL-TIME EQUIVALENT TRAINEES: Medical and Dental Residents	Other Trainees	Total Trainees	EXPENSES – LABOR: Payroll (in thousands)	Employee Benefits (in thousands)	Total (in thousands)	Percent of Total	EXPENSES – TOTAL: Amount (in thousands)	Adjusted, per Admission	Adjusted, per Inpatient Day
VIRGINIA	1,397	19,835	5,661	65,539	92,432	1,537	48	1,585	$ 2,301,678	$ 432,009	$ 2,733,687	55.0	$ 4,973,288		
6-24 beds	1	31	12	100	144	0	0	0	3,190	638	3,827	52.5	7,286		
25-49	78	269	119	1,345	1,811	0	2	2	52,851	10,686	63,537	64.0	99,201		
50-99	222	1,181	432	4,854	6,689	16	1	17	150,564	26,013	176,577	56.1	314,817		
100-199	29	4,096	1,560	12,437	18,122	22	0	22	436,589	80,177	516,766	53.7	962,117		
200-299	32	3,031	983	10,111	14,157	27	0	27	334,587	59,647	394,235	53.4	738,347		
300-399	212	4,736	968	14,376	20,292	223	33	256	502,008	80,597	582,605	54.2	1,074,235		
400-499	2	390	56	809	1,257	6	0	6	37,059	7,940	44,999	43.6	103,259		
500 or more	821	6,101	1,531	21,507	29,960	1,243	12	1,255	784,831	166,311	951,143	56.8	1,674,026		
Psychiatric	144	993	453	8,410	10,000	5	0	5	233,532	57,789	291,321	70.0	416,460		
Hospitals	128	905	422	5,884	7,339	5	0	5	179,822	44,865	224,686	67.3	333,869		
Institutions for mentally retarded	16	88	31	2,526	2,661	0	0	0	53,710	12,924	66,634	80.7	82,591		
General	1,222	18,481	5,056	55,451	80,210	1,532	46	1,578	2,006,544	361,923	2,368,467	53.4	4,433,360		
Hospitals	1,215	18,466	5,041	55,409	80,131	1,532	46	1,578	2,005,060	361,498	2,366,557	53.4	4,428,138		
Hospital units of institutions	7	15	15	42	79	0	0	0	1,484	426	1,910	36.6	5,222		
TB and other respiratory diseases	0	0	0	0	0	0	0	0	0	0	0	0.0	0		
Obstetrics and gynecology	0	0	0	0	0	0	0	0	0	0	0	0.0	0		
Eye, ear, nose, and throat	0	41	13	82	136	0	0	0	3,247	663	3,909	44.3	8,832		
Rehabilitation	15	81	32	487	615	0	0	0	24,034	5,302	29,335	64.3	45,650		
Orthopedic	7	160	6	441	614	0	2	2	19,185	3,164	22,349	55.6	40,168		
Chronic disease	0	24	48	320	392	0	0	0	5,517	720	6,237	51.3	12,162		
All other	9	55	53	348	465	0	0	0	9,620	2,449	12,069	72.5	16,656		
Federal	682	1,239	486	7,379	9,786	312	29	341	243,394	36,828	280,222	70.5	397,559		
Psychiatric	0	0	0	0	0	0	0	0	0	0	0	0.0	0		
General and other special	682	1,239	486	7,379	9,786	312	29	341	243,394	36,828	280,222	70.5	397,559		
Nonfederal	715	18,596	5,175	58,160	82,646	1,225	19	1,244	2,058,285	395,180	2,453,465	53.6	4,575,728		
Psychiatric	144	993	453	8,410	10,000	5	0	5	233,532	57,789	291,321	70.0	416,460		
Hospitals	128	905	422	5,884	7,339	5	0	5	179,822	44,865	224,686	67.3	333,869		
Institutions for mentally retarded	16	88	31	2,526	2,661	0	0	0	53,710	12,924	66,634	80.7	82,591		
TB and other respiratory diseases	0	0	0	0	0	0	0	0	0	0	0	0.0	0		
Long-term general and other special	23	142	125	1,084	1,374	0	0	0	37,058	8,044	45,102	64.6	69,810		
Short-term general and other special	548	17,461	4,597	48,666	71,272	1,220	19	1,239	1,787,695	329,348	2,117,043	51.8	4,089,459		
Hospital units of institutions	7	15	15	42	79	0	0	0	1,484	426	1,910	36.6	5,222		
Community hospitals*	541	17,446	4,582	48,624	71,193	1,220	19	1,239	1,786,210	328,922	2,115,132	51.8	4,084,237	$4,408.21	$ 635.09
6-24 beds	1	31	12	100	144	0	0	0	3,190	638	3,827	52.5	7,286	2,042.55	1,161.82
25-49	6	145	50	557	758	0	2	2	13,979	2,513	16,492	53.1	31,069	3,548.74	681.33
50-99	5	734	311	2,109	3,159	0	0	0	71,683	13,041	84,724	50.1	169,173	3,185.82	557.26
100-199	17	3,780	1,504	11,077	16,378	19	0	19	386,542	69,155	455,697	53.4	853,394	3,605.18	549.21
200-299	8	2,894	887	9,151	12,940	27	0	27	307,961	51,553	359,514	51.7	694,884	3,987.03	504.41
300-399	53	4,427	817	12,359	17,656	16	8	24	452,947	75,399	528,345	53.3	991,837	4,261.75	610.23
400-499	2	390	56	809	1,257	6	0	6	37,059	7,940	44,999	43.6	103,259	5,301.07	771.22
500 or more	449	5,045	945	12,462	18,901	1,152	9	1,161	512,850	108,683	621,534	50.4	1,233,335	6,232.87	890.64
Nongovernment not-for-profit	141	12,360	3,430	34,969	50,900	191	10	201	1,303,295	215,990	1,519,286	54.3	2,799,151	4,050.48	583.51
Investor-owned (for-profit)	5	2,346	528	6,012	8,891	24	0	24	211,972	44,714	256,686	43.6	588,521	4,606.93	691.04
State and local government	395	2,740	624	7,643	11,402	1,005	9	1,014	270,943	68,218	339,161	48.7	696,565	6,467.94	890.47

*For information on community hospitals that excludes nursing-home-type data, refer to Hospital Units columns in tables 4A through 4D, pages 14 through 17.

(continued on next page)

Table
5C (Continued) Washington

Utilization, Personnel, and Finances in States
Excludes AHA nonregistered hospitals (see Table 14, page 240).

CLASSIFICATION	HOSPITALS	BEDS	ADMISSIONS	INPATIENT DAYS	ADJUSTED PATIENT DAYS	OCCUPANCY, percent	AVERAGE DAILY CENSUS	ADJUSTED AVERAGE DAILY CENSUS	AVERAGE STAY, days	SURGICAL OPERATIONS	OUTPATIENT VISITS Emergency	OUTPATIENT VISITS Other	OUTPATIENT VISITS Total	NEWBORNS Bassinets	NEWBORNS Births
WASHINGTON	110	15,773	551,655	3,773,497		65.5	10,335			409,206	1,710,384	5,321,562	7,031,946	1,043	74,756
6-24 beds	9	175	5,554	19,196		30.3	53			3,455	23,052	63,023	86,075	13	202
25-49	27	978	26,019	141,744		39.6	387			19,513	141,581	456,444	598,025	129	4,460
50-99	23	1,568	41,262	329,998		57.6	903			32,322	201,988	253,492	455,480	126	6,190
100-199	24	3,544	131,796	748,626		57.9	2,052			96,361	534,658	1,199,035	1,733,693	243	17,038
200-299	13	3,142	157,159	783,949		68.3	2,146			128,493	462,065	979,247	1,441,312	295	24,852
300-399	9	3,107	123,804	850,017		75.0	2,329			81,329	285,744	1,839,218	2,124,962	189	15,641
400-499	1	488	9,586	110,719		62.1	303			3,693	0	194,849	194,849	0	0
500 or more	4	2,771	56,475	789,248		78.0	2,162			44,040	61,296	336,254	397,550	48	6,373
Psychiatric	8	1,775	10,049	582,397		89.9	1,596			0	1,854	16,196	18,050	0	0
Hospitals	8	1,775	10,049	582,397		89.9	1,596			0	1,854	16,196	18,050	0	0
Institutions for mentally retarded	0	0	0	0		00.0	0			0	0	0	0	0	0
General	101	13,968	540,952	3,184,795		62.4	8,722			408,882	1,705,872	5,299,614	7,005,486	1,043	74,756
Hospitals	100	13,937	540,672	3,184,019		62.6	8,720			408,482	1,705,469	5,292,856	6,998,325	1,043	74,756
Hospital units of institutions	1	31	280	776		06.5	2			400	403	6,758	7,161	0	0
TB and other respiratory diseases	0	0	0	0		00.0	0			0	0	0	0	0	0
Obstetrics and gynecology	0	0	0	0		00.0	0			0	0	0	0	0	0
Eye, ear, nose, and throat	0	0	0	0		00.0	0			0	0	0	0	0	0
Rehabilitation	0	0	0	0		00.0	0			0	0	0	0	0	0
Orthopedic	1	30	654	6,305		56.7	17			324	2,658	5,752	8,410	0	0
Chronic disease	0	0	0	0		00.0	0			0	0	0	0	0	0
All other	0	0	0	0		00.0	0			0	0	0	0	0	0
Federal	8	1,903	49,035	421,260		60.7	1,155			29,044	135,692	1,963,663	2,099,355	64	4,088
Psychiatric	0	0	0	0		00.0	0			0	0	0	0	0	0
General and other special	8	1,903	49,035	421,260		60.7	1,155			29,044	135,692	1,963,663	2,099,355	64	4,088
Nonfederal	102	13,870	502,620	3,352,237		66.2	9,180			380,162	1,574,692	3,357,899	4,932,591	979	70,668
Psychiatric	8	1,775	10,049	582,397		89.9	1,596			0	1,854	16,196	18,050	0	0
Hospitals	8	1,775	10,049	582,397		89.9	1,596			0	1,854	16,196	18,050	0	0
Institutions for mentally retarded	0	0	0	0		00.0	0			0	0	0	0	0	0
TB and other respiratory diseases	0	0	0	0		00.0	0			0	0	0	0	0	0
Long-term general and other special	2	149	773	42,702		78.5	117			306	1,580	4,781	6,361	4	25
Short-term general and other special	92	11,946	491,798	2,727,138		62.5	7,467			379,856	1,571,258	3,336,922	4,908,180	975	70,643
Hospital units of institutions	1	31	280	776		06.5	2			400	403	6,758	7,161	0	0
Community hospitals*	91	11,915	491,518	2,726,362	3,747,213	62.7	7,465	10,275	5.5	379,456	1,570,855	3,330,164	4,901,019	975	70,643
6-24 beds	9	175	5,554	19,196	34,574	30.3	53	95	3.5	3,455	23,052	63,023	86,075	13	202
25-49	22	814	20,362	112,882	191,120	37.8	308	527	5.5	15,629	96,198	200,047	296,245	108	3,529
50-99	18	1,223	37,555	253,399	387,379	56.7	693	1,063	6.7	32,016	200,004	246,414	446,418	122	6,165
100-199	20	2,983	120,284	619,861	911,460	56.9	1,698	2,498	5.2	88,960	509,204	902,558	1,411,762	228	16,398
200-299	13	3,142	157,159	783,949	1,041,194	68.3	2,146	2,855	5.0	128,493	462,065	979,247	1,441,312	295	24,852
300-399	7	2,384	100,342	624,174	802,574	71.7	1,710	2,199	6.2	69,586	219,036	724,164	943,200	161	13,124
400-499	0	0	0	0	0	00.0	0	0	0.0	0	0	0	0	0	0
500 or more	2	1,194	50,262	312,901	378,912	71.8	857	1,038	6.2	41,317	61,296	214,711	276,007	48	6,373
Nongovernment not-for-profit	49	8,458	366,137	1,971,614	2,662,263	63.8	5,398	7,300	5.4	279,957	1,099,734	2,389,553	3,489,287	671	53,238
Investor-owned (for-profit)	5	587	20,334	118,018	177,895	55.2	324	487	5.8	14,367	79,370	96,512	175,882	12	833
State and local government	37	2,870	105,047	636,730	907,055	60.7	1,743	2,488	6.1	85,132	391,751	844,099	1,235,850	292	16,572

*For information on community hospitals that excludes nursing-home-type data, refer to Hospital Units columns in tables 4A through 4D, pages 14 through 17.

Table 5C (Continued) Washington

CLASSIFICATION	FULL-TIME EQUIVALENT PERSONNEL					FULL-TIME EQUIVALENT TRAINEES			EXPENSES: LABOR				EXPENSES: TOTAL		
	Physicians and Dentists	Registered Nurses	Licensed Practical Nurses	Other Salaried Personnel	Total Personnel	Medical and Dental Residents	Other Trainees	Total Trainees	Payroll (in thousands)	Employee Benefits (in thousands)	Total (in thousands)	Percent of Total	Amount (in thousands)	Adjusted, per Admission	Adjusted, per Inpatient Day
WASHINGTON	1,352	14,928	2,573	41,150	60,003	757	66	823	$ 1,719,907	$ 330,445	$ 2,050,352	57.6	$ 3,561,465		
6-24 beds	2	93	40	435	570	0	0	0	14,164	2,685	16,849	54.1	31,132		
25-49	68	603	130	2,176	2,977	4	1	5	76,343	14,401	90,745	58.6	154,895		
50-99	15	969	214	3,199	4,397	0	0	0	113,777	23,951	137,728	52.1	264,378		
100-199	274	3,394	498	9,191	13,357	9	1	10	367,022	72,445	439,467	55.4	793,876		
200-299	25	3,893	350	9,047	13,315	90	33	123	397,017	74,048	471,065	52.6	896,372		
300-399	743	3,634	611	10,512	15,500	478	0	478	453,051	83,967	537,019	62.0	866,075		
400-499	111	287	65	1,060	1,523	97	24	121	59,215	9,596	68,811	77.4	88,891		
500 or more	114	2,055	665	5,530	8,364	79	7	86	239,319	49,350	288,669	62.0	465,845		
Psychiatric	86	491	437	2,297	3,311	1	0	1	85,482	23,685	109,167	76.0	143,613		
Hospitals	86	491	437	2,297	3,311	1	0	1	85,482	23,685	109,167	76.0	143,613		
Institutions for mentally retarded	0	0	0	0	0	0	0	0	0	0	0	0.0	0		
General	1,265	14,418	2,135	38,788	56,606	756	66	822	1,632,029	306,307	1,938,336	56.8	3,412,423		
Hospitals	1,255	14,400	2,126	38,746	56,527	756	65	821	1,630,879	305,977	1,936,855	56.8	3,408,377		
Hospital units of institutions	10	18	9	42	79	0	1	1	1,150	330	1,481	36.6	4,047		
TB and other respiratory diseases	0	0	0	0	0	0	0	0	0	0	0	0.0	0		
Obstetrics and gynecology	0	0	0	0	0	0	0	0	0	0	0	0.0	0		
Eye, ear, nose, and throat	0	0	0	0	0	0	0	0	0	0	0	0.0	0		
Rehabilitation	0	0	0	0	0	0	0	0	0	0	0	0.0	0		
Orthopedic	1	19	1	65	86	0	0	0	2,396	453	2,850	52.5	5,429		
Chronic disease	0	0	0	0	0	0	0	0	0	0	0	0.0	0		
All other	0	0	0	0	0	0	0	0	0	0	0	0.0	0		
Federal	510	1,071	392	5,142	7,115	307	32	339	241,368	37,705	279,074	82.6	337,761		
Psychiatric	0	0	0	0	0	0	0	0	0	0	0	0.0	0		
General and other special	510	1,071	392	5,142	7,115	307	32	339	241,368	37,705	279,074	82.6	337,761		
Nonfederal	842	13,857	2,181	36,008	52,888	450	34	484	1,478,539	292,739	1,771,278	54.9	3,223,704		
Psychiatric	86	491	437	2,297	3,311	1	0	1	85,482	23,685	109,167	76.0	143,613		
Hospitals	86	491	437	2,297	3,311	1	0	1	85,482	23,685	109,167	76.0	143,613		
Institutions for mentally retarded	0	0	0	0	0	0	0	0	0	0	0	0.0	0		
TB and other respiratory diseases	0	0	0	0	0	0	0	0	0	0	0	0.0	0		
Long-term general and other special	3	30	13	212	258	0	0	0	6,691	1,406	8,097	63.2	12,812		
Short-term general and other special	753	13,336	1,731	33,499	49,319	449	34	483	1,386,366	267,648	1,654,014	53.9	3,067,279		
Hospital units of institutions	10	18	9	42	79	0	1	1	1,150	330	1,481	36.6	4,047		
Community hospitals*	743	13,318	1,722	33,457	49,240	449	33	482	1,385,216	267,318	1,652,534	53.9	3,063,232	$4,518.91	$ 817.47
6-24 beds	2	93	40	435	570	0	0	0	14,164	2,685	16,849	54.1	31,132	3,132.96	900.45
25-49	5	497	106	1,589	2,197	4	0	4	51,781	9,176	60,957	53.8	113,318	3,272.82	592.92
50-99	9	901	191	2,764	3,865	0	0	0	99,663	21,188	120,851	51.5	234,611	3,990.11	605.64
100-199	188	3,032	456	7,633	11,309	3	0	3	312,874	58,972	371,845	54.2	686,226	3,898.86	752.89
200-299	25	3,893	350	9,047	13,315	90	33	123	397,017	74,048	471,065	52.6	896,372	4,291.92	860.91
300-399	494	3,238	326	8,390	12,448	280	0	280	344,647	71,209	415,856	55.2	753,096	5,843.98	938.35
400-499	0	0	0	0	0	0	0	0	0	0	0	0.0	0	0.00	0.00
500 or more	20	1,664	253	3,599	5,536	72	0	72	165,070	30,040	195,110	56.0	348,478	5,732.95	919.68
Nongovernment not-for-profit	316	9,703	1,339	24,241	35,599	197	33	230	1,010,506	189,673	1,200,180	53.7	2,236,305	4,514.83	840.00
Investor-owned (for-profit)	3	512	48	1,257	1,820	4	0	4	55,739	9,063	64,803	48.6	133,288	4,322.33	749.25
State and local government	424	3,103	335	7,959	11,821	248	0	248	318,970	68,581	387,551	55.9	693,640	4,572.20	764.72

*For information on community hospitals that excludes nursing-home-type data, refer to Hospital Units columns in tables 4A through 4D, pages 14 through 17.

(continued on next page)

Table

5C (Continued) West Virginia

Utilization, Personnel, and Finances in States

Excludes AHA nonregistered hospitals (see Table 14, page 240).

CLASSIFICATION	HOSPITALS	BEDS	ADMISSIONS	INPATIENT DAYS	ADJUSTED PATIENT DAYS	OCCUPANCY, percent	AVERAGE DAILY CENSUS	ADJUSTED AVERAGE DAILY CENSUS	AVERAGE STAY, days	SURGICAL OPERATIONS	OUTPATIENT VISITS			NEWBORNS	
											Emergency	Other	Total	Bassinets	Births
WEST VIRGINIA	68	10,175	298,941	2,411,347		64.9	6,608			223,111	990,553	2,076,659	3,067,212	579	22,820
6-24 beds	2	41	1,023	6,557		43.9	18			70	4,324	20,956	25,280	0	0
25-49	14	554	10,164	98,797		48.7	270			7,232	53,872	97,850	151,722	14	82
50-99	20	1,439	39,547	288,058		54.9	790			22,105	198,789	331,193	529,982	82	2,217
100-199	10	1,323	37,874	344,828		71.4	945			28,574	141,141	317,143	458,284	59	2,999
200-299	15	3,733	123,769	833,227		61.2	2,283			102,285	396,949	738,125	1,135,074	288	10,798
300-399	4	1,282	33,976	362,506		77.5	994			26,734	91,096	292,028	383,124	65	2,657
400-499	2	937	19,897	243,722		71.3	668			10,215	36,323	125,431	161,754	21	288
500 or more	1	866	32,691	233,652		73.9	640			25,896	68,059	153,933	221,992	50	3,779
Psychiatric	5	699	5,436	199,519		78.3	547			21	133	2,933	3,066	0	0
Hospitals	4	559	5,358	155,589		76.4	427			0	43	2,598	2,641	0	0
Institutions for mentally retarded	1	140	78	43,930		85.7	120			21	90	335	425	0	0
General	59	9,330	291,779	2,180,217		64.0	5,975			220,134	990,420	2,063,812	3,054,232	579	22,820
Hospitals	59	9,330	291,779	2,180,217		64.0	5,975			220,134	990,420	2,063,812	3,054,232	579	22,820
Hospital units of institutions	0	0	0	0		00.0	0			0	0	0	0	0	0
TB and other respiratory diseases	0	0	0	0		00.0	0			0	0	0	0	0	0
Obstetrics and gynecology	0	0	0	0		00.0	0			0	0	0	0	0	0
Eye, ear, nose, and throat	1	26	425	632		07.7	2			2,956	0	3,483	3,483	0	0
Rehabilitation	3	120	1,301	30,979		70.0	84			0	0	6,431	6,431	0	0
Orthopedic	0	0	0	0		00.0	0			0	0	0	0	0	0
Chronic disease	0	0	0	0		00.0	0			0	0	0	0	0	0
All other	0	0	0	0		00.0	0			0	0	0	0	0	0
Federal	4	1,041	16,766	282,839		74.4	775			10,264	32,302	219,239	251,541	0	0
Psychiatric	0	0	0	0		00.0	0			0	0	0	0	0	0
General and other special	4	1,041	16,766	282,839		74.4	775			10,264	32,302	219,239	251,541	0	0
Nonfederal	64	9,134	282,175	2,128,508		63.9	5,833			212,847	958,251	1,857,420	2,815,671	579	22,820
Psychiatric	5	699	5,436	199,519		78.3	547			21	133	2,933	3,066	0	0
Hospitals	4	559	5,358	155,589		76.4	427			0	43	2,598	2,641	0	0
Institutions for mentally retarded	1	140	78	43,930		85.7	120			21	90	335	425	0	0
TB and other respiratory diseases	0	0	0	0		00.0	0			0	0	0	0	0	0
Long-term general and other special	0	0	0	0		00.0	0			0	0	0	0	0	0
Short-term general and other special	59	8,435	276,739	1,928,989		62.7	5,286			212,826	958,118	1,854,487	2,812,605	579	22,820
Hospital units of institutions	0	0	0	0		00.0	0			0	0	0	0	0	0
Community hospitals*	59	8,435	276,739	1,928,989	2,638,292	62.7	5,286	7,230	7.0	212,826	958,118	1,854,487	2,812,605	579	22,820
6-24 beds	2	41	1,023	6,557	12,663	43.9	18	35	6.4	70	4,324	20,956	25,280	0	0
25-49	14	554	10,164	98,797	150,587	48.7	270	414	9.7	7,232	53,872	97,850	151,722	14	82
50-99	18	1,289	37,996	259,249	398,574	55.2	711	1,091	6.8	22,105	198,789	330,598	529,387	82	2,217
100-199	6	755	28,598	184,360	275,560	66.9	505	755	6.4	25,110	111,144	221,639	332,783	59	2,999
200-299	14	3,521	120,135	776,135	1,047,030	60.4	2,127	2,869	6.5	97,313	396,949	704,537	1,101,486	288	10,798
300-399	3	969	31,326	260,084	340,803	73.6	713	934	8.3	26,734	91,053	291,323	382,376	65	2,657
400-499	1	440	14,806	110,155	131,339	68.6	302	360	7.4	8,366	33,928	33,651	67,579	21	288
500 or more	1	866	32,691	233,652	281,736	73.9	640	772	7.1	25,896	68,059	153,933	221,992	50	3,779
Nongovernment not-for-profit	33	6,400	214,566	1,480,968	2,000,198	63.4	4,058	5,480	6.9	168,717	690,397	1,478,903	2,169,300	473	18,291
Investor-owned (for-profit)	15	1,105	32,557	230,561	307,294	57.2	632	844	7.1	23,541	119,236	144,832	264,068	58	2,364
State and local government	11	930	29,616	217,460	330,800	64.1	596	906	7.3	20,568	148,485	230,752	379,237	48	2,165

*For information on community hospitals that excludes nursing-home-type data, refer to Hospital Units columns in tables 4A through 4D, pages 14 through 17.

CLASSIFICATION	FULL-TIME EQUIVALENT PERSONNEL					FULL-TIME EQUIVALENT TRAINEES			EXPENSES						
									LABOR				TOTAL		
	Physicians and Dentists	Registered Nurses	Licensed Practical Nurses	Other Salaried Personnel	Total Personnel	Medical and Dental Residents	Other Trainees	Total Trainees	Payroll (in thousands)	Employee Benefits (in thousands)	Total (in thousands)	Percent of Total	Amount (in thousands)	Adjusted, per Admission	Adjusted, per Inpatient Day
WEST VIRGINIA	339	6,518	2,170	22,652	31,679	417	41	458	$ 737,747	$ 153,040	$ 890,787	52.7	$ 1,690,949		
6-24 beds	2	25	24	82	133	0	0	0	2,023	372	2,395	55.4	4,320		
25-49	14	198	97	976	1,285	0	0	0	23,846	4,332	28,178	47.4	59,503		
50-99	28	735	352	2,860	3,975	1	0	1	78,276	16,401	94,677	48.9	193,525		
100-199	98	798	295	2,989	4,180	32	12	44	107,324	19,742	127,066	53.9	235,727		
200-299	99	2,368	917	8,068	11,452	14	22	36	268,026	51,956	319,982	53.9	593,835		
300-399	32	907	210	3,478	4,627	243	0	243	93,656	21,512	115,168	48.8	235,946		
400-499	45	531	141	1,707	2,424	23	0	23	68,723	13,459	82,181	61.0	134,759		
500 or more	21	956	134	2,492	3,603	104	7	111	95,872	25,267	121,138	51.9	233,334		
Psychiatric	9	108	64	1,124	1,305	0	7	7	24,694	5,960	30,654	65.7	46,670		
Hospitals	7	97	53	842	999	0	0	0	18,099	4,374	22,472	61.5	36,529		
Institutions for mentally retarded	2	11	11	282	306	0	7	7	6,595	1,587	8,182	80.7	10,141		
General	325	6,351	2,073	21,246	29,995	417	34	451	704,792	145,728	850,519	52.5	1,620,700		
Hospitals	325	6,351	2,073	21,246	29,995	417	34	451	704,792	145,728	850,519	52.5	1,620,700		
Hospital units of institutions	0	0	0	0	0	0	0	0	0	0	0	0.0	0		
TB and other respiratory diseases	0	0	0	0	0	0	0	0	0	0	0	0.0	0		
Obstetrics and gynecology	0	0	0	0	0	0	0	0	0	0	0	0.0	0		
Eye, ear, nose, and throat	0	16	0	55	71	0	0	0	1,892	295	2,187	44.9	4,874		
Rehabilitation	5	43	33	227	308	0	0	0	6,369	1,057	7,426	39.7	18,704		
Orthopedic	0	0	0	0	0	0	0	0	0	0	0	0.0	0		
Chronic disease	0	0	0	0	0	0	0	0	0	0	0	0.0	0		
All other	0	0	0	0	0	0	0	0	0	0	0	0.0	0		
Federal	114	408	132	1,938	2,592	35	2	37	78,752	15,017	93,768	60.9	154,073		
Psychiatric	0	0	0	0	0	0	0	0	0	0	0	0.0	0		
General and other special	114	408	132	1,938	2,592	35	2	37	78,752	15,017	93,768	60.9	154,073		
Nonfederal	225	6,110	2,038	20,714	29,087	382	39	421	658,995	138,023	797,018	51.9	1,536,877		
Psychiatric	9	108	64	1,124	1,305	0	7	7	24,694	5,960	30,654	65.7	46,670		
Hospitals	7	97	53	842	999	0	0	0	18,099	4,374	22,472	61.5	36,529		
Institutions for mentally retarded	2	11	11	282	306	0	7	7	6,595	1,587	8,182	80.7	10,141		
TB and other respiratory diseases	0	0	0	0	0	0	0	0	0	0	0	0.0	0		
Long-term general and other special	0	0	0	0	0	0	0	0	0	0	0	0.0	0		
Short-term general and other special	216	6,002	1,974	19,590	27,782	382	32	414	634,301	132,063	766,364	51.4	1,490,207		
Hospital units of institutions	0	0	0	0	0	0	0	0	0	0	0	0.0	0		
Community hospitals*	216	6,002	1,974	19,590	27,782	382	32	414	634,301	132,063	766,364	51.4	1,490,207	$3,918.34	$ 564.84
6-24 beds	2	25	24	82	133	0	0	0	2,023	372	2,395	55.4	4,320	2,206.41	341.16
25-49	14	198	97	976	1,285	0	0	0	23,846	4,332	28,178	47.4	59,503	3,408.13	395.14
50-99	27	701	344	2,684	3,756	1	0	1	72,817	15,149	87,966	48.2	182,513	3,119.35	457.92
100-199	47	555	224	1,752	2,578	2	4	6	62,450	10,910	73,360	53.9	136,081	3,205.53	493.84
200-299	79	2,296	888	7,821	11,084	14	21	35	256,693	49,857	306,550	53.3	575,401	3,566.90	549.56
300-399	26	880	176	2,941	4,023	243	0	243	84,770	19,274	104,044	47.0	221,430	5,329.50	649.73
400-499	0	391	87	842	1,320	18	0	18	35,831	6,902	42,733	55.1	77,624	4,397.21	591.02
500 or more	21	956	134	2,492	3,603	104	7	111	95,872	25,267	121,138	51.9	233,334	5,919.34	828.20
Nongovernment not-for-profit	177	4,954	1,320	15,177	21,628	379	32	411	508,802	107,750	616,553	52.2	1,181,363	4,054.12	590.62
Investor-owned (for-profit)	6	513	350	2,112	2,981	3	0	3	60,872	12,285	73,157	41.5	176,094	3,957.26	573.05
State and local government	33	535	304	2,301	3,173	0	0	0	64,627	12,028	76,655	57.7	132,749	2,988.57	401.30

*For information on community hospitals that excludes nursing-home-type data, refer to Hospital Units columns in tables 4A through 4D, pages 14 through 17.

(continued on next page)

Table

5C (Continued) Wisconsin

Utilization, Personnel, and Finances in States

Excludes AHA nonregistered hospitals (see Table 14, page 240).

CLASSIFICATION	HOSPITALS	BEDS	ADMISSIONS	INPATIENT DAYS	ADJUSTED PATIENT DAYS	OCCUPANCY, percent	AVERAGE DAILY CENSUS	ADJUSTED AVERAGE DAILY CENSUS	AVERAGE STAY, days	SURGICAL OPERATIONS	OUTPATIENT VISITS Emergency	OUTPATIENT VISITS Other	OUTPATIENT VISITS Total	NEWBORNS Bassinets	NEWBORNS Births
WISCONSIN	148	23,756	629,243	5,947,290		68.6	16,296			474,664	1,533,039	5,128,398	6,661,437	1,523	71,630
6-24 beds	4	82	1,910	16,573		54.9	45			730	4,078	45,649	49,727	10	157
25-49	24	874	27,265	154,656		48.6	425			15,890	82,267	256,213	338,480	122	3,098
50-99	40	3,004	68,761	655,334		59.8	1,797			48,242	227,303	659,251	886,554	255	6,994
100-199	41	5,884	149,608	1,342,398		62.5	3,677			123,242	418,225	1,049,991	1,468,216	408	16,877
200-299	17	4,029	129,644	999,753		67.9	2,737			101,991	320,287	1,135,509	1,455,796	296	15,548
300-399	11	3,656	116,531	935,658		70.1	2,564			78,227	251,709	734,498	986,207	233	14,645
400-499	5	2,265	81,799	666,818		80.7	1,828			78,067	140,773	582,967	723,740	157	12,257
500 or more	6	3,962	53,725	1,176,100		81.3	3,223			28,275	88,397	664,320	752,717	42	2,054
Psychiatric	17	4,060	18,683	1,274,547		86.0	3,490			1,054	13,929	475,124	489,053	0	0
Hospitals	16	3,386	18,643	1,040,794		84.2	2,850			1,051	13,536	473,998	487,534	0	0
Institutions for mentally retarded	1	674	40	233,753		95.0	640			3	393	1,126	1,519	0	0
General	130	19,600	609,751	4,652,868		65.1	12,752			473,610	1,519,110	4,631,063	6,150,173	1,523	71,630
Hospitals	130	19,600	609,751	4,652,868		65.1	12,752			473,610	1,519,110	4,631,063	6,150,173	1,523	71,630
Hospital units of institutions	0	0	0	0		00.0	0			0	0	0	0	0	0
TB and other respiratory diseases	0	0	0	0		00.0	0			0	0	0	0	0	0
Obstetrics and gynecology	0	0	0	0		00.0	0			0	0	0	0	0	0
Eye, ear, nose, and throat	0	0	0	0		00.0	0			0	0	0	0	0	0
Rehabilitation	1	96	809	19,875		56.3	54			0	0	22,211	22,211	0	0
Orthopedic	0	0	0	0		00.0	0			0	0	0	0	0	0
Chronic disease	0	0	0	0		00.0	0			0	0	0	0	0	0
All other	0	0	0	0		00.0	0			0	0	0	0	0	0
Federal	3	1,673	16,610	466,469		76.4	1,278			9,898	10,197	290,350	300,547	0	0
Psychiatric	1	664	2,704	202,293		83.4	554			1,051	0	54,985	54,985	0	0
General and other special	2	1,009	13,906	264,176		71.8	724			8,847	10,197	235,365	245,562	0	0
Nonfederal	145	22,083	612,633	5,480,821		68.0	15,018			464,766	1,522,842	4,838,048	6,360,890	1,523	71,630
Psychiatric	16	3,396	15,979	1,072,254		86.5	2,936			3	13,929	420,139	434,068	0	0
Hospitals	15	2,722	15,939	838,501		84.3	2,296			0	13,536	419,013	432,549	0	0
Institutions for mentally retarded	1	674	40	233,753		95.0	640			3	393	1,126	1,519	0	0
TB and other respiratory diseases	0	0	0	0		00.0	0			0	0	0	0	0	0
Long-term general and other special	0	0	0	0		00.0	0			0	0	0	0	0	0
Short-term general and other special	129	18,687	596,654	4,408,567		64.7	12,082			464,763	1,508,913	4,417,909	5,926,822	1,523	71,630
Hospital units of institutions	0	0	0	0		00.0	0			0	0	0	0	0	0
Community hospitals*	129	18,687	596,654	4,408,567	6,096,589	64.7	12,082	16,711	7.4	464,763	1,508,913	4,417,909	5,926,822	1,523	71,630
6-24 beds	2	46	1,247	6,162	10,333	37.0	17	29	4.9	730	4,078	20,124	24,202	10	157
25-49	21	770	26,020	130,125	211,477	46.5	358	580	5.0	15,890	82,242	255,760	338,002	122	3,098
50-99	36	2,693	64,874	581,456	869,215	59.2	1,595	2,382	9.0	48,242	227,303	578,683	805,986	255	6,994
100-199	40	5,750	148,228	1,303,916	1,854,191	62.1	3,572	5,082	8.8	123,242	415,730	1,026,106	1,441,836	408	16,877
200-299	15	3,488	122,323	852,114	1,202,429	66.9	2,333	3,295	7.0	99,208	320,287	1,048,798	1,369,085	296	15,548
300-399	9	3,051	115,102	741,580	967,719	66.6	2,032	2,651	6.4	78,227	251,709	722,583	974,292	233	14,645
400-499	4	1,833	80,357	516,940	658,946	77.3	1,417	1,807	6.4	78,067	140,773	549,028	689,801	157	12,257
500 or more	2	1,056	38,503	276,274	322,279	71.8	758	885	7.2	21,157	66,791	216,827	283,618	42	2,054
Nongovernment not-for-profit	122	17,427	560,107	4,074,408	5,647,661	64.1	11,167	15,481	7.3	421,438	1,412,303	3,831,816	5,244,119	1,475	69,855
Investor-owned (for-profit)	0	0	0	0	0	00.0	0	0	0.0	0	0	0	0	0	0
State and local government	7	1,260	36,547	334,159	448,928	72.6	915	1,230	9.1	43,325	96,610	586,093	682,703	48	1,775

*For information on community hospitals that excludes nursing-home-type data, refer to Hospital Units columns in tables 4A through 4D, pages 14 through 17.

Table 5C (Continued) Wisconsin

CLASSIFICATION	FULL-TIME EQUIVALENT PERSONNEL: Physicians and Dentists	Registered Nurses	Licensed Practical Nurses	Other Salaried Personnel	Total Personnel	FULL-TIME EQUIVALENT TRAINEES: Medical and Dental Residents	Other Trainees	Total Trainees	EXPENSES — LABOR: Payroll (in thousands)	Employee Benefits (in thousands)	Total (in thousands)	Percent of Total	EXPENSES — TOTAL: Amount (in thousands)	Adjusted, per Admission	Adjusted, per Inpatient Day
WISCONSIN	397	16,902	2,295	52,143	71,737	748	138	886	$ 1,826,540	$ 350,345	$ 2,176,885	56.4	$ 3,859,060		
6-24 beds	1	41	16	132	190	0	0	0	5,958	1,071	7,029	55.9	12,577		
25-49	9	587	121	1,924	2,641	0	0	0	56,114	10,559	66,673	55.0	121,228		
50-99	14	1,480	349	5,412	7,255	0	2	2	160,137	29,497	189,635	55.4	342,009		
100-199	12	3,622	584	11,200	15,418	11	3	14	361,014	66,525	427,539	54.5	784,473		
200-299	93	3,387	552	10,274	14,306	87	30	117	366,393	62,915	429,308	56.3	762,511		
300-399	97	3,530	413	9,469	13,509	33	1	34	351,521	69,607	421,127	57.6	731,270		
400-499	13	2,549	46	6,513	9,121	504	41	545	252,904	55,987	308,891	54.2	570,129		
500 or more	158	1,706	214	7,219	9,297	113	61	174	272,499	54,183	326,682	61.1	534,863		
Psychiatric	114	717	134	5,943	6,908	20	9	29	191,547	41,627	233,175	69.8	334,161		
Hospitals	108	682	106	4,768	5,664	20	9	29	164,792	35,189	199,981	68.2	293,018		
Institutions for mentally retarded	6	35	28	1,175	1,244	0	0	0	26,756	6,438	33,194	80.7	41,143		
General	281	16,137	2,149	45,950	64,517	728	129	857	1,627,369	307,577	1,934,946	55.1	3,511,920		
Hospitals	281	16,137	2,149	45,950	64,517	728	129	857	1,627,369	307,577	1,934,946	55.1	3,511,920		
Hospital units of institutions	0	0	0	0	0	0	0	0	0	0	0	0.0	0		
TB and other respiratory diseases	0	0	0	0	0	0	0	0	0	0	0	0.0	0		
Obstetrics and gynecology	0	0	0	0	0	0	0	0	0	0	0	0.0	0		
Eye, ear, nose, and throat	0	0	0	0	0	0	0	0	0	0	0	0.0	0		
Rehabilitation	2	48	12	250	312	0	0	0	7,623	1,141	8,764	67.5	12,979		
Orthopedic	0	0	0	0	0	0	0	0	0	0	0	0.0	0		
Chronic disease	0	0	0	0	0	0	0	0	0	0	0	0.0	0		
All other	0	0	0	0	0	0	0	0	0	0	0	0.0	0		
Federal	173	573	174	2,561	3,481	129	24	153	115,446	15,678	131,124	66.2	198,088		
Psychiatric	21	126	26	754	927	0	0	0	30,516	5,575	36,091	70.4	51,288		
General and other special	152	447	148	1,807	2,554	129	24	153	84,930	10,104	95,033	64.7	146,800		
Nonfederal	224	16,329	2,121	49,582	68,256	619	114	733	1,711,094	334,667	2,045,761	55.9	3,660,972		
Psychiatric	93	591	108	5,189	5,981	20	9	29	161,031	36,053	197,084	69.7	282,873		
Hospitals	87	556	80	4,014	4,737	20	9	29	134,276	29,614	163,890	67.8	241,730		
Institutions for mentally retarded	6	35	28	1,175	1,244	0	0	0	26,756	6,438	33,194	80.7	41,143		
TB and other respiratory diseases	0	0	0	0	0	0	0	0	0	0	0	0.0	0		
Long-term general and other special	0	0	0	0	0	0	0	0	0	0	0	0.0	0		
Short-term general and other special	131	15,738	2,013	44,393	62,275	599	105	704	1,550,062	298,614	1,848,677	54.7	3,378,099		
Hospital units of institutions	0	0	0	0	0	0	0	0	0	0	0	0.0	0		
Community hospitals*	131	15,738	2,013	44,393	62,275	599	105	704	1,550,062	298,614	1,848,677	54.7	3,378,099	$4,082.52	$ 554.10
6-24 beds	0	33	12	81	126	0	0	0	2,442	385	2,828	49.6	5,696	2,725.44	551.26
25-49	9	566	119	1,790	2,484	0	0	0	51,628	9,536	61,164	55.2	110,765	2,615.48	523.77
50-99	8	1,416	335	4,875	6,634	0	0	0	143,172	26,661	169,833	54.3	312,585	3,131.11	359.62
100-199	11	3,573	579	10,964	15,127	11	3	14	354,539	65,152	419,692	54.5	770,247	3,621.57	415.41
200-299	35	3,183	482	9,373	13,073	11	17	28	318,652	59,254	377,906	55.4	681,594	3,937.92	566.85
300-399	58	3,374	368	8,522	12,322	24	1	25	319,323	59,892	379,215	55.6	681,779	4,536.27	704.52
400-499	10	2,531	41	5,947	8,529	504	41	545	240,910	53,567	294,477	53.8	547,236	5,360.28	830.47
500 or more	0	1,062	77	2,841	3,980	49	43	92	119,396	24,166	143,562	53.5	268,195	5,956.05	832.18
Nongovernment not-for-profit	127	14,373	1,955	40,517	56,972	261	105	366	1,404,710	260,281	1,664,991	54.8	3,039,574	3,905.55	538.20
Investor-owned (for-profit)	0	0	0	0	0	0	0	0	0	0	0	0.0	0	0.00	0.00
State and local government	4	1,365	58	3,876	5,303	338	0	338	145,352	38,333	183,686	54.3	338,525	6,882.82	754.07

*For information on community hospitals that excludes nursing-home-type data, refer to Hospital Units columns in tables 4A through 4D, pages 14 through 17.

(continued on next page)

Table

5C (Continued) Wyoming

Utilization, Personnel, and Finances in States

Excludes AHA nonregistered hospitals (see Table 14, page 240).

CLASSIFICATION	HOSPI-TALS	BEDS	ADMISSIONS	INPATIENT DAYS	ADJUSTED PATIENT DAYS	OCCU-PANCY, percent	AVERAGE DAILY CENSUS	ADJUSTED AVERAGE DAILY CENSUS	AVERAGE STAY, days	SURGICAL OPERATIONS	OUTPATIENT VISITS			NEWBORNS	
											Emergency	Other	Total	Bassinets	Births
WYOMING	32	2,925	54,821	629,874		58.9	1,724			38,481	181,704	485,244	666,948	244	6,399
6-24 beds	3	57	2,512	7,648		36.8	21			1,529	18,901	91,788	110,689	19	477
25-49	7	294	5,673	44,323		40.8	120			3,653	16,855	43,447	60,302	29	562
50-99	11	790	15,966	166,226		57.7	456			9,140	55,205	142,208	197,413	93	1,829
100-199	8	985	21,735	211,107		58.7	578			18,964	68,399	168,923	237,322	65	2,510
200-299	2	460	7,009	125,253		74.6	343			5,195	22,344	16,132	38,476	38	1,021
300-399	1	339	1,926	75,317		60.8	206			0	0	22,746	22,746	0	0
400-499	0	0	0	0		00.0	0			0	0	0	0	0	0
500 or more	0	0	0	0		00.0	0			0	0	0	0	0	0
Psychiatric	3	622	3,032	168,651		74.3	462			0	0	22,746	22,746	0	0
Hospitals	3	622	3,032	168,651		74.3	462			0	0	22,746	22,746	0	0
Institutions for mentally retarded	0	0	0	0		00.0	0			0	0	0	0	0	0
General	29	2,303	51,789	461,223		54.8	1,262			38,481	181,704	462,498	644,202	244	6,399
Hospitals	29	2,303	51,789	461,223		54.8	1,262			38,481	181,704	462,498	644,202	244	6,399
Hospital units of institutions	0	0	0	0		00.0	0			0	0	0	0	0	0
TB and other respiratory diseases	0	0	0	0		00.0	0			0	0	0	0	0	0
Obstetrics and gynecology	0	0	0	0		00.0	0			0	0	0	0	0	0
Eye, ear, nose, and throat	0	0	0	0		00.0	0			0	0	0	0	0	0
Rehabilitation	0	0	0	0		00.0	0			0	0	0	0	0	0
Orthopedic	0	0	0	0		00.0	0			0	0	0	0	0	0
Chronic disease	0	0	0	0		00.0	0			0	0	0	0	0	0
All other	0	0	0	0		00.0	0			0	0	0	0	0	0
Federal	3	499	5,742	115,630		63.3	316			3,049	15,469	140,532	156,001	8	305
Psychiatric	1	339	1,926	75,317		60.8	206			0	0	22,746	22,746	0	0
General and other special	2	160	3,816	40,313		68.8	110			3,049	15,469	117,786	133,255	8	305
Nonfederal	29	2,426	49,079	514,244		58.0	1,408			35,432	166,235	344,712	510,947	236	6,094
Psychiatric	2	283	1,106	93,334		90.5	256			0	0	0	0	0	0
Hospitals	2	283	1,106	93,334		90.5	256			0	0	0	0	0	0
Institutions for mentally retarded	0	0	0	0		00.0	0			0	0	0	0	0	0
TB and other respiratory diseases	0	0	0	0		00.0	0			0	0	0	0	0	0
Long-term general and other special	0	0	0	0		00.0	0			0	0	0	0	0	0
Short-term general and other special	27	2,143	47,973	420,910		53.8	1,152			35,432	166,235	344,712	510,947	236	6,094
Hospital units of institutions	0	0	0	0		00.0	0			0	0	0	0	0	0
Community hospitals*	27	2,143	47,973	420,910	584,129	53.8	1,152	1,598	8.8	35,432	166,235	344,712	510,947	236	6,094
6-24 beds	2	33	619	2,540	5,188	21.2	7	14	4.1	358	3,432	5,429	8,861	11	172
25-49	6	246	5,101	33,421	51,684	36.6	90	141	6.6	3,653	16,855	43,447	60,302	29	562
50-99	11	790	15,966	166,226	231,505	57.7	456	633	10.4	9,140	55,205	142,208	197,413	93	1,829
100-199	7	849	19,812	175,902	242,385	56.8	482	664	8.9	17,086	68,399	137,496	205,895	65	2,510
200-299	1	225	6,475	42,821	53,367	52.0	117	146	6.6	5,195	22,344	16,132	38,476	38	1,021
300-399	0	0	0	0	0	00.0	0	0	0.0	0	0	0	0	0	0
400-499	0	0	0	0	0	00.0	0	0	0.0	0	0	0	0	0	0
500 or more	0	0	0	0	0	00.0	0	0	0.0	0	0	0	0	0	0
Nongovernment not-for-profit	9	718	15,576	143,421	193,091	54.6	392	529	9.2	11,745	56,438	96,701	153,139	88	1,985
Investor-owned (for-profit)	2	172	4,535	18,670	25,154	29.7	51	68	4.1	2,867	12,514	24,205	36,719	26	542
State and local government	16	1,253	27,862	258,819	365,884	56.6	709	1,001	9.3	20,820	97,283	223,806	321,089	122	3,567

*For information on community hospitals that excludes nursing-home-type data, refer to Hospital Units columns in tables 4A through 4D, pages 14 through 17.

CLASSIFICATION	FULL-TIME EQUIVALENT PERSONNEL					FULL-TIME EQUIVALENT TRAINEES			EXPENSES						
									LABOR				TOTAL		
	Physicians and Dentists	Registered Nurses	Licensed Practical Nurses	Other Salaried Personnel	Total Personnel	Medical and Dental Residents	Other Trainees	Total Trainees	Payroll (in thousands)	Employee Benefits (in thousands)	Total (in thousands)	Percent of Total	Amount (in thousands)	Adjusted, per Admission	Adjusted, per Inpatient Day
WYOMING	70	1,448	311	5,161	6,990	0	12	12	$ 155,838	$ 29,618	$ 185,456	55.0	$ 337,133		
6-24 beds	26	48	10	244	328	0	0	0	6,073	1,287	7,360	62.0	11,876		
25-49	0	102	26	426	554	0	0	0	12,954	2,581	15,535	49.7	31,245		
50-99	0	314	76	1,283	1,673	0	0	0	36,035	6,684	42,719	54.7	78,036		
100-199	23	609	129	1,962	2,723	0	8	8	59,922	10,928	70,850	52.3	135,496		
200-299	9	285	44	931	1,269	0	4	4	27,496	5,762	33,258	56.1	59,312		
300-399	12	90	26	315	443	0	0	0	13,358	2,377	15,735	74.3	21,168		
400-499	0	0	0	0	0	0	0	0	0	0	0	0.0	0		
500 or more	0	0	0	0	0	0	0	0	0	0	0	0.0	0		
Psychiatric	21	119	52	749	941	0	0	0	23,450	4,850	28,300	72.9	38,832		
Hospitals	21	119	52	749	941	0	0	0	23,450	4,850	28,300	72.9	38,832		
Institutions for mentally retarded	0	0	0	0	0	0	0	0	0	0	0	0.0	0		
General	49	1,329	259	4,412	6,049	0	12	12	132,388	24,769	157,157	52.7	298,301		
Hospitals	49	1,329	259	4,412	6,049	0	12	12	132,388	24,769	157,157	52.7	298,301		
Hospital units of institutions	0	0	0	0	0	0	0	0	0	0	0	0.0	0		
TB and other respiratory diseases	0	0	0	0	0	0	0	0	0	0	0	0.0	0		
Obstetrics and gynecology	0	0	0	0	0	0	0	0	0	0	0	0.0	0		
Eye, ear, nose, and throat	0	0	0	0	0	0	0	0	0	0	0	0.0	0		
Rehabilitation	0	0	0	0	0	0	0	0	0	0	0	0.0	0		
Orthopedic	0	0	0	0	0	0	0	0	0	0	0	0.0	0		
Chronic disease	0	0	0	0	0	0	0	0	0	0	0	0.0	0		
All other	0	0	0	0	0	0	0	0	0	0	0	0.0	0		
Federal	48	173	42	765	1,028	0	6	6	27,096	5,102	32,199	65.1	49,491		
Psychiatric	12	90	26	315	443	0	0	0	13,358	2,377	15,735	74.3	21,168		
General and other special	36	83	16	450	585	0	6	6	13,738	2,725	16,464	58.1	28,322		
Nonfederal	22	1,275	269	4,396	5,962	0	6	6	128,742	24,516	153,258	53.3	287,643		
Psychiatric	9	29	26	434	498	0	0	0	10,092	2,473	12,565	71.1	17,664		
Hospitals	9	29	26	434	498	0	0	0	10,092	2,473	12,565	71.1	17,664		
Institutions for mentally retarded	0	0	0	0	0	0	0	0	0	0	0	0.0	0		
TB and other respiratory diseases	0	0	0	0	0	0	0	0	0	0	0	0.0	0		
Long-term general and other special	0	0	0	0	0	0	0	0	0	0	0	0.0	0		
Short-term general and other special	13	1,246	243	3,962	5,464	0	6	6	118,650	22,043	140,693	52.1	269,979		
Hospital units of institutions	0	0	0	0	0	0	0	0	0	0	0	0.0	0		
Community hospitals*	13	1,246	243	3,962	5,464	0	6	6	118,650	22,043	140,693	52.1	269,979	$3,990.47	$ 462.19
6-24 beds	3	15	7	66	91	0	0	0	1,981	376	2,357	49.7	4,738	3,925.52	913.28
25-49	0	91	24	358	473	0	0	0	10,635	2,089	12,724	48.7	26,149	3,267.80	505.94
50-99	0	314	76	1,283	1,673	0	0	0	36,035	6,684	42,719	54.7	78,036	3,437.25	337.08
100-199	10	559	116	1,690	2,375	0	2	2	50,276	9,113	59,389	52.0	114,312	4,130.66	471.61
200-299	0	267	20	565	852	0	4	4	19,723	3,781	23,505	50.3	46,744	5,792.34	875.90
300-399	0	0	0	0	0	0	0	0	0	0	0	0.0	0	0.00	0.00
400-499	0	0	0	0	0	0	0	0	0	0	0	0.0	0	0.00	0.00
500 or more	0	0	0	0	0	0	0	0	0	0	0	0.0	0	0.00	0.00
Nongovernment not-for-profit	5	475	76	1,339	1,895	0	4	4	42,415	7,814	50,229	51.4	97,785	4,517.46	506.42
Investor-owned (for-profit)	0	104	17	241	362	0	0	0	7,671	1,516	9,187	41.0	22,433	3,657.74	891.82
State and local government	8	667	150	2,382	3,207	0	2	2	68,564	12,713	81,277	54.3	149,761	3,755.58	409.31

*For information on community hospitals that excludes nursing-home-type data, refer to Hospital Units columns n tables 4A through 4D, pages 14 through 17.

Table

5D

Utilization, Personnel, and Finances in U.S. Associated Areas

CLASSIFICATION	HOSPITALS	BEDS	ADMISSIONS	INPATIENT DAYS	ADJUSTED PATIENT DAYS	OCCUPANCY, percent	AVERAGE DAILY CENSUS	ADJUSTED AVERAGE DAILY CENSUS	AVERAGE STAY, days	SURGICAL OPERATIONS	OUTPATIENT VISITS			NEWBORNS	
											Emergency	Other	Total	Bassinets	Births
U.S. ASSOCIATED AREAS	62	10,334	410,976	2,461,715		65.3	6,749			275,425	1,221,019	2,978,841	4,199,860	1,177	64,635
6-24 beds	1	24	1,420	4,215		50.0	12			997	16,638	98,424	115,062	2	216
25-49	5	178	5,354	22,963		36.0	64			6,925	62,668	179,379	242,047	39	650
50-99	15	1,158	50,862	243,302		57.7	668			34,830	99,686	270,449	370,135	142	6,191
100-199	25	3,467	145,994	791,699		62.6	2,171			111,374	498,803	909,894	1,408,697	450	22,290
200-299	6	1,500	69,368	342,177		62.5	938			45,881	179,910	363,207	543,117	199	12,795
300-399	6	2,023	87,890	519,582		70.4	1,424			50,678	251,359	458,184	709,543	190	12,307
400-499	3	1,233	36,594	321,963		71.5	881			19,658	111,955	291,385	403,340	155	10,186
500 or more	1	751	13,494	215,814		78.7	591			5,082	0	407,919	407,919	0	0
Psychiatric	4	850	4,728	230,723		74.4	632			0	1,897	19,300	21,197	0	0
Hospitals	4	850	4,728	230,723		74.4	632			0	1,897	19,300	21,197	0	0
Institutions for mentally retarded	0	0	0	0		00.0	0			0	0	0	0	0	0
General	57	9,405	404,110	2,216,471		64.6	6,077			274,368	1,213,016	2,947,123	4,160,139	1,177	64,635
Hospitals	57	9,405	404,110	2,216,471		64.6	6,077			274,368	1,213,016	2,947,123	4,160,139	1,177	64,635
Hospital units of institutions	0	0	0	0		00.0	0			0	0	0	0	0	0
TB and other respiratory diseases	0	0	0	0		00.0	0			0	0	0	0	0	0
Obstetrics and gynecology	0	0	0	0		00.0	0			0	0	0	0	0	0
Eye, ear, nose, and throat	0	0	0	0		00.0	0			0	0	0	0	0	0
Rehabilitation	0	0	0	0		00.0	0			0	0	0	0	0	0
Orthopedic	0	0	0	0		00.0	0			0	0	0	0	0	0
Chronic disease	0	0	0	0		00.0	0			0	0	0	0	0	0
All other	1	79	2,138	14,521		50.6	40			1,057	6,106	12,418	18,524	0	0
Federal	4	865	19,865	243,566		77.2	668			10,510	48,577	705,270	753,847	22	1,276
Psychiatric	0	0	0	0		00.0	0			0	0	0	0	0	0
General and other special	4	865	19,865	243,566		77.2	668			10,510	48,577	705,270	753,847	22	1,276
Nonfederal	58	9,469	391,111	2,218,149		64.2	6,081			264,915	1,172,442	2,273,571	3,446,013	1,155	63,359
Psychiatric	4	850	4,728	230,723		74.4	632			0	1,897	19,300	21,197	0	0
Hospitals	4	850	4,728	230,723		74.4	632			0	1,897	19,300	21,197	0	0
Institutions for mentally retarded	0	0	0	0		00.0	0			0	0	0	0	0	0
TB and other respiratory diseases	0	0	0	0		00.0	0			0	0	0	0	0	0
Long-term general and other special	0	0	0	0		00.0	0			0	0	0	0	0	0
Short-term general and other special	54	8,619	386,383	1,987,426		63.2	5,449			264,915	1,170,545	2,254,271	3,424,816	1,155	63,359
Hospital units of institutions	0	0	0	0		00.0	0			0	0	0	0	0	0
Community hospitals	54	8,619	386,383	1,987,426	2,522,954	63.2	5,449	6,913	5.1	264,915	1,170,545	2,254,271	3,424,816	1,155	63,359
6-24 beds	0	0	0	0	0	00.0	0	0	0.0	0	0	0	0	0	0
25-49	4	143	3,747	15,321	24,214	30.1	43	66	4.1	4,063	53,169	112,274	165,443	31	409
50-99	13	1,033	46,683	211,509	277,584	56.1	580	761	4.5	33,261	76,736	133,738	210,474	130	5,372
100-199	23	3,112	142,698	711,711	902,490	62.7	1,952	2,473	5.0	111,374	497,600	898,370	1,395,970	450	22,290
200-299	6	1,500	69,368	342,177	402,425	62.5	938	1,102	4.9	45,881	179,910	363,207	543,117	199	12,795
300-399	6	2,023	87,890	519,582	680,324	70.4	1,424	1,865	5.9	50,678	251,359	458,184	709,543	190	12,307
400-499	2	808	35,997	187,126	235,917	63.4	512	646	5.2	19,658	111,771	288,498	400,269	155	10,186
500 or more	0	0	0	0	0	00.0	0	0	0.0	0	0	0	0	0	0
Nongovernment not-for-profit	17	2,811	121,798	637,361	860,103	62.1	1,747	2,355	5.2	69,313	307,372	608,560	915,932	235	10,556
Investor-owned (for-profit)	17	2,108	104,427	483,267	614,275	62.9	1,325	1,685	4.6	67,269	177,878	281,932	459,810	258	13,843
State and local government	20	3,700	160,158	866,798	1,048,576	64.2	2,377	2,873	5.4	128,333	685,295	1,363,779	2,049,074	662	38,960

Table 5D (Continued) U.S. Associated Areas

CLASSIFICATION	FULL-TIME EQUIVALENT PERSONNEL					FULL-TIME EQUIVALENT TRAINEES			EXPENSES						
									LABOR				TOTAL		
	Physicians and Dentists	Registered Nurses	Licensed Practical Nurses	Other Salaried Personnel	Total Personnel	Medical and Dental Residents	Other Trainees	Total Trainees	Payroll (in thousands)	Employee Benefits (in thousands)	Total (in thousands)	Percent of Total	Amount (in thousands)	Adjusted, per Admission	Adjusted, per Inpatient Day
U.S. ASSOCIATED AREAS	1,117	6,872	3,397	20,268	31,654	691	11	702	$ 486,088	$ 99,758	$ 585,846	52.2	$ 1,123,112		
6-24 beds	23	32	7	233	295	0	0	0	4,092	911	5,003	70.1	7,138		
25-49	47	153	69	625	894	0	0	0	11,093	2,013	13,106	62.3	21,033		
50-99	102	665	319	2,217	3,303	0	0	0	52,920	8,930	61,851	51.1	121,134		
100-199	292	2,448	1,271	7,008	11,019	85	0	85	149,934	28,852	178,786	48.6	367,669		
200-299	176	1,182	520	3,005	4,883	75	0	75	71,021	12,616	83,637	58.3	143,541		
300-399	161	1,328	778	3,564	5,831	268	0	268	87,556	18,018	105,573	43.6	241,915		
400-499	153	712	322	2,134	3,321	150	1	151	50,232	12,383	62,616	63.3	98,859		
500 or more	163	352	111	1,482	2,108	113	10	123	59,240	16,035	75,275	61.8	121,821		
Psychiatric	36	178	95	985	1,294	2	1	3	35,861	7,903	43,763	64.6	67,780		
Hospitals	36	178	95	985	1,294	2	1	3	35,861	7,903	43,763	64.6	67,780		
Institutions for mentally retarded	0	0	0	0	0	0	0	0	0	0	0	0.0	0		
General	1,081	6,664	3,293	19,171	30,209	689	10	699	447,832	91,385	539,217	51.4	1,049,991		
Hospitals	1,081	6,664	3,293	19,171	30,209	689	10	699	447,832	91,385	539,217	51.4	1,049,991		
Hospital units of institutions	0	0	0	0	0	0	0	0	0	0	0	0.0	0		
TB and other respiratory diseases	0	0	0	0	0	0	0	0	0	0	0	0.0	0		
Obstetrics and gynecology	0	0	0	0	0	0	0	0	0	0	0	0.0	0		
Eye, ear, nose, and throat	0	0	0	0	0	0	0	0	0	0	0	0.0	0		
Rehabilitation	0	0	0	0	0	0	0	0	0	0	0	0.0	0		
Orthopedic	0	0	0	0	0	0	0	0	0	0	0	0.0	0		
Chronic disease	0	0	0	0	0	0	0	0	0	0	0	0.0	0		
All other	0	30	9	112	151	0	0	0	2,395	471	2,866	53.7	5,341		
Federal	253	471	131	2,370	3,225	113	10	123	77,414	19,637	97,051	63.6	152,578		
Psychiatric	0	0	0	0	0	0	0	0	0	0	0	0.0	0		
General and other special	253	471	131	2,370	3,225	113	10	123	77,414	19,637	97,051	63.6	152,578		
Nonfederal	864	6,401	3,266	17,898	28,429	578	1	579	408,674	80,122	488,795	50.4	970,534		
Psychiatric	36	178	95	985	1,294	2	1	3	35,861	7,903	43,763	64.6	67,780		
Hospitals	36	178	95	985	1,294	2	1	3	35,861	7,903	43,763	64.6	67,780		
Institutions for mentally retarded	0	0	0	0	0	0	0	0	0	0	0	0.0	0		
TB and other respiratory diseases	0	0	0	0	0	0	0	0	0	0	0	0.0	0		
Long-term general and other special	0	0	0	0	0	0	0	0	0	0	0	0.0	0		
Short-term general and other special	828	6,223	3,171	16,913	27,135	576	0	576	372,813	72,219	445,032	49.3	902,754		
Hospital units of institutions	0	0	0	0	0	0	0	0	0	0	0	0.0	0		
Community hospitals	828	6,223	3,171	16,913	27,135	576	0	576	372,813	72,219	445,032	49.3	902,754	$1,853.08	$ 357.82
6-24 beds	0	0	0	0	0	0	0	0	0	0	0	0.0	0	0.00	0.00
25-49	23	116	60	401	600	0	0	0	5,192	760	5,952	52.3	11,390	1,915.19	470.38
50-99	58	598	312	1,687	2,655	0	0	0	41,357	6,775	48,132	48.3	99,728	1,639.24	359.27
100-199	275	2,351	1,211	6,649	10,486	84	0	84	136,652	27,161	163,813	48.6	337,043	1,869.31	373.46
200-299	176	1,182	520	3,005	4,883	75	0	75	71,021	12,616	83,637	58.3	143,541	1,754.16	356.69
300-399	161	1,328	778	3,564	5,831	268	0	268	87,556	18,018	105,573	43.6	241,915	2,143.40	355.59
400-499	135	648	290	1,607	2,680	149	0	149	31,036	6,889	37,924	54.9	69,137	1,523.41	293.06
500 or more	0	0	0	0	0	0	0	0	0	0	0	0.0	0	0.00	0.00
Nongovernment not-for-profit	107	1,552	856	4,773	7,288	95	0	95	109,781	15,611	125,392	48.8	257,091	1,579.49	298.91
Investor-owned (for-profit)	55	1,385	635	3,543	5,618	12	0	12	71,949	15,428	87,377	40.6	215,059	1,621.34	350.10
State and local government	666	3,286	1,680	8,597	14,229	469	0	469	191,083	41,179	232,262	53.9	430,604	2,245.61	410.66

Table

5E

Utilization, Personnel, and Finances in Puerto Rico

CLASSIFICATION	HOSPITALS	BEDS	ADMISSIONS	INPATIENT DAYS	ADJUSTED PATIENT DAYS	OCCUPANCY, percent	AVERAGE DAILY CENSUS	ADJUSTED AVERAGE DAILY CENSUS	AVERAGE STAY, days	SURGICAL OPERATIONS	OUTPATIENT VISITS Emergency	OUTPATIENT VISITS Other	OUTPATIENT VISITS Total	NEWBORNS Bassinets	NEWBORNS Births
PUERTO RICO	56	9,762	388,706	2,339,593		65.7	6,413			258,672	1,066,496	2,612,629	3,679,125	1,071	60,149
6-24 beds	0	0	0	0		00.0	0			0	0	0	0	0	0
25-49	5	178	5,354	22,963		36.0	64			6,925	62,668	179,379	242,047	39	650
50-99	13	1,016	44,188	208,393		56.3	572			33,115	68,386	121,528	189,914	108	4,395
100-199	22	3,061	131,818	708,701		63.5	1,943			97,333	392,218	791,027	1,183,245	380	19,816
200-299	6	1,500	69,368	342,177		62.5	938			45,881	179,910	363,207	543,117	199	12,795
300-399	6	2,023	87,890	519,582		70.4	1,424			50,678	251,359	458,184	709,543	190	12,307
400-499	3	1,233	36,594	321,963		71.5	881			19,658	111,955	291,385	403,340	155	10,186
500 or more	1	751	13,494	215,814		78.7	591			5,082	0	407,919	407,919	0	0
Psychiatric	4	850	4,728	230,723		74.4	632			0	1,897	19,300	21,197	0	0
Hospitals	4	850	4,728	230,723		74.4	632			0	1,897	19,300	21,197	0	0
Institutions for mentally retarded	0	0	0	0		00.0	0			0	0	0	0	0	0
General	51	8,833	381,840	2,094,349		65.0	5,741			257,615	1,058,493	2,580,911	3,639,404	1,071	60,149
Hospitals	51	8,833	381,840	2,094,349		65.0	5,741			257,615	1,058,493	2,580,911	3,639,404	1,071	60,149
Hospital units of institutions	0	0	0	0		00.0	0			0	0	0	0	0	0
TB and other respiratory diseases	0	0	0	0		00.0	0			0	0	0	0	0	0
Obstetrics and gynecology	0	0	0	0		00.0	0			0	0	0	0	0	0
Eye, ear, nose, and throat	0	0	0	0		00.0	0			0	0	0	0	0	0
Rehabilitation	0	0	0	0		00.0	0			0	0	0	0	0	0
Orthopedic	0	0	0	0		00.0	0			0	0	0	0	0	0
Chronic disease	0	0	0	0		00.0	0			0	0	0	0	0	0
All other	1	79	2,138	14,521		50.6	40			1,057	6,106	12,418	18,524	0	0
Federal	2	786	15,101	223,456		77.9	612			7,944	9,499	475,024	484,523	8	241
Psychiatric	0	0	0	0		00.0	0			0	0	0	0	0	0
General and other special	2	786	15,101	223,456		77.9	612			7,944	9,499	475,024	484,523	8	241
Nonfederal	54	8,976	373,605	2,116,137		64.6	5,801			250,728	1,056,997	2,137,605	3,194,602	1,063	59,908
Psychiatric	4	850	4,728	230,723		74.4	632			0	1,897	19,300	21,197	0	0
Hospitals	4	850	4,728	230,723		74.4	632			0	1,897	19,300	21,197	0	0
Institutions for mentally retarded	0	0	0	0		00.0	0			0	0	0	0	0	0
TB and other respiratory diseases	0	0	0	0		00.0	0			0	0	0	0	0	0
Long-term general and other special	0	0	0	0		00.0	0			0	0	0	0	0	0
Short-term general and other special	50	8,126	368,877	1,885,414		63.6	5,169			250,728	1,055,100	2,118,305	3,173,405	1,063	59,908
Hospital units of institutions	0	0	0	0		00.0	0			0	0	0	0	0	0
Community hospitals	50	8,126	368,877	1,885,414	2,406,314	63.6	5,169	6,593	5.1	250,728	1,055,100	2,118,305	3,173,405	1,063	59,908
6-24 beds	0	0	0	0	0	00.0	0	0	0.0	0	0	0	0	0	0
25-49	4	143	3,747	15,321	24,214	30.1	43	66	4.1	4,063	53,169	112,274	165,443	31	409
50-99	12	946	43,353	192,495	258,570	55.8	528	709	4.4	33,115	67,876	116,639	184,515	108	4,395
100-199	20	2,706	128,522	628,713	804,864	63.7	1,724	2,205	4.9	97,333	391,015	779,503	1,170,518	380	19,816
200-299	6	1,500	69,368	342,177	402,425	62.5	938	1,102	4.9	45,881	179,910	363,207	543,117	199	12,795
300-399	6	2,023	87,890	519,582	680,324	70.4	1,424	1,865	5.9	50,678	251,359	458,184	709,543	190	12,307
400-499	2	808	35,997	187,126	235,917	63.4	512	646	5.2	19,658	111,771	288,498	400,269	155	10,186
500 or more	0	0	0	0	0	00.0	0	0	0.0	0	0	0	0	0	0
Nongovernment not-for-profit	17	2,811	121,798	637,361	860,103	62.1	1,747	2,355	5.2	69,313	307,372	608,560	915,932	235	10,556
Investor-owned (for-profit)	17	2,108	104,427	483,267	614,275	62.9	1,325	1,685	4.6	67,269	177,878	281,932	459,810	258	13,843
State and local government	16	3,207	142,652	764,786	931,936	65.4	2,097	2,553	5.4	114,146	569,850	1,227,813	1,797,663	570	35,509

CLASSIFICATION	FULL-TIME EQUIVALENT PERSONNEL					FULL-TIME EQUIVALENT TRAINEES			EXPENSES						
									LABOR				TOTAL		
	Physicians and Dentists	Registered Nurses	Licensed Practical Nurses	Other Salaried Personnel	Total Personnel	Medical and Dental Residents	Other Trainees	Total Trainees	Payroll (in thousands)	Employee Benefits (in thousands)	Total (in thousands)	Percent of Total	Amount (in thousands)	Adjusted, per Admission	Adjusted, per Inpatient Day
PUERTO RICO	965	6,567	3,231	18,418	29,181	676	11	687	$ 435,069	$ 91,571	$ 526,640	51.3	$ 1,026,197		
6-24 beds	0	0	0	0	0	0	0	0	0	0	0	0.0	0		
25-49	47	153	69	625	894	0	0	0	11,093	2,013	13,106	62.3	21,033		
50-99	59	579	298	1,618	2,554	0	0	0	33,686	6,247	39,933	45.3	88,061		
100-199	206	2,261	1,133	5,990	9,590	70	0	70	122,241	24,259	146,500	47.1	310,965		
200-299	176	1,182	520	3,005	4,883	75	0	75	71,021	12,616	83,637	58.3	143,541		
300-399	161	1,328	778	3,564	5,831	268	0	268	87,556	18,018	105,573	43.6	241,915		
400-499	153	712	322	2,134	3,321	150	1	151	50,232	12,383	62,616	63.3	98,859		
500 or more	163	352	111	1,482	2,108	113	10	123	59,240	16,035	75,275	61.8	121,821		
Psychiatric	36	178	95	985	1,294	2	1	3	35,861	7,903	43,763	64.6	67,780		
Hospitals	36	178	95	985	1,294	2	1	3	35,861	7,903	43,763	64.6	67,780		
Institutions for mentally retarded	0	0	0	0	0	0	0	0	0	0	0	0.0	0		
General	929	6,359	3,127	17,321	27,736	674	10	684	396,813	83,197	480,010	50.4	953,075		
Hospitals	929	6,359	3,127	17,321	27,736	674	10	684	396,813	83,197	480,010	50.4	953,075		
Hospital units of institutions	0	0	0	0	0	0	0	0	0	0	0	0.0	0		
TB and other respiratory diseases	0	0	0	0	0	0	0	0	0	0	0	0.0	0		
Obstetrics and gynecology	0	0	0	0	0	0	0	0	0	0	0	0.0	0		
Eye, ear, nose, and throat	0	0	0	0	0	0	0	0	0	0	0	0.0	0		
Rehabilitation	0	0	0	0	0	0	0	0	0	0	0	0.0	0		
Orthopedic	0	0	0	0	0	0	0	0	0	0	0	0.0	0		
Chronic disease	0	0	0	0	0	0	0	0	0	0	0	0.0	0		
All other	0	30	9	112	151	0	0	0	2,395	471	2,866	53.7	5,341		
Federal	187	389	120	1,706	2,402	113	10	123	65,141	17,287	82,429	62.7	131,465		
Psychiatric	0	0	0	0	0	0	0	0	0	0	0	0.0	0		
General and other special	187	389	120	1,706	2,402	113	10	123	65,141	17,287	82,429	62.7	131,465		
Nonfederal	778	6,178	3,111	16,712	26,779	563	1	564	369,928	74,283	444,211	49.6	894,731		
Psychiatric	36	178	95	985	1,294	2	1	3	35,861	7,903	43,763	64.6	67,780		
Hospitals	36	178	95	985	1,294	2	1	3	35,861	7,903	43,763	64.6	67,780		
Institutions for mentally retarded	0	0	0	0	0	0	0	0	0	0	0	0.0	0		
TB and other respiratory diseases	0	0	0	0	0	0	0	0	0	0	0	0.0	0		
Long-term general and other special	0	0	0	0	0	0	0	0	0	0	0	0.0	0		
Short-term general and other special	742	6,000	3,016	15,727	25,485	561	0	561	334,067	66,380	400,448	48.4	826,951		
Hospital units of institutions	0	0	0	0	0	0	0	0	0	0	0	0.0	0		
Community hospitals	742	6,000	3,016	15,727	25,485	561	0	561	334,067	66,380	400,448	48.4	826,951	$1,767.38	$ 343.66
6-24 beds	0	0	0	0	0	0	0	0	0	0	0	0.0	0	0.00	0.00
25-49	23	116	60	401	600	0	0	0	5,192	760	5,952	52.3	11,390	1,915.19	470.38
50-99	58	562	295	1,519	2,434	0	0	0	30,304	5,530	35,833	44.4	80,630	1,402.06	311.83
100-199	189	2,164	1,073	5,631	9,057	69	0	69	108,959	22,568	131,528	46.9	280,339	1,705.59	348.31
200-299	176	1,182	520	3,005	4,883	75	0	75	71,021	12,616	83,637	58.3	143,541	1,754.16	356.69
300-399	161	1,328	778	3,564	5,831	268	0	268	87,556	18,018	105,573	43.6	241,915	2,143.40	355.59
400-499	135	648	290	1,607	2,680	149	0	149	31,036	6,889	37,924	54.9	69,137	1,523.41	293.06
500 or more	0	0	0	0	0	0	0	0	0	0	0	0.0	0	0.00	0.00
Nongovernment not-for-profit	107	1,552	856	4,773	7,288	95	0	95	109,781	15,611	125,392	48.8	257,091	1,579.49	298.91
Investor-owned (for-profit)	55	1,385	635	3,543	5,618	12	0	12	71,949	15,428	87,377	40.6	215,059	1,621.34	350.10
State and local government	580	3,063	1,525	7,411	12,579	454	0	454	152,337	35,341	187,678	52.9	354,801	2,056.99	380.71

Tables

6-7

Metropolitan Statistical Areas

The U.S. Office of Management and Budget, in cooperation with the Federal Committee on Metropolitan Statistical Areas, announced modifications in June 1983 to the standard metropolitan statistical area (SMSA) classification system. As a result of updated statistical information collected by the 1980 census, SMSAs have been officially redesignated as metropolitan statistical areas (MSAs).

An MSA is a geographical designation that represents an integrated social and economic unit with a large population nucleus. Under the new standards, an area qualifies for recognition as an MSA if there is a city within the area of at least 50,000 population or an urban area of at least 50,000 with a total metropolitan population of at least 100,000. MSAs are defined as entire counties, except in the six New England states where they are defined in terms of cities and towns. In addition to the county containing the main city, an MSA also includes additional counties having strong economic and social ties to the central county. Such counties must have a specified level of commuting to the central counties and must meet certain standards regarding metropolitan character, such as population density.

When an MSA encompasses two or more central cities, up to three cities may be specified in the MSA title. They will be listed in order of population size. When a single central city exists, the MSA is named for that particular city. The official MSA title will also include a list of each of the states it covers.

Separate MSA maps for each of the 9 U.S. census divisions may be found immediately preceding the data for those divisions. A map of the 9 U.S. census divisions is found on page 19.

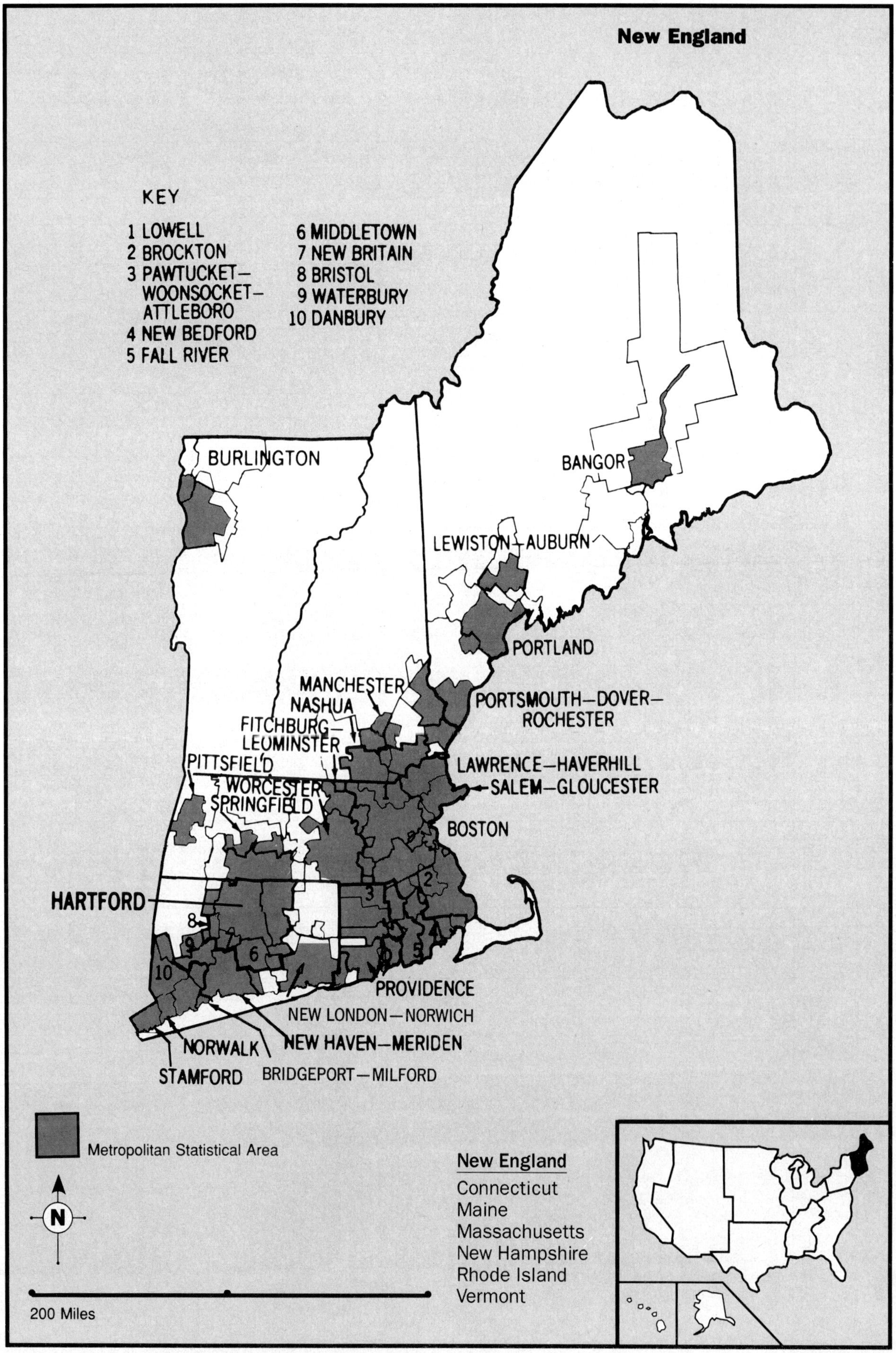
New England
KEY
1 LOWELL
2 BROCKTON
3 PAWTUCKET–WOONSOCKET–ATTLEBORO
4 NEW BEDFORD
5 FALL RIVER
6 MIDDLETOWN
7 NEW BRITAIN
8 BRISTOL
9 WATERBURY
10 DANBURY
BURLINGTON
BANGOR
LEWISTON–AUBURN
PORTLAND
MANCHESTER
NASHUA
PORTSMOUTH–DOVER–ROCHESTER
FITCHBURG–LEOMINSTER
PITTSFIELD
LAWRENCE–HAVERHILL
SALEM–GLOUCESTER
WORCESTER
SPRINGFIELD
BOSTON
HARTFORD
PROVIDENCE
NEW LONDON–NORWICH
NORWALK
NEW HAVEN–MERIDEN
STAMFORD
BRIDGEPORT–MILFORD
Metropolitan Statistical Area
N
200 Miles
New England
Connecticut
Maine
Massachusetts
New Hampshire
Rhode Island
Vermont

Table

6

Utilization, Personnel, and Finances in Community Hospitals, by Metropolitan Statistical Area

Where an MSA is located in multiple states, the MSA will be listed for each state, with hospital data for only that state.

CLASSIFICATION	HOSPITALS	BEDS	ADMISSIONS	INPATIENT DAYS	ADJUSTED PATIENT DAYS	OCCUPANCY, percent	AVERAGE DAILY CENSUS	ADJUSTED AVERAGE DAILY CENSUS	AVERAGE STAY, days	SURGICAL OPERATIONS	OUTPATIENT VISITS			NEWBORNS	
											Emergency	Other	Total	Bassinets	Births
UNITED STATES	5,384	927,360	31,181,046	225,971,653	296,569,640	66.8	619,275	812,752	7.2	21,914,868	86,692,503	214,636,259	301,328,762	68,412	3,958,263
Nonmetropolitan	2,460	206,219	5,690,792	43,373,914	61,255,496	57.6	118,872	167,881	7.6	3,629,283	19,267,235	40,008,084	59,275,319	18,876	623,452
Metropolitan	2,924	721,141	25,490,254	182,597,739	235,314,144	69.4	500,403	644,871	7.2	18,285,585	67,425,268	174,628,175	242,053,443	49,536	3,334,811
CENSUS DIVISION 1, NEW ENGLAND	229	44,363	1,620,584	11,987,553	16,557,977	74.0	32,846	45,371	7.4	1,213,685	5,746,618	13,738,809	19,485,427	3,422	200,883
Nonmetropolitan	79	7,532	250,189	1,822,846	2,707,788	66.3	4,994	7,421	7.3	186,776	1,147,445	2,723,041	3,870,486	822	29,554
Metropolitan	150	36,831	1,370,395	10,164,707	13,850,189	75.6	27,852	37,950	7.4	1,026,909	4,599,173	11,015,768	15,614,941	2,600	171,329
Connecticut	35	9,627	355,057	2,704,095	3,586,130	77.0	7,408	9,825	7.6	265,965	1,217,326	2,940,565	4,157,891	742	50,428
Nonmetropolitan	5	572	20,287	130,006	191,114	62.2	356	523	6.4	15,221	95,251	401,261	496,512	66	2,340
Metropolitan	30	9,055	334,770	2,574,089	3,395,016	77.9	7,052	9,302	7.7	250,744	1,122,075	2,539,304	3,661,379	676	48,088
Bridgeport-Milford	5	1,362	46,328	363,184	455,297	73.1	995	1,247	7.8	32,356	144,164	261,113	405,277	123	7,018
Bristol	1	205	8,976	59,453	89,572	79.5	163	245	6.6	9,090	28,475	104,387	132,862	12	954
Danbury	2	535	20,299	150,670	205,079	77.2	413	561	7.4	14,812	65,028	93,958	158,986	36	3,250
Hartford	8	2,508	87,353	704,744	933,963	77.0	1,930	2,561	8.1	67,664	272,219	737,516	1,009,735	167	12,237
Middletown	1	266	10,634	71,717	104,672	73.7	196	287	6.7	11,672	58,184	170,103	228,287	27	1,170
New Britain	2	409	16,782	118,613	171,326	79.5	325	469	7.1	15,071	56,981	182,731	239,712	24	2,506
New Haven-Meriden	3	1,524	57,697	474,378	588,574	85.3	1,300	1,613	8.2	38,963	180,920	306,429	487,349	88	8,570
New London-Norwich	2	499	21,677	146,312	213,151	80.4	401	584	6.7	18,094	116,997	103,305	220,302	56	3,627
Norwalk	1	406	14,192	103,980	139,344	70.2	285	382	7.3	10,304	32,844	82,683	115,527	20	1,835
Stamford	3	698	25,244	183,816	235,694	72.2	504	646	7.3	16,736	71,868	233,396	305,264	61	3,912
Waterbury	2	643	25,588	197,222	258,344	84.0	540	707	7.7	15,982	94,395	263,683	358,078	62	3,009
Maine	39	4,495	145,569	1,173,342	1,600,755	71.5	3,214	4,386	8.1	108,105	610,472	1,323,947	1,934,419	398	16,377
Nonmetropolitan	30	2,494	74,269	609,408	882,789	66.9	1,668	2,419	8.2	60,215	385,287	829,745	1,215,032	267	8,667
Metropolitan	9	2,001	71,300	563,934	717,966	77.3	1,546	1,967	7.9	47,890	225,185	494,202	719,387	131	7,710
Bangor	2	507	17,763	146,241	190,474	79.1	401	522	8.2	14,973	61,703	226,219	287,922	26	1,985
Lewiston-Auburn	2	468	14,823	109,826	150,609	64.3	301	412	7.4	9,725	56,564	136,466	193,030	47	1,495
Portland	4	947	35,578	285,667	346,412	82.7	783	950	8.0	21,794	94,746	118,262	213,008	55	4,057
Portsmouth-Dover-Rochester	1	79	3,136	22,200	30,471	77.2	61	83	7.1	1,398	12,172	13,255	25,427	3	173
Massachusetts	101	21,875	810,991	5,921,378	8,300,125	74.2	16,225	22,744	7.3	614,734	2,764,029	7,136,865	9,900,894	1,550	93,578
Nonmetropolitan	13	1,449	54,101	367,176	590,770	69.4	1,006	1,619	6.8	38,759	254,235	463,044	717,279	147	6,060
Metropolitan	88	20,426	756,890	5,554,202	7,709,355	74.5	15,219	21,125	7.3	575,975	2,509,794	6,673,821	9,183,615	1,403	87,518
Boston	50	11,921	449,821	3,285,376	4,490,444	75.5	9,004	12,303	7.3	340,002	1,343,423	4,365,040	5,708,463	748	47,666
Brockton	2	576	18,733	153,347	221,591	72.9	420	607	8.2	11,084	84,356	73,617	157,973	29	1,209
Fall River	2	493	18,402	148,792	212,104	82.8	408	581	8.1	16,890	69,680	76,241	145,921	31	2,190
Fitchburg-Leominster	2	337	12,728	76,202	116,149	62.0	209	318	6.0	9,275	57,622	14,507	72,129	41	2,488
Lawrence-Haverhill	5	1,010	34,982	249,591	346,181	67.6	683	950	7.1	29,384	154,323	205,216	359,539	92	4,881
Lowell	3	650	21,758	162,608	262,625	68.5	445	720	7.5	21,614	103,747	303,430	407,177	52	3,183
New Bedford	1	475	16,765	132,681	199,963	76.6	364	548	7.9	14,173	71,688	68,974	140,662	35	2,312
Pawtucket-Woonsocket-Attleboro	1	150	6,432	42,041	73,466	76.7	115	201	6.5	5,900	32,737	48,552	81,289	22	970
Pittsfield	2	429	15,079	120,328	156,336	76.7	329	429	8.0	13,873	34,716	96,935	131,651	26	1,411
Salem-Gloucester	4	794	30,617	211,976	311,960	73.2	581	854	6.9	21,131	111,367	161,052	272,419	82	5,144
Springfield	9	1,906	69,751	503,202	697,007	72.3	1,378	1,911	7.2	49,366	276,461	669,985	946,446	144	8,946
Worcester	7	1,685	61,822	468,058	621,529	76.1	1,283	1,703	7.6	43,283	169,674	590,272	759,946	101	7,118
New Hampshire	27	3,470	124,532	846,149	1,200,534	66.9	2,320	3,289	6.8	83,726	485,949	1,127,355	1,613,304	350	16,807
Nonmetropolitan	17	1,717	58,936	408,015	581,162	65.2	1,119	1,594	6.9	41,674	240,605	605,348	845,953	181	6,717
Metropolitan	10	1,753	65,596	438,134	619,372	68.5	1,201	1,695	6.7	42,052	245,344	522,007	767,351	169	10,090
Lawrence-Haverhill	2	185	4,853	44,867	63,487	66.5	123	173	9.2	3,103	22,621	61,050	83,671	12	541
Lowell	0	0	0	0	0	00.0	0	0	0.0	0	0	0	0	0	0
Manchester	2	584	22,300	149,078	199,600	70.0	409	547	6.7	12,597	67,690	137,181	204,871	35	2,978
Nashua	2	389	16,370	89,621	131,346	63.0	245	360	5.5	9,549	60,852	146,793	207,645	66	3,034
Portsmouth-Dover-Rochester	4	595	22,073	154,568	224,939	71.3	424	615	7.0	16,803	94,181	176,983	271,164	56	3,537
Rhode Island	12	3,180	126,730	921,295	1,273,481	79.4	2,524	3,491	7.3	101,267	472,999	680,688	1,153,687	195	15,896
Nonmetropolitan	1	151	6,355	47,818	68,459	86.8	131	188	7.5	5,728	28,735	53,074	81,809	12	812
Metropolitan	11	3,029	120,375	873,477	1,205,022	79.0	2,393	3,303	7.3	95,539	444,264	627,614	1,071,878	183	15,084
Fall River	0	0	0	0	0	00.0	0	0	0.0	0	0	0	0	0	0
New London-Norwich	1	141	4,751	27,328	42,337	53.2	75	116	5.8	2,795	34,490	56,298	90,788	18	681
Pawtucket-Woonsocket-Attleboro	2	572	20,441	160,568	229,728	76.9	440	630	7.9	13,290	86,807	176,722	263,529	46	1,597
Providence	8	2,316	95,183	685,581	932,957	81.1	1,878	2,557	7.2	79,454	322,967	394,594	717,561	119	12,806

CLASSIFICATION	FULL-TIME EQUIVALENT PERSONNEL: Physicians and Dentists	Registered Nurses	Licensed Practical Nurses	Other Salaried Personnel	Total Personnel	FULL-TIME EQUIVALENT TRAINEES: Medical and Dental Residents	Other Trainees	Total Trainees	EXPENSES — LABOR: Payroll (in thousands)	Employee Benefits (in thousands)	Total (in thousands)	Percent of Total	EXPENSES — TOTAL: Amount (in thousands)	Adjusted, per Admission	Adjusted, per Inpatient Day
UNITED STATES	37,262	809,927	167,933	2,404,397	3,419,519	64,995	4,124	69,119	$90,925,393	$18,186,698	$109,112,090	53.6	$203,692,591	$4,946.68	$ 686.83
Nonmetropolitan	1,878	115,239	44,765	389,387	551,269	1,203	293	1,496	11,683,085	2,280,778	13,963,863	53.3	26,212,966	3,221.89	427.93
Metropolitan	35,384	694,688	123,168	2,015,010	2,868,250	63,792	3,831	67,623	79,242,308	15,905,920	95,148,228	53.6	177,479,624	5,371.38	754.22
CENSUS DIVISION 1, NEW ENGLAND	4,662	46,372	6,966	139,689	197,689	5,773	168	5,941	6,074,538	1,207,241	7,281,779	58.6	12,425,400	5,513.56	750.42
Nonmetropolitan	218	6,725	1,491	19,500	27,934	237	0	237	774,745	155,405	930,150	60.4	1,540,521	4,121.75	568.92
Metropolitan	4,444	39,647	5,475	120,189	169,755	5,536	168	5,704	5,299,794	1,051,836	6,351,629	58.4	10,884,879	5,790.28	785.90
Connecticut	843	10,487	1,366	31,682	44,378	1,325	54	1,379	1,547,787	328,954	1,876,742	63.5	2,957,637	6,237.82	824.74
Nonmetropolitan	51	581	79	1,606	2,317	0	0	0	80,026	19,935	99,961	65.2	153,375	5,135.27	802.53
Metropolitan	792	9,906	1,287	30,076	42,061	1,325	54	1,379	1,467,762	309,019	1,776,781	63.4	2,804,262	6,311.94	825.99
Bridgeport-Milford	86	1,061	162	4,062	5,371	115	0	115	177,648	32,934	210,582	60.4	348,402	5,980.01	765.22
Bristol	7	165	22	668	862	0	0	0	30,698	5,435	36,134	67.8	53,333	3,943.84	595.42
Danbury	85	558	73	1,828	2,544	54	14	68	79,301	18,963	98,264	60.5	162,390	5,859.27	791.84
Hartford	263	2,937	365	8,915	12,480	343	15	358	420,614	77,106	497,721	62.2	800,384	6,884.43	856.98
Middletown	31	263	54	883	1,231	21	2	23	46,454	11,238	57,692	67.5	85,521	5,510.38	817.04
New Britain	24	443	58	1,544	2,069	21	0	21	70,954	14,278	85,233	68.9	123,791	5,102.47	722.55
New Haven-Meriden	68	2,094	204	5,033	7,399	542	20	562	276,679	68,146	344,825	62.5	552,028	7,652.82	937.91
New London-Norwich	45	528	124	1,526	2,223	0	0	0	85,932	15,883	101,815	69.7	145,986	4,622.45	684.90
Norwalk	42	379	36	1,334	1,791	52	0	52	64,303	11,848	76,151	65.4	116,430	6,121.78	835.56
Stamford	74	732	62	2,065	2,933	64	3	67	101,533	23,626	125,159	63.9	195,988	6,032.62	831.53
Waterbury	67	746	127	2,218	3,158	113	0	113	113,645	29,562	143,206	65.1	220,009	6,564.31	851.61
Maine	193	4,154	1,017	12,341	17,705	196	0	196	446,880	81,937	528,817	57.6	918,199	4,603.63	573.60
Nonmetropolitan	68	1,957	580	6,247	8,852	0	0	0	213,127	37,187	250,314	59.2	423,151	3,903.36	479.33
Metropolitan	125	2,197	437	6,094	8,853	196	0	196	233,753	44,750	278,503	56.3	495,048	5,437.45	689.51
Bangor	30	648	142	1,653	2,473	25	0	25	65,996	11,941	77,936	57.2	136,327	5,901.34	715.72
Lewiston-Auburn	17	375	116	1,105	1,613	10	0	10	41,743	9,145	50,888	58.3	87,324	4,302.50	579.80
Portland	74	1,084	178	3,135	4,471	161	0	161	117,514	22,168	139,682	54.9	254,290	5,866.91	734.07
Portsmouth-Dover-Rochester	4	90	1	201	296	0	0	0	8,501	1,495	9,996	58.4	17,108	3,974.84	561.44
Massachusetts	3,205	23,189	2,916	71,635	100,945	3,350	92	3,442	3,108,408	601,122	3,709,529	56.7	6,543,022	5,708.88	788.30
Nonmetropolitan	34	1,211	263	3,731	5,239	0	0	0	179,394	37,919	217,312	62.8	346,286	3,934.13	586.16
Metropolitan	3,171	21,978	2,653	67,904	95,706	3,350	92	3,442	2,929,014	563,203	3,492,217	56.4	6,196,736	5,856.52	803.79
Boston	2,424	14,133	1,083	44,250	61,890	2,792	91	2,883	1,915,136	375,063	2,290,199	54.5	4,202,174	6,771.44	935.80
Brockton	21	429	97	1,468	2,015	5	0	5	62,144	9,127	71,271	57.9	122,996	4,512.45	555.06
Fall River	1	343	89	1,385	1,818	0	0	0	55,563	10,758	66,321	56.9	116,543	4,447.36	549.46
Fitchburg-Leominster	1	268	49	698	1,016	0	0	0	34,968	3,191	38,159	60.4	63,154	3,249.14	543.73
Lawrence-Haverhill	12	761	188	2,062	3,023	0	0	0	94,194	16,590	110,784	61.3	180,763	3,711.70	522.16
Lowell	0	468	127	1,840	2,435	0	1	1	70,164	13,209	83,374	62.7	133,020	3,768.28	506.50
New Bedford	22	355	110	1,267	1,754	0	0	0	52,905	13,177	66,082	69.1	95,628	3,784.71	478.23
Pawtucket-Woonsocket-Attleboro	8	146	26	524	704	0	0	0	19,462	3,927	23,388	66.4	35,223	3,133.73	479.45
Pittsfield	27	413	65	1,266	1,771	53	0	53	49,769	8,035	57,804	58.6	98,720	5,051.16	631.46
Salem-Gloucester	39	985	106	2,551	3,681	19	0	19	107,598	19,277	126,875	62.3	203,641	4,528.07	652.78
Springfield	170	1,920	405	5,882	8,377	160	0	160	236,586	43,664	280,250	60.4	464,289	4,802.92	666.12
Worcester	446	1,757	308	4,711	7,222	321	0	321	230,526	47,184	277,710	57.8	480,585	5,795.27	773.23
New Hampshire	38	3,654	497	9,356	13,545	237	6	243	372,317	75,398	447,715	55.6	805,208	4,543.65	670.71
Nonmetropolitan	11	1,836	243	4,787	6,877	237	0	237	182,517	38,422	220,939	58.1	380,109	4,553.02	654.05
Metropolitan	27	1,818	254	4,569	6,668	0	6	6	189,799	36,976	226,776	53.3	425,099	4,535.31	686.34
Lawrence-Haverhill	0	145	30	449	624	0	0	0	16,254	3,928	20,182	44.9	44,953	5,786.89	708.06
Lowell	0	0	0	0	0	0	0	0	0	0	0	0.0	0		
Manchester	8	641	51	1,444	2,144	0	0	0	63,686	11,804	75,489	52.5	143,830	4,797.21	720.59
Nashua	10	413	77	1,207	1,707	0	0	0	49,696	8,889	58,585	59.9	97,788	4,075.33	744.50
Portsmouth-Dover-Rochester	9	619	96	1,469	2,193	0	6	6	60,163	12,356	72,519	52.3	138,529	4,330.93	615.85
Rhode Island	326	3,295	739	10,339	14,699	469	0	469	427,227	87,891	515,118	61.0	844,596	4,838.68	663.22
Nonmetropolitan	3	163	22	501	689	0	0	0	20,982	3,877	24,859	65.5	37,948	4,170.98	554.31
Metropolitan	323	3,132	717	9,838	14,010	469	0	469	406,245	84,014	490,260	60.8	806,648	4,875.39	669.41
Fall River	0	0	0	0	0	0	0	0	0	0	0	0.0	0		
New London-Norwich	8	67	14	340	429	0	0	0	14,351	3,357	17,708	66.8	26,525	3,603.90	626.51
Pawtucket-Woonsocket-Attleboro	54	451	114	1,502	2,121	70	0	70	64,200	14,708	78,909	60.0	131,563	4,502.04	572.69
Providence	261	2,614	589	7,996	11,460	399	0	399	327,694	65,949	393,643	60.7	648,561	5,032.67	695.17

(continued on next page)

Table

6

(Continued)

Utilization, Personnel, and Finances in Community Hospitals, by Metropolitan Statistical Area

Where an MSA is located in multiple states, the MSA will be listed for each state, with hospital data for only that state.

CLASSIFICATION	HOSPITALS	BEDS	ADMISSIONS	INPATIENT DAYS	ADJUSTED PATIENT DAYS	OCCUPANCY, percent	AVERAGE DAILY CENSUS	ADJUSTED AVERAGE DAILY CENSUS	AVERAGE STAY, days	SURGICAL OPERATIONS	OUTPATIENT VISITS			NEWBORNS	
											Emergency	Other	Total	Bassinets	Births
Vermont	15	1,716	57,705	421,294	596,952	67.3	1,155	1,636	7.3	39,888	195,843	529,389	725,232	187	7,797
Nonmetropolitan	13	1,149	36,241	260,423	393,494	62.1	714	1,078	7.2	25,179	143,332	370,569	513,901	149	4,958
Metropolitan	2	567	21,464	160,871	203,458	77.8	441	558	7.5	14,709	52,511	158,820	211,331	38	2,839
Burlington	2	567	21,464	160,871	203,458	77.8	441	558	7.5	14,709	52,511	158,820	211,331	38	2,839

Table 6 (Continued) **Census Division 1, New England**

CLASSIFICATION	FULL-TIME EQUIVALENT PERSONNEL					FULL-TIME EQUIVALENT TRAINEES			EXPENSES						
									LABOR				TOTAL		
	Physicians and Dentists	Registered Nurses	Licensed Practical Nurses	Other Salaried Personnel	Total Personnel	Medical and Dental Residents	Other Trainees	Total Trainees	Payroll (in thousands)	Employee Benefits (in thousands)	Total (in thousands)	Percent of Total	Amount (in thousands)	Adjusted, per Admission	Adjusted, per Inpatient Day
Vermont	57	1,593	431	4,336	6,417	196	16	212	$ 171,919	$ 31,939	$ 203,858	57.1	$ 356,738	$4,343.47	$ 597.60
Nonmetropolitan	51	977	304	2,628	3,960	0	0	0	98,699	18,066	116,765	58.5	199,653	3,638.25	507.38
Metropolitan	6	616	127	1,708	2,457	196	16	212	73,220	13,873	87,093	55.4	157,086	5,763.34	772.08
Burlington	6	616	127	1,708	2,457	196	16	212	73,220	13,873	87,093	55.4	157,086	5,763.34	772.08

(continued on next page)

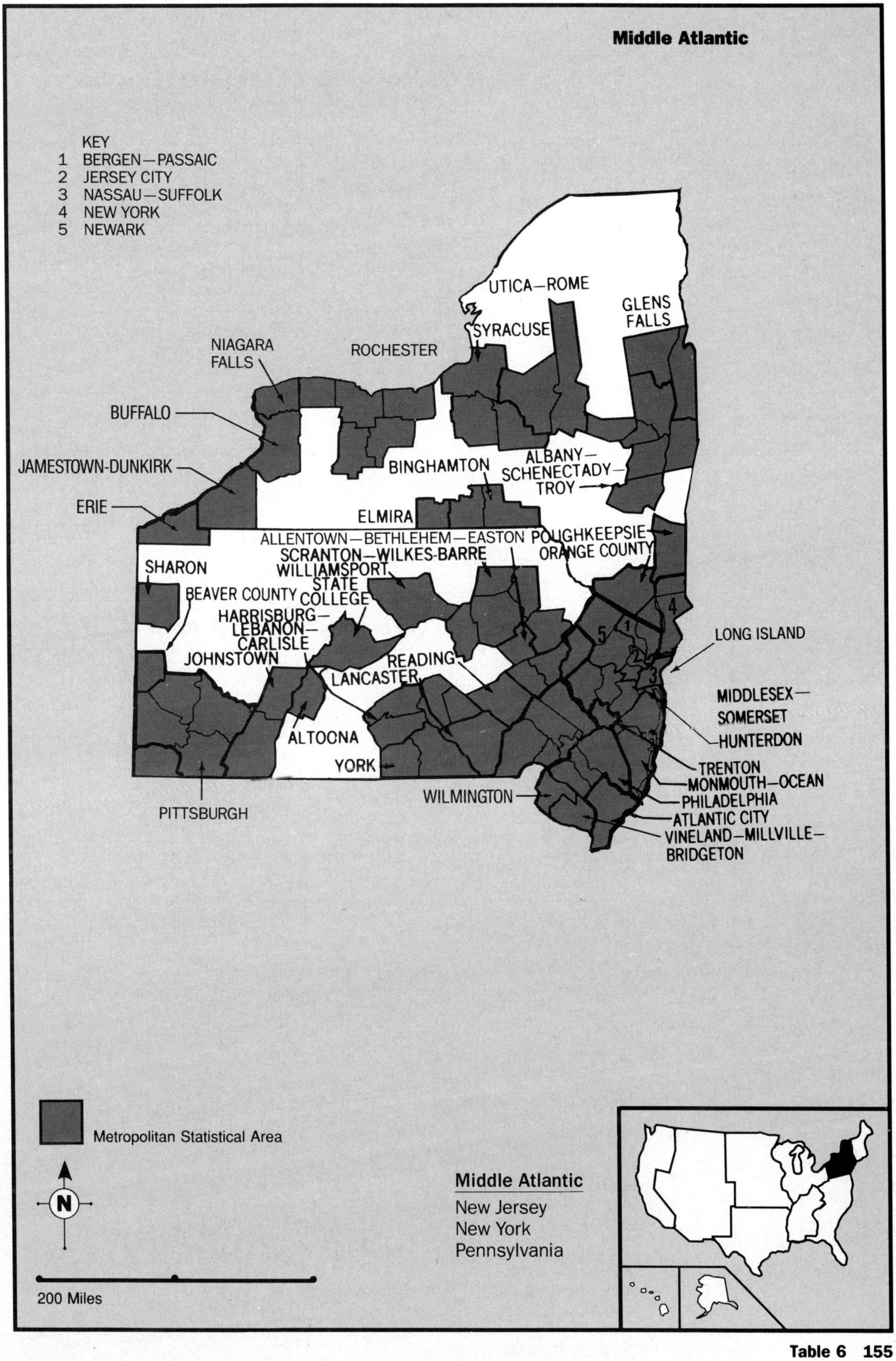
Middle Atlantic
KEY
1 BERGEN—PASSAIC
2 JERSEY CITY
3 NASSAU—SUFFOLK
4 NEW YORK
5 NEWARK
UTICA—ROME
GLENS FALLS
SYRACUSE
NIAGARA FALLS
ROCHESTER
BUFFALO
JAMESTOWN-DUNKIRK
BINGHAMTON
ALBANY—SCHENECTADY—TROY
ERIE
ELMIRA
ALLENTOWN—BETHLEHEM—EASTON
POUGHKEEPSIE
SCRANTON—WILKES-BARRE
ORANGE COUNTY
SHARON
WILLIAMSPORT
STATE COLLEGE
BEAVER COUNTY
HARRISBURG—LEBANON—CARLISLE
LONG ISLAND
JOHNSTOWN
READING
LANCASTER
MIDDLESEX—SOMERSET—HUNTERDON
ALTOONA
YORK
TRENTON
MONMOUTH—OCEAN
WILMINGTON
PHILADELPHIA
PITTSBURGH
ATLANTIC CITY
VINELAND—MILLVILLE—BRIDGETON
Metropolitan Statistical Area
N
Middle Atlantic
New Jersey
New York
Pennsylvania
200 Miles

Table

6

(Continued)

Utilization, Personnel, and Finances in Community Hospitals, by Metropolitan Statistical Area

Where an MSA is located in multiple states, the MSA will be listed for each state, with hospital data for only that state.

CLASSIFICATION	HOSPITALS	BEDS	ADMISSIONS	INPATIENT DAYS	ADJUSTED PATIENT DAYS	OCCUPANCY, percent	AVERAGE DAILY CENSUS	ADJUSTED AVERAGE DAILY CENSUS	AVERAGE STAY, days	SURGICAL OPERATIONS	OUTPATIENT VISITS			NEWBORNS	
											Emergency	Other	Total	Bassinets	Births
CENSUS DIVISION 2, MIDDLE ATLANTIC	**568**	**155,711**	**5,249,072**	**45,750,807**	**59,441,544**	**80.5**	**125,349**	**162,848**	**8.7**	**3,631,500**	**14,181,348**	**46,060,934**	**60,242,282**	**9,845**	**577,672**
Nonmetropolitan	89	13,085	378,686	3,452,301	4,987,860	72.3	9,456	13,663	9.1	303,532	1,413,274	4,623,880	6,037,154	1,073	37,075
Metropolitan	479	142,626	4,870,386	42,298,506	54,453,684	81.3	115,893	149,185	8.7	3,327,968	12,768,074	41,437,054	54,205,128	8,772	540,597
New Jersey	**95**	**28,846**	**1,131,509**	**8,438,916**	**10,619,506**	**80.2**	**23,124**	**29,094**	**7.5**	**676,716**	**2,407,049**	**7,327,144**	**9,734,193**	**1,995**	**114,045**
Nonmetropolitan	0	0	0	0	0	00.0	0	0	0.0	0	0	0	0	0	0
Metropolitan	95	28,846	1,131,509	8,438,916	10,619,506	80.2	23,124	29,094	7.5	676,716	2,407,049	7,327,144	9,734,193	1,995	114,045
Allentown-Bethlehem	2	320	12,217	79,076	94,072	67.8	217	257	6.5	11,268	33,304	42,137	75,441	27	1,249
Atlantic City	5	1,193	52,593	370,834	482,303	85.1	1,015	1,321	7.1	28,237	127,608	215,870	343,478	74	5,057
Bergen-Passaic	12	4,170	184,292	1,241,493	1,538,817	81.6	3,403	4,217	6.7	98,695	301,544	1,346,981	1,648,525	302	17,877
Jersey City	9	2,433	86,760	714,812	882,549	80.5	1,959	2,417	8.2	43,241	221,289	1,302,785	1,524,074	154	8,852
Middlesex-Somerset-Hunterdon	8	2,430	108,591	732,197	903,024	82.6	2,007	2,474	6.7	68,565	196,294	499,672	695,966	242	11,980
Monmouth-Ocean	10	3,361	133,471	1,025,969	1,338,715	83.6	2,810	3,668	7.7	88,635	333,982	673,870	1,007,852	198	12,914
Newark	28	9,057	326,659	2,637,816	3,303,845	79.8	7,228	9,052	8.1	202,848	647,440	1,958,513	2,605,953	556	30,671
Philadelphia	11	3,335	142,153	965,987	1,180,667	79.4	2,648	3,235	6.8	72,334	327,091	703,280	1,030,371	267	15,957
Trenton	6	1,751	58,605	470,365	619,662	73.6	1,288	1,698	8.0	43,002	139,125	330,750	469,875	117	6,638
Vineland-Millville-Bridgeton	2	553	17,465	136,916	195,396	67.8	375	535	7.8	10,873	56,115	185,589	241,704	42	2,324
Wilmington	2	243	8,703	63,451	80,456	71.6	174	220	7.3	9,018	23,257	67,697	90,954	16	526
New York	**235**	**74,476**	**2,321,509**	**23,372,299**	**30,239,515**	**86.0**	**64,038**	**82,852**	**10.1**	**1,549,997**	**6,694,321**	**22,650,123**	**29,344,444**	**4,683**	**293,794**
Nonmetropolitan	44	6,090	160,283	1,746,637	2,475,592	78.5	4,783	6,782	10.9	117,422	601,644	1,842,838	2,444,482	520	18,218
Metropolitan	191	68,386	2,161,226	21,625,662	27,763,923	86.6	59,255	76,070	10.0	1,432,575	6,092,677	20,807,285	26,899,962	4,163	275,576
Albany-Schenectady-Troy	16	3,527	107,856	1,049,343	1,545,274	81.5	2,875	4,236	9.7	104,525	348,073	808,332	1,156,405	281	13,121
Binghamton	2	899	32,780	283,209	418,746	86.2	775	1,147	8.6	24,086	90,562	313,957	404,519	65	3,862
Buffalo	13	4,609	137,452	1,500,280	1,975,209	89.2	4,112	5,412	10.9	129,861	373,523	1,066,670	1,440,193	273	15,845
Elmira	2	542	15,286	156,874	209,824	79.3	430	575	10.3	9,161	51,105	166,087	217,192	30	1,746
Glens Falls	2	553	16,493	148,492	221,145	73.6	407	606	9.0	13,638	45,237	49,037	94,274	48	2,080
Jamestown-Dunkirk	4	581	19,377	165,281	241,302	78.0	453	660	8.5	14,815	78,384	187,737	266,121	67	1,835
Nassau-Suffolk	27	9,093	306,819	2,873,372	3,537,587	86.6	7,873	9,694	9.4	196,768	718,674	1,765,793	2,484,467	576	39,187
New York	82	38,576	1,215,333	12,342,271	15,480,293	87.7	33,815	42,411	10.2	694,684	3,410,092	13,259,786	16,669,878	2,058	155,528
Niagara Falls	5	868	26,766	262,821	362,644	82.9	720	994	9.8	30,362	95,284	273,387	368,671	91	2,006
Orange County	6	1,016	36,562	289,009	379,949	78.1	793	1,042	7.9	25,045	145,380	177,298	322,678	84	4,608
Poughkeepsie	3	705	24,326	211,868	294,629	82.4	581	807	8.7	19,665	89,504	185,128	274,632	46	3,657
Rochester	15	4,059	111,754	1,293,088	1,687,955	87.3	3,544	4,625	11.6	88,132	317,417	1,379,418	1,696,835	275	16,740
Syracuse	8	2,286	76,168	713,635	937,117	85.6	1,956	2,568	9.4	57,506	201,599	765,478	967,077	169	11,242
Utica-Rome	6	1,072	34,254	336,119	472,249	85.9	921	1,293	9.8	24,327	127,843	409,177	537,020	100	4,119
Pennsylvania	**238**	**52,389**	**1,796,054**	**13,939,592**	**18,582,523**	**72.9**	**38,187**	**50,902**	**7.8**	**1,404,787**	**5,079,978**	**16,083,667**	**21,163,645**	**3,167**	**169,833**
Nonmetropolitan	45	6,995	218,403	1,705,664	2,512,268	66.8	4,673	6,881	7.8	186,110	811,630	2,781,042	3,592,672	553	18,857
Metropolitan	193	45,394	1,577,651	12,233,928	16,070,255	73.8	33,514	44,021	7.8	1,218,677	4,268,348	13,302,625	17,570,973	2,614	150,976
Allentown-Bethlehem	9	2,405	87,641	705,480	908,396	80.3	1,932	2,489	8.0	75,125	237,688	863,582	1,101,270	122	8,567
Altoona	5	684	22,762	165,083	245,886	66.2	453	673	7.3	22,053	69,797	225,138	294,935	54	2,009
Beaver County	2	632	20,096	135,409	206,898	58.5	370	567	6.7	23,822	57,398	171,703	229,101	48	1,679
Erie	8	1,526	46,060	346,092	440,259	62.1	947	1,206	7.5	27,166	118,781	298,307	417,088	77	4,587
Harrisburg-Lebanon-Carlisle	11	2,350	83,040	635,287	869,547	74.1	1,741	2,381	7.7	76,376	202,318	1,288,225	1,490,543	142	9,060
Johnstown	7	1,112	36,614	277,476	408,028	68.4	761	1,118	7.6	35,187	115,803	309,412	425,215	60	2,599
Lancaster	5	1,278	48,293	311,936	409,694	67.0	856	1,123	6.5	38,757	107,073	488,803	595,876	95	6,415
Philadelphia	69	17,420	604,667	4,826,225	6,171,453	75.9	13,221	16,907	8.0	431,366	1,491,246	4,453,744	5,944,990	977	62,803
Pittsburgh	40	10,796	381,575	3,004,502	3,850,630	76.2	8,231	10,547	7.9	283,073	1,060,828	3,081,143	4,141,971	519	28,576
Reading	4	1,064	40,990	277,617	386,706	71.4	760	1,059	6.8	35,840	127,689	274,275	401,964	70	4,567
Scranton-Wilkes-Barre	17	3,369	110,120	882,582	1,198,971	71.8	2,418	3,284	8.0	87,407	335,812	1,049,430	1,385,242	233	9,681
Sharon	4	666	23,528	150,788	226,978	62.2	414	621	6.4	26,477	83,359	184,578	267,937	54	1,766
State College	3	370	10,708	78,362	104,242	57.8	214	286	7.3	9,259	39,825	92,964	132,789	36	1,481
Williamsport	4	675	20,571	143,711	227,859	58.2	393	624	7.0	21,804	95,564	244,646	340,210	52	1,816
York	5	1,047	40,986	293,378	414,708	76.7	803	1,136	7.2	24,965	125,167	276,675	401,842	75	5,370

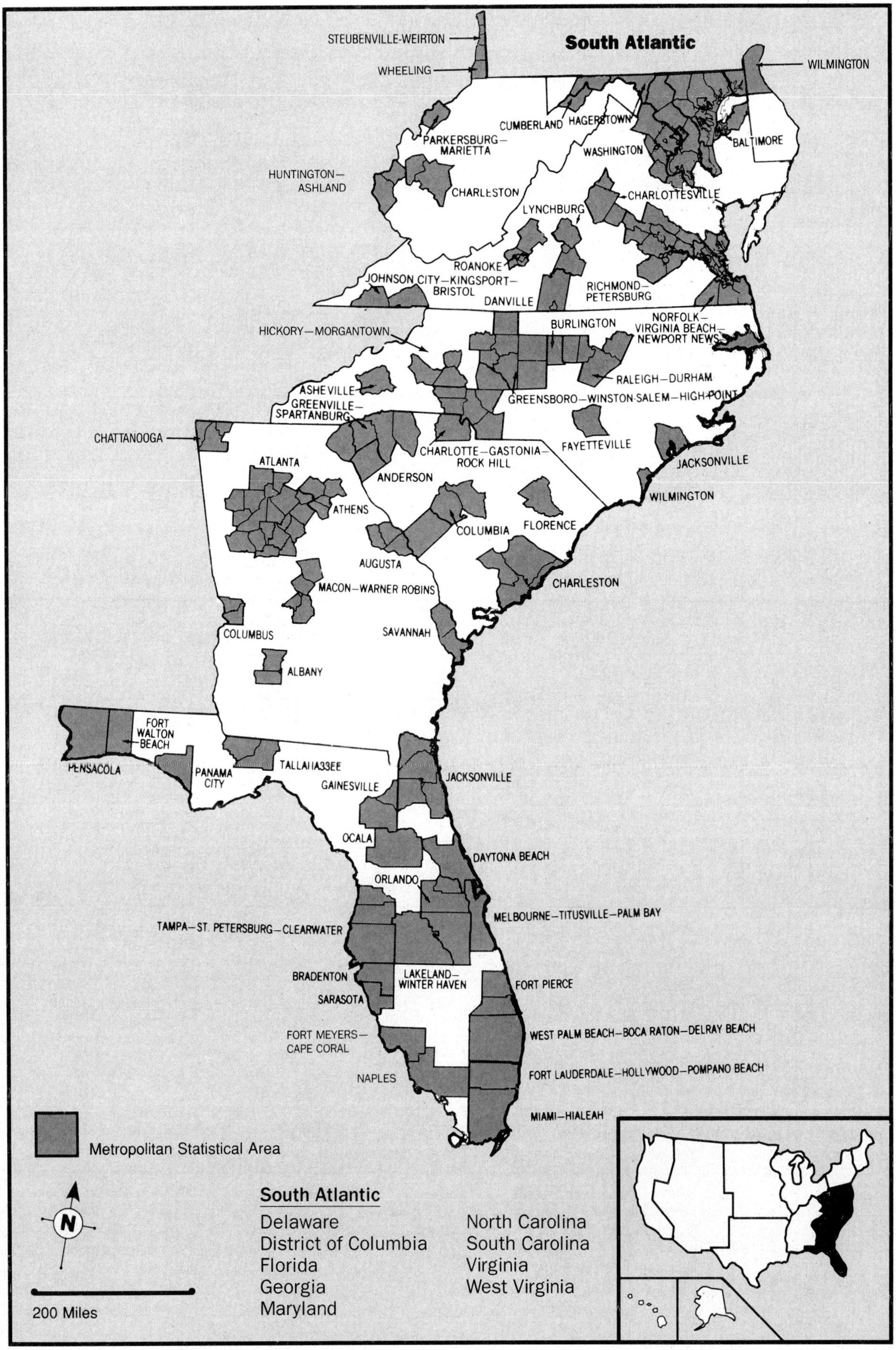
South Atlantic
STEUBENVILLE-WEIRTON
WHEELING
WILMINGTON
CUMBERLAND
HAGERSTOWN
PARKERSBURG–MARIETTA
BALTIMORE
WASHINGTON
HUNTINGTON–ASHLAND
CHARLESTON
CHARLOTTESVILLE
LYNCHBURG
ROANOKE
JOHNSON CITY–KINGSPORT–BRISTOL
DANVILLE
RICHMOND–PETERSBURG
HICKORY–MORGANTOWN
BURLINGTON
NORFOLK–VIRGINIA BEACH–NEWPORT NEWS
ASHEVILLE
RALEIGH–DURHAM
GREENVILLE–SPARTANBURG
GREENSBORO–WINSTON-SALEM–HIGH POINT
CHATTANOOGA
CHARLOTTE–GASTONIA–ROCK HILL
FAYETTEVILLE
ATLANTA
JACKSONVILLE
ANDERSON
WILMINGTON
ATHENS
FLORENCE
COLUMBIA
AUGUSTA
CHARLESTON
MACON–WARNER ROBINS
SAVANNAH
COLUMBUS
ALBANY
FORT WALTON BEACH
PENSACOLA
PANAMA CITY
TALLAHASSEE
GAINESVILLE
JACKSONVILLE
OCALA
DAYTONA BEACH
ORLANDO
MELBOURNE–TITUSVILLE–PALM BAY
TAMPA–ST. PETERSBURG–CLEARWATER
BRADENTON
LAKELAND–WINTER HAVEN
FORT PIERCE
SARASOTA
FORT MEYERS–CAPE CORAL
WEST PALM BEACH–BOCA RATON–DELRAY BEACH
NAPLES
FORT LAUDERDALE–HOLLYWOOD–POMPANO BEACH
MIAMI–HIALEAH
Metropolitan Statistical Area
N
200 Miles
South Atlantic
Delaware
District of Columbia
Florida
Georgia
Maryland
North Carolina
South Carolina
Virginia
West Virginia

Table

6 (Continued)

Utilization, Personnel, and Finances in Community Hospitals, by Metropolitan Statistical Area

Where an MSA is located in multiple states, the MSA will be listed for each state, with hospital data for only that state.

CLASSIFICATION	HOSPITALS	BEDS	ADMISSIONS	INPATIENT DAYS	ADJUSTED PATIENT DAYS	OCCUPANCY, percent	AVERAGE DAILY CENSUS	ADJUSTED AVERAGE DAILY CENSUS	AVERAGE STAY, days	SURGICAL OPERATIONS	OUTPATIENT VISITS: Emergency	OUTPATIENT VISITS: Other	OUTPATIENT VISITS: Total	NEWBORNS: Bassinets	NEWBORNS: Births
CENSUS DIVISION 3, SOUTH ATLANTIC	**803**	**157,711**	**5,511,559**	**38,807,448**	**49,974,178**	**67.4**	**106,359**	**136,951**	**7.0**	**3,919,849**	**16,008,318**	**27,491,383**	**43,499,701**	**10,588**	**660,826**
Nonmetropolitan	336	37,743	1,200,790	8,674,696	11,899,509	63.0	23,782	32,618	7.2	755,040	4,482,842	6,582,422	11,065,264	3,208	123,602
Metropolitan	467	119,968	4,310,769	30,132,752	38,074,669	68.8	82,577	104,333	7.0	3,164,809	11,525,476	20,908,961	32,434,437	7,380	537,224
Delaware	**8**	**2,006**	**84,090**	**560,406**	**745,334**	**76.6**	**1,536**	**2,043**	**6.7**	**77,860**	**254,573**	**711,617**	**966,190**	**139**	**11,259**
Nonmetropolitan	4	583	26,582	160,585	238,710	75.6	441	654	6.0	18,409	103,226	274,447	377,673	63	3,216
Metropolitan	4	1,423	57,508	399,821	506,624	77.0	1,095	1,389	7.0	59,451	151,347	437,170	588,517	76	8,043
Wilmington	4	1,423	57,508	399,821	506,624	77.0	1,095	1,389	7.0	59,451	151,347	437,170	588,517	76	8,043
District of Columbia	**11**	**4,557**	**157,832**	**1,252,183**	**1,514,470**	**75.3**	**3,431**	**4,149**	**7.9**	**118,590**	**384,105**	**887,932**	**1,272,037**	**312**	**20,664**
Nonmetropolitan	0	0	0	0	0	00.0	0	0	0.0	0	0	0	0	0	0
Metropolitan	11	4,557	157,832	1,252,183	1,514,470	75.3	3,431	4,149	7.9	118,590	384,105	887,932	1,272,037	312	20,664
Washington	11	4,557	157,832	1,252,183	1,514,470	75.3	3,431	4,149	7.9	118,590	384,105	887,932	1,272,037	312	20,664
Florida	**224**	**50,594**	**1,638,871**	**11,405,957**	**14,328,466**	**61.8**	**31,260**	**39,258**	**7.0**	**1,107,148**	**4,387,767**	**7,245,758**	**11,633,525**	**2,502**	**185,305**
Nonmetropolitan	38	3,903	110,986	731,124	977,171	51.3	2,001	2,675	6.6	78,649	378,084	516,838	894,922	151	7,413
Metropolitan	186	46,691	1,527,885	10,674,833	13,351,295	62.7	29,259	36,583	7.0	1,028,499	4,009,683	6,728,920	10,738,603	2,351	177,892
Bradenton	2	895	23,599	181,312	217,244	55.5	497	595	7.7	12,096	61,614	35,640	97,254	33	2,371
Daytona Beach	7	1,358	39,354	273,523	377,367	55.2	750	1,034	7.0	28,968	162,827	208,358	371,185	51	4,200
Fort Lauderdale-Hollywood-Pompano Beach	21	5,734	162,447	1,204,346	1,464,107	57.6	3,302	4,014	7.4	88,968	449,388	525,114	974,502	254	17,882
Fort Myers-Cape Coral	4	1,202	47,886	278,463	330,624	63.6	764	906	5.8	39,675	101,020	95,871	196,891	58	4,786
Fort Pierce	3	661	28,456	187,676	240,247	77.8	514	658	6.6	16,512	82,271	162,065	244,336	39	3,455
Fort Walton Beach	4	482	12,776	75,548	99,443	43.2	208	273	5.9	8,314	50,647	56,318	106,965	22	901
Gainesville	5	1,270	45,157	305,199	383,419	65.7	835	1,050	6.8	28,915	77,078	268,330	345,408	59	5,803
Jacksonville	15	3,158	116,802	767,916	996,021	66.7	2,106	2,727	6.6	88,823	344,459	529,244	873,703	218	15,104
Lakeland-Winter Haven	7	1,338	46,968	325,545	435,614	66.6	891	1,192	6.9	35,431	151,493	198,950	350,443	113	6,228
Melbourne-Titusville-Palm Bay	4	966	45,583	280,974	365,980	79.6	769	1,003	6.2	35,283	122,149	204,580	326,729	85	5,256
Miami-Hialeah	30	8,931	279,461	2,097,887	2,542,114	64.4	5,748	6,963	7.5	170,369	583,806	1,081,540	1,665,346	423	33,400
Naples	1	436	19,193	110,230	136,821	69.3	302	375	5.7	7,573	79,600	82,501	162,101	28	2,278
Ocala	2	432	19,832	123,791	155,656	78.5	339	427	6.2	13,693	55,927	72,616	128,543	26	2,307
Orlando	12	3,686	126,398	828,129	1,049,291	61.5	2,268	2,876	6.6	93,113	342,347	452,160	794,507	240	18,901
Panama City	2	465	18,562	130,763	166,393	77.0	358	456	7.0	13,623	58,173	64,219	122,392	44	2,160
Pensacola	7	1,754	47,923	355,443	455,513	55.5	974	1,247	7.4	32,596	122,747	318,494	441,241	71	5,592
Sarasota	4	1,309	40,287	290,136	343,340	60.7	795	940	7.2	28,226	84,669	99,965	184,634	49	3,381
Tallahassee	5	1,086	39,899	288,993	372,884	73.0	793	1,022	7.2	25,270	100,552	182,486	283,038	84	4,891
Tampa-St. Petersburg-Clearwater	36	8,288	258,059	1,843,594	2,282,499	61.1	5,060	6,261	7.1	183,819	690,217	1,246,270	1,936,487	311	25,925
West Palm Beach-Boca Raton-Delray Beach	15	3,240	109,243	725,365	936,718	61.3	1,986	2,564	6.6	77,232	288,699	844,199	1,132,898	143	13,071
Georgia	**163**	**25,500**	**888,048**	**6,120,975**	**7,937,120**	**65.8**	**16,777**	**21,747**	**6.9**	**573,437**	**2,802,663**	**4,046,177**	**6,848,840**	**1,999**	**106,216**
Nonmetropolitan	91	9,062	270,198	2,023,293	2,728,777	61.2	5,546	7,474	7.5	142,679	961,078	1,319,630	2,280,708	776	27,515
Metropolitan	72	16,438	617,850	4,097,682	5,208,343	68.3	11,231	14,273	6.6	430,758	1,841,585	2,726,547	4,568,132	1,223	78,701
Albany	2	638	23,418	153,413	199,039	65.8	420	545	6.6	13,862	79,331	81,695	161,026	40	2,909
Athens	3	679	25,432	173,600	221,583	70.1	476	607	6.8	16,740	82,560	71,304	153,864	44	2,590
Atlanta	43	9,467	373,487	2,389,815	3,071,385	69.2	6,549	8,418	6.4	243,365	1,108,284	1,642,384	2,750,668	740	49,754
Augusta	6	1,821	61,017	438,922	524,606	66.1	1,204	1,438	7.2	48,587	147,626	528,437	676,063	137	7,444
Chattanooga	3	310	10,209	78,823	109,861	69.7	216	300	7.7	6,572	37,587	33,385	70,972	20	1,216
Columbus	4	1,071	30,541	205,816	255,265	52.7	564	700	6.7	28,135	78,181	76,294	154,475	48	3,669
Macon-Warner Robins	7	1,278	49,938	301,883	390,760	64.8	828	1,071	6.0	37,822	194,254	170,450	364,704	108	6,051
Savannah	4	1,174	43,808	355,410	435,844	83.0	974	1,194	8.1	35,675	113,762	122,598	236,360	86	5,068
Maryland	**52**	**13,472**	**562,280**	**3,863,982**	**4,938,583**	**78.6**	**10,583**	**13,531**	**6.9**	**480,636**	**1,438,065**	**3,123,024**	**4,561,089**	**859**	**69,420**
Nonmetropolitan	7	963	43,756	264,171	350,270	75.1	723	959	6.0	33,632	137,171	527,911	665,082	97	4,994
Metropolitan	45	12,509	518,524	3,599,811	4,588,313	78.8	9,860	12,572	6.9	447,004	1,300,894	2,595,113	3,896,007	762	64,426
Baltimore	27	8,274	338,170	2,450,465	3,129,124	81.1	6,713	8,574	7.2	283,161	788,408	1,972,251	2,760,659	453	38,398
Cumberland	3	501	19,325	149,037	197,354	81.4	408	541	7.7	19,591	67,417	61,814	129,231	28	1,311
Hagerstown	1	312	13,162	82,172	104,761	72.1	225	287	6.2	10,953	53,659	100,525	154,184	22	1,602
Washington	13	3,283	141,614	887,841	1,114,599	74.0	2,431	3,054	6.3	127,842	371,571	410,834	782,405	245	22,799
Wilmington	1	139	6,253	30,296	42,475	59.7	83	116	4.8	5,457	19,839	49,689	69,528	14	316

CLASSIFICATION	FULL-TIME EQUIVALENT PERSONNEL: Physicians and Dentists	Registered Nurses	Licensed Practical Nurses	Other Salaried Personnel	Total Personnel	FULL-TIME EQUIVALENT TRAINEES: Medical and Dental Residents	Other Trainees	Total Trainees	EXPENSES — LABOR: Payroll (in thousands)	Employee Benefits (in thousands)	Total (in thousands)	Percent of Total	EXPENSES — TOTAL: Amount (in thousands)	Adjusted, per Admission	Adjusted, per Inpatient Day
CENSUS DIVISION 3, SOUTH ATLANTIC	3,891	141,841	30,999	401,568	578,299	9,076	649	9,725	$14,585,955	$ 2,895,080	$17,481,035	51.7	$ 33,812,948	$4,737.15	$ 676.61
Nonmetropolitan	640	24,090	9,623	79,146	113,499	465	72	537	2,384,830	460,585	2,845,415	52.2	5,448,867	3,291.59	457.91
Metropolitan	3,251	117,751	21,376	322,422	464,800	8,611	577	9,188	12,201,124	2,434,495	14,635,620	51.6	28,364,081	5,173.63	744.96
Delaware	101	2,708	412	6,789	10,010	200	0	200	269,581	56,818	326,398	56.8	574,402	5,111.88	770.66
Nonmetropolitan	23	716	164	1,929	2,832	0	0	0	64,656	13,020	77,676	54.5	142,444	3,608.64	596.72
Metropolitan	78	1,992	248	4,860	7,178	200	0	200	204,924	43,798	248,723	57.6	431,958	5,925.92	852.62
Wilmington	78	1,992	248	4,860	7,178	200	0	200	204,924	43,798	248,723	57.6	431,958	5,925.92	852.62
District of Columbia	634	5,036	547	14,055	20,272	1,062	33	1,095	709,635	127,011	836,646	55.5	1,507,467	7,875.55	995.38
Nonmetropolitan	0	0	0	0	0	0	0	0	0	0	0	0.0	0		
Metropolitan	634	5,036	547	14,055	20,272	1,062	33	1,095	709,635	127,011	836,646	55.5	1,507,467	7,875.55	995.38
Washington	634	5,036	547	14,055	20,272	1,062	33	1,095	709,635	127,011	836,646	55.5	1,507,467	7,875.55	995.38
Florida	538	43,497	8,862	119,000	171,897	1,501	97	1,598	4,423,579	964,210	5,387,789	48.9	11,019,208	5,312.36	769.04
Nonmetropolitan	17	2,152	733	7,005	9,907	8	4	12	230,507	53,656	284,163	47.9	593,793	3,938.53	607.67
Metropolitan	521	41,345	8,129	111,995	161,990	1,493	93	1,586	4,193,072	910,554	5,103,626	49.0	10,425,415	5,420.04	780.85
Bradenton	0	579	123	1,486	2,188	0	0	0	53,441	13,338	66,779	43.7	152,721	5,397.28	703.00
Daytona Beach	0	1,069	259	3,270	4,598	20	5	25	108,862	26,273	135,134	49.2	274,444	5,025.90	727.26
Fort Lauderdale-Hollywood-Pompano Beach	36	3,923	985	11,378	16,322	7	32	39	452,133	101,353	553,486	48.1	1,151,265	5,820.99	786.33
Fort Myers-Cape Coral	4	1,236	301	3,274	4,815	0	0	0	116,817	18,276	135,094	49.2	274,520	4,837.27	830.31
Fort Pierce	3	842	139	1,937	2,921	0	0	0	62,503	7,254	69,757	44.7	156,148	4,272.52	649.95
Fort Walton Beach	1	324	75	766	1,166	0	1	1	24,703	5,440	30,143	43.4	69,441	4,126.27	698.30
Gainesville	0	1,527	183	4,272	5,982	0	3	3	139,580	25,194	164,774	47.7	345,174	6,112.29	900.25
Jacksonville	2	3,410	456	8,815	12,683	268	39	307	322,838	76,086	398,924	48.5	822,715	5,407.62	826.00
Lakeland-Winter Haven	23	1,118	330	3,663	5,134	0	0	0	126,834	20,482	147,316	55.6	264,884	4,219.91	608.07
Melbourne-Titusville-Palm Bay	0	929	167	2,935	4,031	0	0	0	112,456	21,212	133,668	51.1	261,328	4,405.32	714.05
Miami-Hialeah	268	8,281	1,219	23,065	32,833	673	3	676	895,439	219,279	1,114,718	51.1	2,180,874	6,310.14	857.90
Naples	24	333	144	1,337	1,838	0	0	0	51,664	10,138	61,801	57.8	106,849	4,485.10	780.94
Ocala	0	452	69	1,203	1,724	0	0	0	37,136	7,282	44,418	49.6	89,591	3,611.08	575.57
Orlando	21	4,399	918	9,185	14,523	148	2	150	379,675	82,666	462,341	49.9	925,929	5,746.43	882.43
Panama City	0	462	122	1,192	1,776	0	0	0	39,496	9,677	49,173	48.0	102,533	4,331.57	616.21
Pensacola	9	1,390	361	3,587	5,347	12	0	12	115,436	21,394	136,830	46.6	293,720	4,772.21	644.81
Sarasota	0	888	280	2,815	3,983	0	0	0	97,642	26,815	124,457	48.2	258,468	5,406.83	752.81
Tallahassee	0	756	222	2,619	3,597	27	3	30	93,730	17,808	111,538	45.3	246,193	4,759.46	660.24
Tampa-St. Petersburg-Clearwater	127	6,360	1,349	17,617	25,453	326	5	331	672,666	147,276	819,942	47.3	1,733,343	5,414.06	759.41
West Palm Beach-Boca Raton-Delray Beach	3	3,067	427	7,579	11,076	12	0	12	290,020	53,311	343,331	48.0	715,277	5,047.79	763.60
Georgia	551	20,066	5,714	63,077	89,408	1,403	86	1,489	2,133,117	425,592	2,558,709	51.2	5,000,289	4,302.95	629.99
Nonmetropolitan	30	4,352	2,414	17,050	23,846	50	44	94	474,332	91,183	565,514	51.3	1,103,215	2,968.41	404.29
Metropolitan	521	15,714	3,300	46,027	65,562	1,353	42	1,395	1,658,785	334,410	1,993,195	51.1	3,897,074	4,930.46	748.24
Albany	0	428	190	1,385	2,003	0	0	0	46,706	8,301	55,007	48.9	112,577	3,705.01	565.60
Athens	0	470	130	1,780	2,380	0	0	0	64,312	11,990	76,301	56.3	135,433	4,214.12	611.21
Atlanta	101	10,141	1,478	26,890	38,610	724	34	758	1,031,869	197,587	1,229,456	51.2	2,401,956	4,964.23	782.04
Augusta	360	1,699	505	5,739	8,303	474	0	474	195,141	49,763	244,904	57.2	427,932	5,803.49	815.72
Chattanooga	2	271	86	749	1,108	3	0	3	24,732	4,723	29,455	53.6	54,913	3,886.29	499.84
Columbus	11	548	263	2,135	3,007	35	8	43	57,345	11,793	69,139	42.2	163,662	4,324.99	641.14
Macon-Warner Robins	23	1,051	281	3,676	5,031	60	0	60	114,123	22,215	136,337	46.6	292,876	4,498.66	749.50
Savannah	24	1,106	367	3,623	5,120	57	0	57	124,557	28,038	152,596	49.6	307,725	5,782.02	706.04
Maryland	619	14,760	1,408	41,955	58,742	1,018	120	1,138	1,578,214	297,836	1,876,050	56.1	3,346,704	4,640.37	677.66
Nonmetropolitan	19	869	161	3,048	4,097	0	3	3	88,049	16,367	104,415	55.4	188,322	3,249.11	537.65
Metropolitan	600	13,891	1,247	38,907	54,645	1,018	117	1,135	1,490,166	281,470	1,771,635	56.1	3,158,383	4,761.95	688.35
Baltimore	554	9,655	832	27,423	38,464	956	55	1,011	1,062,631	201,123	1,263,754	56.3	2,244,012	5,180.01	717.14
Cumberland	1	446	74	1,273	1,794	0	0	0	42,783	8,743	51,526	57.0	90,461	3,520.99	458.37
Hagerstown	6	311	50	1,047	1,414	0	1	1	30,507	5,965	36,472	54.6	66,777	3,979.55	637.42
Washington	37	3,332	247	8,739	12,415	62	61	123	340,240	63,127	403,366	55.3	729,273	4,078.50	654.29
Wilmington	2	147	44	365	558	0	0	0	14,006	2,512	16,518	59.3	27,859	3,177.75	655.90

(continued on next page)

Table

6 (Continued)

Utilization, Personnel, and Finances in Community Hospitals, by Metropolitan Statistical Area

Where an MSA is located in multiple states, the MSA will be listed for each state, with hospital data for only that state.

CLASSIFICATION	HOSPITALS	BEDS	ADMISSIONS	INPATIENT DAYS	ADJUSTED PATIENT DAYS	OCCUPANCY, percent	AVERAGE DAILY CENSUS	ADJUSTED AVERAGE DAILY CENSUS	AVERAGE STAY, days	SURGICAL OPERATIONS	OUTPATIENT VISITS			NEWBORNS	
											Emergency	Other	Total	Bassinets	Births
North Carolina	**120**	**21,934**	**784,414**	**5,856,343**	**7,647,972**	**73.2**	**16,047**	**20,958**	**7.5**	**566,390**	**2,407,273**	**3,712,401**	**6,119,674**	**1,781**	**99,954**
Nonmetropolitan	74	8,981	303,377	2,290,423	3,110,321	69.9	6,278	8,525	7.5	188,514	1,136,653	1,217,192	2,353,845	878	34,445
Metropolitan	46	12,953	481,037	3,565,920	4,537,651	75.4	9,769	12,433	7.4	377,876	1,270,620	2,495,209	3,765,829	903	65,509
Asheville	2	711	30,883	199,753	242,840	76.9	547	665	6.5	27,106	72,586	100,606	173,192	32	3,201
Burlington	2	340	8,271	84,478	121,635	67.9	231	333	10.2	8,623	44,425	39,941	84,366	35	1,123
Charlotte-Gastonia-Rock Hill	11	3,224	118,946	878,723	1,157,178	74.7	2,409	3,171	7.4	91,009	358,532	388,490	747,022	260	18,022
Fayetteville	2	581	21,920	169,154	216,709	79.7	463	594	7.7	12,878	74,903	117,349	192,252	48	4,794
Greensboro-Winston-Salem-High Point	13	3,319	125,732	944,189	1,166,999	77.9	2,586	3,197	7.5	90,775	317,487	363,264	680,751	219	14,372
Hickory	5	794	26,131	164,941	239,028	56.8	451	655	6.3	25,781	90,566	195,232	285,798	84	3,633
Jacksonville	1	133	6,926	32,683	47,748	67.7	90	131	4.7	3,439	28,481	73,028	101,509	22	2,398
Raleigh-Durham	8	3,293	122,729	941,686	1,151,444	78.3	2,580	3,155	7.7	99,269	212,838	1,172,634	1,385,472	165	15,078
Wilmington	2	558	19,499	150,313	194,070	73.8	412	532	7.7	18,996	70,802	44,665	115,467	38	2,888
South Carolina	**69**	**11,208**	**413,045**	**2,899,854**	**3,792,993**	**71.0**	**7,960**	**10,411**	**7.0**	**287,099**	**1,297,569**	**2,139,063**	**3,436,632**	**919**	**53,604**
Nonmetropolitan	37	3,983	132,173	953,683	1,311,879	65.9	2,625	3,611	7.2	82,809	542,167	600,059	1,142,226	424	17,144
Metropolitan	32	7,225	280,872	1,946,171	2,481,114	73.8	5,335	6,800	6.9	204,290	755,402	1,539,004	2,294,406	495	36,460
Anderson	1	468	18,561	115,165	148,770	67.5	316	409	6.2	13,434	43,028	168,638	211,666	30	2,099
Augusta	1	195	8,064	49,884	59,357	70.3	137	163	6.2	5,349	33,000	3,043	36,043	22	1,157
Charleston	7	1,838	68,095	462,308	574,376	68.9	1,267	1,573	6.8	49,388	161,268	304,257	465,525	120	9,013
Charlotte-Gastonia-Rock Hill	2	370	11,470	90,877	122,275	67.3	249	335	7.9	9,056	51,590	32,106	83,696	25	1,737
Columbia	4	1,367	61,786	423,630	520,680	85.0	1,162	1,427	6.9	46,343	161,681	285,058	446,739	107	8,517
Florence	4	689	30,563	200,742	261,566	79.8	550	716	6.6	18,724	71,595	117,059	188,654	28	3,053
Greenville-Spartanburg	13	2,298	82,333	603,565	794,090	72.0	1,654	2,177	7.3	61,996	233,240	628,843	862,083	163	10,884
Virginia	**97**	**20,005**	**706,240**	**4,918,759**	**6,430,948**	**67.4**	**13,479**	**17,624**	**7.0**	**495,863**	**2,078,185**	**3,770,924**	**5,849,109**	**1,498**	**91,584**
Nonmetropolitan	43	5,718	171,650	1,280,690	1,786,371	61.4	3,509	4,896	7.5	105,503	650,440	1,064,277	1,714,717	482	16,919
Metropolitan	54	14,287	534,590	3,638,069	4,644,577	69.8	9,970	12,728	6.8	390,360	1,427,745	2,706,647	4,134,392	1,016	74,665
Charlottesville	2	851	34,614	243,173	303,713	78.3	666	832	7.0	17,627	82,796	340,725	423,521	55	3,626
Danville	1	391	12,899	104,285	131,433	73.1	286	360	8.1	8,176	42,952	31,282	74,234	26	1,398
Johnson City-Kingsport-Bristol	1	147	4,600	28,021	37,586	52.4	77	103	6.1	4,207	16,292	7,174	23,466	12	564
Lynchburg	2	734	21,554	198,061	251,381	74.0	543	689	9.2	17,118	55,237	66,465	121,702	39	2,666
Norfolk-Virginia Beach-Newport News	16	4,055	154,596	1,015,649	1,350,276	68.7	2,784	3,700	6.6	116,126	459,672	863,150	1,322,822	361	22,866
Richmond-Petersburg	15	3,929	140,879	977,926	1,226,143	68.2	2,679	3,360	6.9	94,555	328,720	732,474	1,061,194	229	16,337
Roanoke	4	1,272	43,495	332,606	405,708	71.6	911	1,112	7.6	33,783	110,705	262,164	372,869	67	4,229
Washington	13	2,908	121,953	738,348	938,337	69.6	2,024	2,572	6.1	98,768	331,371	403,213	734,584	227	22,979
West Virginia	**59**	**8,435**	**276,739**	**1,928,989**	**2,638,292**	**62.7**	**5,286**	**7,230**	**7.0**	**212,826**	**958,118**	**1,854,487**	**2,812,605**	**579**	**22,820**
Nonmetropolitan	42	4,550	142,068	970,727	1,396,010	58.4	2,659	3,824	6.8	104,845	574,023	1,062,068	1,636,091	337	11,956
Metropolitan	17	3,885	134,671	958,262	1,242,282	67.6	2,627	3,406	7.1	107,981	384,095	792,419	1,176,514	242	10,864
Charleston	6	1,449	50,438	351,723	449,558	66.6	965	1,233	7.0	46,304	131,070	271,522	402,592	65	4,180
Cumberland	1	51	1,174	8,227	14,198	45.1	23	39	7.0	1,620	10,449	15,032	25,481	0	0
Huntington-Ashland	3	778	29,011	194,921	234,854	68.6	534	644	6.7	16,286	86,450	97,507	183,957	57	2,871
Parkersburg-Marietta	3	593	20,316	141,283	191,485	65.3	387	525	7.0	18,719	68,071	153,185	221,256	30	1,407
Steubenville-Weirton	1	265	8,796	52,734	70,760	54.3	144	194	6.0	4,188	23,750	40,544	64,294	21	344
Wheeling	3	749	24,936	209,374	281,427	76.6	574	771	8.4	20,864	64,305	214,629	278,934	69	2,062

CLASSIFICATION	FULL-TIME EQUIVALENT PERSONNEL					FULL-TIME EQUIVALENT TRAINEES			EXPENSES						
									LABOR				TOTAL		
	Physicians and Dentists	Registered Nurses	Licensed Practical Nurses	Other Salaried Personne	Total Personnel	Medical and Dental Residents	Other Trainees	Total Trainees	Payroll (in thousands)	Employee Benefits (in thousands)	Total (in thousands)	Percent of Total	Amount (in thousands)	Adjusted, per Admission	Adjusted, per Inpatient Day
North Carolina	**584**	**22,563**	**4,626**	**60,188**	**87,961**	**1,494**	**110**	**1,604**	**$ 2,103,497**	**$ 380,323**	**$ 2,483,820**	**54.5**	**$ 4,553,511**	**$4,408.28**	**$ 595.39**
Nonmetropolitan	408	7,372	2,098	21,002	30,880	172	11	183	647,955	114,124	762,078	55.0	1,386,006	3,358.47	445.62
Metropolitan	176	15,191	2,528	39,186	57,081	1,322	99	1,421	1,455,543	266,199	1,721,742	54.4	3,167,505	5,106.78	698.05
Asheville	0	877	175	1,991	3,043	0	0	0	78,607	13,757	92,364	53.3	173,428	4,617.23	714.16
Burlington	0	265	79	734	1,078	0	0	0	22,976	3,995	26,971	55.4	48,684	3,861.03	400.24
Charlotte-Gastonia-Rock Hill	115	3,270	389	9,964	13,738	135	0	135	357,236	65,297	422,533	55.8	756,875	4,793.54	654.07
Fayetteville	2	552	187	1,504	2,245	0	0	0	52,588	9,328	61,916	50.8	121,843	4,343.31	562.24
Greensboro-Winston-Salem-High Point	9	3,632	718	9,823	14,182	445	61	506	358,352	62,187	420,539	55.8	753,330	4,813.64	645.53
Hickory	36	831	109	1,758	2,734	0	0	0	62,457	13,216	75,673	50.1	150,904	3,981.64	631.32
Jacksonville	0	134	60	398	592	0	0	0	11,956	2,208	14,164	57.1	24,794	2,450.19	519.26
Raleigh-Durham	13	4,890	720	11,241	16,864	710	38	748	444,689	83,155	527,844	52.4	1,008,078	6,546.09	875.49
Wilmington	1	740	91	1,773	2,605	32	0	32	66,681	13,056	79,737	61.5	129,570	5,056.99	667.65
South Carolina	**107**	**9,763**	**2,874**	**28,290**	**41,034**	**796**	**152**	**948**	**947,820**	**182,305**	**1,130,126**	**50.5**	**2,236,923**	**4,167.57**	**589.75**
Nonmetropolitan	16	2,309	1,067	8,003	11,395	18	4	22	231,084	44,351	275,435	50.6	544,043	3,014.84	414.70
Metropolitan	91	7,454	1,807	20,287	29,639	778	148	926	716,737	137,954	854,691	50.5	1,692,881	4,751.41	682.31
Anderson	9	306	98	1,438	1,851	19	15	34	35,997	5,408	41,405	51.0	81,177	3,385.60	545.65
Augusta	0	179	67	447	693	0	0	0	14,992	3,245	18,237	52.9	34,507	3,596.38	581.35
Charleston	1	1,737	548	4,730	7,016	400	1	401	169,793	33,985	203,777	44.5	457,447	5,426.87	796.42
Charlotte-Gastonia-Rock Hill	0	269	40	727	1,036	0	0	0	19,980	5,959	25,940	41.8	62,108	4,082.59	507.94
Columbia	19	1,812	381	4,745	6,957	183	83	266	178,502	30,928	209,429	53.2	393,967	5,169.77	756.64
Florence	6	756	192	2,080	3,034	17	25	42	72,889	14,672	87,561	52.1	168,047	4,220.80	642.47
Greenville-Spartanburg	56	2,395	481	6,120	9,052	159	24	183	224,584	43,757	268,340	54.1	495,627	4,623.73	624.14
Virginia	**541**	**17,446**	**4,582**	**48,624**	**71,193**	**1,220**	**19**	**1,239**	**1,786,210**	**328,922**	**2,115,132**	**51.8**	**4,084,237**	**4,408.21**	**635.09**
Nonmetropolitan	11	3,544	1,770	11,378	16,703	7	0	7	346,248	63,133	409,381	53.1	771,553	3,227.04	431.91
Metropolitan	530	13,902	2,812	37,246	54,490	1,213	19	1,232	1,439,963	265,789	1,705,752	51.5	3,312,684	4,819.02	713.24
Charlottesville	395	1,274	186	3,039	4,894	540	9	549	110,800	27,318	138,118	42.0	328,719	7,451.25	1,082.34
Danville	0	259	147	980	1,386	0	0	0	29,773	5,244	35,017	56.6	61,824	3,802.90	470.38
Johnson City-Kingsport-Bristol	1	114	53	273	441	0	0	0	8,305	1,409	9,715	52.2	18,608	3,015.81	495.07
Lynchburg	3	543	95	1,438	2,079	0	0	0	56,359	10,280	66,639	59.9	111,184	4,062.87	442.29
Norfolk-Virginia Beach-Newport News	17	4,007	851	10,343	15,218	76	0	76	397,079	60,950	458,029	52.4	874,149	4,249.03	647.39
Richmond-Petersburg	29	3,570	948	10,252	14,799	496	2	498	361,594	79,930	441,524	49.9	885,456	4,971.60	722.15
Roanoke	37	969	304	3,352	4,662	85	0	85	112,424	20,931	133,355	49.9	267,138	4,909.62	658.45
Washington	48	3,166	228	7,569	11,011	16	8	24	363,628	59,726	423,354	55.3	765,606	4,930.93	815.92
West Virginia	**216**	**6,002**	**1,974**	**19,590**	**27,782**	**382**	**32**	**414**	**634,301**	**132,063**	**766,364**	**51.4**	**1,490,207**	**3,918.34**	**564.84**
Nonmetropolitan	116	2,776	1,216	9,737	13,839	210	6	216	302,001	64,752	366,753	51.0	719,492	3,539.01	515.39
Metropolitan	100	3,226	758	9,859	13,943	172	26	198	332,301	67,311	399,611	51.8	770,714	4,354.00	620.40
Charleston	34	1,257	233	3,918	5,442	104	7	111	140,874	32,030	172,904	50.3	343,442	5,228.15	763.96
Cumberland	0	26	3	128	149	0	0	0	3,105	721	3,826	55.3	6,921	3,415.85	487.43
Huntington-Ashland	1	742	164	1,588	2,495	18	19	37	67,330	13,889	81,219	57.0	142,516	4,043.69	606.83
Parkersburg-Marietta	25	407	189	1,597	2,218	0	0	0	50,371	8,025	58,395	55.4	105,427	3,775.91	550.58
Steubenville-Weirton	13	140	5	526	684	0	0	0	15,089	2,195	17,284	53.2	32,461	2,750.22	458.75
Wheeling	27	654	164	2,110	2,955	50	0	50	55,532	10,451	65,982	47.1	139,948	4,076.78	497.28

(continued on next page)

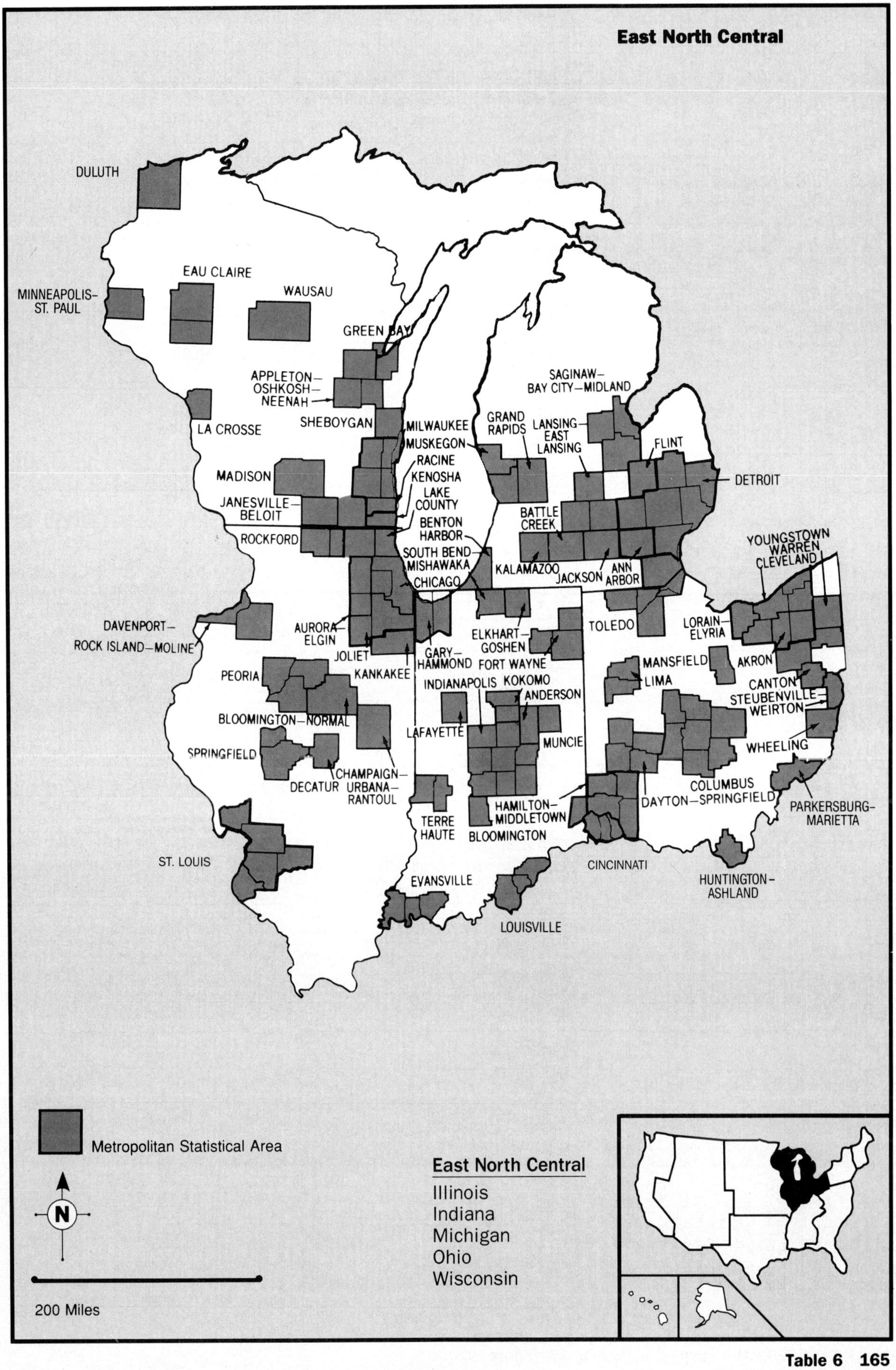
East North Central
DULUTH
EAU CLAIRE
WAUSAU
MINNEAPOLIS-
ST. PAUL
GREEN BAY
APPLETON–
OSHKOSH–
NEENAH
SHEBOYGAN
LA CROSSE
MILWAUKEE
MUSKEGON
RACINE
KENOSHA
LAKE
COUNTY
MADISON
JANESVILLE–
BELOIT
ROCKFORD
BENTON
HARBOR
SOUTH BEND–
MISHAWAKA
CHICAGO
GRAND
RAPIDS
LANSING–
EAST
LANSING
SAGINAW–
BAY CITY–MIDLAND
FLINT
DETROIT
BATTLE
CREEK
KALAMAZOO
JACKSON
ANN
ARBOR
YOUNGSTOWN
WARREN
CLEVELAND
TOLEDO
LORAIN–
ELYRIA
AKRON
CANTON
STEUBENVILLE–
WEIRTON
WHEELING
MANSFIELD
LIMA
DAVENPORT–
ROCK ISLAND–MOLINE
AURORA–
ELGIN
JOLIET
GARY–
HAMMOND
ELKHART–
GOSHEN
FORT WAYNE
KANKAKEE
PEORIA
INDIANAPOLIS
KOKOMO
ANDERSON
BLOOMINGTON–NORMAL
LAFAYETTE
MUNCIE
SPRINGFIELD
CHAMPAIGN–
URBANA–
RANTOUL
DECATUR
TERRE
HAUTE
BLOOMINGTON
HAMILTON–
MIDDLETOWN
DAYTON–SPRINGFIELD
COLUMBUS
PARKERSBURG–
MARIETTA
ST. LOUIS
CINCINNATI
HUNTINGTON–
ASHLAND
EVANSVILLE
LOUISVILLE
Metropolitan Statistical Area
N
200 Miles
East North Central
Illinois
Indiana
Michigan
Ohio
Wisconsin

Table
6 (Continued)

Utilization, Personnel, and Finances in Community Hospitals, by Metropolitan Statistical Area

Where an MSA is located in multiple states, the MSA will be listed for each state, with hospital data for only that state.

CLASSIFICATION	HOSPITALS	BEDS	ADMISSIONS	INPATIENT DAYS	ADJUSTED PATIENT DAYS	OCCUPANCY, percent	AVERAGE DAILY CENSUS	ADJUSTED AVERAGE DAILY CENSUS	AVERAGE STAY, days	SURGICAL OPERATIONS	OUTPATIENT VISITS			NEWBORNS	
											Emergency	Other	Total	Bassinets	Births
CENSUS DIVISION 4, EAST NORTH CENTRAL	818	163,712	5,404,346	38,598,241	52,104,001	64.6	105,770	142,774	7.1	4,057,133	15,553,424	47,882,338	63,435,762	12,687	654,562
Nonmetropolitan	338	32,460	903,878	6,444,712	9,600,862	54.4	17,654	26,311	7.1	628,712	3,265,164	8,656,735	11,921,899	3,126	98,776
Metropolitan	480	131,252	4,500,468	32,153,529	42,503,139	67.1	88,116	116,463	7.1	3,428,421	12,288,260	39,225,603	51,513,863	9,561	555,786
Illinois	210	46,065	1,499,435	11,053,001	14,305,703	65.8	30,292	39,201	7.4	1,021,673	4,057,815	12,366,581	16,424,396	3,405	185,275
Nonmetropolitan	79	7,770	214,252	1,515,777	2,157,428	53.4	4,147	5,909	7.1	134,150	689,004	1,712,351	2,401,355	622	18,806
Metropolitan	131	38,295	1,285,183	9,537,224	12,148,275	68.3	26,145	33,292	7.4	887,523	3,368,811	10,654,230	14,023,041	2,783	166,469
Aurora-Elgin	5	1,292	41,541	256,649	345,235	54.4	703	946	6.2	36,156	153,216	331,748	484,964	121	6,382
Bloomington-Normal	2	617	15,627	137,157	196,122	60.9	376	537	8.8	15,358	44,436	99,571	144,007	43	2,055
Champaign-Urbana-Rantoul	2	892	26,084	202,195	247,568	62.1	554	679	7.8	19,427	38,512	66,129	104,641	31	3,302
Chicago	76	24,122	834,353	6,227,997	7,701,618	70.8	17,076	21,110	7.5	531,220	2,120,082	7,181,908	9,301,990	1,756	112,322
Davenport-Rock Island-Moline	5	951	28,278	184,556	275,327	53.1	505	754	6.5	16,047	83,694	304,412	388,106	98	2,700
Decatur	2	725	22,460	177,633	253,771	67.2	487	696	7.9	20,391	78,735	167,472	246,207	64	2,139
Joliet	3	863	33,166	205,248	270,590	65.2	563	741	6.2	17,909	75,250	253,856	329,106	74	3,644
Kankakee	2	558	15,919	135,489	184,063	66.5	371	504	8.5	10,718	58,612	218,766	277,378	42	1,803
Lake County	7	1,538	53,908	352,443	481,016	62.7	965	1,318	6.5	44,180	154,981	435,522	590,503	130	8,926
Peoria	5	1,558	50,985	404,297	544,108	71.1	1,107	1,490	7.9	48,640	132,686	369,070	501,756	119	5,375
Rockford	5	1,110	37,755	256,877	335,466	63.4	704	919	6.8	35,219	112,256	306,130	418,386	83	5,214
St. Louis	12	2,401	70,080	551,672	745,279	63.1	1,514	2,042	7.9	50,665	196,142	585,467	781,609	156	7,997
Springfield	5	1,668	55,027	445,011	568,112	73.1	1,220	1,556	8.1	41,593	120,209	334,179	454,388	66	4,610
Indiana	113	21,866	727,241	4,832,689	6,585,205	60.6	13,240	18,044	6.6	579,242	2,018,370	6,641,361	8,659,731	1,832	83,915
Nonmetropolitan	55	5,225	161,091	948,102	1,450,930	49.7	2,596	3,975	5.9	118,271	578,430	1,786,090	2,364,520	643	18,332
Metropolitan	58	16,641	566,150	3,884,587	5,134,275	64.0	10,644	14,069	6.9	460,971	1,439,940	4,855,271	6,295,211	1,189	65,583
Anderson	3	621	16,655	121,881	194,286	53.8	334	533	7.3	14,082	60,005	199,068	259,073	41	1,659
Bloomington	1	285	13,127	69,613	102,019	67.0	191	280	5.3	10,070	49,751	203,543	253,294	20	1,878
Cincinnati	1	109	3,412	20,148	32,094	50.5	55	88	5.9	3,183	17,269	58,147	75,416	14	353
Elkhart-Goshen	2	527	17,164	104,123	142,115	54.1	285	389	6.1	14,748	54,464	124,549	179,013	49	3,144
Evansville	5	1,570	45,324	317,581	396,840	55.5	871	1,088	7.0	27,793	135,966	320,758	456,724	70	4,558
Fort Wayne	5	1,458	52,108	342,288	428,060	64.3	937	1,173	6.6	48,851	96,643	463,362	560,005	124	7,088
Gary-Hammond	7	2,785	100,692	731,889	917,122	72.0	2,005	2,512	7.3	65,765	195,687	759,611	955,298	185	9,910
Indianapolis	18	5,497	196,998	1,369,267	1,823,909	68.3	3,752	4,998	7.0	167,637	484,673	1,808,769	2,293,442	386	22,568
Kokomo	3	486	14,094	90,782	141,634	51.2	249	388	6.4	12,428	68,400	219,284	287,684	47	1,700
Lafayette	2	619	17,618	119,826	170,096	53.0	328	466	6.8	16,979	50,705	145,474	196,179	36	2,718
Louisville	4	614	20,541	131,031	177,926	58.5	359	487	6.4	14,438	65,953	121,039	186,992	47	1,814
Muncie	1	542	16,816	120,589	152,373	60.9	330	417	7.2	18,937	39,236	134,836	174,072	55	1,888
South Bend-Mishawaka	3	879	31,893	206,511	267,798	64.4	566	735	6.5	28,159	72,210	133,405	205,615	54	3,975
Terre Haute	3	649	19,708	139,058	188,003	58.9	382	515	7.1	17,901	48,978	163,426	212,404	61	2,330
Michigan	176	33,951	1,069,361	8,116,557	11,467,395	65.5	22,246	31,419	7.6	889,408	3,345,541	11,974,009	15,319,550	2,838	148,879
Nonmetropolitan	71	6,106	161,492	1,216,696	1,908,178	54.7	3,338	5,231	7.5	122,147	669,097	1,978,493	2,647,590	597	19,557
Metropolitan	105	27,845	907,869	6,899,861	9,559,217	67.9	18,908	26,188	7.6	767,261	2,676,444	9,995,516	12,671,960	2,241	129,322
Ann Arbor	5	1,783	66,898	506,208	682,131	77.8	1,387	1,870	7.6	55,230	134,869	935,515	1,070,384	121	7,357
Battle Creek	4	580	15,018	119,759	178,377	56.4	327	490	8.0	15,264	60,348	112,822	173,170	56	2,261
Benton Harbor	4	765	18,644	170,693	234,906	61.2	468	643	9.2	14,820	77,992	180,350	258,342	40	2,717
Detroit	55	15,015	491,439	3,785,299	5,271,294	69.1	10,372	14,439	7.7	408,589	1,570,068	6,067,853	7,637,921	1,216	71,809
Flint	6	1,789	64,723	440,881	583,197	67.5	1,208	1,598	6.8	49,619	155,681	475,194	630,875	153	8,380
Grand Rapids	9	2,286	76,787	573,900	765,314	68.9	1,575	2,096	7.5	68,376	184,047	522,589	706,636	260	13,774
Jackson	3	589	18,455	113,537	160,730	52.8	311	440	6.2	14,475	40,073	389,425	429,498	52	1,808
Kalamazoo	3	872	31,093	208,585	276,224	65.6	572	757	6.7	26,486	85,523	331,481	417,004	72	4,704
Lansing-East Lansing	7	1,627	45,317	371,431	554,290	62.6	1,018	1,518	8.2	39,729	161,147	409,789	570,936	131	7,304
Muskegon	3	667	18,545	129,530	210,522	53.2	355	577	7.0	23,783	60,267	199,419	259,686	44	2,600
Saginaw-Bay City-Midland	6	1,872	60,950	480,038	642,232	70.2	1,315	1,760	7.9	50,890	146,429	371,079	517,508	96	6,608

CLASSIFICATION	FULL-TIME EQUIVALENT PERSONNEL					FULL-TIME EQUIVALENT TRAINEES			EXPENSES						
									LABOR				TOTAL		
	Physicians and Dentists	Registered Nurses	Licensed Practical Nurses	Other Salaried Personnel	Total Personnel	Medical and Dental Residents	Other Trainees	Total Trainees	Payroll (in thousands)	Employee Benefits (in thousands)	Total (in thousands)	Percent of Total	Amount (in thousands)	Adjusted, per Admission	Adjusted, per Inpatient Day
CENSUS DIVISION 4, EAST NORTH CENTRAL	5,560	148,600	24,478	448,496	627,134	13,335	931	14,266	$16,294,569	$ 3,218,782	$19,513,352	54.1	$ 36,057,873	$4,900.01	$ 692.04
Nonmetropolitan	167	19,578	5,654	65,115	90,514	82	46	128	1,977,279	391,978	2,369,257	54.4	4,352,638	3,180.79	453.36
Metropolitan	5,393	129,022	18,824	383,381	536,620	13,253	885	14,138	14,317,290	2,826,805	17,144,095	54.1	31,705,235	5,292.75	745.95
Illinois	1,797	40,996	5,056	125,662	173,511	3,790	107	3,897	4,615,536	857,240	5,472,776	53.4	10,254,113	5,252.56	716.79
Nonmetropolitan	32	4,336	1,165	14,581	20,114	36	10	46	407,105	76,757	483,862	53.7	901,510	2,925.38	417.86
Metropolitan	1,765	36,660	3,891	111,081	153,397	3,754	97	3,851	4,208,431	780,483	4,988,914	53.3	9,352,603	5,688.78	769.87
Aurora-Elgin	29	1,205	25	3,169	4,428	0	0	0	121,827	21,201	143,028	55.5	257,833	4,589.32	746.83
Bloomington-Normal	4	390	57	1,390	1,841	0	0	0	44,172	8,962	53,134	52.7	100,778	4,471.49	513.86
Champaign-Urbana-Rantoul	1	681	57	1,846	2,585	0	0	0	55,455	10,988	66,442	48.0	138,301	4,293.20	558.64
Chicago	1,608	24,587	2,118	74,088	102,401	3,516	90	3,606	2,985,519	535,307	3,520,826	53.1	6,624,509	6,391.41	860.15
Davenport-Rock Island-Moline	1	824	42	2,045	2,912	0	0	0	63,610	13,935	77,545	54.7	141,883	3,364.70	515.32
Decatur	4	461	266	1,978	2,709	7	0	7	54,559	10,545	65,104	57.2	113,791	3,532.88	448.40
Joliet	4	851	51	1,995	2,901	0	0	0	83,246	17,881	101,127	58.3	173,606	3,941.21	641.58
Kankakee	5	455	63	1,290	1,813	0	0	0	40,848	8,632	49,481	49.8	99,435	4,589.01	540.22
Lake County	9	1,442	103	4,177	5,731	0	0	0	149,109	27,333	176,442	53.1	332,037	4,532.86	690.28
Peoria	66	1,759	248	4,781	6,854	142	1	143	167,764	33,246	201,010	51.3	391,954	5,694.44	720.36
Rockford	17	1,075	167	3,289	4,548	0	6	6	116,108	23,660	139,768	52.2	267,996	5,426.56	798.88
St. Louis	5	1,635	302	5,813	7,755	16	0	16	170,742	35,950	206,693	55.6	372,057	3,933.20	499.22
Springfield	12	1,295	392	5,220	6,919	73	0	73	155,473	32,842	188,315	55.6	338,424	4,801.29	595.70
Indiana	197	19,769	3,205	60,699	83,870	645	171	816	1,949,445	378,589	2,328,034	53.0	4,393,563	4,389.62	667.19
Nonmetropolitan	15	3,374	895	11,886	16,170	0	24	24	338,473	61,696	400,169	53.5	748,547	3,024.60	515.91
Metropolitan	182	16,395	2,310	48,813	67,700	645	147	792	1,610,972	316,893	1,927,866	52.9	3,645,015	4,838.01	709.94
Anderson	1	369	88	1,41[illegible]	1,869	0	0	0	39,300	11,683	50,983	52.6	96,942	3,651.01	498.96
Bloomington	1	291	102	986	1,380	0	0	0	33,407	6,581	39,988	58.0	68,968	3,585.01	676.03
Cincinnati	0	96	28	225	349	0	0	0	8,598	1,722	10,320	56.9	18,141	3,337.75	565.24
Elkhart-Goshen	4	364	55	1,134	1,557	2	0	2	36,202	4,775	40,977	53.0	77,249	3,293.62	543.56
Evansville	16	1,346	83	3,807	5,252	25	0	25	123,337	22,141	145,478	54.4	267,354	4,670.43	673.71
Fort Wayne	2	1,502	227	3,961	5,692	8	0	8	147,991	26,628	174,620	51.3	340,560	5,172.46	795.59
Gary-Hammond	16	2,597	231	7,503	10,353	12	76	88	248,327	53,879	302,205	52.7	573,385	4,523.53	625.20
Indianapolis	101	6,734	997	20,121	27,953	495	59	554	658,728	127,154	785,883	53.0	1,483,355	5,604.84	813.28
Kokomo	11	401	23	1,226	1,661	0	0	0	37,618	8,858	46,476	56.1	82,888	3,777.61	585.23
Lafayette	3	521	94	1,740	2,358	0	10	10	48,278	10,173	58,451	55.5	105,321	4,210.49	619.19
Louisville	0	359	106	1,531	1,996	0	0	0	47,947	8,635	56,583	55.8	101,445	3,623.55	570.15
Muncie	22	240	31	1,247	1,540	45	0	45	44,090	8,227	52,317	56.6	92,497	4,353.22	607.04
South Bend-Mishawaka	1	953	93	2,444	3,491	45	0	45	88,409	17,739	106,148	48.3	219,677	5,322.28	820.31
Terre Haute	4	622	152	1,471	2,249	13	2	15	48,741	8,698	57,439	49.0	117,234	4,380.79	623.58
Michigan	2,211	30,308	6,434	96,209	135,162	3,598	266	3,864	3,724,291	727,684	4,451,975	54.2	8,210,713	5,357.51	716.01
Nonmetropolitan	79	3,717	1,420	12,722	17,938	25	0	25	420,795	83,040	503,835	55.9	901,475	3,476.61	472.43
Metropolitan	2,132	26,591	5,014	83,487	117,224	3,573	266	3,839	3,303,496	644,643	3,948,139	54.0	7,309,238	5,740.55	764.63
Ann Arbor	108	2,754	191	8,241	11,294	689	0	689	372,794	58,036	430,830	53.4	806,338	8,882.53	1,182.09
Battle Creek	1	471	127	1,287	1,886	0	0	0	49,953	6,677	56,631	56.8	99,696	4,370.74	558.91
Benton Harbor	3	487	75	1,611	2,176	0	0	0	48,108	9,908	58,016	54.4	106,563	4,071.47	453.64
Detroit	1,791	13,603	2,339	46,879	64,612	2,151	180	2,331	1,797,083	365,881	2,162,964	53.1	4,076,125	5,909.27	773.27
Flint	47	1,616	538	4,660	6,861	234	57	291	206,339	46,185	252,525	60.7	416,350	4,743.65	713.91
Grand Rapids	55	2,580	402	5,700	8,737	303	14	317	224,205	40,297	264,502	54.2	488,441	4,642.54	638.22
Jackson	22	448	172	1,344	1,986	0	0	0	61,633	11,460	73,093	60.1	121,638	4,452.17	756.78
Kalamazoo	26	1,164	161	2,386	3,737	0	0	0	122,559	22,844	145,403	50.7	286,966	6,975.01	1,038.89
Lansing-East Lansing	30	1,477	284	4,624	6,415	147	0	147	164,776	31,895	196,670	54.4	361,532	5,403.01	652.24
Muskegon	2	487	170	1,558	2,217	8	0	8	63,919	12,317	76,236	52.7	144,663	4,853.00	687.16
Saginaw-Bay City-Midland	47	1,504	555	5,197	7,303	41	15	56	192,127	39,143	231,270	57.7	400,926	4,686.23	624.27

(continued on next page)

Table
6 (Continued)

Utilization, Personnel, and Finances in Community Hospitals, by Metropolitan Statistical Area

Where an MSA is located in multiple states, the MSA will be listed for each state, with hospital data for only that state.

CLASSIFICATION	HOSPITALS	BEDS	ADMISSIONS	INPATIENT DAYS	ADJUSTED PATIENT DAYS	OCCUPANCY, percent	AVERAGE DAILY CENSUS	ADJUSTED AVERAGE DAILY CENSUS	AVERAGE STAY, days	SURGICAL OPERATIONS	OUTPATIENT VISITS			NEWBORNS	
											Emergency	Other	Total	Bassinets	Births
Ohio	190	43,143	1,511,655	10,187,427	13,649,109	64.7	27,910	37,399	6.7	1,102,047	4,622,785	12,482,478	17,105,263	3,089	164,863
Nonmetropolitan	64	6,754	216,725	1,238,980	1,908,255	50.3	3,394	5,232	5.7	154,135	880,623	2,106,565	2,987,188	742	25,444
Metropolitan	126	36,389	1,294,930	8,948,447	11,740,854	67.4	24,516	32,167	6.9	947,912	3,742,162	10,375,913	14,118,075	2,347	139,419
Akron	8	2,555	93,533	660,875	868,716	70.8	1,810	2,379	7.1	60,604	266,683	1,105,342	1,372,025	162	9,527
Canton	5	1,536	55,148	362,401	481,675	64.6	992	1,320	6.6	32,938	146,819	397,990	544,809	106	6,124
Cincinnati	14	4,745	173,047	1,226,108	1,615,642	70.8	3,359	4,428	7.1	140,841	468,190	1,012,512	1,480,702	272	21,379
Cleveland	30	8,861	301,784	2,199,480	2,799,937	68.0	6,026	7,671	7.3	219,600	843,993	2,724,605	3,568,598	602	31,415
Columbus	14	4,756	193,936	1,252,752	1,626,775	72.2	3,433	4,455	6.5	132,866	582,962	1,401,488	1,984,450	305	23,567
Dayton-Springfield	11	4,146	138,184	964,176	1,268,869	63.7	2,643	3,478	7.0	118,566	379,278	1,155,345	1,534,623	254	15,454
Hamilton-Middletown	4	892	32,716	200,066	287,577	61.4	548	788	6.1	25,055	136,771	221,151	357,922	75	3,309
Huntington-Ashland	1	117	3,569	21,503	29,981	50.4	59	82	6.0	2,252	9,253	17,083	26,336	16	435
Lima	4	651	27,779	159,203	230,549	67.0	436	631	5.7	18,599	67,991	240,356	308,347	47	3,487
Lorain-Elyria	5	969	31,908	191,445	271,499	54.0	523	745	6.0	28,042	121,839	319,021	440,860	83	3,305
Mansfield	3	463	13,669	84,869	118,085	50.3	233	323	6.2	10,372	53,574	142,613	196,187	44	1,899
Parkersburg-Marietta	2	279	7,534	43,921	67,300	43.0	120	185	5.8	7,052	26,744	99,134	125,878	21	969
Steubenville-Weirton	2	385	11,868	85,479	120,434	61.0	235	330	7.2	6,843	47,576	146,702	194,278	28	870
Toledo	11	3,254	112,993	815,486	1,072,939	68.7	2,235	2,940	7.2	87,268	325,300	654,684	979,984	172	11,327
Wheeling	3	336	8,952	86,119	121,754	69.9	235	333	9.6	4,893	28,830	57,724	86,554	14	252
Youngstown-Warren	9	2,444	88,310	594,564	759,122	66.7	1,629	2,079	6.7	52,121	236,359	680,163	916,522	146	6,100
Wisconsin	129	18,687	596,654	4,408,567	6,096,589	64.7	12,082	16,711	7.4	464,763	1,508,913	4,417,909	5,926,822	1,523	71,630
Nonmetropolitan	69	6,605	150,318	1,525,157	2,176,071	63.3	4,179	5,964	10.1	100,009	448,010	1,073,236	1,521,246	522	16,637
Metropolitan	60	12,082	446,336	2,883,410	3,920,518	65.4	7,903	10,747	6.5	364,754	1,060,903	3,344,673	4,405,576	1,001	54,993
Appleton-Oshkosh-Neenah	7	1,117	37,429	241,567	347,614	59.4	663	954	6.5	33,097	124,275	415,581	539,856	119	4,946
Duluth	1	55	1,907	9,454	15,708	47.3	26	43	5.0	1,315	9,727	36,242	45,969	10	165
Eau Claire	5	874	21,420	176,723	247,327	55.4	484	678	8.3	14,758	49,879	158,891	208,770	60	2,180
Green Bay	3	768	29,050	172,898	248,998	61.7	474	682	6.0	26,506	72,560	155,847	228,407	51	3,984
Janesville-Beloit	3	495	16,668	110,524	157,898	61.2	303	432	6.6	13,272	55,078	108,828	163,906	43	2,226
Kenosha	2	336	12,044	70,773	104,694	57.7	194	287	5.9	6,580	57,347	81,656	139,003	34	1,533
La Crosse	2	625	24,232	144,396	176,263	63.4	396	484	6.0	21,489	46,268	140,430	186,698	43	2,546
Madison	4	1,334	54,880	335,002	436,258	68.7	917	1,196	6.1	57,010	74,062	432,161	506,223	79	6,153
Milwaukee	22	5,089	201,471	1,304,295	1,742,167	70.3	3,576	4,775	6.5	153,259	457,197	1,519,644	1,976,841	427	24,596
Minneapolis-St. Paul	4	196	4,888	49,465	72,888	68.9	135	200	10.1	2,864	9,600	37,455	47,055	31	737
Racine	3	543	19,895	124,524	177,227	62.8	341	486	6.3	14,667	63,700	119,402	183,102	39	2,945
Sheboygan	3	397	10,924	81,797	113,232	56.4	224	310	7.5	10,084	19,166	80,314	99,480	40	1,410
Wausau	1	253	11,528	61,992	80,244	67.2	170	220	5.4	9,853	22,044	58,222	80,266	25	1,572

CLASSIFICATION	FULL-TIME EQUIVALENT PERSONNEL					FULL-TIME EQUIVALENT TRAINEES			EXPENSES						
									LABOR				TOTAL		
	Physicians and Dentists	Registered Nurses	Licensed Practical Nurses	Other Salaried Personnel	Total Personnel	Medical and Dental Residents	Other Trainees	Total Trainees	Payroll (in thousands)	Employee Benefits (in thousands)	Total (in thousands)	Percent of Total	Amount (in thousands)	Adjusted, per Admission	Adjusted, per Inpatient Day
Ohio	1,224	41,789	7,770	121,533	172,316	4,703	282	4,985	$ 4,455,235	$ 956,656	$ 5,411,891	55.1	$ 9,821,385	$4,801.23	$ 719.56
Nonmetropolitan	20	4,856	1,479	14,843	21,198	21	2	23	472,692	105,545	578,238	54.1	1,068,137	3,189.66	559.75
Metropolitan	1,204	36,933	6,291	106,690	151,118	4,682	280	4,962	3,982,543	851,110	4,833,653	55.2	8,753,249	5,116.69	745.54
Akron	108	2,608	593	7,352	10,661	413	13	426	284,463	65,832	350,295	56.8	616,594	4,943.47	709.78
Canton	25	1,272	416	4,253	5,966	89	58	147	142,376	29,300	171,676	54.7	313,654	4,269.20	651.17
Cincinnati	182	4,992	676	14,895	20,745	614	27	641	552,993	113,347	666,339	52.3	1,274,258	5,563.62	788.70
Cleveland	587	8,659	1,618	26,408	37,272	1,646	111	1,757	1,033,015	220,059	1,253,074	57.3	2,187,060	5,662.64	781.11
Columbus	130	5,283	433	16,203	22,049	970	11	981	580,445	132,242	712,687	54.5	1,307,490	5,145.17	803.73
Dayton-Springfield	23	4,447	407	11,483	16,360	349	15	364	421,331	75,370	496,701	53.8	923,726	5,059.49	727.99
Hamilton-Middletown	1	832	133	2,198	3,164	0	1	1	80,471	16,111	96,581	51.6	187,337	3,965.65	651.43
Huntington-Ashland	2	73	30	267	372	1	0	1	7,200	1,429	8,629	54.0	15,970	3,209.45	532.68
Lima	0	821	140	2,099	3,060	0	7	7	75,201	13,068	88,269	55.0	160,634	3,992.59	696.75
Lorain-Elyria	13	864	286	2,268	3,431	0	0	0	82,894	16,240	99,134	53.6	185,097	4,081.25	681.76
Mansfield	0	395	101	1,037	1,533	0	0	0	35,198	6,769	41,967	55.7	75,289	3,942.66	637.58
Parkersburg-Marietta	4	152	84	490	730	0	0	0	16,491	3,207	19,698	50.7	38,853	3,357.79	577.31
Steubenville-Weirton	6	347	55	983	1,391	6	0	6	33,613	6,297	39,910	57.4	69,495	4,181.40	577.04
Toledo	41	3,602	601	9,934	14,178	362	18	380	372,401	86,049	458,450	55.7	823,581	5,516.65	767.59
Wheeling	15	223	89	637	964	0	0	0	20,222	3,529	23,751	56.4	42,118	3,394.94	345.92
Youngstown-Warren	67	2,363	629	6,183	9,242	232	19	251	244,229	62,263	306,492	57.6	532,093	4,676.18	700.93
Wisconsin	131	15,738	2,013	44,393	62,275	599	105	704	1,550,062	298,614	1,848,677	54.7	3,378,099	4,082.52	554.10
Nonmetropolitan	21	3,295	695	11,083	15,094	0	10	10	338,214	64,939	403,153	55.0	732,970	3,353.20	336.83
Metropolitan	110	12,443	1,318	33,310	47,181	599	95	694	1,211,848	233,675	1,445,523	54.6	2,645,129	4,344.35	674.69
Appleton-Oshkosh-Neenah	13	959	195	3,094	4,261	16	0	16	98,303	18,611	116,915	54.9	213,097	3,944.27	613.03
Duluth	0	36	18	116	170	0	0	0	4,921	878	5,799	48.6	11,939	3,767.45	760.06
Eau Claire	3	477	87	1,551	2,118	0	0	0	51,623	8,356	59,979	58.1	103,250	3,521.60	417.46
Green Bay	0	927	169	2,294	3,390	0	0	0	82,025	15,410	97,435	56.6	171,996	4,095.34	690.75
Janesville-Beloit	7	379	57	1,095	1,538	0	0	0	34,870	6,278	41,147	57.0	72,141	3,003.77	456.89
Kenosha	0	277	37	877	1,191	0	0	0	30,246	6,126	36,372	54.3	66,931	3,700.90	639.30
La Crosse	16	675	81	1,920	2,692	8	0	8	63,877	10,438	74,316	57.2	130,021	4,404.65	737.65
Madison	13	1,784	71	4,336	6,204	380	0	380	168,147	41,014	209,161	54.2	386,251	5,426.09	885.37
Milwaukee	58	5,690	408	14,855	21,011	195	91	286	572,055	107,062	679,118	54.3	1,250,445	4,608.02	717.75
Minneapolis-St. Paul	0	97	17	360	474	0	0	0	9,821	1,637	11,458	55.0	20,833	2,752.09	285.83
Racine	0	563	114	1,314	1,991	0	4	4	46,047	7,279	53,325	50.6	105,480	3,692.25	595.17
Sheboygan	0	259	56	670	985	0	0	0	23,771	4,808	28,579	53.6	53,304	3,523.99	470.75
Wausau	0	320	8	828	1,156	0	0	0	26,143	5,778	31,921	53.7	59,440	3,983.40	740.75

(continued on next page)

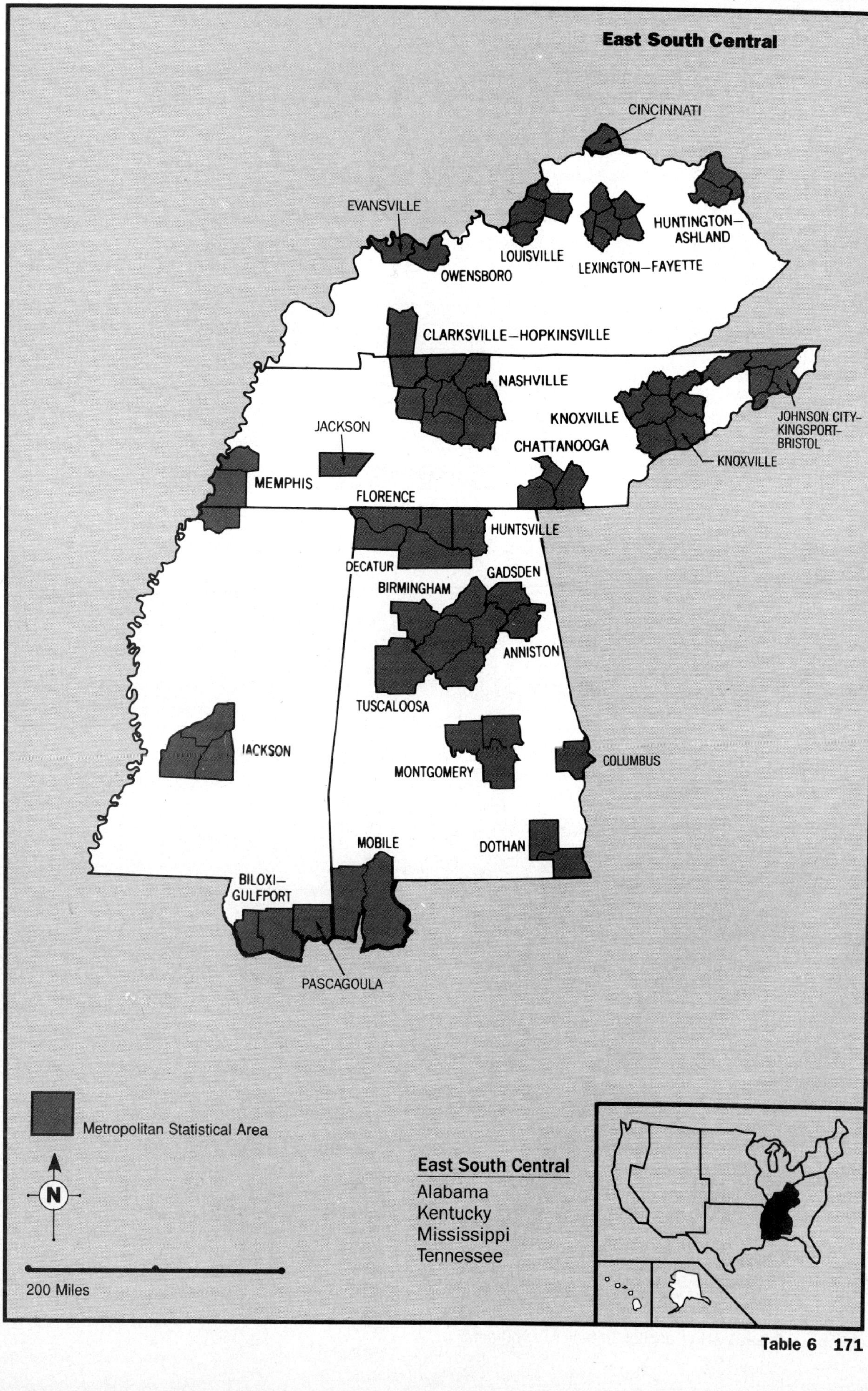
East South Central
CINCINNATI
EVANSVILLE
HUNTINGTON–
ASHLAND
LOUISVILLE
OWENSBORO
LEXINGTON–FAYETTE
CLARKSVILLE–HOPKINSVILLE
NASHVILLE
KNOXVILLE
JOHNSON CITY-
KINGSPORT-
BRISTOL
JACKSON
CHATTANOOGA
KNOXVILLE
MEMPHIS
FLORENCE
HUNTSVILLE
DECATUR
GADSDEN
BIRMINGHAM
ANNISTON
TUSCALOOSA
JACKSON
MONTGOMERY
COLUMBUS
MOBILE
DOTHAN
BILOXI–
GULFPORT
PASCAGOULA
Metropolitan Statistical Area
N
200 Miles
East South Central
Alabama
Kentucky
Mississippi
Tennessee

Table

6 (Continued)

Utilization, Personnel, and Finances in Community Hospitals, by Metropolitan Statistical Area

Where an MSA is located in multiple states, the MSA will be listed for each state, with hospital data for only that state.

CLASSIFICATION	HOSPI-TALS	BEDS	ADMISSIONS	INPATIENT DAYS	ADJUSTED PATIENT DAYS	OCCU-PANCY, percent	AVERAGE DAILY CENSUS	ADJUSTED AVERAGE DAILY CENSUS	AVERAGE STAY, days	SURGICAL OPERATIONS	OUTPATIENT VISITS			NEWBORNS	
											Emergency	Other	Total	Bassinets	Births
CENSUS DIVISION 5, EAST SOUTH CENTRAL	**464**	**70,780**	**2,322,816**	**16,159,889**	**20,738,062**	**62.6**	**44,284**	**56,830**	**7.0**	**1,489,107**	**6,286,308**	**10,110,057**	**16,396,365**	**4,835**	**227,454**
Nonmetropolitan	288	28,322	824,508	5,863,310	7,977,908	56.8	16,074	21,869	7.1	445,925	2,605,559	3,646,173	6,251,732	2,079	75,611
Metropolitan	176	42,458	1,498,308	10,296,579	12,760,154	66.4	28,210	34,961	6.9	1,043,182	3,680,749	6,463,884	10,144,633	2,756	151,843
Alabama	**120**	**18,638**	**597,023**	**4,254,741**	**5,374,854**	**62.5**	**11,656**	**14,727**	**7.1**	**375,365**	**1,619,940**	**3,027,927**	**4,647,867**	**1,383**	**59,117**
Nonmetropolitan	59	5,218	133,985	1,074,701	1,456,635	56.4	2,944	3,993	8.0	73,860	507,484	613,477	1,120,961	381	12,690
Metropolitan	61	13,420	463,038	3,180,040	3,918,219	64.9	8,712	10,734	6.9	301,505	1,112,456	2,414,450	3,526,906	1,002	46,427
Anniston	4	484	16,203	101,028	139,756	57.0	276	383	6.2	9,320	59,767	63,172	122,939	47	1,532
Birmingham	19	5,038	180,049	1,233,359	1,504,772	67.1	3,378	4,124	6.9	118,768	346,281	1,328,396	1,674,677	361	14,656
Columbus	1	234	3,908	35,864	43,190	41.9	98	118	9.2	2,954	15,573	13,353	28,926	0	0
Decatur	4	522	16,941	103,070	140,170	54.2	283	385	6.1	12,844	59,155	85,145	144,300	35	2,012
Dothan	3	693	28,038	180,132	225,243	71.3	494	617	6.4	17,424	72,873	110,493	183,366	63	2,644
Florence	4	904	23,760	229,158	285,068	69.5	628	781	9.6	16,808	69,490	87,438	156,928	60	2,049
Gadsden	2	503	16,464	115,697	146,537	63.0	317	401	7.0	10,940	35,778	91,604	127,382	39	1,626
Huntsville	3	930	34,071	213,412	257,116	62.9	585	704	6.3	21,236	105,550	42,423	147,973	67	4,736
Mobile	10	2,123	72,512	475,913	576,174	61.4	1,304	1,578	6.6	50,707	141,520	393,640	535,160	205	8,601
Montgomery	8	1,265	43,977	279,737	339,741	60.6	767	930	6.4	26,949	100,665	128,679	229,344	77	5,444
Tuscaloosa	3	724	27,115	212,670	260,452	80.4	582	713	7.8	13,555	105,804	70,107	175,911	48	3,127
Kentucky	**107**	**15,718**	**531,817**	**3,580,816**	**4,693,845**	**62.4**	**9,815**	**12,861**	**6.7**	**376,531**	**1,512,828**	**2,884,352**	**4,397,180**	**1,106**	**52,334**
Nonmetropolitan	73	7,641	242,256	1,629,985	2,227,267	58.5	4,469	6,103	6.7	150,476	789,054	1,448,066	2,237,120	606	21,811
Metropolitan	34	8,077	289,561	1,950,831	2,466,578	66.2	5,346	6,758	6.7	226,055	723,774	1,436,286	2,160,060	500	30,523
Cincinnati	4	997	38,237	257,181	339,653	70.7	705	930	6.7	23,500	110,098	172,146	282,244	66	4,405
Clarksville-Hopkinsville	1	194	5,857	31,642	45,985	44.8	87	126	5.4	4,306	14,950	26,255	41,205	20	857
Evansville	1	213	8,524	42,527	57,972	54.9	117	159	5.0	4,539	22,567	67,430	89,997	8	906
Huntington-Ashland	2	468	19,047	119,401	162,291	69.9	327	445	6.3	12,328	48,012	83,819	131,831	25	1,164
Lexington-Fayette	11	2,062	67,557	477,972	585,205	63.6	1,311	1,604	7.1	54,990	151,248	438,698	589,946	130	6,784
Louisville	13	3,649	131,732	908,382	1,132,119	68.2	2,488	3,102	6.9	114,709	316,133	599,801	915,934	217	14,624
Owensboro	2	494	18,607	113,726	143,353	63.0	311	392	6.1	11,683	60,766	48,137	108,903	34	1,783
Mississippi	**103**	**12,907**	**395,804**	**2,799,572**	**3,633,316**	**59.4**	**7,670**	**9,957**	**7.1**	**205,704**	**969,770**	**1,185,178**	**2,154,948**	**819**	**40,778**
Nonmetropolitan	86	9,115	265,306	1,912,132	2,539,212	57.5	5,239	6,960	7.2	128,723	674,202	777,424	1,451,626	576	26,942
Metropolitan	17	3,792	130,498	887,440	1,094,104	64.1	2,431	2,997	6.8	76,981	295,568	407,754	703,322	243	13,836
Biloxi-Gulfport	5	824	28,215	178,725	229,303	59.5	490	628	6.3	16,242	71,829	102,942	174,771	75	2,739
Jackson	11	2,623	88,796	620,225	756,477	64.8	1,699	2,072	7.0	52,252	175,984	264,460	440,444	140	10,052
Memphis	0	0	0	0	0	00.0	0	0	0.0	0	0	0	0	0	0
Pascagoula	1	345	13,487	88,490	108,324	70.1	242	297	6.6	8,487	47,755	40,352	88,107	28	1,045
Tennessee	**134**	**23,517**	**798,172**	**5,524,760**	**7,036,047**	**64.4**	**15,143**	**19,285**	**6.9**	**531,507**	**2,183,770**	**3,012,600**	**5,196,370**	**1,527**	**75,225**
Nonmetropolitan	70	6,348	182,961	1,246,492	1,754,794	53.9	3,422	4,813	6.8	92,866	634,819	807,206	1,442,025	516	14,168
Metropolitan	64	17,169	615,211	4,278,268	5,281,253	68.3	11,721	14,472	7.0	438,641	1,548,951	2,205,394	3,754,345	1,011	61,057
Chattanooga	10	1,732	59,578	376,746	474,657	59.6	1,032	1,301	6.3	45,953	213,632	132,542	346,174	62	6,113
Clarksville-Hopkinsville	1	200	8,491	42,720	62,978	58.5	117	173	5.0	5,976	25,548	78,143	103,691	28	1,369
Jackson	2	828	26,549	177,560	218,736	58.7	486	599	6.7	18,711	47,489	45,299	92,788	32	2,950
Johnson City-Kingsport-Bristol	9	1,814	63,335	415,546	536,642	62.8	1,139	1,470	6.6	47,159	209,707	211,878	421,585	161	5,103
Knoxville	11	2,771	110,847	747,484	947,865	74.0	2,050	2,597	6.7	97,447	258,861	376,932	635,793	145	9,607
Memphis	11	4,914	161,248	1,347,639	1,574,307	75.1	3,691	4,314	8.4	107,176	348,002	483,601	831,603	243	19,019
Nashville	20	4,910	185,163	1,170,573	1,466,068	65.3	3,206	4,018	6.3	116,219	445,712	876,999	1,322,711	340	16,896

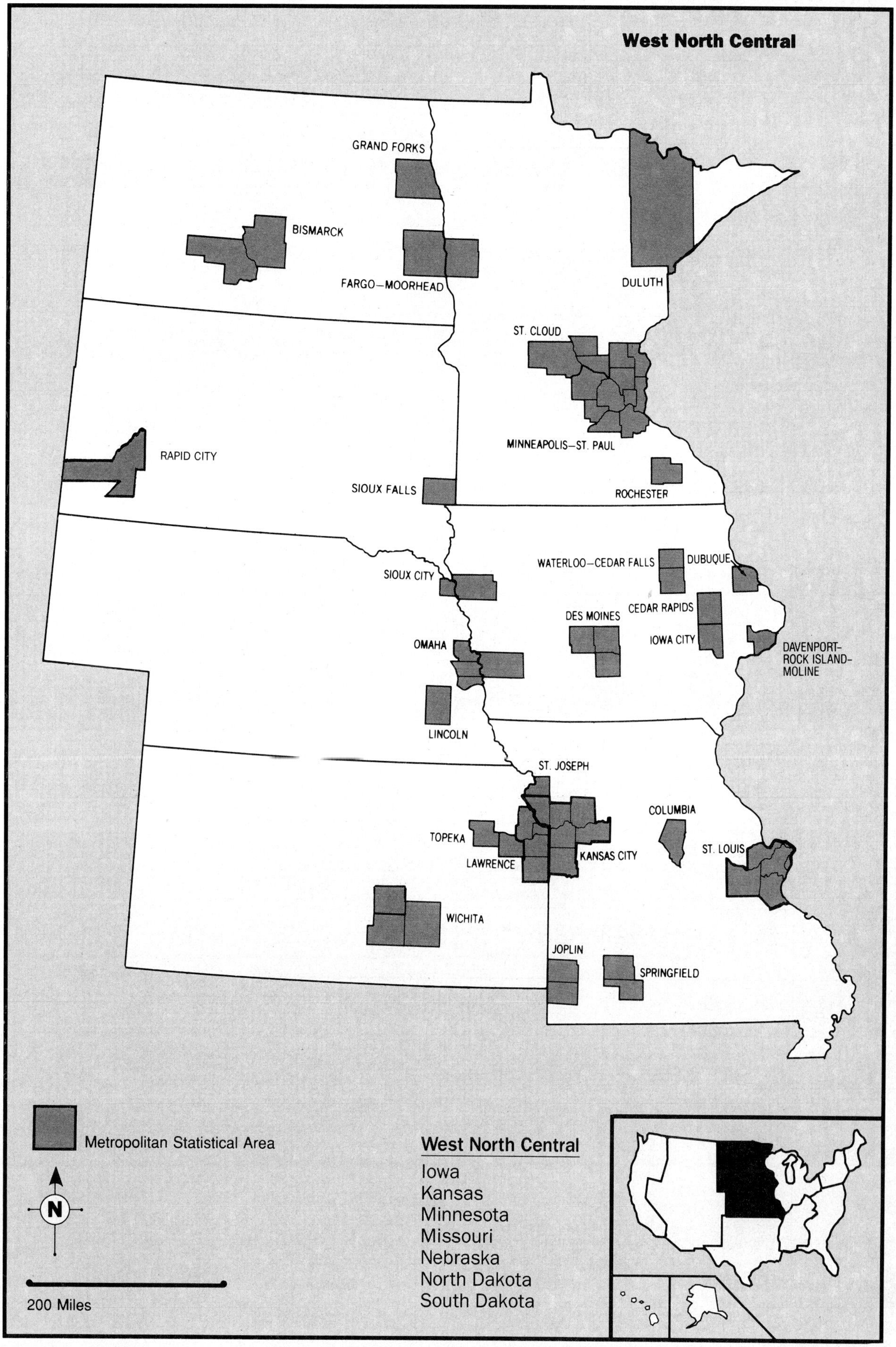
West North Central
GRAND FORKS
BISMARCK
FARGO—MOORHEAD
DULUTH
ST. CLOUD
MINNEAPOLIS—ST. PAUL
RAPID CITY
SIOUX FALLS
ROCHESTER
WATERLOO—CEDAR FALLS
DUBUQUE
SIOUX CITY
CEDAR RAPIDS
DES MOINES
IOWA CITY
DAVENPORT-ROCK ISLAND-MOLINE
OMAHA
LINCOLN
ST. JOSEPH
COLUMBIA
TOPEKA
ST. LOUIS
LAWRENCE
KANSAS CITY
WICHITA
JOPLIN
SPRINGFIELD
Metropolitan Statistical Area
N
200 Miles
West North Central
Iowa
Kansas
Minnesota
Missouri
Nebraska
North Dakota
South Dakota

Table
6 (Continued)

Utilization, Personnel, and Finances in Community Hospitals, by Metropolitan Statistical Area

Where an MSA is located in multiple states, the MSA will be listed for each state, with hospital data for only that state.

CLASSIFICATION	HOSPITALS	BEDS	ADMISSIONS	INPATIENT DAYS	ADJUSTED PATIENT DAYS	OCCUPANCY, percent	AVERAGE DAILY CENSUS	ADJUSTED AVERAGE DAILY CENSUS	AVERAGE STAY, days	SURGICAL OPERATIONS	OUTPATIENT VISITS			NEWBORNS	
											Emergency	Other	Total	Bassinets	Births
CENSUS DIVISION 6, WEST NORTH CENTRAL	**742**	**87,047**	**2,335,033**	**19,621,868**	**26,104,823**	**61.8**	**53,763**	**71,532**	**8.4**	**1,740,822**	**5,313,256**	**15,331,351**	**20,644,607**	**6,833**	**265,847**
Nonmetropolitan	556	37,532	745,823	7,811,436	10,969,655	57.0	21,406	30,055	10.5	474,639	1,862,072	5,633,433	7,495,505	3,686	80,687
Metropolitan	186	49,515	1,589,210	11,810,432	15,135,168	65.3	32,357	41,477	7.4	1,266,183	3,451,184	9,697,918	13,149,102	3,147	185,160
Iowa	**124**	**14,239**	**385,138**	**3,206,410**	**4,390,469**	**61.7**	**8,787**	**12,028**	**8.3**	**320,555**	**927,876**	**3,184,404**	**4,112,280**	**1,101**	**39,016**
Nonmetropolitan	99	6,852	148,908	1,426,900	2,070,062	57.1	3,912	5,670	9.6	98,005	410,954	1,295,766	1,706,720	642	16,007
Metropolitan	25	7,387	236,230	1,779,510	2,320,407	66.0	4,875	6,358	7.5	222,550	516,922	1,888,638	2,405,560	459	23,009
Cedar Rapids	2	919	28,189	220,081	305,449	65.6	603	836	7.8	25,078	75,766	194,634	270,400	61	3,145
Davenport-Rock Island-Moline	3	632	21,149	147,686	184,967	63.9	404	508	7.0	16,034	52,937	119,139	172,076	55	2,482
Des Moines	7	2,082	69,285	534,676	698,166	70.3	1,464	1,912	7.7	48,424	161,725	510,183	671,908	127	6,834
Dubuque	2	558	15,636	120,471	153,327	59.1	330	420	7.7	14,745	35,887	52,337	88,224	42	1,730
Iowa City	2	1,119	42,374	309,775	390,828	75.9	849	1,071	7.3	77,997	40,625	501,283	541,908	46	3,024
Omaha	2	539	12,386	107,452	137,916	54.7	295	378	8.7	8,627	30,091	84,394	114,485	36	1,143
Sioux City	2	807	23,622	177,263	218,146	60.2	486	598	7.5	16,228	50,851	117,379	168,230	45	2,159
Waterloo-Cedar Falls	5	731	23,589	162,106	231,608	60.7	444	635	6.9	15,417	69,040	309,289	378,329	47	2,492
Kansas	**138**	**11,796**	**304,551**	**2,393,809**	**3,213,322**	**55.6**	**6,563**	**8,806**	**7.9**	**205,457**	**693,498**	**2,190,791**	**2,884,289**	**1,055**	**36,746**
Nonmetropolitan	117	6,426	129,731	1,182,968	1,666,379	50.5	3,246	4,567	9.1	81,024	310,418	1,093,161	1,403,579	691	13,552
Metropolitan	21	5,370	174,820	1,210,841	1,546,943	61.8	3,317	4,239	6.9	124,433	383,080	1,097,630	1,480,710	364	23,194
Kansas City	10	2,189	67,532	446,215	567,815	55.9	1,223	1,556	6.6	52,164	159,231	624,786	784,017	161	9,464
Lawrence	1	165	6,350	34,006	50,392	56.4	93	138	5.4	4,704	16,279	58,808	75,087	24	1,079
Topeka	2	700	23,023	164,866	208,501	64.4	451	572	7.2	19,194	58,495	51,988	110,483	54	3,209
Wichita	8	2,316	77,915	565,754	720,235	66.9	1,550	1,973	7.3	48,371	149,075	362,048	511,123	125	9,442
Minnesota	**152**	**19,434**	**529,744**	**4,735,154**	**6,292,515**	**66.8**	**12,973**	**17,238**	**8.9**	**375,777**	**1,156,055**	**3,215,539**	**4,371,594**	**1,609**	**67,458**
Nonmetropolitan	106	8,363	130,218	1,944,581	2,717,996	63.7	5,328	7,444	14.9	80,028	328,158	975,016	1,303,174	806	16,622
Metropolitan	46	11,071	399,526	2,790,573	3,574,519	69.1	7,645	9,794	7.0	295,749	827,897	2,240,523	3,068,420	803	50,836
Duluth	9	1,390	33,351	334,165	437,686	66.0	918	1,199	10.0	26,024	70,577	246,954	317,531	69	3,162
Fargo-Moorhead	0	0	0	0	0	00.0	0	0	0.0	0	0	0	0	0	0
Minneapolis-St. Paul	29	7,480	294,110	1,875,267	2,475,766	68.7	5,136	6,784	6.4	205,379	694,012	1,869,678	2,563,690	619	42,290
Rochester	3	1,541	55,359	414,923	440,030	73.8	1,137	1,205	7.5	55,845	31,477	58,134	89,611	47	2,872
St. Cloud	5	660	16,706	166,218	221,037	68.8	454	606	9.9	8,501	31,831	65,757	97,588	68	2,512
Missouri	**135**	**24,355**	**737,219**	**5,489,754**	**7,237,715**	**61.7**	**15,038**	**19,842**	**7.4**	**549,601**	**1,834,707**	**4,625,247**	**6,459,954**	**1,569**	**79,304**
Nonmetropolitan	69	5,595	165,035	1,104,876	1,567,267	54.0	3,023	4,298	6.7	102,078	478,929	1,099,026	1,577,955	484	15,241
Metropolitan	66	18,760	572,184	4,384,878	5,670,448	64.0	12,015	15,544	7.7	447,523	1,355,778	3,526,221	4,881,999	1,085	64,063
Columbia	4	1,082	30,456	232,466	290,898	58.9	637	797	7.6	27,716	52,452	290,973	343,425	46	3,365
Joplin	5	739	24,939	162,671	215,852	60.2	445	591	6.5	19,510	84,263	166,294	250,557	46	2,359
Kansas City	24	4,812	144,592	1,116,930	1,429,665	63.7	3,065	3,925	7.7	118,072	331,021	1,090,331	1,421,352	269	17,438
St. Joseph	1	580	14,844	135,765	178,275	64.1	372	488	9.1	13,460	36,785	100,982	137,767	40	1,705
St. Louis	29	9,765	302,517	2,320,388	3,038,053	65.1	6,355	8,325	7.7	225,313	744,223	1,697,383	2,441,606	598	33,857
Springfield	3	1,782	54,836	416,658	517,705	64.0	1,141	1,418	7.6	43,452	107,034	180,258	287,292	86	5,339
Nebraska	**90**	**8,611**	**187,977**	**1,810,607**	**2,431,589**	**57.6**	**4,960**	**6,663**	**9.6**	**168,584**	**365,012**	**1,239,014**	**1,604,026**	**757**	**23,453**
Nonmetropolitan	76	4,562	81,339	865,246	1,250,102	52.0	2,370	3,427	10.6	62,863	149,742	594,833	744,575	508	10,053
Metropolitan	14	4,049	106,638	945,361	1,181,487	64.0	2,590	3,236	8.9	105,721	215,270	644,181	859,451	249	13,400
Lincoln	3	742	26,745	174,387	220,713	64.4	478	605	6.5	24,484	55,236	233,819	289,055	75	3,738
Omaha	11	3,307	79,893	770,974	960,774	63.9	2,112	2,631	9.7	81,237	160,034	410,362	570,396	174	9,662
Sioux City	0	0	0	0	0	00.0	0	0	0.0	0	0	0	0	0	0
North Dakota	**50**	**4,412**	**95,983**	**1,033,620**	**1,323,463**	**64.3**	**2,835**	**3,626**	**10.8**	**65,330**	**165,125**	**375,088**	**540,213**	**340**	**9,803**
Nonmetropolitan	41	2,766	39,815	634,256	833,746	62.9	1,741	2,283	15.9	22,463	72,025	217,358	289,383	241	3,826
Metropolitan	9	1,646	56,168	399,364	489,717	66.5	1,094	1,343	7.1	42,867	93,100	157,730	250,830	99	5,977
Bismarck	3	547	17,244	121,597	154,981	61.1	334	425	7.1	16,757	27,056	59,801	86,857	31	1,776
Fargo-Moorhead	3	634	25,854	161,894	189,657	69.9	443	520	6.3	16,503	46,736	29,181	75,917	46	2,736
Grand Forks	3	465	13,070	115,873	145,079	68.2	317	398	8.9	9,607	19,308	68,748	88,056	22	1,465
South Dakota	**53**	**4,200**	**94,421**	**952,514**	**1,215,750**	**62.1**	**2,607**	**3,329**	**10.1**	**55,518**	**170,983**	**501,268**	**672,251**	**402**	**10,067**
Nonmetropolitan	48	2,968	50,777	652,609	864,103	60.2	1,786	2,366	12.9	28,178	111,846	358,273	470,119	314	5,386
Metropolitan	5	1,232	43,644	299,905	351,647	66.6	821	963	6.9	27,340	59,137	142,995	202,132	88	4,681
Rapid City	2	340	12,668	78,967	100,475	63.5	216	275	6.2	7,824	24,099	34,849	58,948	28	1,759
Sioux Falls	3	892	30,976	220,938	251,172	67.8	605	688	7.1	19,516	35,038	108,146	143,184	60	2,922

CLASSIFICATION	FULL-TIME EQUIVALENT PERSONNEL: Physicians and Dentists	Registered Nurses	Licensed Practical Nurses	Other Salaried Personnel	Total Personnel	FULL-TIME EQUIVALENT TRAINEES: Medical and Dental Residents	Other Trainees	Total Trainees	EXPENSES — LABOR: Payroll (in thousands)	Employee Benefits (in thousands)	Total (in thousands)	Percent of Total	EXPENSES — TOTAL: Amount (in thousands)	Adjusted, per Admission	Adjusted, per Inpatient Day
CENSUS DIVISION 6, WEST NORTH CENTRAL	**1,547**	**64,419**	**12,511**	**190,501**	**268,978**	**3,037**	**259**	**3,296**	**$ 6,513,183**	**$ 1,184,063**	**$ 7,697,246**	**53.4**	**$ 14,407,136**	**$4,611.03**	**$ 551.90**
Nonmetropolitan	159	16,422	5,771	58,701	81,053	61	44	105	1,570,921	283,458	1,854,379	54.8	3,385,737	3,127.93	308.65
Metropolitan	1,388	47,997	6,740	131,800	187,925	2,976	215	3,191	4,942,262	900,605	5,842,867	53.0	11,021,399	5,397.17	728.20
Iowa	**61**	**10,967**	**1,477**	**31,141**	**43,646**	**581**	**52**	**633**	**971,798**	**188,349**	**1,160,147**	**53.4**	**2,174,443**	**4,135.35**	**495.26**
Nonmetropolitan	23	3,768	764	11,771	16,326	17	2	19	315,593	56,698	372,291	56.2	662,955	3,037.96	320.26
Metropolitan	38	7,199	713	19,370	27,320	564	50	614	656,206	131,651	787,857	52.1	1,511,489	4,913.89	651.39
Cedar Rapids	3	1,012	67	2,053	3,175	24	28	52	71,560	10,803	82,363	56.5	145,904	3,793.96	477.67
Davenport-Rock Island-Moline	0	658	37	1,426	2,121	6	0	6	53,079	8,394	61,473	47.6	129,194	4,872.31	698.47
Des Moines	20	1,772	221	6,464	8,497	108	10	118	203,181	34,453	237,634	51.0	466,270	5,179.11	667.85
Dubuque	0	483	38	1,133	1,654	0	0	0	37,203	7,218	44,422	53.1	83,670	4,156.69	545.70
Iowa City	10	1,567	74	3,739	5,390	426	12	438	142,605	36,229	178,834	51.6	346,910	6,479.81	887.63
Omaha	0	281	72	927	1,280	0	0	0	32,622	5,427	38,050	53.6	71,052	4,466.40	515.18
Sioux City	0	819	60	1,839	2,718	0	0	0	57,602	15,959	73,562	51.7	142,234	4,877.89	652.01
Waterloo-Cedar Falls	5	607	144	1,729	2,485	0	0	0	58,353	13,167	71,520	56.6	126,254	3,728.72	545.12
Kansas	**392**	**8,078**	**1,555**	**24,921**	**34,946**	**307**	**49**	**356**	**776,748**	**128,953**	**905,701**	**53.0**	**1,710,015**	**4,160.57**	**532.16**
Nonmetropolitan	20	2,992	722	10,046	13,780	2	10	12	265,604	47,651	313,255	54.7	572,748	3,066.18	343.71
Metropolitan	372	5,086	833	14,875	21,166	305	39	344	511,143	81,302	592,446	52.1	1,137,267	5,072.33	735.17
Kansas City	296	2,034	315	5,707	8,352	296	0	296	203,241	37,741	240,982	54.4	442,627	5,087.67	779.53
Lawrence	0	119	16	373	513	0	0	0	12,959	2,049	15,008	53.9	27,867	2,961.39	553.00
Topeka	7	769	121	2,052	2,949	0	0	0	75,369	11,507	86,876	54.2	160,224	5,497.49	768.46
Wichita	69	2,164	381	6,738	9,352	9	39	48	219,575	30,005	249,579	49.3	506,549	5,134.55	703.31
Minnesota	**183**	**14,045**	**2,677**	**38,643**	**55,553**	**295**	**40**	**335**	**1,612,875**	**306,651**	**1,919,526**	**56.9**	**3,375,761**	**4,781.88**	**536.47**
Nonmetropolitan	8	2,541	1,092	10,720	14,361	0	0	0	310,583	58,032	368,615	57.6	639,870	3,322.24	235.42
Metropolitan	175	11,504	1,585	27,923	41,192	295	40	335	1,302,293	248,619	1,550,911	56.7	2,735,890	5,329.52	765.39
Duluth	4	864	322	2,813	4,009	0	0	0	102,515	17,042	119,557	59.2	201,935	4,631.32	461.37
Fargo-Moorhead	0	0	0	0	0	0	0	0	0	0	0	0.0	0		
Minneapolis-St. Paul	171	8,566	747	21,332	30,816	295	40	335	1,010,666	186,693	1,197,359	56.0	2,139,147	5,517.22	864.03
Rochester	0	1,648	399	2,423	4,476	0	0	0	141,153	34,664	175,818	58.6	299,815	5,041.70	681.35
St. Cloud	0	426	117	1,343	1,891	0	0	0	47,958	10,220	58,178	61.2	94,994	4,211.64	429.76
Missouri	**828**	**20,367**	**4,293**	**63,760**	**89,248**	**1,472**	**62**	**1,534**	**2,167,588**	**387,067**	**2,554,655**	**52.0**	**4,916,508**	**5,021.87**	**679.29**
Nonmetropolitan	85	3,234	1,776	12,090	17,185	41	14	55	315,817	60,836	376,653	51.2	735,498	3,114.72	469.29
Metropolitan	743	17,133	2,517	51,670	72,063	1,431	48	1,479	1,851,771	326,231	2,178,002	52.1	4,181,010	5,628.08	737.33
Columbia	18	1,126	231	3,610	4,985	201	0	201	115,478	24,044	139,522	53.1	262,726	6,905.30	903.16
Joplin	20	690	156	1,882	2,748	3	0	3	55,161	10,664	65,825	46.7	141,055	4,208.20	653.48
Kansas City	98	4,047	684	13,186	18,015	227	17	244	490,797	86,056	576,853	54.4	1,060,695	5,710.98	741.92
St. Joseph	0	353	72	1,216	1,641	0	0	0	37,709	6,788	44,496	46.3	96,205	4,935.63	539.65
St. Louis	588	9,239	1,186	27,519	38,532	986	31	1,017	1,012,993	175,214	1,188,206	51.4	2,310,130	5,805.28	760.40
Springfield	19	1,678	188	4,257	6,142	14	0	14	139,633	23,465	163,098	52.6	310,198	4,550.97	599.18
Nebraska	**51**	**5,255**	**1,476**	**17,144**	**23,926**	**352**	**15**	**367**	**509,873**	**91,743**	**601,616**	**50.5**	**1,191,070**	**4,675.43**	**489.83**
Nonmetropolitan	8	1,878	818	6,469	9,173	1	13	14	168,000	26,692	194,692	53.4	364,758	2,996.85	291.78
Metropolitan	43	3,377	658	10,675	14,753	351	2	353	341,873	65,052	406,925	49.2	826,312	6,211.15	699.38
Lincoln	13	874	240	2,197	3,318	0	2	2	76,775	12,153	88,928	49.9	178,054	5,250.93	806.72
Omaha	30	2,503	418	8,484	11,435	351	0	351	265,097	52,899	317,996	49.1	648,258	6,539.61	674.73
Sioux City	0	0	0	0	0	0	0	0	0	0	0	0.0	0		
North Dakota	**26**	**2,680**	**655**	**7,514**	**10,875**	**0**	**21**	**21**	**248,293**	**43,509**	**291,801**	**51.7**	**564,565**	**4,468.16**	**426.58**
Nonmetropolitan	9	854	350	3,642	4,855	0	3	3	94,463	15,689	110,151	55.4	198,789	3,510.43	238.43
Metropolitan	17	1,826	305	3,872	6,020	0	18	18	153,830	27,820	181,650	49.7	365,776	5,245.98	746.91
Bismarck	12	570	125	1,378	2,085	0	0	0	47,960	7,805	55,765	46.2	120,812	5,491.45	779.53
Fargo-Moorhead	1	900	128	1,602	2,631	0	0	0	69,979	12,710	82,690	49.9	165,582	5,376.03	873.06
Grand Forks	4	356	52	892	1,304	0	18	18	35,890	7,305	43,195	54.4	79,383	4,690.26	547.17
South Dakota	**6**	**3,027**	**378**	**7,373**	**10,784**	**30**	**20**	**50**	**226,009**	**37,791**	**263,800**	**55.6**	**474,773**	**3,904.51**	**390.52**
Nonmetropolitan	6	1,155	249	3,963	5,373	0	2	2	100,863	17,860	118,723	56.2	211,119	3,002.13	244.32
Metropolitan	0	1,872	129	3,410	5,411	30	18	48	125,147	19,931	145,078	55.0	263,654	5,142.17	749.77
Rapid City	0	323	53	851	1,227	0	0	0	31,880	4,208	36,088	53.8	67,029	4,191.93	667.12
Sioux Falls	0	1,549	76	2,559	4,184	30	18	48	93,267	15,723	108,990	55.4	196,625	5,572.81	782.83

(continued on next page)

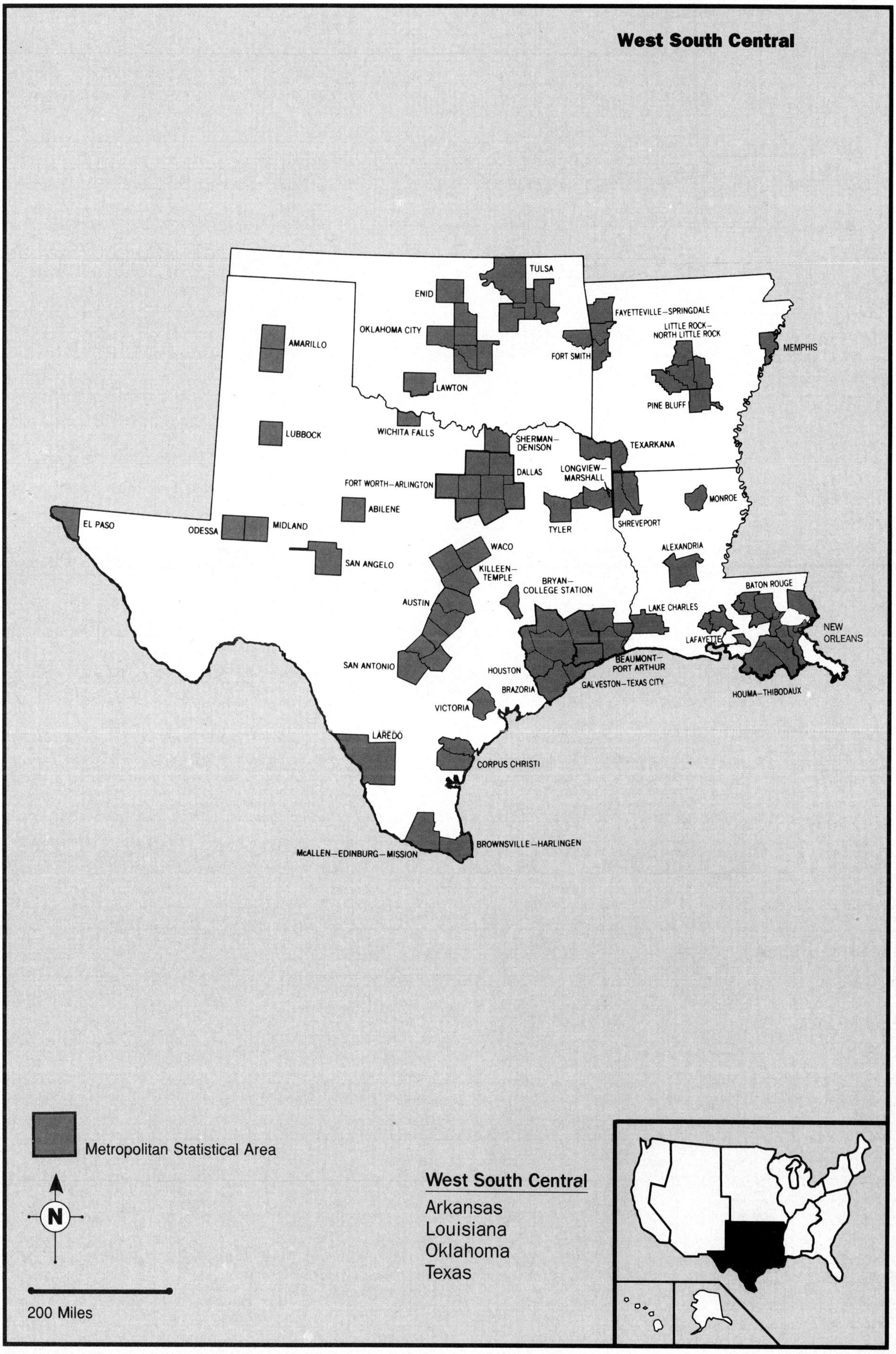
West South Central
TULSA
ENID
OKLAHOMA CITY
AMARILLO
LAWTON
FAYETTEVILLE–SPRINGDALE
LITTLE ROCK–
NORTH LITTLE ROCK
FORT SMITH
MEMPHIS
PINE BLUFF
LUBBOCK
WICHITA FALLS
SHERMAN–
DENISON
TEXARKANA
DALLAS
LONGVIEW–
MARSHALL
FORT WORTH–ARLINGTON
MONROE
ABILENE
EL PASO
ODESSA
MIDLAND
TYLER
SHREVEPORT
WACO
ALEXANDRIA
SAN ANGELO
KILLEEN–
TEMPLE
BRYAN–
COLLEGE STATION
BATON ROUGE
AUSTIN
LAKE CHARLES
NEW
ORLEANS
LAFAYETTE
BEAUMONT–
PORT ARTHUR
SAN ANTONIO
HOUSTON
GALVESTON–TEXAS CITY
BRAZORIA
HOUMA–THIBODAUX
VICTORIA
LAREDO
CORPUS CHRISTI
BROWNSVILLE–HARLINGEN
McALLEN–EDINBURG–MISSION
Metropolitan Statistical Area
N
200 Miles
West South Central
Arkansas
Louisiana
Oklahoma
Texas

Table

6 (Continued)

Utilization, Personnel, and Finances in Community Hospitals, by Metropolitan Statistical Area

Where an MSA is located in multiple states, the MSA will be listed for each state, with hospital data for only that state.

CLASSIFICATION	HOSPITALS	BEDS	ADMISSIONS	INPATIENT DAYS	ADJUSTED PATIENT DAYS	OCCUPANCY, percent	AVERAGE DAILY CENSUS	ADJUSTED AVERAGE DAILY CENSUS	AVERAGE STAY, days	SURGICAL OPERATIONS	OUTPATIENT VISITS: Emergency	OUTPATIENT VISITS: Other	OUTPATIENT VISITS: Total	NEWBORNS: Bassinets	NEWBORNS: Births
CENSUS DIVISION 7, WEST SOUTH CENTRAL	**765**	**101,698**	**3,321,869**	**21,468,716**	**27,555,732**	**57.9**	**58,893**	**75,594**	**6.5**	**2,188,907**	**8,353,038**	**15,095,350**	**23,448,388**	**8,509**	**444,391**
Nonmetropolitan	390	24,921	699,703	4,348,989	5,960,992	47.9	11,931	16,347	6.2	380,990	2,031,436	2,695,306	4,726,742	2,342	75,104
Metropolitan	375	76,777	2,622,166	17,119,727	21,594,740	61.2	46,962	59,247	6.5	1,807,917	6,321,602	12,400,044	18,721,646	6,167	369,287
Arkansas	**86**	**10,843**	**346,819**	**2,453,917**	**3,158,232**	**62.0**	**6,728**	**8,651**	**7.1**	**212,225**	**896,514**	**1,273,915**	**2,170,429**	**809**	**34,260**
Nonmetropolitan	65	5,446	165,792	1,074,832	1,455,610	54.1	2,949	3,988	6.5	87,262	464,953	643,406	1,108,359	472	16,926
Metropolitan	21	5,397	181,027	1,379,085	1,702,622	70.0	3,779	4,663	7.6	124,963	431,561	630,509	1,062,070	337	17,334
Fayetteville-Springdale	3	591	17,436	143,256	180,542	66.3	392	494	8.2	11,905	55,336	39,551	94,887	36	2,148
Fort Smith	4	975	33,653	249,828	312,814	70.3	685	858	7.4	30,063	84,014	70,130	154,144	65	3,193
Little Rock-North Little Rock	11	2,972	102,588	752,086	913,791	69.3	2,060	2,502	7.3	61,548	217,936	436,673	654,609	168	9,784
Memphis	1	146	4,216	31,326	44,552	58.9	86	122	7.4	4,432	13,889	9,520	23,409	18	280
Pine Bluff	1	475	14,195	127,937	157,730	73.9	351	432	9.0	10,787	38,965	31,944	70,909	50	1,929
Texarkana	1	238	8,939	74,652	93,193	86.1	205	255	8.4	6,228	21,421	42,691	64,112	0	0
Louisiana	**140**	**19,085**	**606,863**	**3,998,692**	**5,102,977**	**57.4**	**10,958**	**13,982**	**6.6**	**384,083**	**1,703,268**	**3,691,255**	**5,394,523**	**1,486**	**70,023**
Nonmetropolitan	63	4,288	122,147	789,154	1,065,342	50.5	2,165	2,920	6.5	61,526	363,755	476,709	840,464	349	11,764
Metropolitan	77	14,797	484,716	3,209,538	4,037,635	59.4	8,793	11,062	6.6	322,557	1,339,513	3,214,546	4,554,059	1,137	58,259
Alexandria	3	738	26,494	165,721	204,479	61.5	454	560	6.3	16,691	86,388	201,413	287,801	91	3,272
Baton Rouge	11	2,016	65,799	434,934	557,646	59.2	1,193	1,528	6.6	41,016	163,910	297,569	461,479	113	8,926
Houma-Thibodaux	5	630	25,898	132,699	185,115	57.5	362	508	5.1	20,051	86,848	120,554	207,402	89	3,613
Lafayette	6	977	35,154	231,039	300,625	64.7	632	823	6.6	29,141	102,451	149,113	251,564	119	5,203
Lake Charles	6	849	27,121	164,447	206,685	53.2	452	567	6.1	18,087	74,959	136,898	211,857	70	2,902
Monroe	5	1,060	37,803	254,471	297,168	65.8	697	815	6.7	18,049	91,151	159,143	250,294	97	4,523
New Orleans	31	6,377	197,630	1,379,737	1,703,278	59.3	3,779	4,666	7.0	139,908	541,351	1,366,274	1,907,625	429	23,136
Shreveport	10	2,150	68,817	446,490	582,639	56.9	1,224	1,595	6.5	39,614	192,455	783,582	976,037	129	6,684
Oklahoma	**111**	**12,425**	**381,928**	**2,617,927**	**3,308,489**	**57.7**	**7,173**	**9,063**	**6.9**	**246,780**	**874,782**	**1,402,793**	**2,277,575**	**1,052**	**41,386**
Nonmetropolitan	71	4,658	123,647	784,441	1,069,409	46.1	2,149	2,929	6.3	66,332	310,961	426,950	737,911	474	12,281
Metropolitan	40	7,767	258,281	1,833,486	2,239,080	64.7	5,024	6,134	7.1	180,448	563,821	975,843	1,539,664	578	29,105
Enid	3	371	10,760	73,575	96,497	54.4	202	265	6.8	8,594	19,200	48,232	67,432	30	1,067
Fort Smith	1	50	1,602	8,263	12,200	46.0	23	33	5.2	526	3,780	7,295	11,075	5	104
Lawton	2	347	11,346	77,878	99,113	61.7	214	271	6.9	7,545	42,243	30,592	72,835	43	1,609
Oklahoma City	20	4,101	142,291	989,694	1,212,223	66.1	2,712	3,322	7.0	100,393	327,481	570,106	897,587	344	15,338
Tulsa	14	2,898	92,282	684,076	819,047	64.6	1,873	2,243	7.4	63,390	171,117	319,618	490,735	156	10,987
Texas	**428**	**59,345**	**1,986,259**	**12,398,180**	**15,986,034**	**57.3**	**34,034**	**43,898**	**6.2**	**1,345,819**	**4,878,474**	**8,727,387**	**13,605,861**	**5,162**	**298,722**
Nonmetropolitan	191	10,529	288,117	1,700,562	2,370,631	44.3	4,668	6,510	5.9	165,870	891,767	1,148,241	2,040,008	1,047	34,133
Metropolitan	237	48,816	1,698,142	10,697,618	13,615,403	60.2	29,366	37,388	6.3	1,179,949	3,986,707	7,579,146	11,565,853	4,115	264,589
Abilene	2	456	17,537	116,749	147,636	70.2	320	405	6.7	14,495	34,122	36,353	70,475	49	2,616
Amarillo	5	1,048	34,577	218,791	288,688	57.2	599	791	6.3	31,351	75,724	163,472	239,196	57	4,193
Austin	10	1,756	79,750	429,322	525,250	67.3	1,182	1,450	5.4	48,428	190,327	315,020	505,347	154	14,502
Beaumont-Port Arthur	10	2,007	60,617	407,675	522,179	55.7	1,118	1,431	6.7	37,408	156,053	272,419	428,472	132	5,236
Brazoria	4	314	9,883	51,052	74,602	44.6	140	204	5.2	5,750	43,448	49,927	93,375	34	1,178
Brownsville-Harlingen	5	803	28,237	179,459	225,203	61.3	492	617	6.4	20,957	60,455	65,290	125,745	50	5,562
Bryan-College Station	2	279	12,627	60,358	76,965	59.1	165	211	4.8	7,495	38,794	22,505	61,299	50	2,597
Corpus Christi	9	1,454	49,923	319,618	409,562	62.8	913	1,172	6.4	40,017	94,995	206,959	301,954	131	7,338
Dallas	38	7,343	274,848	1,662,412	2,115,140	62.1	4,559	5,803	6.0	185,850	659,936	1,442,644	2,102,580	641	45,451
El Paso	7	1,721	66,148	391,869	484,517	62.3	1,072	1,328	5.9	35,096	147,404	117,198	264,602	153	14,124
Fort Worth-Arlington	22	3,837	145,714	830,386	1,089,813	59.6	2,288	3,001	5.7	94,092	409,429	753,291	1,162,720	400	23,971
Galveston-Texas City	6	1,572	41,869	329,229	438,194	57.3	901	1,200	7.9	28,092	108,687	405,656	514,343	111	5,837
Houston	51	13,356	415,270	2,801,512	3,563,359	57.4	7,673	9,763	6.7	289,240	816,576	2,161,274	2,977,850	870	62,872
Killeen-Temple	4	626	24,577	148,886	184,732	65.2	408	507	6.1	16,492	53,499	52,328	105,827	71	3,969
Laredo	2	383	17,217	97,097	121,000	69.5	266	331	5.6	8,244	43,598	38,706	82,304	40	4,003
Longview-Marshall	5	505	21,525	119,804	162,059	65.1	329	444	5.6	17,680	68,505	101,224	169,729	70	3,028
Lubbock	6	1,562	49,684	361,408	424,056	63.3	989	1,161	7.3	38,073	88,854	143,243	232,097	346	5,630
McAllen-Edinburg-Mission	5	864	38,463	188,259	232,460	59.7	516	637	4.9	21,568	59,023	88,842	147,865	92	8,902
Midland	2	282	11,328	68,041	89,536	66.0	186	246	6.0	7,880	42,999	68,170	111,169	35	1,960
Odessa	2	372	14,309	83,221	103,854	61.3	228	284	5.8	9,038	43,133	41,788	84,921	36	2,851
San Angelo	3	486	17,476	107,951	145,755	60.9	296	399	6.2	16,128	71,337	61,916	133,253	56	2,113
San Antonio	18	4,417	149,995	991,646	1,243,992	61.5	2,716	3,409	6.6	119,386	374,889	666,837	1,041,726	323	22,919
Sherman-Denison	3	562	16,965	102,494	140,751	50.0	281	386	6.0	11,970	44,848	46,229	91,077	46	1,724
Texarkana	2	429	17,176	107,368	135,092	68.8	295	370	6.3	13,611	44,025	30,988	75,013	29	2,259
Tyler	5	868	28,892	202,554	259,385	63.9	555	710	7.0	18,315	85,193	78,183	163,376	43	2,814
Victoria	3	531	16,209	106,887	132,405	55.4	294	363	6.6	12,050	36,153	31,871	68,024	22	1,621
Waco	3	541	20,055	108,966	145,892	55.3	299	400	5.4	16,590	49,884	60,337	110,221	44	3,069
Wichita Falls	3	442	17,271	104,604	133,326	64.7	286	365	6.1	14,653	44,817	56,476	101,293	30	2,250

Table 6 (Continued) Census Division 7, West South Central

CLASSIFICATION	FULL-TIME EQUIVALENT PERSONNEL: Physicians and Dentists	FULL-TIME EQUIVALENT PERSONNEL: Registered Nurses	FULL-TIME EQUIVALENT PERSONNEL: Licensed Practical Nurses	FULL-TIME EQUIVALENT PERSONNEL: Other Salaried Personnel	FULL-TIME EQUIVALENT PERSONNEL: Total Personnel	FULL-TIME EQUIVALENT TRAINEES: Medical and Dental Residents	FULL-TIME EQUIVALENT TRAINEES: Other Trainees	FULL-TIME EQUIVALENT TRAINEES: Total Trainees	EXPENSES, LABOR: Payroll (in thousands)	EXPENSES, LABOR: Employee Benefits (in thousands)	EXPENSES, LABOR: Total (in thousands)	EXPENSES, LABOR: Percent of Total	EXPENSES, TOTAL: Amount (in thousands)	EXPENSES, TOTAL: Adjusted, per Admission	EXPENSES, TOTAL: Adjusted, per Inpatient Day
CENSUS DIVISION 7, WEST SOUTH CENTRAL	**780**	**72,898**	**29,099**	**238,323**	**341,100**	**4,685**	**774**	**5,459**	**$ 7,962,159**	**$ 1,544,797**	**$ 9,506,955**	**49.1**	**$ 19,368,316**	**$4,508.20**	**$ 702.88**
Nonmetropolitan	75	10,413	8,350	41,401	60,239	0	19	19	1,163,725	230,684	1,394,409	49.5	2,815,706	2,915.73	472.36
Metropolitan	705	62,485	20,749	196,922	280,861	4,685	755	5,440	6,798,434	1,314,112	8,112,547	49.0	16,552,611	4,969.94	766.51
Arkansas	**20**	**7,004**	**3,994**	**22,382**	**33,400**	**279**	**49**	**328**	**716,536**	**131,549**	**848,084**	**50.3**	**1,685,047**	**3,729.58**	**533.54**
Nonmetropolitan	8	2,449	2,058	9,258	13,773	0	1	1	254,694	48,546	303,240	49.3	615,567	2,728.69	422.89
Metropolitan	12	4,555	1,936	13,124	19,627	279	48	327	461,841	83,003	544,844	50.9	1,069,479	4,727.71	628.14
Fayetteville-Springdale	4	412	186	1,298	1,900	0	5	5	36,600	6,059	42,659	53.1	80,405	3,525.76	445.35
Fort Smith	0	665	303	1,936	2,904	0	2	2	61,346	13,576	74,922	52.7	142,088	3,331.10	454.23
Little Rock-North Little Rock	8	2,942	1,094	7,745	11,789	279	0	279	296,977	53,251	350,228	50.4	695,222	5,513.31	760.81
Memphis	0	74	47	291	412	0	0	0	8,385	1,436	9,821	52.3	18,769	3,130.23	421.28
Pine Bluff	0	268	179	1,063	1,510	0	0	0	33,415	5,279	38,694	49.8	77,671	4,438.10	492.43
Texarkana	0	194	127	791	1,112	0	41	41	25,119	3,402	28,521	51.6	55,324	4,957.79	593.65
Louisiana	**153**	**12,903**	**5,006**	**44,847**	**62,909**	**1,279**	**15**	**1,294**	**1,448,100**	**266,659**	**1,714,759**	**48.0**	**3,575,006**	**4,574.56**	**700.57**
Nonmetropolitan	12	1,673	1,379	7,332	10,396	0	0	0	200,238	38,237	238,475	48.6	490,894	2,946.26	460.79
Metropolitan	141	11,230	3,627	37,515	52,513	1,279	15	1,294	1,247,861	228,423	1,476,284	47.9	3,084,111	5,015.79	763.84
Alexandria	12	578	181	1,871	2,642	31	0	31	58,265	10,766	69,031	47.0	146,851	4,483.59	718.17
Baton Rouge	3	1,541	507	4,669	6,720	55	0	55	158,032	30,686	188,718	50.2	376,245	4,431.47	674.70
Houma-Thibodaux	4	476	199	1,753	2,432	0	0	0	53,535	8,548	62,083	48.8	127,301	3,485.20	687.68
Lafayette	10	729	324	2,394	3,457	29	0	29	78,813	13,811	92,624	47.5	195,046	4,272.17	648.80
Lake Charles	8	554	210	1,737	2,509	7	0	7	60,660	10,978	71,638	45.8	156,370	4,561.55	756.56
Monroe	0	681	417	2,647	3,745	25	3	28	71,091	12,490	83,581	47.7	175,057	3,932.54	589.08
New Orleans	87	5,178	1,310	17,133	23,708	916	12	928	569,816	109,908	679,724	45.7	1,485,947	6,037.17	872.40
Shreveport	17	1,493	479	5,311	7,300	216	0	216	197,650	31,234	228,885	54.3	421,295	4,675.03	723.08
Oklahoma	**63**	**8,074**	**3,071**	**30,357**	**41,565**	**516**	**128**	**644**	**888,778**	**167,124**	**1,055,903**	**50.5**	**2,091,066**	**4,301.98**	**632.03**
Nonmetropolitan	16	1,851	1,299	7,910	11,076	0	6	6	210,185	38,879	249,064	51.7	482,039	2,840.85	450.75
Metropolitan	47	6,223	1,772	22,447	30,489	516	122	638	678,593	128,246	806,838	50.1	1,609,027	5,085.58	718.61
Enid	0	216	86	806	1,108	0	0	0	28,841	5,922	34,763	44.6	77,924	5,519.11	807.53
Fort Smith	0	19	9	76	104	0	0	0	1,903	385	2,288	54.5	4,195	1,773.82	343.86
Lawton	0	135	90	829	1,054	0	0	0	23,882	4,435	28,316	42.8	66,200	4,576.88	667.92
Oklahoma City	20	3,586	1,232	12,033	16,871	499	40	539	380,953	72,848	453,802	50.9	891,077	5,098.07	735.08
Tulsa	27	2,267	355	8,703	11,352	17	82	99	243,014	44,656	287,669	50.5	569,631	5,147.81	695.48
Texas	**544**	**44,917**	**17,028**	**140,737**	**203,226**	**2,611**	**582**	**3,193**	**4,908,745**	**979,464**	**5,888,210**	**49.0**	**12,017,198**	**4,663.50**	**751.73**
Nonmetropolitan	39	4,440	3,614	16,901	24,994	0	12	12	498,607	105,022	603,629	49.2	1,227,205	3,039.10	517.67
Metropolitan	505	40,477	13,414	123,836	178,232	2,611	570	3,181	4,410,139	874,442	5,284,580	49.0	10,789,993	4,965.35	792.48
Abilene	0	544	176	1,591	2,311	0	28	28	47,569	9,323	56,892	50.5	112,686	5,076.19	763.27
Amarillo	1	1,013	267	2,552	3,833	0	0	0	101,681	16,034	117,715	53.9	218,241	4,780.44	755.98
Austin	7	1,713	408	4,285	6,413	0	8	8	168,152	31,116	199,268	50.0	398,788	4,057.75	759.23
Beaumont-Port Arthur	1	1,122	696	3,886	5,705	2	2	4	140,602	30,175	170,777	47.8	357,493	4,574.80	684.62
Brazoria	0	215	80	573	868	0	0	0	19,648	4,860	24,508	48.3	50,729	3,478.65	680.00
Brownsville-Harlingen	6	496	305	1,909	2,716	0	0	0	53,228	10,877	64,106	50.6	126,705	3,521.33	562.62
Bryan-College Station	0	246	97	768	1,111	0	0	0	25,616	4,554	30,171	52.0	58,038	3,601.69	754.08
Corpus Christi	7	996	570	3,778	5,351	48	0	48	111,573	24,959	136,532	48.4	282,372	4,434.24	689.45
Dallas	97	7,377	1,066	20,441	28,981	1,064	10	1,074	679,857	120,669	800,526	46.7	1,715,463	4,865.98	811.04
El Paso	0	1,138	259	4,276	5,673	0	3	3	131,216	28,417	159,632	48.6	328,717	4,017.91	678.44
Fort Worth-Arlington	29	4,099	1,085	9,948	15,161	155	0	155	375,807	75,701	451,508	49.0	921,299	4,790.27	845.37
Galveston-Texas City	0	1,186	304	4,279	5,769	431	0	431	160,096	24,802	184,898	52.6	351,634	6,214.93	802.46
Houston	305	10,429	2,982	33,928	47,644	367	419	786	1,323,288	285,342	1,608,631	49.3	3,262,723	6,155.67	915.63
Killeen-Temple	0	596	213	2,100	2,909	158	0	158	60,676	14,727	75,403	57.0	132,309	4,298.95	716.22
Laredo	0	200	155	1,265	1,620	0	0	0	25,328	5,893	31,221	49.5	63,096	2,931.83	521.45
Longview-Marshall	0	477	225	1,303	2,005	0	0	0	42,373	8,453	50,826	47.8	106,260	3,619.46	655.69
Lubbock	0	1,042	575	3,492	5,109	0	12	12	127,952	27,444	155,396	49.6	313,071	5,268.16	738.28
McAllen-Edinburg-Mission	1	547	389	1,673	2,610	0	9	9	61,898	9,255	71,154	41.3	172,204	3,619.41	740.79
Midland	0	265	124	763	1,152	0	0	0	27,659	7,208	34,867	46.4	75,138	5,040.79	839.19
Odessa	0	281	120	894	1,295	0	0	0	31,537	5,814	37,350	50.8	73,477	4,098.20	707.50
San Angelo	0	346	159	1,193	1,698	0	10	10	38,974	8,049	47,023	51.5	91,349	3,861.90	626.73
San Antonio	5	3,642	1,892	10,914	16,453	368	45	413	387,840	64,052	451,892	49.5	913,492	4,827.75	734.32
Sherman-Denison	0	487	177	1,018	1,682	0	0	0	39,167	8,848	48,015	50.2	95,640	4,101.04	679.50
Texarkana	0	314	205	865	1,384	0	0	0	35,091	7,467	42,558	47.7	89,204	4,127.51	660.32
Tyler	45	714	272	2,647	3,678	18	4	22	85,235	18,850	104,086	48.3	215,647	5,888.79	831.38
Victoria	0	298	196	907	1,401	0	12	12	32,449	6,376	38,824	45.4	85,533	4,263.22	645.99
Waco	0	382	132	1,387	1,901	0	0	0	37,680	6,821	44,501	46.2	96,306	3,563.85	660.12
Wichita Falls	1	312	285	1,201	1,799	0	8	8	37,947	8,355	46,303	56.2	82,379	3,723.86	617.88

(continued on next page)

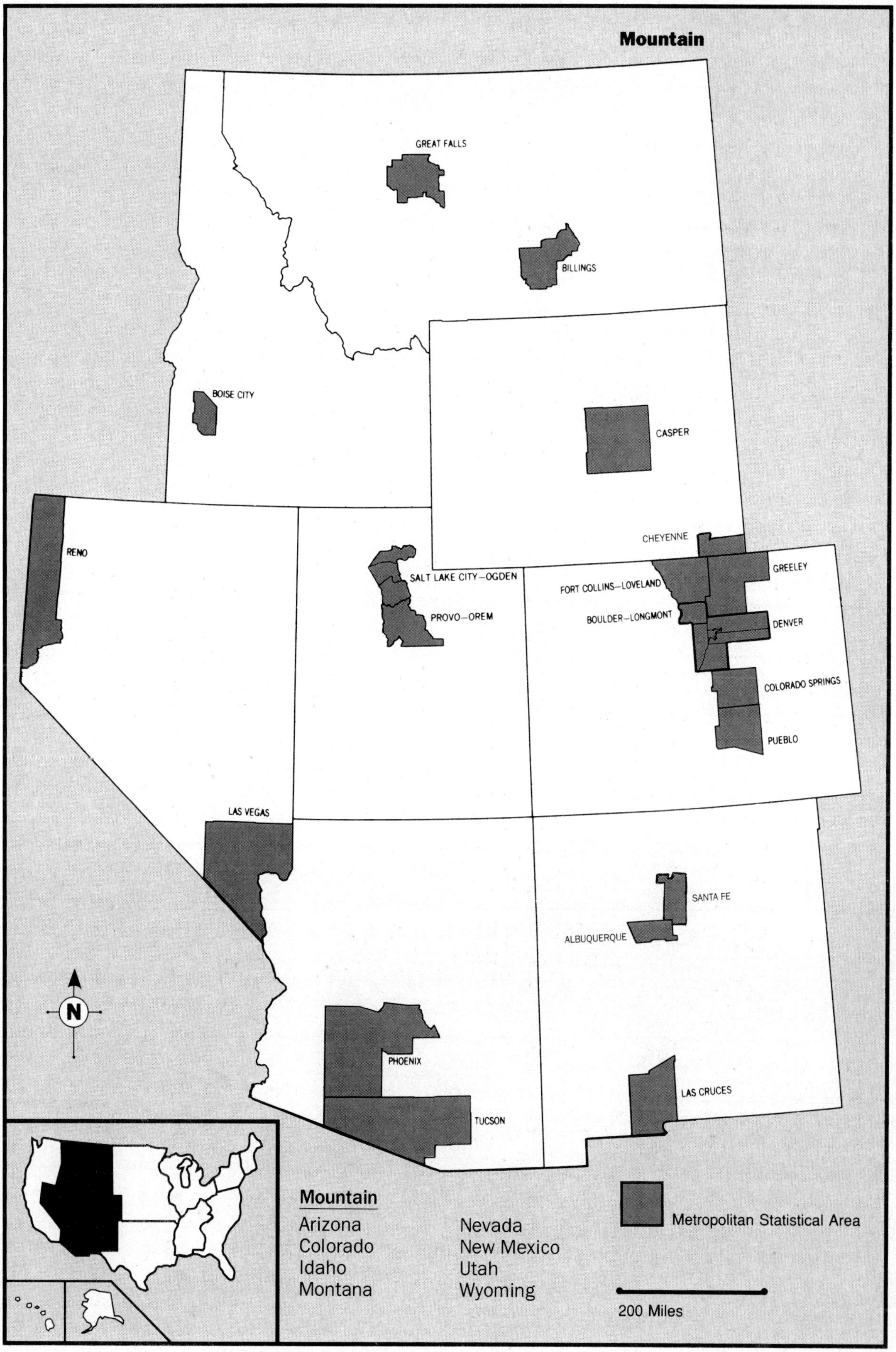
Mountain
GREAT FALLS
BILLINGS
BOISE CITY
CASPER
CHEYENNE
RENO
SALT LAKE CITY–OGDEN
PROVO–OREM
FORT COLLINS–LOVELAND
GREELEY
BOULDER–LONGMONT
DENVER
COLORADO SPRINGS
PUEBLO
LAS VEGAS
SANTA FE
ALBUQUERQUE
PHOENIX
TUCSON
LAS CRUCES
N
Mountain
Arizona
Colorado
Idaho
Montana
Nevada
New Mexico
Utah
Wyoming
Metropolitan Statistical Area
200 Miles

Table

6

(Continued)

Utilization, Personnel, and Finances in Community Hospitals, by Metropolitan Statistical Area

Where an MSA is located in multiple states, the MSA will be listed for each state, with hospital data for only that state.

CLASSIFICATION	HOSPITALS	BEDS	ADMISSIONS	INPATIENT DAYS	ADJUSTED PATIENT DAYS	OCCUPANCY, percent	AVERAGE DAILY CENSUS	ADJUSTED AVERAGE DAILY CENSUS	AVERAGE STAY, days	SURGICAL OPERATIONS	OUTPATIENT VISITS			NEWBORNS	
											Emergency	Other	Total	Bassinets	Births
CENSUS DIVISION 8, MOUNTAIN	**355**	**42,238**	**1,425,988**	**9,331,969**	**12,452,759**	**60.5**	**25,572**	**34,129**	**6.5**	**1,017,703**	**3,781,390**	**10,168,519**	**13,949,909**	**3,728**	**219,514**
Nonmetropolitan	238	15,343	393,800	3,138,155	4,459,394	56.0	8,595	12,217	8.0	237,388	1,228,739	3,114,522	4,343,261	1,598	57,316
Metropolitan	117	26,895	1,032,188	6,193,814	7,993,365	63.1	16,977	21,912	6.0	780,315	2,552,651	7,053,997	9,606,648	2,130	162,198
Arizona	**61**	**9,973**	**396,422**	**2,249,577**	**2,902,911**	**61.8**	**6,165**	**7,953**	**5.7**	**248,500**	**933,071**	**1,802,683**	**2,735,754**	**776**	**60,780**
Nonmetropolitan	26	1,840	63,760	376,227	539,431	56.0	1,030	1,475	5.9	33,318	188,165	402,973	591,138	194	9,999
Metropolitan	35	8,133	332,662	1,873,350	2,363,480	63.1	5,135	6,478	5.6	215,182	744,906	1,399,710	2,144,616	582	50,781
Phoenix	27	6,153	247,180	1,403,710	1,768,478	62.5	3,848	4,849	5.7	168,674	560,103	942,480	1,502,583	432	39,189
Tucson	8	1,980	85,482	469,640	595,002	65.0	1,287	1,629	5.5	46,508	184,803	457,230	642,033	150	11,592
Colorado	**69**	**10,316**	**334,781**	**2,409,593**	**3,203,958**	**64.0**	**6,605**	**8,790**	**7.2**	**262,374**	**871,857**	**2,639,072**	**3,510,929**	**811**	**49,179**
Nonmetropolitan	40	2,478	54,114	556,625	794,638	61.5	1,523	2,179	10.3	35,072	169,400	564,419	733,819	228	7,248
Metropolitan	29	7,838	280,667	1,852,968	2,409,320	64.8	5,082	6,611	6.6	227,302	702,457	2,074,653	2,777,110	583	41,931
Boulder-Longmont	3	395	15,593	73,801	104,867	52.7	208	297	4.7	10,789	49,708	126,875	176,583	49	3,083
Colorado Springs	2	1,006	35,004	215,801	274,549	58.7	591	753	6.2	24,859	91,971	167,993	259,964	70	5,673
Denver	18	5,208	182,683	1,284,478	1,659,940	67.6	3,519	4,547	7.0	156,304	447,882	1,429,724	1,877,606	346	26,889
Fort Collins-Loveland	3	407	16,509	92,726	134,762	62.4	254	369	5.6	13,045	49,015	87,217	136,232	44	2,709
Greeley	1	281	12,003	57,998	73,288	56.6	159	201	4.8	9,017	25,650	89,871	115,521	23	1,725
Pueblo	2	541	18,875	128,164	161,914	64.9	351	444	6.8	13,288	38,231	172,973	211,204	51	1,852
Idaho	**43**	**3,200**	**96,621**	**650,658**	**936,588**	**55.7**	**1,783**	**2,568**	**6.7**	**69,805**	**284,812**	**769,847**	**1,054,659**	**316**	**15,203**
Nonmetropolitan	40	2,636	70,923	514,402	743,735	53.5	1,409	2,039	7.3	48,352	228,487	538,121	766,608	275	11,606
Metropolitan	3	564	25,698	136,256	192,853	66.3	374	529	5.3	21,453	56,325	231,726	288,051	41	3,597
Boise City	3	564	25,698	136,256	192,853	66.3	374	529	5.3	21,453	56,325	231,726	288,051	41	3,597
Montana	**55**	**4,633**	**105,405**	**1,035,165**	**1,364,420**	**61.2**	**2,836**	**3,741**	**9.8**	**59,696**	**236,542**	**606,925**	**843,467**	**307**	**10,579**
Nonmetropolitan	51	3,449	69,717	764,654	1,036,507	60.7	2,095	2,842	11.0	37,756	165,002	473,422	638,424	254	7,299
Metropolitan	4	1,184	35,688	270,511	327,913	62.6	741	899	7.6	21,940	71,540	133,503	205,043	53	3,280
Billings	2	560	20,307	134,147	157,550	65.7	368	432	6.6	13,031	37,086	43,331	80,417	24	1,922
Great Falls	2	624	15,381	136,364	170,363	59.8	373	467	8.9	8,909	34,454	90,172	124,626	29	1,358
Nevada	**21**	**3,373**	**115,995**	**741,705**	**925,916**	**60.3**	**2,033**	**2,535**	**6.4**	**87,847**	**368,815**	**717,436**	**1,086,251**	**243**	**19,517**
Nonmetropolitan	10	470	11,402	81,135	129,524	47.4	223	354	7.1	5,951	70,520	102,680	173,200	57	2,187
Metropolitan	11	2,903	104,593	660,570	796,392	62.3	1,810	2,181	6.3	81,896	298,295	614,756	913,051	186	17,330
Las Vegas	8	1,946	69,680	456,598	551,029	64.3	1,251	1,509	6.6	59,091	191,753	406,585	598,338	112	11,741
Reno	3	957	34,913	203,972	245,363	58.4	559	672	5.8	22,805	106,542	208,171	314,713	74	5,589
New Mexico	**37**	**4,192**	**153,319**	**879,852**	**1,222,121**	**57.5**	**2,410**	**3,347**	**5.7**	**112,652**	**394,350**	**1,443,023**	**1,837,373**	**407**	**22,783**
Nonmetropolitan	24	1,829	58,584	342,144	468,057	51.2	937	1,282	5.8	32,690	171,129	356,122	527,251	206	8,292
Metropolitan	13	2,363	94,735	537,708	754,064	62.3	1,473	2,065	5.7	79,962	223,221	1,086,901	1,310,122	201	14,491
Albuquerque	10	1,844	71,368	417,728	600,331	62.0	1,144	1,644	5.9	62,425	152,676	1,039,708	1,192,384	137	10,432
Las Cruces	1	240	11,268	60,915	74,454	69.6	167	204	5.4	7,408	31,260	25,006	56,266	34	2,315
Santa Fe	2	279	12,099	59,065	79,279	58.1	162	217	4.9	10,129	39,285	22,187	61,472	30	1,744
Utah	**42**	**4,408**	**175,472**	**944,509**	**1,312,716**	**58.7**	**2,588**	**3,597**	**5.4**	**141,397**	**525,708**	**1,844,821**	**2,370,529**	**632**	**35,379**
Nonmetropolitan	23	970	31,868	175,201	284,254	49.6	481	779	5.5	19,473	115,595	406,525	522,120	194	6,456
Metropolitan	19	3,438	143,604	769,308	1,028,462	61.3	2,107	2,818	5.4	121,924	410,113	1,438,296	1,848,409	438	28,923
Provo-Orem	4	574	26,583	123,271	161,346	58.9	338	442	4.6	18,172	87,858	271,550	359,408	83	6,979
Salt Lake City-Ogden	15	2,864	117,021	646,037	867,116	61.8	1,769	2,376	5.5	103,752	322,255	1,166,746	1,489,001	355	21,944
Wyoming	**27**	**2,143**	**47,973**	**420,910**	**584,129**	**53.8**	**1,152**	**1,598**	**8.8**	**35,432**	**166,235**	**344,712**	**510,947**	**236**	**6,094**
Nonmetropolitan	24	1,671	33,432	327,767	463,248	53.7	897	1,267	9.8	24,776	120,441	270,260	390,701	190	4,229
Metropolitan	3	472	14,541	93,143	120,881	54.0	255	331	6.4	10,656	45,794	74,452	120,246	46	1,865
Casper	1	225	6,475	42,821	53,367	52.0	117	146	6.6	5,195	22,344	16,132	38,476	38	1,021
Cheyenne	2	247	8,066	50,322	67,514	55.9	138	185	6.2	5,461	23,450	58,320	81,770	8	844

Table 6 (Continued) Census Division 8, Mountain

CLASSIFICATION	FULL-TIME EQUIVALENT PERSONNEL: Physicians and Dentists	Registered Nurses	Licensed Practical Nurses	Other Salaried Personnel	Total Personnel	FULL-TIME EQUIVALENT TRAINEES: Medical and Dental Residents	Other Trainees	Total Trainees	EXPENSES — LABOR: Payroll (in thousands)	Employee Benefits (in thousands)	Total (in thousands)	Percent of Total	EXPENSES — TOTAL: Amount (in thousands)	Adjusted, per Admission	Adjusted, per Inpatient Day
CENSUS DIVISION 8, MOUNTAIN	1,304	36,790	5,875	101,226	145,195	955	95	1,050	$ 3,771,887	$ 750,649	$ 4,522,537	50.5	$ 8,954,950	$4,680.06	$ 719.11
Nonmetropolitan	97	8,260	2,242	27,739	38,338	12	44	56	831,361	164,586	995,946	51.8	1,921,253	3,372.02	430.83
Metropolitan	1,207	28,530	3,633	73,487	106,857	943	51	994	2,940,527	586,064	3,526,590	50.1	7,033,698	5,234.72	879.94
Arizona	132	9,556	1,204	24,988	35,880	505	0	505	1,007,621	191,394	1,199,015	47.6	2,516,625	4,877.48	866.93
Nonmetropolitan	18	1,230	238	4,096	5,582	0	0	0	129,412	26,801	156,213	49.7	314,120	3,390.32	582.32
Metropolitan	114	8,326	966	20,892	30,298	505	0	505	878,209	164,593	1,042,802	47.3	2,202,505	5,202.98	931.89
Phoenix	105	6,145	690	15,032	21,972	501	0	501	659,985	125,075	785,059	46.5	1,688,207	5,366.20	954.61
Tucson	9	2,181	276	5,860	8,326	4	0	4	218,224	39,519	257,743	50.1	514,299	4,730.66	864.36
Colorado	1,009	9,929	980	27,239	39,157	270	20	290	1,063,495	189,791	1,253,286	54.0	2,322,897	5,208.83	725.01
Nonmetropolitan	27	1,284	316	4,567	6,194	12	0	12	132,624	23,374	155,998	55.3	282,219	3,506.18	355.15
Metropolitan	982	8,645	664	22,672	32,963	258	20	278	930,871	166,417	1,097,288	53.8	2,040,678	5,583.83	846.99
Boulder-Longmont	0	547	22	1,411	1,980	0	1	1	49,058	7,475	56,533	56.5	100,018	4,496.59	953.76
Colorado Springs	0	1,320	76	2,812	4,208	6	0	6	108,975	18,728	127,703	57.3	222,914	5,002.44	811.93
Denver	973	5,635	449	14,953	22,010	204	19	223	646,782	116,993	763,775	53.0	1,441,973	6,080.68	868.69
Fort Collins-Loveland	5	402	36	1,257	1,700	12	0	12	44,742	10,038	54,780	55.6	98,510	4,378.60	730.99
Greeley	4	312	15	766	1,097	19	0	19	32,074	5,439	37,514	55.4	67,716	4,464.69	923.97
Pueblo	0	429	66	1,473	1,968	17	0	17	49,239	7,744	56,983	52.0	109,548	4,592.64	676.58
Idaho	4	2,456	680	6,522	9,662	0	13	13	219,375	41,165	260,540	50.9	512,279	3,700.85	546.96
Nonmetropolitan	1	1,627	590	4,686	6,904	0	1	1	150,905	31,133	182,038	50.8	358,286	3,509.20	481.74
Metropolitan	3	829	90	1,836	2,758	0	12	12	68,470	10,032	78,502	51.0	153,993	4,239.56	798.50
Boise City	3	829	90	1,836	2,758	0	12	12	68,470	10,032	78,502	51.0	153,993	4,239.56	798.50
Montana	8	2,505	578	8,160	11,251	0	14	14	249,500	46,407	295,907	53.5	552,973	3,972.79	405.28
Nonmetropolitan	7	1,456	331	5,458	7,252	0	14	14	148,766	28,164	176,930	53.7	329,239	3,432.25	317.64
Metropolitan	1	1,049	247	2,702	3,999	0	0	0	100,734	18,243	118,977	53.2	223,734	5,171.24	682.30
Billings	1	589	135	1,458	2,183	0	0	0	55,482	9,952	65,433	48.8	134,086	5,625.60	851.07
Great Falls	0	460	112	1,244	1,816	0	0	0	45,252	8,291	53,544	59.7	89,648	4,613.87	526.22
Nevada	23	3,278	567	7,538	11,406	11	4	15	318,738	71,692	390,430	49.4	790,498	5,510.96	853.75
Nonmetropolitan	4	202	73	898	1,177	0	4	4	27,924	6,432	34,356	54.9	62,573	3,678.83	483.10
Metropolitan	19	3,076	494	6,640	10,229	11	0	11	290,814	65,260	356,074	48.9	727,925	5,757.44	914.03
Las Vegas	19	2,067	388	3,860	6,334	11	0	11	177,008	38,380	215,388	47.1	456,886	5,421.44	829.15
Reno	0	1,009	106	2,780	3,895	0	0	0	113,807	26,879	140,686	51.9	271,038	6,429.11	1,104.64
New Mexico	24	3,286	760	10,311	14,381	10	28	38	352,063	72,949	425,012	47.4	897,073	4,172.47	734.03
Nonmetropolitan	10	1,099	330	3,297	4,736	0	25	25	101,675	18,627	120,302	48.4	248,606	3,058.41	531.14
Metropolitan	14	2,187	430	7,014	9,645	10	3	13	250,388	54,322	304,710	47.0	648,467	4,849.73	859.96
Albuquerque	4	1,727	362	5,725	7,818	4	3	7	203,325	43,969	247,294	46.1	536,221	5,173.39	893.21
Las Cruces	3	229	23	575	830	0	0	0	20,627	3,802	24,429	49.9	49,005	3,558.02	658.19
Santa Fe	7	231	45	714	997	6	0	6	26,436	6,551	32,987	52.2	63,241	3,882.45	797.70
Utah	91	4,534	863	12,506	17,994	159	10	169	442,447	115,207	557,654	51.0	1,092,626	4,409.36	832.34
Nonmetropolitan	18	606	180	1,886	2,690	0	0	0	59,271	14,532	73,803	51.1	144,460	2,804.67	508.21
Metropolitan	73	3,928	683	10,620	15,304	159	10	169	383,176	100,675	483,851	51.0	948,165	4,830.43	921.93
Provo-Orem	7	492	183	1,518	2,200	0	0	0	59,848	15,040	74,888	59.0	126,900	3,586.58	786.51
Salt Lake City-Ogden	66	3,436	500	9,102	13,104	159	10	169	323,328	85,635	408,963	49.8	821,265	5,103.94	947.12
Wyoming	13	1,246	243	3,962	5,464	0	6	6	118,650	22,043	140,693	52.1	269,979	3,990.47	462.19
Nonmetropolitan	12	756	184	2,851	3,803	0	0	0	80,784	15,522	96,306	53.0	181,750	3,724.91	392.34
Metropolitan	1	490	59	1,111	1,661	0	6	6	37,865	6,522	44,387	50.3	88,229	4,677.38	729.89
Casper	0	267	20	565	852	0	4	4	19,723	3,781	23,505	50.3	46,744	5,792.34	875.90
Cheyenne	1	223	39	546	809	0	2	2	18,142	2,741	20,882	50.3	41,485	3,843.72	614.47

(continued on next page)

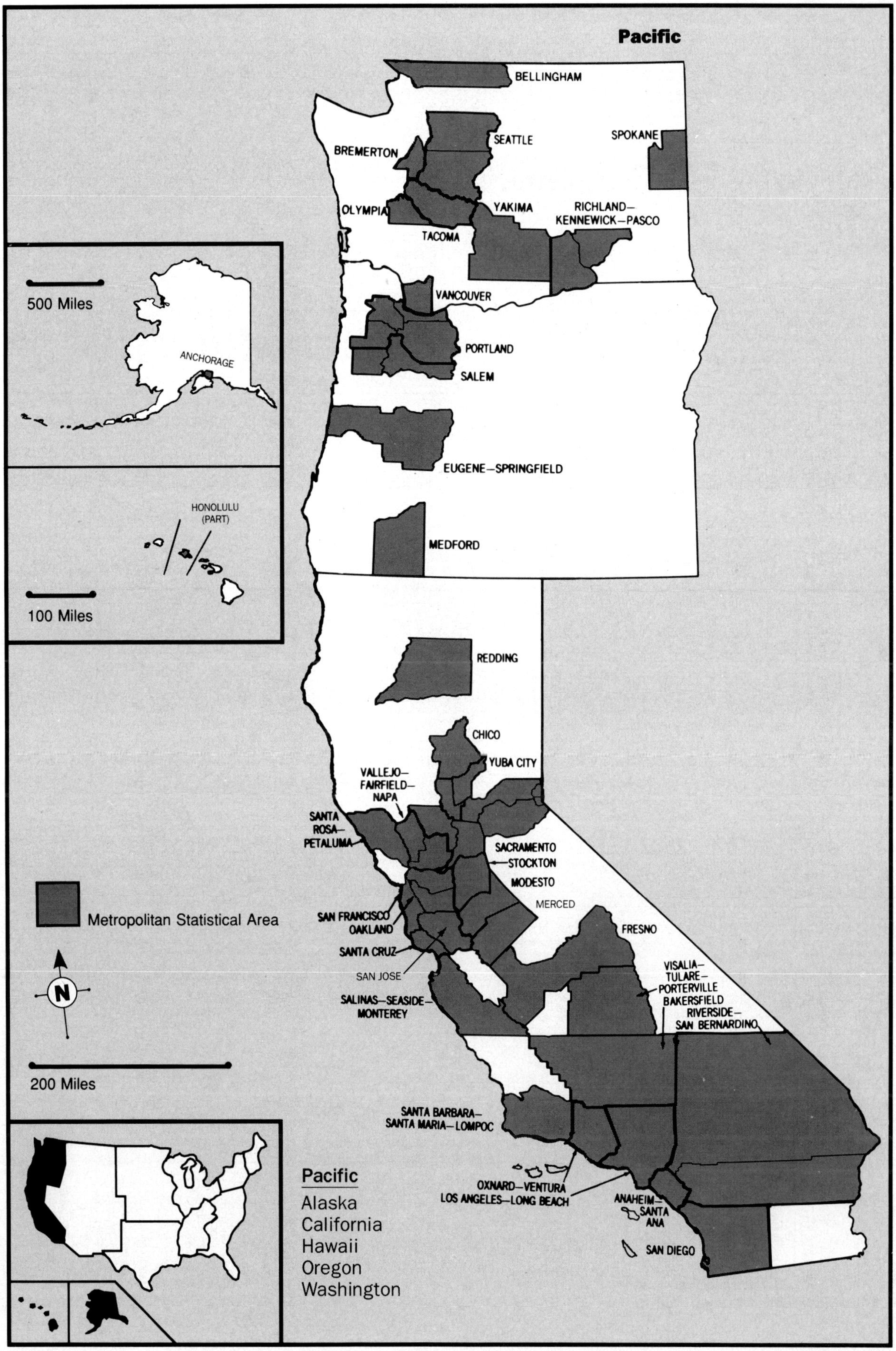
Pacific
BELLINGHAM
SEATTLE
SPOKANE
BREMERTON
OLYMPIA
YAKIMA
RICHLAND–KENNEWICK–PASCO
TACOMA
VANCOUVER
PORTLAND
SALEM
EUGENE–SPRINGFIELD
MEDFORD
REDDING
CHICO
YUBA CITY
VALLEJO–FAIRFIELD–NAPA
SANTA ROSA–PETALUMA
SACRAMENTO
STOCKTON
MODESTO
MERCED
SAN FRANCISCO
OAKLAND
FRESNO
SANTA CRUZ
SAN JOSE
VISALIA–TULARE–PORTERVILLE
BAKERSFIELD
RIVERSIDE–SAN BERNARDINO
SALINAS–SEASIDE–MONTEREY
SANTA BARBARA–SANTA MARIA–LOMPOC
OXNARD–VENTURA
LOS ANGELES–LONG BEACH
ANAHEIM–SANTA ANA
SAN DIEGO
500 Miles
ANCHORAGE
HONOLULU (PART)
100 Miles
Metropolitan Statistical Area
N
200 Miles
Pacific
Alaska
California
Hawaii
Oregon
Washington

Table 6 (Continued)

Utilization, Personnel, and Finances in Community Hospitals, by Metropolitan Statistical Area

Where an MSA is located in multiple states, the MSA will be listed for each state, with hospital data for only that state.

CLASSIFICATION	HOSPITALS	BEDS	ADMISSIONS	INPATIENT DAYS	ADJUSTED PATIENT DAYS	OCCUPANCY, percent	AVERAGE DAILY CENSUS	ADJUSTED AVERAGE DAILY CENSUS	AVERAGE STAY, days	SURGICAL OPERATIONS	OUTPATIENT VISITS Emergency	OUTPATIENT VISITS Other	OUTPATIENT VISITS Total	NEWBORNS Bassinets	NEWBORNS Births
CENSUS DIVISION 9, PACIFIC	640	104,100	3,989,779	24,245,162	31,640,564	63.8	66,439	86,723	6.1	2,656,162	11,468,803	28,757,518	40,226,321	7,965	707,114
Nonmetropolitan	146	9,281	293,415	1,817,469	2,691,528	53.7	4,980	7,380	6.2	216,281	1,230,704	2,332,572	3,563,276	942	45,727
Metropolitan	494	94,819	3,696,364	22,427,693	28,949,036	64.8	61,459	79,343	6.1	2,439,881	10,238,099	26,424,946	36,663,045	7,023	661,387
Alaska	16	1,194	37,201	215,935	297,512	49.4	590	816	5.8	23,749	139,300	303,160	442,460	129	7,366
Nonmetropolitan	10	480	14,357	84,814	131,295	48.1	231	361	5.9	9,214	60,454	113,015	173,469	67	2,830
Metropolitan	6	714	22,844	131,121	166,217	50.3	359	455	5.7	14,535	78,846	190,145	268,991	62	4,536
Anchorage	6	714	22,844	131,121	166,217	50.3	359	455	5.7	14,535	78,846	190,145	268,991	62	4,536
California	445	80,031	3,063,199	18,734,637	24,076,492	64.2	51,344	65,990	6.1	1,945,575	8,598,304	21,088,868	29,687,172	5,925	569,847
Nonmetropolitan	51	3,012	99,307	580,686	880,013	52.8	1,591	2,411	5.8	69,429	512,122	944,905	1,457,027	251	16,607
Metropolitan	394	77,019	2,963,892	18,153,951	23,196,479	64.6	49,753	63,579	6.1	1,876,146	8,086,182	20,143,963	28,230,145	5,674	553,240
Anaheim-Santa Ana	35	6,284	243,526	1,276,399	1,633,625	55.6	3,497	4,475	5.2	155,368	564,941	1,184,649	1,749,590	545	50,729
Bakersfield	10	1,212	48,769	274,759	364,276	62.0	752	997	5.6	28,575	182,478	243,294	425,772	107	10,048
Chico	5	595	22,889	142,045	195,408	65.4	389	536	6.2	16,795	88,572	156,812	245,384	38	3,039
Fresno	10	1,621	71,006	380,209	517,775	64.1	1,039	1,419	5.4	52,906	257,142	574,291	831,433	122	15,487
Los Angeles-Long Beach	127	28,010	1,025,123	6,390,452	8,014,927	62.6	17,525	21,990	6.2	632,445	2,335,328	5,967,691	8,303,019	1,976	197,932
Merced	5	337	13,934	67,284	93,101	54.6	184	255	4.8	9,813	50,138	96,022	146,160	38	3,444
Modesto	7	1,244	39,282	329,177	437,552	72.5	902	1,198	8.4	25,884	164,360	216,528	380,888	79	5,335
Oakland	28	5,063	207,092	1,269,752	1,641,426	68.7	3,479	4,497	6.1	119,413	832,149	2,189,751	3,021,900	432	35,734
Oxnard-Ventura	8	1,427	50,717	331,013	433,689	63.6	907	1,187	6.5	36,437	175,155	273,282	448,437	133	11,044
Redding	3	455	17,079	117,898	150,636	71.2	324	413	6.9	11,502	62,466	40,506	102,972	22	2,216
Riverside-San Bernardino	32	5,653	245,911	1,308,218	1,706,945	63.4	3,582	4,675	5.3	144,406	682,663	1,377,418	2,060,081	386	46,164
Sacramento	17	3,621	151,721	945,722	1,175,206	71.6	2,593	3,221	6.2	96,271	399,570	1,232,913	1,632,483	297	25,825
Salinas-Seaside-Monterey	4	600	28,243	147,306	198,578	67.3	404	544	5.2	16,610	74,192	178,238	252,430	80	5,899
San Diego	25	6,247	237,446	1,525,700	1,900,389	66.9	4,180	5,205	6.4	164,588	541,530	1,222,734	1,764,264	334	45,686
San Francisco	23	5,520	200,302	1,370,880	1,791,294	68.1	3,758	4,907	6.8	135,075	579,949	2,606,242	3,186,191	317	22,972
San Jose	14	3,485	149,880	884,245	1,147,128	69.5	2,422	3,142	5.9	88,219	378,277	898,018	1,276,295	360	31,883
Santa Barbara-Santa Maria-Lompoc	8	1,031	33,432	240,940	318,623	64.1	661	873	7.2	25,334	92,293	156,883	249,176	89	6,560
Santa Cruz	2	392	16,790	94,001	119,810	65.8	258	329	5.6	11,314	47,164	68,795	115,959	38	3,247
Santa Rosa-Petaluma	8	804	34,859	180,243	231,438	61.4	494	634	5.2	20,628	100,042	232,338	332,380	46	5,658
Stockton	7	1,023	45,152	244,606	341,992	65.5	670	938	5.4	30,301	178,877	501,846	680,723	98	9,124
Vallejo-Fairfield-Napa	7	1,495	40,290	401,899	473,500	73.6	1,100	1,297	10.0	26,384	174,024	556,721	730,745	61	6,385
Visalia-Tulare-Porterville	7	648	28,040	168,911	228,124	71.3	462	625	6.0	18,852	93,110	125,713	218,823	60	6,611
Yuba City	2	252	12,409	62,292	81,037	67.9	171	222	5.0	9,026	31,762	43,278	75,040	16	2,218
Hawaii	18	2,887	95,958	896,665	1,126,889	85.1	2,456	3,089	9.3	61,624	221,875	1,560,500	1,782,375	221	16,462
Nonmetropolitan	9	786	25,264	227,950	263,103	79.4	624	721	9.0	15,450	64,448	77,110	141,558	76	4,453
Metropolitan	9	2,101	70,694	668,715	863,786	87.2	1,832	2,368	9.5	46,174	157,427	1,483,390	1,640,817	145	12,009
Honolulu	9	2,101	70,694	668,715	863,786	87.2	1,832	2,368	9.5	46,174	157,427	1,483,390	1,640,817	145	12,009
Oregon	70	8,073	301,903	1,671,563	2,392,458	56.8	4,584	6,553	5.5	245,758	938,469	2,474,826	3,413,295	715	42,796
Nonmetropolitan	37	2,581	81,175	485,801	744,382	51.6	1,333	2,039	6.0	66,672	322,574	625,843	948,417	293	11,253
Metropolitan	33	5,492	220,728	1,185,762	1,648,076	59.2	3,251	4,514	5.4	179,086	615,895	1,848,983	2,464,878	422	31,543
Eugene-Springfield	5	698	29,668	167,579	227,956	65.9	460	625	5.6	20,638	79,097	172,553	251,650	47	3,854
Medford	3	519	16,497	94,201	129,847	49.7	258	355	5.7	15,518	45,289	120,793	166,082	28	2,169
Portland	21	3,742	151,856	811,726	1,134,534	59.5	2,225	3,107	5.3	128,035	421,917	1,486,289	1,908,206	293	21,660
Salem	4	533	22,707	112,256	155,739	57.8	308	427	4.9	14,895	69,592	69,348	138,940	54	3,860
Washington	91	11,915	491,518	2,726,362	3,747,213	62.7	7,465	10,275	5.5	379,456	1,570,855	3,330,164	4,901,019	975	70,643
Nonmetropolitan	39	2,422	73,312	438,218	672,735	49.6	1,201	1,848	6.0	55,516	271,106	571,699	842,805	255	10,584
Metropolitan	52	9,493	418,206	2,288,144	3,074,478	66.0	6,264	8,427	5.5	323,940	1,299,749	2,758,465	4,058,214	720	60,059
Bellingham	1	211	10,191	50,274	70,532	65.4	138	193	4.9	6,859	40,124	16,412	56,536	24	1,632
Bremerton	1	244	13,171	65,013	76,951	73.0	178	211	4.9	7,495	31,745	16,511	48,256	28	1,948
Olympia	2	463	17,457	93,889	126,322	55.5	257	346	5.4	13,651	43,734	92,972	136,706	35	2,103
Richland-Kennewick-Pasco	4	385	12,469	59,237	96,801	42.1	162	265	4.8	10,542	81,099	86,443	167,542	50	2,989
Seattle	24	4,756	225,644	1,238,838	1,641,489	71.3	3,392	4,500	5.5	178,977	657,148	1,762,644	2,419,792	347	31,585
Spokane	6	1,359	49,177	304,717	383,935	61.4	834	1,052	6.2	37,084	120,061	127,683	247,744	69	5,722
Tacoma	8	1,253	54,647	297,598	414,425	65.0	814	1,136	5.4	43,535	160,294	395,207	555,501	88	7,806
Vancouver	1	290	13,455	72,003	106,446	67.9	197	292	5.4	10,943	49,924	57,593	107,517	35	2,546
Yakima	5	532	21,995	106,575	157,577	54.9	292	432	4.8	14,854	115,620	203,000	318,620	44	3,728

CLASSIFICATION	Full-Time Equivalent Personnel: Physicians and Dentists	Registered Nurses	Licensed Practical Nurses	Other Salaried Personnel	Total Personnel	Full-Time Equivalent Trainees: Medical and Dental Residents	Other Trainees	Total Trainees	Expenses, Labor: Payroll (in thousands)	Employee Benefits (in thousands)	Total (in thousands)	Percent of Total	Expenses, Total: Amount (in thousands)	Adjusted, per Admission	Adjusted, per Inpatient Day
CENSUS DIVISION 9, PACIFIC	**4,755**	**102,745**	**15,734**	**285,527**	**408,761**	**5,902**	**441**	**6,343**	**$12,373,461**	**$ 2,784,761**	**$15,158,221**	**52.9**	**$ 28,630,179**	**$5,462.70**	**$ 904.86**
Nonmetropolitan	58	6,988	1,430	20,514	28,990	2	3	5	728,957	156,826	885,783	53.5	1,655,274	3,789.63	614.99
Metropolitan	4,697	95,757	14,304	265,013	379,771	5,900	438	6,338	11,644,504	2,627,934	14,272,438	52.9	26,974,905	5,614.81	931.81
Alaska	**16**	**1,092**	**91**	**2,581**	**3,780**	**0**	**0**	**0**	**137,102**	**30,547**	**167,649**	**52.7**	**318,243**	**6,249.37**	**1,069.68**
Nonmetropolitan	16	360	49	1,016	1,441	0	0	0	50,263	11,267	61,531	56.8	108,321	4,915.63	825.02
Metropolitan	0	732	42	1,565	2,339	0	0	0	86,838	19,280	106,118	50.6	209,922	7,266.76	1,262.94
Anchorage	0	732	42	1,565	2,339	0	0	0	86,838	19,280	106,118	50.6	209,922	7,266.76	1,262.94
California	**3,400**	**76,175**	**12,536**	**218,445**	**310,556**	**5,038**	**392**	**5,430**	**9,671,480**	**2,241,375**	**11,912,854**	**52.7**	**22,617,379**	**5,708.83**	**939.40**
Nonmetropolitan	4	2,258	487	7,079	9,828	0	0	0	246,292	60,639	306,931	50.9	603,077	4,024.41	685.30
Metropolitan	3,396	73,917	12,049	211,366	300,728	5,038	392	5,430	9,425,188	2,180,736	11,605,923	52.7	22,014,301	5,775.05	949.04
Anaheim-Santa Ana	20	6,680	704	15,533	22,937	273	9	282	721,913	178,777	900,691	49.3	1,825,425	5,826.09	1,117.41
Bakersfield	54	1,024	361	3,933	5,372	85	0	85	149,062	37,578	186,640	55.5	336,397	5,126.52	923.47
Chico	0	715	211	1,722	2,648	0	0	0	72,594	16,345	88,939	55.5	160,307	5,107.12	820.37
Fresno	0	1,726	329	5,849	7,904	134	0	134	205,637	56,158	261,795	53.8	486,699	5,001.02	939.98
Los Angeles-Long Beach	1,845	24,694	4,113	75,021	105,673	2,204	212	2,416	3,398,611	762,776	4,161,387	52.4	7,941,278	6,155.97	990.81
Merced	0	284	95	878	1,257	18	4	22	31,417	8,133	39,550	52.1	75,926	3,948.53	815.53
Modesto	0	1,321	262	2,595	4,178	21	42	63	83,714	26,167	109,881	48.5	226,440	4,343.84	517.52
Oakland	141	4,855	781	13,864	19,641	230	31	261	685,844	161,815	847,660	55.1	1,537,085	5,710.12	936.43
Oxnard-Ventura	0	1,162	169	3,369	4,700	37	0	37	125,850	30,782	156,632	49.0	319,697	4,798.81	737.16
Redding	1	696	136	1,126	1,959	11	0	11	51,439	11,441	62,880	50.2	125,185	5,834.76	831.04
Riverside-San Bernardino	610	6,158	1,069	16,215	24,052	492	21	513	676,278	148,649	824,927	51.5	1,602,275	4,954.07	938.68
Sacramento	159	4,460	539	10,233	15,391	374	9	383	463,324	120,880	584,204	54.4	1,073,363	5,682.72	913.34
Salinas-Seaside-Monterey	33	652	131	2,058	2,874	34	2	36	86,765	20,562	107,326	55.5	193,297	5,081.69	973.41
San Diego	75	5,825	717	16,151	22,768	176	3	179	705,307	152,367	857,674	52.2	1,643,544	5,545.13	864.85
San Francisco	286	5,715	651	16,918	23,570	568	50	618	837,930	182,678	1,020,607	55.2	1,849,409	7,083.36	1,032.44
San Jose	118	3,396	581	12,398	16,493	241	0	241	564,397	117,522	681,919	52.6	1,295,712	6,625.08	1,129.53
Santa Barbara-Santa Maria-Lompoc	3	858	162	2,383	3,406	44	0	44	96,314	25,820	122,134	52.5	232,737	5,382.32	730.45
Santa Cruz	3	338	45	1,025	1,411	2	0	2	42,599	15,960	58,559	57.3	102,239	4,752.67	853.35
Santa Rosa-Petaluma	18	606	154	1,884	2,662	34	0	34	89,722	22,295	112,016	51.4	217,814	4,760.55	941.13
Stockton	1	1,072	367	3,076	4,516	55	9	64	130,755	31,602	162,357	55.8	291,019	4,638.42	850.95
Vallejo-Fairfield-Napa	27	838	156	2,821	3,842	5	0	5	116,347	31,891	148,238	53.8	275,611	5,012.58	582.07
Visalia-Tulare-Porterville	1	636	208	1,816	2,661	0	0	0	66,970	14,663	81,633	54.9	148,650	3,895.85	651.62
Yuba City	1	206	108	498	813	0	0	0	22,400	5,874	28,274	52.2	54,190	3,410.10	668.71
Hawaii	**26**	**2,667**	**497**	**8,988**	**12,178**	**28**	**7**	**35**	**313,353**	**61,641**	**374,994**	**52.2**	**718,524**	**6,048.48**	**637.62**
Nonmetropolitan	1	520	175	1,570	2,266	0	0	0	58,348	9,697	68,045	52.5	129,582	4,582.90	492.51
Metropolitan	25	2,147	322	7,418	9,912	28	7	35	255,005	51,945	306,950	52.1	588,942	6,506.28	681.81
Honolulu	25	2,147	322	7,418	9,912	28	7	35	255,005	51,945	306,950	52.1	588,942	6,506.28	681.81
Oregon	**570**	**9,493**	**888**	**22,056**	**33,007**	**387**	**9**	**396**	**866,310**	**183,880**	**1,050,190**	**54.9**	**1,912,802**	**4,431.64**	**799.51**
Nonmetropolitan	25	2,208	315	5,985	8,533	0	3	3	198,756	41,749	240,505	56.0	429,329	3,456.84	576.76
Metropolitan	545	7,285	573	16,071	24,474	387	6	393	667,554	142,131	809,685	54.6	1,483,473	4,825.45	900.12
Eugene-Springfield	2	762	89	2,077	2,930	0	0	0	77,235	17,116	94,351	52.6	179,223	4,484.83	786.22
Medford	14	522	67	1,442	2,045	0	0	0	50,964	10,513	61,477	60.2	102,125	4,447.19	786.51
Portland	526	5,239	292	11,110	17,167	387	6	393	479,983	102,979	582,962	53.7	1,085,132	5,099.57	956.46
Salem	3	762	125	1,442	2,332	0	0	0	59,372	11,523	70,895	60.6	116,993	3,689.24	751.21
Washington	**743**	**13,318**	**1,722**	**33,457**	**49,240**	**449**	**33**	**482**	**1,385,216**	**267,318**	**1,652,534**	**53.9**	**3,063,232**	**4,518.91**	**817.47**
Nonmetropolitan	12	1,642	404	4,864	6,922	2	0	2	175,297	33,475	208,772	54.2	384,966	3,424.11	572.24
Metropolitan	731	11,676	1,318	28,593	42,318	447	33	480	1,209,919	233,844	1,443,762	53.9	2,678,267	4,736.60	871.13
Bellingham	0	271	20	572	863	0	0	0	25,232	4,684	29,915	50.4	59,329	4,149.73	841.16
Bremerton	0	247	63	442	752	0	20	20	21,284	4,587	25,872	57.5	44,957	2,883.91	584.23
Olympia	1	590	81	1,215	1,887	0	0	0	46,740	9,267	56,007	54.0	103,741	4,405.90	821.25
Richland-Kennewick-Pasco	0	299	46	809	1,154	0	0	0	31,143	5,893	37,035	51.1	72,436	3,480.98	748.29
Seattle	676	6,856	322	16,074	23,928	384	13	397	668,688	130,698	799,386	52.6	1,519,761	5,053.19	925.84
Spokane	20	1,430	331	3,140	4,921	46	0	46	162,439	29,663	192,102	58.0	331,129	5,342.16	862.46
Tacoma	25	1,084	270	4,143	5,527	17	0	17	165,636	32,667	198,303	55.5	357,551	4,696.71	862.76
Vancouver	4	339	36	664	1,043	0	0	0	36,151	6,679	42,830	57.8	74,145	3,727.55	696.55
Yakima	5	560	149	1,523	2,243	0	0	0	52,606	9,707	62,312	54.1	115,218	3,551.30	731.19

Table
7

Utilization, Personnel, and Finances in Community Hospitals, for the 100 Largest Central Cities

City rank is based on *1980 Census of Population for Cities of 100,000 and Over by Rank Order* (final counts as published in 1980 Census Advance Reports by State, Series PH030-V). Figures for Nashville-Davidson include the city of Nashville and the County of Davidson, Tennessee. Virginia Beach is consolidated with Princess Anne County, Virginia.

CLASSIFICATION	HOSPITALS	BEDS	ADMISSIONS	INPATIENT DAYS	ADJUSTED PATIENT DAYS	OCCUPANCY, percent	AVERAGE DAILY CENSUS	ADJUSTED AVERAGE DAILY CENSUS	AVERAGE STAY, days	SURGICAL OPERATIONS	OUTPATIENT VISITS			NEWBORNS	
											Emergency	Other	Total	Bassinets	Births
New York, NY	64	34,148	1,062,116	11,040,115	13,784,477	88.6	30,246	37,763	10.4	589,192	3,016,869	11,771,358	14,788,227	1,769	138,379
Chicago, IL	43	13,199	433,258	3,489,232	4,296,322	72.5	9,569	11,780	8.1	261,514	1,121,105	4,129,346	5,250,451	890	55,738
Los Angeles, CA	51	12,630	480,581	3,020,532	3,824,124	65.5	8,278	10,482	6.3	294,691	1,085,121	2,884,275	3,969,396	867	91,811
Philadelphia, PA	37	10,357	349,085	2,968,355	3,764,980	78.5	8,131	10,314	8.5	246,979	839,306	2,500,121	3,339,427	487	33,391
Houston, TX	33	10,431	332,806	2,294,294	2,898,651	60.2	6,284	7,942	6.9	238,537	589,554	1,857,602	2,447,156	654	51,595
Detroit, MI	18	5,938	199,552	1,535,229	2,050,923	70.9	4,208	5,619	7.7	143,435	707,939	3,202,210	3,910,149	420	32,013
Dallas, TX	24	5,698	211,753	1,335,537	1,675,553	64.3	3,664	4,598	6.3	136,917	461,144	1,240,061	1,701,205	434	35,015
San Diego, CA	14	3,678	139,027	893,945	1,124,888	66.6	2,448	3,081	6.4	109,585	261,583	910,535	1,172,118	178	23,465
Phoenix, AZ	14	3,732	152,304	873,436	1,088,481	64.1	2,393	2,985	5.7	101,488	334,995	719,039	1,054,034	270	25,149
Baltimore, MD	20	6,785	267,129	2,034,096	2,606,038	82.1	5,572	7,140	7.6	229,050	579,276	1,740,213	2,319,489	350	31,672
San Antonio, TX	16	4,245	141,978	953,681	1,189,032	61.5	2,612	3,258	6.7	112,650	353,985	637,282	991,267	297	21,562
Indianapolis, IN	9	4,264	152,370	1,103,683	1,435,610	70.9	3,024	3,934	7.2	130,094	347,469	1,219,507	1,566,976	254	17,236
San Francisco, CA	13	3,374	125,203	858,854	1,103,702	69.8	2,355	3,023	6.9	75,846	335,893	1,409,797	1,745,690	207	14,919
Memphis, TN	10	4,814	158,241	1,332,208	1,551,773	75.8	3,649	4,252	8.4	105,531	336,162	475,115	811,277	233	18,881
Washington, DC	11	4,557	157,832	1,252,183	1,514,470	75.3	3,431	4,149	7.9	118,590	384,105	887,932	1,272,037	312	20,664
San Jose, CA	6	1,930	79,323	494,798	635,166	70.2	1,355	1,740	6.2	41,733	246,188	535,633	781,821	192	17,674
Milwaukee, WI	13	3,697	149,610	1,003,177	1,288,854	74.4	2,751	3,533	6.7	101,927	315,323	1,027,123	1,342,446	273	17,342
Cleveland, OH	14	5,606	182,577	1,447,431	1,804,229	70.7	3,965	4,944	7.9	120,328	506,779	1,956,350	2,463,129	298	18,601
Columbus, OH	7	3,889	159,101	1,074,470	1,356,642	75.7	2,945	3,716	6.8	108,625	430,953	1,004,792	1,435,745	176	16,667
Boston, MA	18	5,763	226,052	1,663,725	2,151,544	79.1	4,560	5,896	7.4	162,567	477,730	2,235,890	2,713,620	285	22,152
New Orleans, LA	17	3,969	119,263	889,496	1,076,698	61.4	2,437	2,950	7.5	74,153	356,635	1,067,771	1,424,406	201	12,663
Jacksonville, FL	9	2,565	97,731	659,521	848,362	70.5	1,808	2,324	6.7	72,287	260,359	411,435	671,794	172	12,909
Seattle, WA	11	3,060	134,793	818,299	1,056,433	73.3	2,242	2,895	6.1	103,395	309,501	1,409,014	1,718,515	161	14,128
Denver, CO	11	3,976	130,095	1,015,652	1,300,803	70.0	2,783	3,564	7.8	109,570	277,735	1,151,789	1,429,524	200	18,430
Nashville-Davidson, TN	11	3,767	141,167	927,142	1,137,161	67.4	2,540	3,116	6.6	90,039	311,514	720,743	1,032,257	236	11,917
St. Louis, MO	20	7,654	239,973	1,871,695	2,428,762	67.0	5,127	6,655	7.8	177,351	578,595	1,371,665	1,950,260	418	25,639
Kansas City, MO	12	3,243	99,413	790,166	986,723	66.9	2,170	2,711	7.9	76,827	206,443	818,085	1,024,528	169	13,163
El Paso, TX	7	1,721	66,148	391,869	484,517	62.3	1,072	1,328	5.9	35,096	147,404	117,198	264,602	153	14,124
Atlanta, GA	15	4,823	190,929	1,296,521	1,640,873	73.7	3,554	4,495	6.8	119,955	479,183	957,516	1,436,699	384	25,992
Pittsburgh, PA	20	6,671	231,472	1,883,826	2,322,219	77.3	5,159	6,360	8.1	175,927	549,725	1,876,366	2,426,091	278	18,420
Oklahoma City, OK	10	3,112	108,907	776,398	932,842	68.4	2,128	2,556	7.1	80,843	220,355	439,969	660,324	223	11,960
Cincinnati, OH	13	4,594	167,332	1,188,230	1,563,096	70.9	3,255	4,284	7.1	137,956	442,703	967,195	1,409,898	272	21,379
Fort Worth, TX	10	2,283	91,056	544,059	715,107	65.3	1,491	1,958	6.0	50,643	254,141	567,578	821,719	259	15,268
Minneapolis, MN	7	3,643	142,521	916,538	1,176,861	68.9	2,511	3,224	6.4	103,446	280,922	982,421	1,263,343	213	16,760
Portland, OR	12	2,864	113,114	641,842	881,039	61.5	1,760	2,413	5.7	93,083	264,341	1,215,824	1,480,165	219	16,204
Honolulu, HI	6	1,757	61,214	567,238	726,863	88.4	1,554	1,993	9.3	39,498	126,024	1,404,174	1,530,198	106	10,575
Long Beach, CA	8	2,135	72,720	484,700	596,540	62.2	1,328	1,636	6.7	44,036	160,667	566,520	727,187	170	15,444
Tulsa, OK	6	2,429	81,682	616,729	727,038	69.5	1,689	1,992	7.6	57,501	133,280	274,825	408,105	127	10,343
Buffalo, NY	9	3,789	115,306	1,224,338	1,597,640	88.5	3,355	4,378	10.6	98,081	293,361	887,888	1,181,249	261	14,675
Toledo, OH	6	2,112	77,855	536,014	690,536	69.6	1,469	1,892	6.9	59,105	228,942	459,340	688,282	115	9,007
Miami, FL	16	5,108	175,100	1,263,647	1,539,347	67.8	3,462	4,216	7.2	106,934	364,135	714,877	1,079,012	317	27,383
Austin, TX	6	1,461	69,912	386,350	462,333	72.9	1,065	1,278	5.5	39,932	144,441	282,238	426,679	115	12,844
Oakland, CA	7	1,296	61,030	347,381	451,009	73.5	952	1,235	5.7	34,482	214,938	382,113	597,051	116	11,063
Albuquerque, NM	10	1,844	71,368	417,728	600,331	62.0	1,144	1,644	5.9	62,425	152,676	1,039,708	1,192,384	137	10,432
Tucson, AZ	8	1,980	85,482	469,640	595,002	65.0	1,287	1,629	5.5	46,508	184,803	457,230	642,033	150	11,592
Newark, NJ	6	2,238	80,482	654,035	800,470	80.1	1,792	2,193	8.1	41,993	188,148	483,142	671,290	131	8,707
Charlotte, NC	6	2,014	72,658	542,177	703,241	73.8	1,486	1,927	7.5	65,250	186,793	240,693	427,486	136	12,255
Omaha, NE	9	3,101	75,353	741,037	917,209	65.5	2,030	2,512	9.8	77,744	146,451	393,985	540,436	148	9,135
Louisville, KY	11	3,488	127,239	872,929	1,083,790	68.5	2,391	2,969	6.9	111,155	295,949	579,038	874,987	207	14,212
Birmingham, AL	12	3,975	147,344	1,015,974	1,209,761	70.0	2,782	3,315	6.9	101,756	247,312	927,524	1,174,836	301	13,345

CLASSIFICATION	FULL-TIME EQUIVALENT PERSONNEL: Physicians and Dentists	Registered Nurses	Licensed Practical Nurses	Other Salaried Personnel	Total Personnel	FULL-TIME EQUIVALENT TRAINEES: Medical and Dental Residents	Other Trainees	Total Trainees
New York, NY	7,016	32,407	4,071	114,863	158,357	10,641	251	10,892
Chicago, IL	1,200	12,666	1,733	43,698	59,297	2,628	80	2,708
Los Angeles, CA	1,283	11,920	1,706	38,175	53,084	1,615	152	1,767
Philadelphia, PA	1,236	10,850	1,240	33,703	47,029	2,413	87	2,500
Houston, TX	305	8,814	2,333	28,924	40,376	349	411	760
Detroit, MI	1,212	5,736	1,073	20,623	28,644	1,022	159	1,181
Dallas, TX	97	5,974	717	16,577	23,365	1,064	10	1,074
San Diego, CA	73	3,517	370	9,996	13,956	174	3	177
Phoenix, AZ	102	3,902	461	9,739	14,204	474	0	474
Baltimore, MD	529	8,121	637	23,210	32,497	956	55	1,011
San Antonio, TX	5	3,529	1,780	10,445	15,759	368	45	413
Indianapolis, IN	95	5,623	846	16,176	22,740	477	59	536
San Francisco, CA	134	3,437	444	11,541	15,556	564	40	604
Memphis, TN	34	3,932	988	13,687	18,641	211	171	382
Washington, DC	634	5,036	547	14,055	20,272	1,062	33	1,095
San Jose, CA	75	1,766	267	5,823	7,937	159	0	159
Milwaukee, WI	57	4,475	190	11,283	16,011	192	88	280
Cleveland, OH	490	5,849	733	18,271	25,346	1,612	111	1,723
Columbus, OH	129	4,345	340	13,815	18,630	967	11	978
Boston, MA	2,217	8,282	387	26,967	37,853	2,560	62	2,622
New Orleans, LA	82	3,364	773	11,372	15,591	915	12	927
Jacksonville, FL	2	2,922	317	7,497	10,738	268	39	307
Seattle, WA	497	4,527	156	10,837	16,017	367	13	380
Denver, CO	973	3,968	324	11,382	16,647	200	19	219
Nashville-Davidson, TN	44	4,160	953	10,513	15,675	286	13	299
St. Louis, MO	416	7,505	976	22,436	31,333	932	31	963
Kansas City, MO	93	2,737	435	9,633	12,904	227	1	228
El Paso, TX	0	1,138	259	4,275	5,673	0	3	3
Atlanta, GA	99	5,335	611	15,583	21,628	707	22	729
Pittsburgh, PA	491	8,318	876	22,155	31,841	1,229	0	1,229
Oklahoma City, OK	19	2,825	877	9,655	13,376	499	40	539
Cincinnati, OH	182	4,888	651	14,503	20,224	614	27	641
Fort Worth, TX	18	2,788	709	6,813	10,328	137	0	137
Minneapolis, MN	73	5,024	324	11,271	16,692	223	31	254
Portland, OR	326	4,104	224	9,098	13,752	387	2	389
Honolulu, HI	24	1,888	269	6,587	8,768	28	7	35
Long Beach, CA	185	1,904	281	5,043	7,413	72	34	106
Tulsa, OK	24	2,030	282	7,801	10,137	16	82	98
Buffalo, NY	390	3,753	551	11,266	15,960	212	6	218
Toledo, OH	25	2,638	362	7,252	10,277	345	18	363
Miami, FL	203	5,840	664	14,193	20,900	536	0	536
Austin, TX	7	1,528	314	3,742	5,591	0	8	8
Oakland, CA	98	1,437	211	3,940	5,686	194	0	194
Albuquerque, NM	4	1,727	362	5,725	7,818	4	3	7
Tucson, AZ	9	2,181	276	5,860	8,326	4	0	4
Newark, NJ	436	2,124	316	6,405	9,281	234	31	265
Charlotte, NC	114	2,394	203	6,837	9,548	135	0	135
Omaha, NE	30	2,357	393	8,079	10,859	351	0	351
Louisville, KY	10	3,480	446	9,553	13,489	12	15	27
Birmingham, AL	653	4,043	833	11,659	17,228	563	0	563

CLASSIFICATION	EXPENSES — LABOR: Payroll (in thousands)	Employee Benefits (in thousands)	Total (in thousands)	Percent of Total	EXPENSES — TOTAL: Amount (in thousands)	Adjusted, per Admission	Adjusted, per Inpatient Day
New York, NY	$ 5,565,147	$ 1,135,380	$ 6,700,526	60.1	$ 11,150,814	$8,338.90	$ 808.94
Chicago, IL	1,743,097	296,031	2,039,128	54.4	3,746,843	7,011.52	872.10
Los Angeles, CA	1,704,149	383,005	2,087,154	52.7	3,963,092	6,486.65	1,036.34
Philadelphia, PA	1,467,712	285,301	1,753,013	55.0	3,188,735	7,299.57	846.95
Houston, TX	1,132,805	246,016	1,378,821	49.8	2,766,253	6,571.50	954.32
Detroit, MI	730,169	150,173	880,341	49.8	1,766,465	6,582.96	861.30
Dallas, TX	565,948	95,677	661,624	47.1	1,405,743	5,243.28	838.97
San Diego, CA	436,592	90,886	527,478	51.4	1,026,596	5,872.20	912.62
Phoenix, AZ	432,352	82,395	514,747	46.3	1,112,689	5,831.67	1,022.24
Baltimore, MD	908,422	169,349	1,077,771	56.1	1,922,555	5,596.08	737.73
San Antonio, TX	373,887	61,390	435,277	49.3	883,065	4,972.27	742.68
Indianapolis, IN	533,722	105,629	639,351	52.2	1,224,854	6,167.50	853.19
San Francisco, CA	582,902	120,879	703,781	55.7	1,262,797	7,859.67	1,144.15
Memphis, TN	455,427	83,482	538,909	50.7	1,063,242	5,696.45	685.18
Washington, DC	709,635	127,011	836,646	55.5	1,507,467	7,875.55	995.38
San Jose, CA	290,175	57,812	347,987	54.6	637,874	6,237.40	1,004.26
Milwaukee, WI	442,110	83,525	525,635	54.0	972,812	5,042.26	754.79
Cleveland, OH	722,594	154,883	877,477	57.7	1,519,795	6,703.04	842.35
Columbus, OH	496,164	115,648	611,812	54.7	1,118,406	5,561.02	824.39
Boston, MA	1,169,736	239,002	1,408,738	52.7	2,674,939	9,031.37	1,243.26
New Orleans, LA	382,161	67,130	449,291	46.8	960,397	6,598.67	891.98
Jacksonville, FL	279,338	66,323	345,661	48.8	708,105	5,609.64	834.67
Seattle, WA	441,229	87,861	529,090	52.5	1,007,580	5,791.59	953.76
Denver, CO	498,487	90,818	589,305	53.9	1,092,317	6,548.39	839.73
Nashville-Davidson, TN	391,161	84,414	475,574	48.9	972,161	5,560.32	854.90
St. Louis, MO	818,804	143,476	962,279	51.1	1,883,667	6,041.89	775.57
Kansas City, MO	360,387	63,202	423,589	54.4	779,009	6,286.74	789.49
El Paso, TX	131,216	28,417	159,632	48.6	328,717	4,017.91	678.44
Atlanta, GA	611,987	113,155	725,143	51.9	1,397,243	5,710.00	851.52
Pittsburgh, PA	846,861	169,214	1,016,075	50.9	1,995,947	6,925.39	859.50
Oklahoma City, OK	307,130	58,262	365,393	50.4	724,588	5,537.04	776.75
Cincinnati, OH	540,741	109,025	649,766	52.1	1,246,528	5,637.69	797.47
Fort Worth, TX	261,139	54,348	315,488	49.4	638,151	5,301.75	892.39
Minneapolis, MN	563,061	107,909	670,970	55.0	1,220,085	6,660.47	1,036.73
Portland, OR	403,558	87,660	491,217	54.6	900,433	5,802.62	1,022.01
Honolulu, HI	223,707	44,879	268,586	51.3	523,348	6,714.07	720.01
Long Beach, CA	246,507	49,165	295,672	53.1	557,090	6,204.64	933.87
Tulsa, OK	220,836	39,779	260,615	50.6	514,927	5,353.23	708.25
Buffalo, NY	378,804	65,135	443,939	54.9	808,803	5,369.76	506.25
Toledo, OH	275,827	66,408	342,235	55.7	614,235	6,089.74	889.51
Miami, FL	585,767	156,019	741,786	53.2	1,394,561	6,402.47	905.94
Austin, TX	150,355	26,018	176,372	50.2	351,512	4,190.50	760.30
Oakland, CA	203,478	53,815	257,293	54.5	472,216	5,915.56	1,047.02
Albuquerque, NM	203,325	43,969	247,294	46.1	536,221	5,173.39	893.21
Tucson, AZ	218,224	39,519	257,743	50.1	514,299	4,730.66	864.36
Newark, NJ	303,026	67,896	370,922	58.1	637,985	6,502.03	797.01
Charlotte, NC	254,063	48,702	302,766	54.5	555,928	5,851.75	790.52
Omaha, NE	252,722	51,291	304,012	48.9	622,117	6,730.61	678.27
Louisville, KY	322,650	64,939	387,589	48.4	800,836	5,072.69	738.92
Birmingham, AL	403,495	80,765	484,260	48.2	1,004,943	5,646.99	830.70

(continued on next page)

Table

7

(Continued)

Utilization, Personnel, and Finances in Community Hospitals, for the 100 Largest Central Cities

City rank is based on *1980 Census of Population for Cities of 100,000 and Over by Rank Order* (final counts as published in 1980 Census Advance Reports by State, Series PH030-V). Figures for Nashville-Davidson include the city of Nashville and the County of Davidson, Tennessee. Virginia Beach is consolidated with Princess Anne County, Virginia.

CLASSIFICATION	HOSPITALS	BEDS	ADMISSIONS	INPATIENT DAYS	ADJUSTED PATIENT DAYS	OCCUPANCY, percent	AVERAGE DAILY CENSUS	ADJUSTED AVERAGE DAILY CENSUS	AVERAGE STAY, days	SURGICAL OPERATIONS	OUTPATIENT VISITS			NEWBORNS	
											Emergency	Other	Total	Bassinets	Births
Wichita, KS	4	1,857	68,622	471,121	594,162	69.5	1,290	1,627	6.9	40,572	127,076	307,925	435,001	107	8,712
Sacramento, CA	7	2,410	101,048	659,816	800,196	75.0	1,808	2,193	6.5	60,122	208,047	944,882	1,152,929	178	16,991
Tampa, FL	10	2,599	85,867	618,016	757,229	65.2	1,694	2,075	7.2	53,622	171,215	300,667	471,882	117	12,648
St. Paul, MN	5	997	43,101	259,437	341,128	71.2	710	934	6.0	27,258	135,148	398,449	533,597	60	4,129
Norfolk, VA	5	1,460	56,627	398,417	505,140	74.9	1,093	1,384	7.0	45,893	118,843	289,488	408,331	100	7,997
Virginia Beach, VA	2	480	19,788	115,009	150,642	65.6	315	413	5.8	11,226	71,626	84,330	155,956	46	2,912
Rochester, NY	7	3,002	86,308	986,796	1,235,386	90.1	2,704	3,385	11.4	65,192	215,529	933,687	1,149,216	169	13,592
Akron, OH	5	1,827	67,634	492,823	634,795	73.9	1,350	1,739	7.3	44,863	191,501	582,063	773,564	103	7,280
St. Petersburg, FL	8	2,111	57,972	421,661	513,604	54.8	1,156	1,407	7.3	38,394	152,419	379,762	532,181	64	5,167
Corpus Christi, TX	8	1,379	47,256	305,609	391,507	63.5	875	1,123	6.5	38,270	86,068	195,867	281,935	125	6,993
Jersey City, NJ	4	1,189	42,803	347,213	442,260	80.0	951	1,212	8.1	18,583	127,269	295,700	422,969	57	4,415
Anaheim, CA	6	1,099	37,601	211,786	270,213	52.8	580	741	5.6	21,273	121,249	80,752	202,001	105	8,715
Baton Rouge, LA	7	1,751	58,752	377,414	475,681	59.1	1,035	1,303	6.4	37,424	132,940	225,966	358,906	99	8,697
Richmond, VA	13	3,523	123,855	863,636	1,069,890	67.2	2,366	2,932	7.0	84,359	288,569	638,501	927,070	185	14,293
Fresno, CA	5	1,301	62,864	347,111	464,225	73.0	950	1,272	5.5	47,238	203,217	490,567	693,784	88	12,714
Colorado Springs, CO	2	1,006	35,004	215,801	274,549	58.7	591	753	6.2	24,859	91,971	167,993	259,964	70	5,673
Shreveport, LA	7	1,850	61,512	404,726	527,103	59.9	1,109	1,443	6.6	34,359	172,588	764,408	936,996	116	6,191
Lexington-Fayette, KY	7	1,779	60,959	433,395	519,002	66.8	1,189	1,423	7.1	51,705	112,102	393,830	505,932	95	6,361
Santa Ana, CA	4	589	24,621	99,441	126,692	46.3	273	347	4.0	17,632	41,608	108,969	150,577	53	6,142
Dayton, OH	5	2,374	80,175	582,888	743,675	67.3	1,598	2,039	7.3	73,106	206,272	759,375	965,647	123	9,411
Jackson, MS	8	2,363	83,247	563,803	676,020	65.3	1,544	1,852	6.8	50,461	154,424	227,623	382,047	130	9,697
Mobile, AL	7	1,883	64,427	436,946	521,319	63.6	1,198	1,428	6.8	45,641	112,555	363,844	476,399	170	7,614
Yonkers, NY	3	639	22,925	192,224	257,565	82.3	526	706	8.4	16,046	66,996	322,535	389,531	28	1,829
Des Moines, IA	6	2,029	68,607	530,864	690,144	71.7	1,454	1,890	7.7	48,188	155,198	498,069	653,267	121	6,793
Knoxville, TN	7	2,120	87,762	588,899	722,875	76.2	1,615	1,981	6.7	78,566	170,331	287,564	457,895	89	7,418
Grand Rapids, MI	6	1,950	64,458	513,286	666,649	72.2	1,408	1,826	8.0	57,327	144,639	330,562	475,201	206	11,388
Montgomery, AL	4	1,000	38,106	221,788	269,490	60.8	608	738	5.8	24,638	78,573	92,967	171,540	77	5,444
Lubbock, TX	6	1,562	49,684	361,408	424,056	63.3	989	1,161	7.3	38,073	88,854	143,243	232,097	346	5,630
Anchorage, AK	2	579	18,741	107,770	133,145	50.9	295	365	5.8	13,088	59,741	158,523	218,264	42	3,711
Fort Wayne, IN	3	1,347	47,448	319,899	388,954	65.0	876	1,066	6.7	45,450	79,114	396,039	475,153	103	6,289
Lincoln, NE	3	742	26,745	174,387	220,713	64.4	478	605	6.5	24,484	55,236	233,819	289,055	75	3,738
Spokane, WA	6	1,359	49,177	304,717	383,935	61.4	834	1,052	6.2	37,084	120,061	127,683	247,744	69	5,722
Riverside, CA	4	954	46,749	227,126	312,731	65.2	622	856	4.9	25,897	139,904	179,495	319,399	56	11,535
Madison, WI	3	1,298	53,591	328,541	425,069	69.3	899	1,165	6.1	56,252	69,604	422,515	492,119	79	6,153
Huntington Beach, CA	2	242	6,759	36,698	48,500	41.7	101	132	5.4	4,779	13,539	20,013	33,552	25	401
Syracuse, NY	4	1,726	64,545	548,525	664,835	87.1	1,503	1,822	8.5	46,346	141,819	543,970	685,789	118	9,631
Chattanooga, TN	8	1,623	57,335	361,048	455,527	60.9	989	1,248	6.3	45,660	203,616	128,140	331,756	62	6,113
Columbus, GA	4	1,071	30,541	205,816	255,265	52.7	564	700	6.7	28,135	78,181	76,294	154,475	48	3,669
Las Vegas, NV	5	1,711	63,236	413,761	491,909	66.3	1,134	1,347	6.5	53,353	153,397	356,922	510,319	100	10,974
Salt Lake City, UT	6	1,521	65,382	403,904	512,801	72.7	1,106	1,405	6.2	52,528	125,114	688,544	813,658	156	10,510
Worcester, MA	5	1,576	58,122	439,465	574,158	76.4	1,204	1,573	7.6	41,603	146,547	511,572	658,119	101	7,118
Warren, MI	2	224	7,375	58,955	89,412	72.3	162	245	8.0	6,718	22,670	125,175	147,845	35	1,041
Kansas City, KS	3	1,096	34,042	255,162	313,116	63.8	699	858	7.5	22,628	71,232	382,672	453,904	62	3,644
Arlington, TX	3	628	22,890	129,465	158,270	58.3	366	448	5.7	20,102	52,441	62,348	114,789	68	3,677
Flint, MI	5	1,758	63,947	437,215	575,488	68.1	1,198	1,577	6.8	48,795	147,748	464,278	612,026	153	8,380
Aurora, CO	2	325	13,367	62,575	82,291	52.6	171	225	4.7	14,000	53,182	75,481	128,663	40	2,146
Tacoma, WA	7	1,054	45,016	243,532	331,174	63.2	666	908	5.4	37,194	117,331	247,070	364,401	68	6,316
Little Rock, AR	7	2,445	80,704	624,469	743,964	69.9	1,710	2,038	7.7	49,557	153,950	376,320	530,270	112	7,544
Providence, RI	5	1,778	73,311	526,156	694,832	81.0	1,441	1,904	7.2	53,931	221,021	275,687	496,708	72	10,646
Greensboro, NC	3	879	34,849	271,088	331,607	84.5	743	909	7.8	24,219	83,750	168,410	252,160	72	4,851

Table 7 (Continued)

CLASSIFICATION	FULL-TIME EQUIVALENT PERSONNEL					FULL-TIME EQUIVALENT TRAINEES			EXPENSES						
									LABOR				TOTAL		
	Physicians and Dentists	Registered Nurses	Licensed Practical Nurses	Other Salaried Personnel	Total Personnel	Medical and Dental Residents	Other Trainees	Total Trainees	Payroll (in thousands)	Employee Benefits (in thousands)	Total (in thousands)	Percent of Total	Amount (in thousands)	Adjusted, per Admission	Adjusted, per Inpatient Day
Wichita, KS	68	1,936	340	6,007	8,351	9	39	48	$ 198,317	$ 26,316	$ 224,633	49.0	$ 458,677	$5,306.18	$ 771.97
Sacramento, CA	157	3,192	376	7,057	10,782	374	9	383	321,636	82,936	404,572	54.5	742,023	6,073.30	927.30
Tampa, FL	117	2,358	483	6,858	9,816	262	3	265	257,188	62,603	319,792	49.1	650,827	6,194.28	859.48
St. Paul, MN	12	1,121	112	2,983	4,228	55	0	55	146,513	27,671	174,184	56.2	309,809	5,485.39	908.19
Norfolk, VA	2	1,844	330	4,125	6,301	16	0	16	165,944	24,193	190,138	53.4	356,318	4,955.41	705.39
Virginia Beach, VA	0	340	85	1,120	1,545	0	0	0	39,969	7,078	47,047	48.1	97,890	3,757.33	649.82
Rochester, NY	260	2,891	436	8,392	11,979	444	0	444	318,936	59,816	378,752	59.4	637,617	5,610.26	516.13
Akron, OH	81	2,054	377	5,522	8,034	352	3	355	216,006	48,441	264,447	55.7	475,083	5,362.35	748.40
St. Petersburg, FL	6	1,586	371	4,264	6,227	54	1	55	157,056	26,255	183,311	46.2	396,776	5,641.07	772.53
Corpus Christi, TX	7	956	553	3,645	5,161	48	0	48	107,046	23,419	130,466	48.6	268,192	4,451.84	685.03
Jersey City, NJ	95	767	175	3,079	4,116	105	0	105	121,262	23,652	144,914	60.7	238,588	4,374.88	539.48
Anaheim, CA	0	1,136	146	2,113	3,395	12	9	21	95,847	22,289	118,136	47.5	248,467	5,119.12	919.52
Baton Rouge, LA	3	1,412	421	4,065	5,901	55	0	55	142,054	27,468	169,522	50.4	336,423	4,505.46	707.25
Richmond, VA	29	3,254	738	8,920	12,941	496	2	498	326,167	73,833	400,000	49.3	811,126	5,242.03	758.14
Fresno, CA	0	1,571	299	5,267	7,137	134	0	134	187,243	52,034	239,277	54.8	436,853	5,202.43	941.04
Colorado Springs, CO	0	1,320	76	2,812	4,208	6	0	6	108,975	18,728	127,703	57.3	222,914	5,002.44	811.93
Shreveport, LA	17	1,352	438	4,798	6,605	216	0	216	180,346	27,553	207,899	55.0	377,912	4,697.77	716.96
Lexington-Fayette, KY	6	1,846	224	4,852	6,928	13	22	35	164,091	24,697	188,788	51.4	367,277	4,997.58	707.66
Santa Ana, CA	4	428	65	1,038	1,535	0	0	0	61,783	18,109	79,892	45.1	177,000	5,616.19	1,397.09
Dayton, OH	20	2,706	201	6,707	9,634	286	15	301	260,999	41,397	302,395	54.2	557,956	5,455.40	750.27
Jackson, MS	42	1,570	483	5,785	7,880	318	0	318	170,956	29,785	200,741	53.4	375,569	3,764.57	555.56
Mobile, AL	3	1,553	547	4,618	6,721	166	0	166	152,660	30,133	182,794	44.5	410,970	5,369.21	788.33
Yonkers, NY	63	511	100	2,035	2,709	23	0	23	75,904	15,927	91,830	61.0	150,538	4,935.01	584.46
Des Moines, IA	20	1,747	219	6,414	8,400	108	10	118	201,455	34,064	235,519	51.0	461,762	5,211.64	669.08
Knoxville, TN	98	2,415	549	6,372	9,434	98	34	132	224,543	48,390	272,934	49.2	554,748	5,127.39	767.42
Grand Rapids, MI	54	2,274	302	4,958	7,588	303	14	317	194,600	35,589	230,189	53.9	427,014	5,017.26	640.54
Montgomery, AL	0	926	215	2,180	3,321	0	0	0	76,029	12,983	89,012	47.6	186,966	4,046.52	693.78
Lubbock, TX	0	1,042	575	3,492	5,109	0	12	12	127,952	27,444	155,396	49.6	313,071	5,268.16	738.28
Anchorage, AK	0	635	33	1,290	1,958	0	0	0	75,181	16,270	91,451	49.6	184,251	7,963.13	1,383.84
Fort Wayne, IN	2	1,388	216	3,594	5,200	8	0	8	137,043	24,348	161,391	51.0	316,599	5,486.14	813.98
Lincoln, NE	13	874	240	2,191	3,318	0	2	2	76,775	12,153	88,928	49.9	178,054	5,250.93	806.72
Spokane, WA	20	1,430	331	3,140	4,921	46	0	46	162,439	29,663	192,102	58.0	331,129	5,342.16	862.46
Riverside, CA	0	954	189	2,601	3,744	20	1	21	106,279	21,933	128,212	52.5	244,167	3,800.97	780.76
Madison, WI	12	1,746	70	4,229	6,057	380	0	380	164,642	40,388	205,031	54.1	379,153	5,498.79	891.98
Huntington Beach, CA	0	107	31	453	591	0	0	0	20,485	4,323	24,808	44.7	55,509	6,213.89	1,144.51
Syracuse, NY	98	1,732	330	5,517	7,677	343	0	343	225,777	47,952	273,729	59.7	458,401	5,844.94	689.50
Chattanooga, TN	19	1,677	277	4,102	6,075	91	0	91	160,534	22,893	183,427	49.1	373,627	5,166.02	820.21
Columbus, GA	11	548	263	2,185	3,007	35	8	43	57,345	11,793	69,139	42.2	163,662	4,324.99	641.14
Las Vegas, NV	19	1,929	354	3,445	5,747	11	0	11	159,188	35,324	194,513	47.4	410,725	5,457.48	834.96
Salt Lake City, UT	53	2,173	251	5,722	8,199	159	9	168	204,921	55,747	260,669	49.5	526,176	6,301.96	1,026.08
Worcester, MA	446	1,632	275	4,416	6,769	321	0	321	219,793	44,611	264,404	57.8	457,164	5,956.76	796.23
Warren, MI	2	159	10	724	895	57	0	57	25,096	4,881	29,977	50.8	58,984	5,341.83	659.69
Kansas City, KS	296	1,018	229	3,404	4,947	296	0	296	110,819	21,292	132,112	55.7	237,080	5,667.30	757.16
Arlington, TX	11	444	106	1,325	1,886	18	0	18	43,118	6,831	49,949	45.6	109,653	3,937.28	692.82
Flint, MI	47	1,596	535	4,578	6,756	234	57	291	203,999	45,880	249,879	60.7	411,732	4,779.91	715.45
Aurora, CO	0	283	45	829	1,157	0	0	0	29,990	6,201	36,190	42.6	84,995	4,855.76	1,032.86
Tacoma, WA	23	863	202	3,142	4,230	17	0	17	130,120	25,704	155,823	52.4	297,191	4,848.30	897.39
Little Rock, AR	8	2,499	782	6,597	9,886	279	0	279	258,572	46,184	304,755	50.6	602,287	6,216.64	809.56
Providence, RI	255	1,981	306	6,700	9,242	387	0	387	266,017	53,349	319,366	60.8	525,412	5,471.10	756.17
Greensboro, NC	9	1,205	104	2,705	4,023	34	5	39	102,040	18,003	120,044	56.5	212,580	5,058.42	641.06

Tables

8-11

Approvals and Affiliations

The approvals and affiliations noted in tables 10A and 10B were reported by the approving bodies specified as of the dates below.

1 Accreditation under one of the programs of the Joint Commission on Accreditation of Healthcare Organizations (January 1991).

2 Cancer program approved by the American College of Surgeons (January 1991).

3 Approval to participate in residency training, by the Accreditation Council for Graduate Medical Education (January 1991).*

5 Medical school affiliation, reported by the American Medical Association (January 1991).

6 Hospital-controlled professional nursing school, reported by the National League for Nursing (January 1991).

8 Member of the Council of Teaching Hospitals of the Association of American Medical Colleges (January 1991).

9 Hospital contracting or participating in a Blue Cross Plan, reported by the Blue Cross Association (January 1991).

10 Certified for participation in the Health Insurance for the Aged (Medicare) Program by the U.S. Department of Health and Human Services (January 1991).

*As of June 30, 1975, internship (formerly code 4) was included under residency code 3.

Table

8

Utilization, Personnel, and Finances in Community Hospitals Affiliated with Medical Schools

CLASSIFICATION	HOSPITALS	BEDS	ADMISSIONS	INPATIENT DAYS	ADJUSTED PATIENT DAYS	OCCUPANCY, percent	AVERAGE DAILY CENSUS	ADJUSTED AVERAGE DAILY CENSUS	AVERAGE STAY, days	SURGICAL OPERATIONS	OUTPATIENT VISITS			NEWBORNS	
											Emergency	Other	Total	Bassinets	Births
UNITED STATES	962	374,461	13,747,704	102,625,966	129,610,231	75.1	281,183	355,125	7.5	9,484,493	33,098,859	107,582,063	140,680,922	24,975	1,886,258
Nongovernment	821	312,365	11,437,876	84,979,528	107,052,209	74.5	232,838	293,320	7.4	8,216,609	25,316,478	83,544,002	108,860,480	20,132	1,469,937
Less than 300 beds	330	61,888	2,328,477	15,777,261	20,990,077	69.9	43,235	57,518	6.8	1,820,881	6,444,108	21,170,581	27,614,689	3,972	259,050
300-399	170	58,694	2,203,010	15,383,017	19,532,659	71.8	42,149	53,516	7.0	1,587,919	5,121,666	13,663,718	18,785,384	4,303	294,994
400-499	131	58,669	2,172,489	16,103,352	20,290,909	75.2	44,124	55,598	7.4	1,572,664	4,693,241	15,060,645	19,753,886	4,321	311,158
500 or more	190	133,114	4,733,900	37,715,898	46,238,564	77.6	103,330	126,688	8.0	3,235,145	9,057,463	33,649,058	42,706,521	7,536	604,735
State and local government	141	62,096	2,309,828	17,646,438	22,558,022	77.9	48,345	61,805	7.6	1,267,884	7,782,381	24,038,061	31,820,442	4,843	416,321
Less than 300 beds	47	9,103	361,596	2,272,230	3,174,838	68.4	6,224	8,697	6.3	209,579	1,527,903	3,543,458	5,071,361	1,129	71,487
300-399	23	7,955	324,037	2,222,611	2,837,235	76.6	6,090	7,771	6.9	159,180	960,394	2,911,995	3,872,389	618	60,655
400-499	22	10,024	387,394	2,898,059	3,735,818	79.2	7,936	10,238	7.5	216,540	1,401,952	5,138,725	6,540,677	754	69,117
500 or more	49	35,014	1,236,801	10,253,538	12,810,131	80.2	28,095	35,099	8.3	682,585	3,892,132	12,443,883	16,336,015	2,342	215,062
CENSUS DIVISION 1, NEW ENGLAND	73	24,309	921,965	6,905,222	9,061,922	77.8	18,920	24,833	7.5	659,121	2,650,088	7,683,966	10,334,054	1,682	118,324
Nongovernment	67	22,868	875,139	6,509,407	8,496,463	78.0	17,835	23,284	7.4	628,713	2,486,269	6,774,779	9,261,048	1,620	115,469
Less than 300 beds	35	7,422	279,601	1,950,344	2,716,037	72.0	5,343	7,444	7.0	221,653	1,018,804	2,603,372	3,622,176	560	36,039
300-399	14	4,824	183,749	1,385,660	1,810,366	78.7	3,796	4,960	7.5	128,398	524,689	1,524,364	2,049,053	333	18,909
400-499	9	4,128	154,892	1,201,931	1,527,632	79.8	3,294	4,187	7.8	108,218	339,722	1,122,532	1,462,254	269	21,346
500 or more	9	6,494	256,897	1,971,472	2,442,428	83.2	5,402	6,693	7.7	170,444	603,054	1,524,511	2,127,565	458	39,175
State and local government	6	1,441	46,826	395,815	565,459	75.3	1,085	1,549	8.5	30,408	163,819	909,187	1,073,006	62	2,855
Less than 300 beds	4	719	20,184	186,764	271,544	71.2	512	744	9.3	12,526	64,572	503,921	568,493	44	1,284
300-399	2	722	26,642	209,051	293,915	79.4	573	805	7.8	17,882	99,247	405,266	504,513	18	1,571
400-499	0	0	0	0	0	00.0	0	0	0.0	0	0	0	0	0	0
500 or more	0	0	0	0	0	00.0	0	0	0.0	0	0	0	0	0	0
CENSUS DIVISION 2, MIDDLE ATLANTIC	212	92,132	3,189,340	28,166,861	35,428,709	83.8	77,168	97,060	8.8	2,085,733	7,767,134	28,707,583	36,474,717	5,788	394,309
Nongovernment	192	80,425	2,863,800	24,363,617	30,685,354	83.0	66,747	84,064	8.5	1,960,315	6,389,665	23,514,662	29,904,327	5,196	345,638
Less than 300 beds	60	11,642	425,370	3,196,706	4,306,694	75.2	8,758	11,796	7.5	349,472	1,225,684	4,041,211	5,266,895	772	43,920
300-399	40	13,817	511,214	4,045,076	5,082,052	80.2	11,084	13,922	7.9	337,894	1,230,248	3,423,168	4,653,416	1,185	60,815
400-499	39	17,317	643,461	5,208,776	6,568,373	82.4	14,270	17,996	8.1	445,100	1,345,261	4,763,138	6,108,399	1,271	82,107
500 or more	53	37,649	1,283,755	11,913,059	14,728,235	86.7	32,635	40,350	9.3	827,849	2,588,472	11,287,145	13,875,617	1,968	158,796
State and local government	20	11,707	325,540	3,803,244	4,743,355	89.0	10,421	12,996	11.7	125,418	1,377,469	5,192,921	6,570,390	592	48,671
Less than 300 beds	1	161	5,834	42,634	59,443	72.7	117	163	7.3	8,434	0	64,909	64,909	0	0
300-399	3	1,062	34,181	326,503	386,051	84.3	895	1,057	9.6	17,193	105,838	397,387	503,225	60	5,390
400-499	5	2,413	81,100	789,923	1,013,420	89.6	2,163	2,777	9.7	33,897	357,854	1,439,583	1,797,437	178	15,823
500 or more	11	8,071	204,425	2,644,184	3,284,441	89.8	7,246	8,999	12.9	65,894	913,777	3,291,042	4,204,819	354	27,458
CENSUS DIVISION 3, SOUTH ATLANTIC	124	53,210	2,003,908	14,608,086	18,130,789	75.2	40,024	49,679	7.3	1,421,998	4,924,119	11,376,516	16,300,635	3,482	287,205
Nongovernment	102	40,154	1,515,729	10,913,318	13,521,085	74.5	29,902	37,049	7.2	1,142,082	3,389,511	8,079,960	11,469,471	2,486	201,232
Less than 300 beds	36	6,027	223,161	1,513,790	1,978,363	68.8	4,148	5,420	6.8	203,383	555,113	1,819,179	2,374,292	316	20,094
300-399	22	7,740	304,209	2,049,139	2,611,450	72.5	5,614	7,154	6.7	247,657	726,513	1,587,203	2,313,716	540	43,936
400-499	16	7,235	278,738	1,981,032	2,479,616	75.1	5,430	6,795	7.1	194,860	719,995	1,213,980	1,933,975	555	45,974
500 or more	28	19,152	709,621	5,369,357	6,451,656	76.8	14,710	17,680	7.6	496,182	1,387,890	3,459,598	4,847,488	1,075	91,228
State and local government	22	13,056	488,179	3,694,768	4,609,704	77.5	10,122	12,630	7.6	279,916	1,534,608	3,296,556	4,831,164	996	85,973
Less than 300 beds	2	312	10,679	91,325	122,627	80.1	250	336	8.6	4,663	87,240	42,303	129,543	18	976
300-399	2	699	29,072	180,278	226,982	70.7	494	622	6.2	15,567	67,854	107,149	175,003	89	4,891
400-499	3	1,408	47,704	363,378	488,126	70.7	995	1,338	7.6	37,017	203,332	286,234	489,566	144	9,616
500 or more	15	10,637	400,724	3,059,787	3,771,969	78.8	8,383	10,334	7.6	222,669	1,176,182	2,860,870	4,037,052	745	70,490
CENSUS DIVISION 4, EAST NORTH CENTRAL	176	74,066	2,652,508	19,432,154	24,982,750	71.9	53,258	68,464	7.3	1,966,292	6,600,431	24,564,930	31,165,361	4,944	337,021
Nongovernment	162	66,843	2,410,774	17,507,540	22,498,372	71.8	47,984	61,655	7.3	1,819,671	5,842,322	21,639,488	27,481,810	4,483	305,648
Less than 300 beds	54	10,924	390,610	2,755,401	3,692,611	69.2	7,556	10,124	7.1	306,629	1,140,621	3,505,726	4,646,347	701	36,864
300-399	31	10,638	385,991	2,621,843	3,475,629	67.6	7,186	9,524	6.8	295,344	1,034,656	2,860,357	3,895,013	737	47,393
400-499	31	13,917	519,141	3,642,174	4,701,529	71.7	9,981	12,884	7.0	401,150	1,165,646	4,318,181	5,483,827	1,113	80,103
500 or more	46	31,364	1,115,032	8,488,122	10,628,603	74.2	23,261	29,123	7.6	816,548	2,501,399	10,955,224	13,456,623	1,932	141,288
State and local government	14	7,223	241,734	1,924,614	2,484,378	73.0	5,274	6,809	8.0	146,621	758,109	2,925,442	3,683,551	461	31,373
Less than 300 beds	4	1,123	37,241	257,328	353,331	62.8	705	968	6.9	28,569	144,205	360,889	505,094	73	3,053
300-399	2	736	26,141	196,795	253,934	73.2	539	695	7.5	5,226	88,339	409,144	497,483	39	4,177
400-499	2	903	31,990	235,578	338,135	71.4	645	927	7.4	39,779	122,420	613,652	736,072	45	3,281
500 or more	6	4,461	146,362	1,234,913	1,538,978	75.9	3,385	4,219	8.4	73,047	403,145	1,541,757	1,944,902	304	20,862

Table 8 (Continued)

CLASSIFICATION	FULL-TIME EQUIVALENT PERSONNEL: Physicians and Dentists	Registered Nurses	Licensed Practical Nurses	Other Salaried Personnel	Total Personnel	FULL-TIME EQUIVALENT TRAINEES: Medical and Dental Residents	Other Trainees	Total Trainees	EXPENSES — LABOR: Payroll (in thousands)	Employee Benefits (in thousands)	Total (in thousands)	Percent of Total	EXPENSES — TOTAL: Amount (in thousands)	Adjusted, per Admission	Adjusted, per Inpatient Day
UNITED STATES	30,073	408,393	60,693	1,208,479	1,707,638	60,882	3,108	63,990	$ 48,576,547	$ 9,697,969	$ 58,274,516	54.7	$ 106,566,509	$ 6,108.35	$ 822.21
Nongovernment	20,440	337,489	47,039	980,963	1,385,936	40,672	2,128	42,800	39,367,105	7,663,949	47,031,055	54.2	86,783,530	5,996.32	810.67
Less than 300 beds	3,672	67,831	10,436	197,403	279,345	3,810	385	4,195	7,594,882	1,482,752	9,077,634	53.5	16,969,018	5,419.06	808.43
300-399	3,333	58,770	9,745	172,984	244,832	4,896	185	5,081	6,899,714	1,328,918	8,228,632	54.6	15,076,551	5,384.81	771.86
400-499	2,926	60,708	8,276	174,753	246,663	6,277	399	6,676	6,994,390	1,347,986	8,342,377	55.1	15,139,698	5,528.29	746.13
500 or more	10,509	150,180	18,582	435,825	615,096	25,689	1,159	26,848	17,878,118	3,504,293	21,382,411	54.0	39,598,263	6,823.74	856.39
State and local government	9,633	70,904	13,654	227,511	321,702	20,210	980	21,190	9,209,442	2,034,019	11,243,461	56.8	19,782,978	6,653.66	876.98
Less than 300 beds	577	8,520	2,588	27,603	39,294	1,369	101	1,470	1,097,470	247,659	1,345,130	53.4	2,518,729	4,991.96	793.34
300-399	1,274	10,755	1,516	30,473	44,024	2,652	58	2,710	1,224,851	260,241	1,485,091	55.6	2,670,187	6,435.27	941.12
400-499	1,615	12,129	2,069	40,935	56,749	3,290	32	3,322	1,747,848	392,151	2,139,999	58.8	3,640,325	7,272.62	974.44
500 or more	6,167	39,500	7,481	128,487	181,635	12,899	789	13,688	5,139,273	1,133,969	6,273,241	57.3	10,953,737	7,052.33	855.08
CENSUS DIVISION 1, NEW ENGLAND	4,109	28,965	3,050	87,482	123,606	5,737	158	5,895	3,914,651	793,197	4,707,848	57.8	8,146,228	6,706.93	898.95
Nongovernment	3,683	27,061	2,809	82,144	115,697	5,207	148	5,355	3,664,059	737,302	4,401,361	57.8	7,614,258	6,635.98	896.17
Less than 300 beds	667	7,666	933	24,288	33,554	638	38	676	1,056,828	214,008	1,270,836	60.4	2,104,447	5,382.92	774.82
300-399	496	5,699	535	17,498	24,228	1,083	55	1,138	817,679	162,789	980,468	58.5	1,676,317	6,974.83	925.95
400-499	275	4,538	591	13,353	18,757	876	30	906	615,687	119,880	735,567	56.7	1,297,180	6,566.34	849.14
500 or more	2,245	9,158	750	27,005	39,158	2,610	25	2,635	1,173,865	240,626	1,414,491	55.8	2,536,315	7,961.24	1,038.44
State and local government	426	1,904	241	5,338	7,909	530	10	540	250,592	55,895	306,487	57.6	531,970	7,918.70	940.78
Less than 300 beds	18	715	120	2,465	3,318	61	10	71	92,332	22,317	114,649	55.6	206,214	7,010.98	759.41
300-399	408	1,189	121	2,873	4,591	469	0	469	158,260	33,578	191,837	58.9	325,756	8,625.65	1,108.33
400-499	0	0	0	0	0	0	0	0	0	0	0	0.0	0	0.00	0.00
500 or more	0	0	0	0	0	0	0	0	0	0	0	0.0	0	0.00	0.00
CENSUS DIVISION 2, MIDDLE ATLANTIC	12,052	95,417	13,108	295,202	415,779	19,788	419	20,207	12,927,075	2,584,241	15,511,317	58.0	26,723,397	6,610.94	754.29
Nongovernment	8,652	84,366	10,927	250,877	354,822	15,681	367	16,048	10,832,942	2,152,826	12,985,769	56.9	22,833,008	6,287.76	744.10
Less than 300 beds	1,051	11,744	1,855	35,904	50,554	1,192	26	1,218	1,443,022	280,317	1,723,339	57.2	3,011,310	5,116.32	699.22
300-399	1,430	13,314	2,236	38,289	55,269	1,473	5	1,478	1,588,670	323,785	1,912,456	56.9	3,363,491	5,240.29	661.84
400-499	1,163	17,532	2,430	52,183	73,308	2,166	21	2,187	2,107,382	408,675	2,516,058	56.9	4,423,410	5,452.32	673.44
500 or more	5,008	41,776	4,406	124,501	175,691	10,850	315	11,165	5,693,867	1,140,049	6,833,916	56.8	12,034,798	7,570.80	817.12
State and local government	3,400	11,051	2,181	44,325	60,957	4,107	52	4,159	2,094,133	431,415	2,525,548	64.9	3,890,389	9,466.63	820.18
Less than 300 beds	42	295	33	1,079	1,449	49	0	49	28,625	5,676	34,300	54.0	63,490	7,805.51	1,068.08
300-399	374	1,295	191	4,435	6,295	459	0	459	205,557	45,535	251,092	62.0	405,207	10,002.14	1,049.62
400-499	757	2,845	398	10,799	14,799	830	0	830	516,197	118,659	634,855	65.6	967,939	9,289.96	955.12
500 or more	2,227	6,616	1,559	28,012	38,414	2,769	52	2,821	1,343,755	261,546	1,605,300	65.4	2,453,753	9,506.25	747.08
CENSUS DIVISION 3, SOUTH ATLANTIC	3,168	60,272	10,126	168,147	241,713	8,715	470	9,185	6,509,085	1,322,512	7,831,596	53.6	14,621,180	5,844.11	806.43
Nongovernment	1,459	45,495	6,929	123,534	177,417	4,606	300	4,906	4,853,694	937,382	5,791,076	53.4	10,844,635	5,734.12	802.05
Less than 300 beds	334	7,121	906	19,628	27,989	335	30	365	748,572	142,552	891,125	51.1	1,742,878	5,822.46	880.97
300-399	198	7,306	1,383	21,504	30,391	538	28	566	802,810	138,886	941,696	54.2	1,736,257	4,469.02	664.86
400-499	555	7,438	1,140	21,010	30,143	1,022	112	1,134	868,989	172,598	1,041,587	56.5	1,844,069	5,282.21	743.69
500 or more	372	23,630	3,500	61,392	88,894	2,711	130	2,841	2,433,323	483,345	2,916,668	52.8	5,521,431	6,463.18	855.82
State and local government	1,709	14,777	3,197	44,613	64,296	4,109	170	4,279	1,655,391	385,130	2,040,520	54.0	3,776,545	6,184.79	819.26
Less than 300 beds	0	181	94	779	994	0	1	1	20,490	3,836	24,327	53.7	45,324	3,163.32	369.61
300-399	9	629	231	2,064	2,933	23	41	64	72,742	13,477	86,219	56.8	151,897	4,150.31	669.20
400-499	166	1,115	393	4,094	5,768	198	0	198	144,967	28,140	173,107	52.3	330,908	5,153.69	677.92
500 or more	1,534	12,852	2,479	37,736	54,601	3,888	128	4,016	1,417,192	339,676	1,756,868	54.1	3,248,416	6,556.06	861.20
CENSUS DIVISION 4, EAST NORTH CENTRAL	4,433	81,987	10,164	244,124	340,708	11,779	806	12,585	9,270,874	1,805,519	11,076,392	53.7	20,608,019	6,026.14	824.89
Nongovernment	3,697	72,543	8,943	217,474	302,657	9,118	675	9,793	8,164,387	1,539,287	9,703,674	53.1	18,280,102	5,883.72	812.51
Less than 300 beds	366	11,247	1,879	33,872	47,304	664	104	768	1,253,484	242,573	1,496,057	53.2	2,811,130	5,310.60	761.29
300-399	463	10,889	1,771	32,679	45,742	663	39	702	1,157,440	209,622	1,367,062	52.8	2,589,467	5,064.39	745.04
400-499	776	14,451	1,563	41,397	58,187	1,618	59	1,677	1,626,423	299,707	1,926,130	55.4	3,475,372	5,181.11	739.20
500 or more	2,092	35,956	3,730	109,646	151,424	6,173	473	6,646	4,127,040	787,384	4,914,425	52.3	9,404,133	6,739.07	884.79
State and local government	736	9,444	1,221	26,650	38,051	2,661	131	2,792	1,106,486	266,232	1,372,718	59.0	2,327,917	7,440.36	937.02
Less than 300 beds	32	1,269	215	3,346	4,862	341	2	343	139,772	38,083	177,855	55.5	320,281	6,173.38	906.46
300-399	44	1,003	137	2,787	3,971	107	0	107	122,945	11,391	134,336	58.8	228,315	6,761.69	899.11
400-499	7	1,220	123	4,277	5,567	338	0	338	138,053	33,240	171,293	54.5	314,014	6,792.12	928.66
500 or more	653	5,952	746	16,300	23,651	1,875	129	2,004	705,717	183,518	889,234	60.7	1,465,307	8,095.71	952.13

(continued on next page)

Table 8 (Continued)

Utilization, Personnel, and Finances in Community Hospitals Affiliated with Medical Schools

CLASSIFICATION	HOSPITALS	BEDS	ADMISSIONS	INPATIENT DAYS	ADJUSTED PATIENT DAYS	OCCUPANCY, percent	AVERAGE DAILY CENSUS	ADJUSTED AVERAGE DAILY CENSUS	AVERAGE STAY, days	SURGICAL OPERATIONS	OUTPATIENT VISITS: Emergency	OUTPATIENT VISITS: Other	OUTPATIENT VISITS: Total	NEWBORNS: Bassinets	NEWBORNS: Births
CENSUS DIVISION 5, EAST SOUTH CENTRAL	49	19,850	740,819	5,201,624	6,239,713	71.8	14,250	17,096	7.0	474,260	1,686,143	3,413,083	5,099,226	1,250	82,342
Nongovernment	37	14,417	522,634	3,729,626	4,472,992	70.9	10,218	12,255	7.1	338,355	1,082,752	2,323,733	3,406,485	833	49,547
Less than 300 beds	17	2,967	107,668	691,512	904,475	63.9	1,895	2,478	6.4	66,243	271,329	762,380	1,033,709	152	6,164
300-399	3	1,046	41,122	268,245	334,041	70.3	735	916	6.5	33,041	107,179	141,995	249,174	99	4,284
400-499	8	3,424	125,187	870,419	1,033,907	69.7	2,385	2,833	7.0	77,484	325,104	572,505	897,609	243	15,177
500 or more	9	6,980	248,657	1,899,450	2,200,569	74.5	5,203	6,028	7.6	161,587	379,140	846,853	1,225,993	339	23,922
State and local government	12	5,433	218,185	1,471,998	1,766,721	74.2	4,032	4,841	6.7	135,905	603,391	1,089,350	1,692,741	417	32,795
Less than 300 beds	3	436	20,013	103,220	139,105	64.7	282	382	5.2	10,395	84,172	163,309	247,481	91	3,251
300-399	1	358	15,552	97,693	110,343	74.9	268	302	6.3	6,606	39,883	20,191	60,074	26	3,911
400-499	2	920	38,658	254,459	302,491	75.8	697	829	6.6	19,990	97,389	264,697	362,086	59	5,716
500 or more	6	3,719	143,962	1,016,626	1,214,782	74.9	2,785	3,328	7.1	98,914	381,947	641,153	1,023,100	241	19,917
CENSUS DIVISION 6, WEST NORTH CENTRAL	83	30,490	1,038,003	7,599,496	9,579,591	68.3	20,818	26,244	7.3	822,044	2,064,860	6,804,646	8,869,506	1,806	123,774
Nongovernment	74	26,850	912,927	6,658,089	8,363,514	67.9	18,240	22,911	7.3	689,668	1,817,302	5,021,865	6,839,167	1,622	113,806
Less than 300 beds	31	5,322	197,474	1,363,088	1,756,204	70.2	3,736	4,812	6.9	151,303	546,067	1,421,657	1,967,724	328	21,518
300-399	19	6,539	225,160	1,562,021	1,964,441	65.4	4,277	5,383	6.9	167,377	489,799	1,505,672	1,995,471	415	29,684
400-499	8	3,599	112,167	853,060	1,067,354	64.9	2,337	2,923	7.6	96,708	213,275	526,653	739,928	205	12,521
500 or more	16	11,390	378,126	2,879,920	3,575,515	69.3	7,890	9,793	7.6	274,280	568,161	1,567,883	2,136,044	674	50,083
State and local government	9	3,640	125,076	941,407	1,216,077	70.8	2,578	3,333	7.5	132,376	247,558	1,782,781	2,030,339	184	9,968
Less than 300 beds	3	637	15,704	134,309	197,459	57.8	368	541	8.6	10,265	56,572	249,093	305,665	45	1,163
300-399	1	313	11,017	78,901	94,442	69.0	216	259	7.2	7,687	24,028	22,720	46,748	18	1,099
400-499	3	1,240	47,148	325,105	418,518	71.8	890	1,147	6.9	32,568	124,372	770,208	894,580	90	5,593
500 or more	2	1,450	51,207	403,092	505,658	76.1	1,104	1,386	7.9	81,856	42,586	740,760	783,346	31	2,113
CENSUS DIVISION 7, WEST SOUTH CENTRAL	91	31,628	1,140,377	7,889,916	9,816,408	68.3	21,616	26,897	6.9	731,041	2,693,877	6,941,623	9,635,500	2,426	171,945
Nongovernment	67	23,141	799,792	5,668,589	6,898,378	67.1	15,530	18,903	7.1	585,242	1,424,090	3,228,745	4,652,835	1,250	87,252
Less than 300 beds	34	5,868	195,860	1,370,048	1,735,417	64.0	3,753	4,755	7.0	155,240	482,201	1,045,350	1,527,551	259	15,169
300-399	13	4,392	148,503	1,019,084	1,261,076	63.6	2,793	3,456	6.9	107,160	286,778	386,416	673,194	293	19,332
400-499	6	2,817	95,469	707,334	866,652	68.8	1,938	2,375	7.4	68,215	180,919	226,203	407,122	213	14,390
500 or more	14	10,064	359,960	2,572,123	3,035,233	70.0	7,046	8,317	7.1	254,627	474,192	1,570,776	2,044,968	485	38,361
State and local government	24	8,487	340,585	2,221,327	2,918,030	71.7	6,086	7,994	6.5	145,799	1,269,787	3,712,878	4,982,665	1,176	84,693
Less than 300 beds	12	2,040	77,513	479,855	629,805	64.5	1,316	1,725	6.2	36,420	365,745	596,393	962,138	517	16,279
300-399	5	1,665	75,961	438,487	569,204	72.1	1,200	1,560	5.8	28,635	252,620	440,573	693,193	196	21,059
400-499	0	0	0	0	0	00.0	0	0	0.0	0	0	0	0	0	0
500 or more	7	4,782	187,111	1,302,985	1,719,021	74.7	3,570	4,709	7.0	80,744	651,422	2,675,912	3,327,334	463	47,355
CENSUS DIVISION 8, MOUNTAIN	41	13,183	526,220	3,277,895	4,203,323	68.1	8,981	11,517	6.2	357,467	1,045,460	4,492,512	5,537,972	989	85,379
Nongovernment	34	11,128	436,464	2,733,840	3,490,008	67.3	7,490	9,564	6.3	310,952	794,941	3,607,423	4,402,364	809	67,138
Less than 300 beds	19	3,665	151,765	892,364	1,201,761	66.8	2,447	3,293	5.9	113,148	311,462	1,990,563	2,302,025	295	24,893
300-399	6	2,039	74,138	486,005	611,939	65.3	1,331	1,676	6.6	51,924	140,603	427,632	568,235	130	7,803
400-499	4	1,819	84,866	454,374	560,014	68.4	1,244	1,535	5.4	72,316	117,678	523,487	641,165	183	15,516
500 or more	5	3,605	125,695	901,097	1,116,294	68.5	2,468	3,060	7.2	73,564	225,198	665,741	890,939	201	18,926
State and local government	7	2,055	89,756	544,055	713,315	72.6	1,491	1,953	6.1	46,515	250,519	885,089	1,135,608	180	18,241
Less than 300 beds	3	474	21,915	108,251	156,738	62.7	297	429	4.9	13,883	67,751	168,748	236,499	55	4,186
300-399	2	667	30,392	196,060	247,716	80.5	537	678	6.5	16,422	62,647	339,639	402,286	52	5,697
400-499	2	914	37,449	239,744	308,861	71.9	657	846	6.4	16,210	120,121	376,702	496,823	73	8,358
500 or more	0	0	0	0	0	00.0	0	0	0.0	0	0	0	0	0	0
CENSUS DIVISION 9, PACIFIC	113	35,593	1,534,564	9,544,712	12,167,026	73.5	26,148	33,335	6.2	966,537	3,666,747	13,597,204	17,263,951	2,608	285,959
Nongovernment	86	26,539	1,100,617	6,895,502	8,626,043	71.2	18,892	23,635	6.3	741,611	2,089,626	9,353,347	11,442,973	1,833	184,207
Less than 300 beds	44	8,051	356,968	2,044,008	2,698,515	69.5	5,599	7,396	5.7	253,810	892,827	3,981,143	4,873,970	589	54,389
300-399	22	7,659	328,924	1,945,944	2,381,665	69.6	5,333	6,525	5.9	219,124	581,201	1,806,911	2,388,112	571	62,838
400-499	10	4,413	158,568	1,184,252	1,485,832	73.5	3,245	4,070	7.5	108,613	285,641	1,793,966	2,079,607	269	24,024
500 or more	10	6,416	256,157	1,721,298	2,060,031	73.5	4,715	5,644	6.7	160,064	329,957	1,771,327	2,101,284	404	42,956
State and local government	27	9,054	433,947	2,649,210	3,540,983	80.1	7,256	9,700	6.1	224,926	1,577,121	4,243,857	5,820,978	775	101,752
Less than 300 beds	15	3,201	152,513	868,544	1,244,786	74.3	2,377	3,409	5.7	84,424	657,646	1,393,893	2,051,539	286	41,295
300-399	5	1,733	75,079	498,843	654,648	78.9	1,368	1,793	6.6	43,962	219,938	769,926	989,864	120	12,860
400-499	5	2,226	103,345	689,872	866,267	84.9	1,889	2,374	6.7	37,079	376,464	1,387,649	1,764,113	165	20,730
500 or more	2	1,894	103,010	591,951	775,282	85.6	1,622	2,124	5.7	59,461	323,073	692,389	1,015,462	204	26,867

Table 8 (Continued)

CLASSIFICATION	FULL-TIME EQUIVALENT PERSONNEL: Physicians and Dentists	Registered Nurses	Licensed Practical Nurses	Other Salaried Personne	Total Personnel	FULL-TIME EQUIVALENT TRAINEES: Medical and Dental Residents	Other Trainees	Total Trainees	EXPENSES — LABOR: Payroll (in thousands)	Employee Benefits (in thousands)	Total (in thousands)	Percent of Total	EXPENSES — TOTAL: Amount (in thousands)	Adjusted, per Admission	Adjusted, per Inpatient Day
CENSUS DIVISION 5, EAST SOUTH CENTRAL	950	20,203	4,508	59,043	84,704	1,769	244	2,013	$ 1,988,826	$ 367,688	$ 2,356,515	50.7	$ 4,645,756	$ 5,190.53	$ 744.55
Nongovernment	159	14,055	3,109	41,848	59,171	645	197	842	1,382,894	256,472	1,639,366	50.5	3,247,317	5,137.23	725.98
Less than 300 beds	103	3,169	675	9,533	13,480	72	27	99	268,909	49,384	318,293	50.9	625,661	4,410.19	691.74
300-399	0	1,036	207	2,977	4,220	0	22	22	94,868	17,629	112,497	45.7	246,128	4,813.68	736.82
400-499	1	3,497	864	9,919	14,281	73	81	154	336,325	60,826	397,151	48.9	811,949	5,441.54	785.32
500 or more	55	6,353	1,363	19,419	27,190	500	67	567	682,792	128,633	811,425	51.9	1,563,580	5,393.44	710.53
State and local government	791	6,148	1,399	17,195	25,533	1,124	47	1,171	605,932	111,216	717,149	51.3	1,398,439	5,318.69	791.54
Less than 300 beds	2	345	206	1,178	1,731	0	13	13	45,103	12,985	58,088	49.0	118,619	4,379.36	852.73
300-399	1	332	80	1,095	1,508	166	0	166	35,032	8,122	43,154	41.7	103,395	5,886.11	937.04
400-499	0	1,098	192	3,039	4,329	0	0	0	106,198	15,839	122,037	51.5	236,870	5,157.76	783.07
500 or more	788	4,373	921	11,883	17,965	958	34	992	419,599	74,270	493,870	52.6	939,554	5,451.37	773.43
CENSUS DIVISION 6, WEST NORTH CENTRAL	1,018	32,807	4,538	87,200	125,563	2,288	154	2,442	3,369,181	621,920	3,991,101	53.3	7,483,341	5,720.92	781.18
Nongovernment	696	27,712	3,908	72,652	104,968	832	112	944	2,818,707	502,491	3,321,199	53.2	6,244,816	5,445.02	746.67
Less than 300 beds	187	6,499	915	15,210	22,811	143	24	167	602,169	96,697	698,866	52.3	1,335,611	5,260.44	760.51
300-399	103	6,656	1,083	18,382	26,224	132	0	132	717,037	129,441	846,478	53.8	1,572,111	5,545.25	800.28
400-499	6	4,120	407	9,964	14,497	54	46	100	341,653	62,902	404,554	52.4	771,673	5,531.71	722.98
500 or more	400	10,437	1,503	29,096	41,436	503	42	545	1,157,849	213,452	1,371,300	53.5	2,565,421	5,458.55	717.50
State and local government	322	5,095	630	14,548	20,595	1,456	42	1,498	550,474	119,429	669,903	54.1	1,238,524	7,684.01	1,018.46
Less than 300 beds	15	376	168	1,531	2,090	26	0	26	51,818	9,128	60,947	55.6	109,655	4,899.70	555.33
300-399	0	475	27	1,496	1,998	319	0	319	47,184	8,653	55,837	47.5	117,630	8,920.18	1,245.53
400-499	297	1,745	316	5,764	8,122	685	30	715	211,805	41,081	252,885	58.4	433,060	7,055.51	1,034.75
500 or more	10	2,499	119	5,757	8,385	426	12	438	239,667	60,567	300,234	51.9	578,178	9,000.84	1,143.42
CENSUS DIVISION 7, WEST SOUTH CENTRAL	603	29,451	8,242	98,550	136,846	4,258	515	4,773	3,385,005	627,243	4,012,248	50.7	7,907,881	5,556.48	805.58
Nongovernment	155	21,361	5,708	67,280	94,504	1,222	144	1,366	2,354,706	446,164	2,800,869	49.9	5,618,118	5,757.03	814.41
Less than 300 beds	53	5,621	1,720	17,323	24,717	293	32	325	607,087	115,491	722,579	48.2	1,500,308	6,010.49	864.52
300-399	25	3,089	1,379	10,597	15,090	181	0	181	350,973	77,736	428,708	48.6	883,013	4,784.11	700.21
400-499	9	2,256	555	7,289	10,109	67	7	74	250,743	43,447	294,189	52.5	560,303	4,789.90	646.51
500 or more	68	10,395	2,054	32,071	44,588	681	105	786	1,145,903	209,490	1,355,393	50.7	2,674,494	6,297.25	881.15
State and local government	448	8,090	2,534	31,270	42,342	3,036	371	3,407	1,030,300	181,079	1,211,379	52.9	2,289,764	5,118.95	784.70
Less than 300 beds	60	1,383	840	5,464	7,747	162	7	169	182,390	25,243	207,633	51.6	402,683	3,956.06	639.38
300-399	15	1,937	420	5,141	7,513	373	8	381	192,386	36,006	228,392	52.1	438,707	4,456.37	770.74
400-499	0	0	0	0	0	0	0	0	0	0	0	0.0	0	0.00	0.00
500 or more	373	4,770	1,274	20,665	27,082	2,501	356	2,857	655,523	119,830	775,353	53.5	1,448,373	5,862.03	842.56
CENSUS DIVISION 8, MOUNTAIN	344	15,283	1,726	41,656	59,009	858	47	905	1,634,241	332,047	1,966,288	51.1	3,844,237	5,665.15	914.57
Nongovernment	308	12,738	1,382	34,303	48,731	481	36	517	1,368,695	273,392	1,642,087	51.1	3,211,255	5,738.08	920.13
Less than 300 beds	199	4,877	498	13,519	19,093	109	34	143	516,397	104,118	620,515	49.3	1,258,940	6,080.43	1,047.58
300-399	12	2,067	175	5,178	7,432	35	0	35	228,465	46,454	274,919	52.7	521,848	5,574.71	852.78
400-499	44	2,041	251	5,599	7,935	111	2	113	238,675	52,601	291,276	53.5	544,121	5,192.98	971.62
500 or more	53	3,753	458	10,007	14,271	226	0	226	385,158	70,220	455,378	51.4	886,346	5,747.99	794.01
State and local government	36	2,545	344	7,353	10,278	377	11	388	265,546	58,655	324,201	51.2	632,982	5,322.00	887.38
Less than 300 beds	11	556	109	1,673	2,349	16	2	18	59,251	9,465	68,716	52.7	130,412	4,123.69	832.04
300-399	5	1,063	108	3,325	4,501	139	9	148	98,434	25,017	123,452	50.8	243,215	6,284.14	981.83
400-499	20	926	127	2,355	3,428	222	0	222	107,861	24,173	132,033	50.9	259,356	5,335.55	839.72
500 or more	0	0	0	0	0	0	0	0	0	0	0	0.0	0	0.00	0.00
CENSUS DIVISION 9, PACIFIC	3,396	44,008	5,231	127,075	179,710	5,690	295	5,985	5,577,609	1,243,603	6,821,211	54.2	12,586,469	6,413.05	1,034.47
Nongovernment	1,631	32,158	3,324	90,856	127,969	2,880	149	3,029	3,927,021	818,633	4,745,654	53.4	8,890,020	6,435.62	1,030.60
Less than 300 beds	712	9,887	1,055	28,189	39,843	364	70	434	1,098,414	237,611	1,336,025	51.8	2,578,733	5,478.11	955.61
300-399	606	8,714	976	25,940	36,236	791	36	827	1,141,772	222,577	1,364,349	54.8	2,487,919	6,142.99	1,044.61
400-499	97	4,835	475	14,039	19,446	290	41	331	608,514	127,351	735,865	52.1	1,411,621	7,079.63	950.05
500 or more	216	8,722	818	22,688	32,444	1,435	2	1,437	1,078,321	231,094	1,309,415	54.3	2,411,748	7,875.07	1,170.73
State and local government	1,765	11,850	1,907	36,219	51,741	2,810	146	2,956	1,650,588	424,969	2,075,557	56.2	3,696,448	6,359.42	1,043.90
Less than 300 beds	397	3,400	803	10,154	14,754	714	66	780	477,689	120,926	598,615	53.4	1,122,051	5,148.89	901.40
300-399	418	2,832	201	7,263	10,714	597	0	597	292,311	78,461	370,772	56.5	656,064	6,668.26	1,002.16
400-499	368	3,180	520	10,668	14,736	1,017	2	1,019	522,768	131,019	653,788	59.5	1,098,178	8,447.07	1,267.71
500 or more	582	2,438	383	8,134	11,537	482	78	560	357,819	94,563	452,382	55.2	820,156	6,077.84	1,057.88

Table

9

Utilization, Personnel Per Census, and Finances Per Inpatient Day in Accredited Hospitals

Expense components may not add to total expenses because of rounding to the nearest thousand.

CLASSIFICATION	HOSPITALS	BEDS	ADMISSIONS	OCCUPANCY, percent	AVERAGE DAILY CENSUS	ADJUSTED AVERAGE DAILY CENSUS	AVG. STAY, days	SURGICAL OPERATIONS	NEWBORNS			OUTPATIENT VISITS		
									Bassinets	Births	Days	Emergency	Other	Total
UNITED STATES	**5,104**	**1,080,203**	**31,734,514**	**69.9**	**754,596**			**21,992,305**	**64,404**	**3,864,297**	**9,922,921**	**85,380,423**	**256,646,930**	**342,027,353**
6-24 beds	58	1,132	32,656	38.0	430			27,757	162	2,538	9,426	203,247	1,134,852	1,338,099
25-49	524	20,567	581,872	45.3	9,316			343,493	2,220	56,413	129,693	2,802,257	9,194,153	11,996,410
50-99	1,190	87,018	2,340,612	55.0	47,877			1,468,502	6,756	251,170	589,826	8,360,307	21,118,366	29,478,673
100-199	1,387	196,468	5,914,115	62.2	122,236			4,285,239	13,880	694,567	1,716,600	19,062,884	47,858,717	66,921,601
200-299	794	193,166	6,385,196	68.1	131,629			4,651,204	13,062	758,307	1,913,170	18,116,021	46,392,742	64,508,763
300-399	473	161,919	5,216,775	72.2	116,899			3,741,184	9,857	666,572	1,699,570	12,692,593	37,001,036	49,693,629
400-499	265	118,889	3,808,265	74.8	88,974			2,613,284	7,111	519,812	1,319,879	8,792,265	30,072,745	38,865,010
500 or more	413	301,044	7,455,023	78.8	237,235			4,861,642	11,356	914,918	2,544,757	15,350,849	63,874,319	79,225,168
Federal	**293**	**93,707**	**1,661,730**	**73.1**	**68,531**			**1,080,478**	**1,831**	**79,109**	**224,682**	**4,365,426**	**49,668,990**	**54,034,416**
Psychiatric	17	11,654	58,674	80.4	9,366			3,897	0	0	0	6,374	1,200,960	1,207,334
General and other special	276	82,053	1,603,056	72.1	59,165			1,076,581	1,831	79,109	224,682	4,359,052	48,468,030	52,827,082
Nonfederal	**4,811**	**986,496**	**30,072,784**	**69.5**	**686,065**			**20,911,827**	**62,573**	**3,785,188**	**9,698,239**	**81,014,997**	**206,977,940**	**287,992,937**
Psychiatric	560	121,229	587,055	80.8	97,993			5,237	5	177	286	219,828	3,934,613	4,154,441
Nongovernment not-for-profit	70	8,150	79,950	74.2	6,050			602	5	177	286	20,389	821,914	842,303
Investor-owned (for-profit)	307	28,296	283,492	63.6	18,009			1,491	0	0	0	48,140	568,269	616,409
State and local government	183	84,783	223,613	87.2	73,934			3,144	0	0	0	151,299	2,544,430	2,695,729
TB and other respiratory diseases	3	278	1,721	66.5	185			2,039	0	0	0	0	16,500	16,500
Nongovernment not-for-profit	1	63	276	55.6	35			230	0	0	0	0	710	710
Investor-owned (for-profit)	0	0	0	00.0	0			0	0	0	0	0	0	0
State and local government	2	215	1,445	69.8	150			1,809	0	0	0	0	15,790	15,790
Long-term general and other special	89	15,896	73,112	84.0	13,347			16,009	22	2,046	5,938	50,028	1,296,511	1,346,539
Nongovernment not-for-profit	37	4,958	34,944	81.4	4,035			8,082	22	2,046	5,938	31,840	741,751	773,591
Investor-owned (for-profit)	16	1,143	7,425	74.2	848			474	0	0	0	866	221,577	222,443
State and local government	36	9,795	30,743	86.4	8,464			7,453	0	0	0	17,322	333,183	350,505
Short-term general and other special	4,159	849,093	29,410,896	67.7	574,540	750,818	7.1	20,888,542	62,546	3,782,965	9,692,015	80,745,141	201,730,316	282,475,457
6-24 beds	35	690	17,269	35.4	244	682	5.1	18,217	103	1,597	6,962	61,943	259,084	321,027
25-49	423	16,784	477,268	42.5	7,129	11,288	5.4	295,229	1,861	44,630	99,044	1,982,452	4,557,970	6,540,422
50-99	922	67,100	2,055,778	52.3	35,122	51,011	6.2	1,412,875	6,418	236,336	551,853	7,692,761	15,226,061	22,918,822
100-199	1,172	166,404	5,477,621	61.0	101,584	140,581	6.8	4,118,842	13,298	670,743	1,648,532	17,990,018	37,253,860	55,243,878
200-299	713	173,458	6,121,887	66.9	116,091	153,595	6.9	4,520,300	12,875	748,871	1,886,846	17,594,518	40,594,375	58,188,893
300-399	395	134,606	4,924,751	70.0	94,220	120,299	7.0	3,554,827	9,740	658,560	1,679,709	12,393,226	30,119,849	42,513,075
400-499	219	97,426	3,590,794	73.4	71,486	90,242	7.3	2,500,487	6,991	509,899	1,285,995	8,359,162	24,306,647	32,665,809
500 or more	280	192,625	6,745,528	77.2	148,664	183,120	8.0	4,467,765	11,260	912,329	2,533,074	14,671,061	49,412,470	64,083,531
Nongovernment not-for-profit	2,706	616,140	21,830,325	69.8	430,140	561,958	7.2	15,874,749	44,440	2,721,991	7,013,674	57,361,798	152,273,246	209,635,044
6-24 beds	18	359	10,112	38.7	139	409	4.9	12,126	63	1,036	5,802	36,048	171,569	207,617
25-49	247	9,743	288,895	44.8	4,367	7,142	5.5	193,085	1,091	27,231	59,738	1,209,641	2,957,782	4,167,423
50-99	485	34,923	1,074,928	55.4	19,346	28,611	6.6	767,990	3,324	117,068	276,864	4,144,723	9,134,350	13,279,073
100-199	698	100,255	3,450,041	63.3	63,468	88,874	6.7	2,644,026	8,074	410,409	1,004,974	11,629,072	26,106,395	37,735,467
200-299	541	131,947	4,734,803	69.1	91,196	121,588	7.0	3,535,081	9,633	563,114	1,453,132	13,553,434	34,243,612	47,797,046
300-399	321	109,864	4,075,133	70.7	77,703	99,539	7.0	3,007,461	8,072	536,495	1,385,975	10,122,951	24,907,261	35,030,212
400-499	177	78,623	2,905,614	74.2	58,345	73,654	7.3	2,071,085	5,636	400,765	1,027,034	6,381,144	18,447,858	24,829,002
500 or more	219	150,426	5,290,799	76.8	115,576	142,141	8.0	3,643,895	8,547	665,873	1,800,155	10,284,785	36,304,419	46,589,204
Investor-owned (for-profit)	631	93,490	2,860,652	53.1	49,641	63,531	6.3	2,191,321	5,943	328,202	777,830	7,422,302	11,194,925	18,617,227
6-24 beds	3	43	1,345	39.5	17	42	3.9	2,934	0	0	0	3,242	9,551	12,793
25-49	34	1,365	34,495	42.9	585	803	6.2	21,404	94	2,013	4,396	107,208	226,420	333,628
50-99	180	13,692	411,588	47.5	6,499	8,716	5.7	289,278	969	47,907	107,658	1,280,178	1,756,505	3,036,683
100-199	272	37,481	1,159,797	52.6	19,698	25,981	6.2	899,372	2,643	137,838	327,839	3,254,003	5,182,247	8,436,250
200-299	95	22,434	685,328	55.1	12,353	15,264	6.6	525,764	1,235	74,421	180,102	1,654,113	2,025,751	3,679,864
300-399	28	9,107	267,951	56.3	5,128	6,200	7.0	220,150	515	31,106	73,408	504,084	900,022	1,404,106
400-499	13	5,706	177,734	53.5	3,055	3,717	6.3	138,626	321	20,545	47,724	377,232	730,492	1,107,724
500 or more	6	3,662	122,414	63.0	2,306	2,808	6.9	93,793	166	14,372	36,703	242,242	363,937	606,179
State and local government	822	139,463	4,719,919	67.9	94,759	125,329	7.3	2,822,472	12,163	732,772	1,900,511	15,961,041	38,262,145	54,223,186
6-24 beds	14	288	5,812	30.6	88	231	5.6	3,157	40	561	1,160	22,653	77,964	100,617
25-49	142	5,676	153,878	38.4	2,177	3,343	5.2	80,740	676	15,386	34,910	665,603	1,373,768	2,039,371
50-99	257	18,485	569,262	50.2	9,277	13,684	5.9	355,607	2,125	71,361	167,331	2,267,860	4,335,206	6,603,066
100-199	202	28,668	867,783	64.2	18,418	25,726	7.7	575,444	2,581	122,496	315,719	3,106,943	5,965,218	9,072,161
200-299	77	19,077	701,756	65.7	12,542	16,743	6.5	459,455	2,007	111,336	253,612	2,386,971	4,325,012	6,711,983
300-399	46	15,635	581,667	72.8	11,389	14,560	7.1	327,216	1,153	90,959	220,326	1,766,191	4,312,566	6,078,757
400-499	29	13,097	507,446	77.0	10,086	12,871	7.3	290,776	1,034	88,589	211,237	1,600,786	5,128,297	6,729,083
500 or more	55	38,537	1,332,315	79.9	30,782	38,171	8.4	730,077	2,547	232,084	696,216	4,144,034	12,744,114	16,888,148
Hospital units of institutions	4	93	1,623	46.2	43	432	9.6	273	25	305	4,028	3,844	22,905	26,749
Community hospitals	4,155	849,000	29,409,273	67.7	574,497	750,386	7.1	20,888,269	62,521	3,782,660	9,687,987	80,741,297	201,707,411	282,448,708

Table 9 (Continued)

CLASSIFICATION	FULL-TIME EQUIVALENT PERSONNEL: TOTAL Number	FULL-TIME EQUIVALENT PERSONNEL: TOTAL Per 100 Adjusted Census	FULL-TIME EQUIVALENT PERSONNEL: RN Number	FULL-TIME EQUIVALENT PERSONNEL: RN Per 100 Adjusted Census	FULL-TIME EQUIVALENT PERSONNEL: LPN Number	FULL-TIME EQUIVALENT PERSONNEL: LPN Per 100 Adjusted Census	EXPENSES: LABOR: PAYROLL Amount (in thousands)	EXPENSES: LABOR: EMPLOYEE BENEFITS Amount (in thousands)	EXPENSES: LABOR: TOTAL Amount (in thousands)	EXPENSES: LABOR: TOTAL Adjusted, per Admission	EXPENSES: LABOR: TOTAL Adjusted Per Inpatient Day	EXPENSES: OTHER Amount (in thousands)	EXPENSES: TOTAL Amount (in thousands)	EXPENSES: TOTAL Adjusted, per Admission	EXPENSES: TOTAL Adjusted per Inpatient Day
UNITED STATES	3,770,255		848,596		179,232		$101,921,288	$20,388,107	$122,309,395			$97,689,608	$220,893,964		
6-24 beds	5,462		785		273		113,773	22,764	136,537			76,780	213,823		
25-49	69,227		12,545		4,693		1,483,678	295,347	1,779,025			1,362,347	3,150,840		
50-99	250,713		51,556		17,643		5,881,730	1,189,177	7,070,907			6,112,484	13,242,307		
100-199	624,352		141,027		36,922		15,653,635	3,152,941	18,806,575			16,554,143	35,657,603		
200-299	674,558		158,552		34,058		18,058,413	3,556,565	21,614,978			18,271,503	40,033,983		
300-399	600,470		140,432		26,479		16,499,917	3,279,677	19,779,594			15,602,456	35,484,075		
400-499	452,919		105,628		18,192		12,918,765	2,566,617	15,485,382			11,801,001	27,362,687		
500 or more	1,092,554		238,071		40,972		31,311,376	6,325,020	37,636,396			27,908,895	65,748,646		
Federal	285,119		43,293		13,440		8,285,882	1,407,719	9,693,601			4,803,674	14,471,447		
Psychiatric	18,773		2,458		824		536,173	94,577	630,750			261,673	892,451		
General and other special	266,346		40,835		12,616		7,749,709	1,313,141	9,062,850			4,542,001	13,578,996		
Nonfederal	3,485,136		805,303		165,792		93,635,406	18,980,389	112,615,794			92,885,934	206,422,517		
Psychiatric	211,672		26,685		9,071		5,684,758	1,316,943	7,001,702			2,912,093	9,952,522		
Nongovernment not-for-profit	20,663		3,211		247		577,350	119,911	697,261			399,712	1,102,434		
Investor-owned (for-profit)	47,554		8,191		1,491		1,351,093	295,469	1,646,561			1,382,981	3,055,039		
State and local government	143,455		15,283		7,333		3,756,316	901,564	4,657,880			1,129,401	5,795,049		
TB and other respiratory diseases	748		91		65		15,417	3,317	18,735			11,073	29,840		
Nongovernment not-for-profit	199		35		27		5,266	1,564	6,829			4,983	11,812		
Investor-owned (for-profit)	0		0		0		0	0	0			0	0		
State and local government	549		56		38		10,152	1,754	11,905			6,090	18,028		
Long-term general and other special	41,041		5,332		2,202		1,166,333	280,016	1,446,349			671,614	2,126,527		
Nongovernment not-for-profit	15,683		2,344		739		438,313	93,082	531,395			287,351	819,334		
Investor-owned (for-profit)	3,489		393		287		96,793	22,274	119,067			77,489	197,185		
State and local government	21,869		2,595		1,176		631,227	164,661	795,888			306,774	1,110,008		
Short-term general and other special	3,231,675	430	773,195	103	154,454	21	86,768,897	17,380,112	104,149,009	$2,692.09	$380.12	89,291,155	194,313,629	$5,022.71	$709.19
6-24 beds	2,002	294	387	57	202	30	46,209	9,111	55,320	1,361.48	222.96	48,851	104,762	2,578.31	422.22
25-49	51,050	452	10,117	90	4,040	36	1,058,089	204,587	1,262,676	1,642.44	306.54	1,131,651	2,401,382	3,123.63	582.98
50-99	199,012	390	43,550	85	15,694	31	4,523,060	919,481	5,442,541	1,796.66	292.39	5,027,262	10,512,717	3,470.39	564.78
100-199	541,765	385	128,839	92	33,657	24	13,446,136	2,722,937	16,169,073	2,124.46	315.35	14,856,291	31,301,412	4,112.70	610.48
200-299	622,396	405	150,960	98	31,591	21	16,529,229	3,291,487	19,820,716	2,447.54	353.56	17,389,276	37,356,673	4,612.95	666.37
300-399	531,885	442	131,155	109	23,381	19	14,565,807	2,880,106	17,445,913	2,773.14	397.33	14,633,695	32,206,972	5,119.51	733.51
400-499	401,825	445	97,796	108	15,540	17	11,390,778	2,271,817	13,662,595	3,014.58	414.84	11,097,205	24,834,432	5,479.59	754.06
500 or more	881,740	482	210,391	115	30,349	17	25,209,589	5,080,586	30,290,175	3,642.38	453.21	25,106,923	55,595,279	6,685.31	831.82
Nongovernment not-for-profit	2,423,517	431	585,332	104	104,502	19	65,829,245	12,834,260	78,663,505	2,743.17	383.53	65,599,275	144,788,044	5,049.08	705.92
6-24 beds	1,206	295	215	53	122	30	26,838	5,298	32,135	1,281.21	215.06	26,952	59,182	2,359.56	396.06
25-49	32,688	458	6,582	92	2,152	30	676,532	127,288	803,820	1,684.75	308.45	727,474	1,536,694	3,220.80	589.68
50-99	110,265	385	24,535	86	7,613	27	2,535,070	503,628	3,038,698	1,875.93	290.83	2,585,240	5,645,095	3,484.98	540.28
100-199	352,948	397	83,753	94	19,227	22	8,958,857	1,738,519	10,697,376	2,202.40	329.80	8,970,264	19,745,583	4,065.27	608.75
200-299	493,451	406	119,308	98	23,192	19	13,117,972	2,548,064	15,666,036	2,483.35	353.03	13,085,447	28,861,477	4,575.07	650.38
300-399	435,409	437	106,715	107	18,557	19	11,965,691	2,337,732	14,303,423	2,739.93	393.70	11,767,051	26,157,411	5,010.66	719.99
400-499	319,688	434	78,986	107	11,920	16	9,021,414	1,752,466	10,773,881	2,938.47	400.80	8,672,753	19,510,525	5,321.30	725.81
500 or more	677,862	477	165,238	116	21,719	15	19,526,871	3,821,265	23,348,136	3,591.08	450.05	19,764,093	43,272,078	6,655.50	834.10
Investor-owned (for-profit)	252,742	398	64,526	102	18,018	28	6,316,643	1,403,994	7,720,637	2,089.03	333.49	9,728,698	17,691,262	4,786.86	764.17
6-24 beds	150	357	44	105	12	29	5,775	966	6,741	1,605.72	501.77	6,560	13,776	3,281.62	1,025.48
25-49	3,383	421	630	78	366	46	72,400	15,437	87,837	1,703.52	300.22	98,359	186,998	3,626.66	639.14
50-99	35,324	405	7,704	88	3,118	36	837,376	187,273	1,024,649	1,823.08	322.79	1,283,323	2,325,151	4,136.96	732.49
100-199	102,302	394	26,390	102	7,403	28	2,511,942	585,458	3,097,401	2,013.14	327.59	3,864,751	7,147,150	4,645.26	755.90
200-299	58,752	385	16,061	105	3,910	26	1,544,531	337,101	1,881,632	2,213.48	337.72	2,379,703	4,286,358	5,042.32	769.32
300-399	25,268	408	6,475	104	1,608	26	671,647	136,141	807,789	2,499.21	357.12	1,032,172	1,849,867	5,723.28	817.82
400-499	15,585	419	4,054	109	963	26	390,836	80,701	471,538	2,174.56	347.62	629,635	1,102,742	5,085.44	812.96
500 or more	11,978	427	3,168	113	638	23	282,135	60,916	343,051	2,298.33	334.56	434,194	779,220	5,220.52	759.93
State and local government	555,416	443	123,337	98	31,934	25	14,623,009	3,141,858	17,764,867	2,813.08	388.43	13,963,182	31,834,322	5,040.99	696.06
6-24 beds	646	280	128	55	68	29	13,596	2,847	16,444	1,448.52	192.87	15,340	31,803	2,801.53	373.03
25-49	14,979	448	2,905	87	1,522	46	309,157	61,862	371,020	1,545.26	303.97	305,818	677,691	2,822.51	555.22
50-99	53,423	390	11,311	83	4,963	36	1,150,614	228,580	1,379,195	1,627.60	276.32	1,158,698	2,542,470	3,000.39	509.39
100-199	86,515	336	18,696	73	7,027	27	1,975,336	398,960	2,374,296	1,953.86	253.07	2,021,276	4,408,679	3,628.00	469.91
200-299	70,193	419	15,591	93	4,489	27	1,866,726	406,322	2,273,048	2,418.87	371.89	1,924,126	4,208,839	4,478.85	688.59
300-399	71,208	489	17,965	123	3,216	22	1,928,468	406,233	2,334,701	3,123.51	439.22	1,834,472	4,199,695	5,618.62	790.08
400-499	66,552	517	14,756	115	2,657	21	1,978,528	438,649	2,417,177	3,725.44	514.65	1,794,816	4,221,165	6,505.82	898.75
500 or more	191,900	503	41,985	110	7,992	21	5,400,584	1,198,404	6,598,987	3,963.18	473.68	4,908,635	11,543,981	6,933.01	828.63
Hospital units of institutions	206	48	36	8	30	7	4,566	907	5,473	319.00	34.68	4,634	10,135	590.70	64.22
Community hospitals	3,231,469	431	773,159	103	154,424	21	86,764,331	17,379,204	104,143,536	2,693.14	380.32	89,286,521	194,303,494	5,024.67	709.57

Table
10A
AHA Membership, Approval, and Affiliation Status in the United States

CLASSIFICATION	TOTAL	AHA MEMBERS Hospitals	AHA MEMBERS Beds	AHA MEMBERS Admissions	ACCREDITATION (A-1)	CANCER PROGRAM (A-2)	RESIDENCY (A-3)	MEDICAL SCHOOL AFFILIATION (A-5)	PROFESSIONAL NURSING SCHOOL (A-6)	COUNCIL OF TEACHING HOSPITALS (A-8)	BLUE CROSS PARTICIPATION (A-9)	MEDICARE CERTIFICATION (A-10)
UNITED STATES	**6,649**	**4,850**	**978,615**	**29,943,448**	**5,104**	**1,207**	**1,249**	**1,238**	**152**	**387**	**5,690**	**6,004**
6-24 beds	301	169	3,221	93,868	58	0	5	5	0	0	234	245
25-49	1,095	690	26,219	694,361	524	6	27	25	0	0	940	986
50-99	1,633	1,068	76,732	2,016,498	1,190	38	64	64	1	1	1,402	1,488
100-199	1,562	1,156	164,532	5,136,009	1,387	205	174	180	13	13	1,373	1,454
200-299	830	711	173,215	5,928,256	794	294	238	235	38	43	748	783
300-399	503	432	147,763	5,046,968	473	249	237	233	33	65	433	453
400-499	276	242	108,522	3,705,801	265	158	174	172	24	67	231	245
500 or more	449	382	278,411	7,321,687	413	257	330	324	43	198	329	350
Federal	**337**	**331**	**97,391**	**1,749,565**	**293**	**74**	**148**	**150**	**0**	**70**	**57**	**42**
Psychiatric	17	17	11,654	58,674	17	0	2	2	0	0	6	0
General and other special	320	314	85,737	1,690,891	276	74	146	148	0	70	51	42
Nonfederal	**6,312**	**4,519**	**881,224**	**28,193,883**	**4,811**	**1,133**	**1,101**	**1,088**	**152**	**317**	**5,633**	**5,962**
Psychiatric	757	280	54,694	268,992	560	2	108	107	0	1	475	561
Nongovernment not-for-profit	127	84	9,610	87,826	70	0	26	25	0	1	82	89
Investor-owned (for-profit)	372	131	12,521	113,830	307	0	12	14	0	0	261	282
State and local government	258	65	32,563	67,336	183	2	70	68	0	0	132	190
TB and other respiratory diseases	4	3	370	1,615	3	0	2	2	0	0	3	4
Nongovernment not-for-profit	1	1	63	276	1	0	1	1	0	0	1	1
Investor-owned (for-profit)	0	0	0	0	0	0	0	0	0	0	0	0
State and local government	3	2	307	1,339	2	0	1	1	0	0	2	3
Long-term general and other special	131	89	19,341	69,967	89	1	20	17	1	0	85	114
Nongovernment not-for-profit	58	46	7,568	37,597	37	1	11	9	1	0	40	48
Investor-owned (for-profit)	18	8	605	4,434	16	0	0	0	0	0	8	17
State and local government	55	35	11,168	27,936	36	0	9	8	0	0	37	49
Short-term general and other special	5,420	4,147	806,819	27,853,309	4,159	1,130	971	962	151	316	5,070	5,283
6-24 beds	241	120	2,388	54,684	35	0	5	5	0	0	221	221
25-49	944	601	22,954	586,334	423	6	19	18	0	0	882	908
50-99	1,270	891	63,738	1,814,619	922	34	35	37	1	1	1,176	1,233
100-199	1,309	1,011	143,779	4,767,526	1,172	193	120	126	13	10	1,219	1,291
200-299	740	654	159,273	5,686,776	713	283	196	191	38	34	702	731
300-399	409	382	130,365	4,789,404	395	238	196	193	32	51	390	398
400-499	222	212	94,577	3,499,982	219	148	155	153	24	60	208	219
500 or more	285	276	189,745	6,653,984	280	228	245	239	43	160	272	282
Nongovernment not-for-profit	3,202	2,748	605,290	21,345,715	2,706	928	803	792	139	243	3,016	3,125
6-24 beds	84	51	1,039	25,921	18	0	4	4	0	0	73	71
25-49	409	305	11,655	319,305	247	5	17	17	0	0	380	390
50-99	635	514	37,060	1,071,003	485	23	31	34	1	1	588	617
100-199	778	653	93,934	3,219,353	698	143	87	88	10	10	733	769
200-299	562	514	125,533	4,525,275	541	239	171	166	37	29	540	555
300-399	331	320	109,543	4,078,016	321	209	168	166	29	35	318	325
400-499	179	173	76,985	2,855,068	177	124	130	128	24	46	171	176
500 or more	224	218	149,541	5,251,774	219	185	195	189	38	122	213	222
Investor-owned (for-profit)	749	383	61,826	1,971,043	631	60	25	29	1	2	663	730
6-24 beds	15	5	76	2,334	3	0	1	1	0	0	15	15
25-49	80	29	1,119	26,352	34	0	0	0	0	0	67	74
50-99	219	77	5,658	174,428	180	5	1	1	0	0	192	212
100-199	287	162	22,543	754,563	272	25	11	15	0	0	260	283
200-299	99	70	16,374	511,203	95	14	4	4	0	0	87	98
300-399	30	23	7,547	228,983	28	8	4	4	1	1	26	29
400-499	13	11	4,847	150,766	13	3	3	3	0	1	10	13
500 or more	6	6	3,662	122,414	6	5	1	1	0	0	6	6
State and local government	1,469	1,016	139,703	4,536,551	822	142	143	141	11	71	1,391	1,428
6-24 beds	142	64	1,273	26,429	14	0	0	0	0	0	133	135
25-49	455	267	10,180	240,677	142	1	2	1	0	0	435	444
50-99	416	300	21,020	569,188	257	6	3	2	0	0	396	404
100-199	244	196	27,302	793,610	202	25	22	23	3	0	226	239
200-299	79	70	17,366	650,298	77	30	21	21	1	5	75	78
300-399	48	39	13,275	482,405	46	21	24	23	2	15	46	44
400-499	30	28	12,745	494,148	29	21	22	22	0	13	27	30
500 or more	55	52	36,542	1,279,796	55	38	49	49	5	38	53	54
Hospital units of institutions	36	4	118	1,481	4	0	1	0	0	0	10	3
Community hospitals	5,384	4,143	806,701	27,851,828	4,155	1,130	970	962	151	316	5,060	5,280

10B

AHA Membership, Approval, and Affiliation Status in States

CLASSIFICATION	TOTAL	AHA MEMBERS Hospitals	AHA MEMBERS Beds	AHA MEMBERS Admissions	ACCREDITATION (A-1)	CANCER PROGRAM (A-2)	RESIDENCY (A-3)	MEDICAL SCHOOL AFFILIATION (A-5)	PROFESSIONAL NURSING SCHOOL (A-6)	COUNCIL OF TEACHING HOSPITALS (A-8)	BLUE CROSS PARTICIPATION (A-9)	MEDICARE CERTIFICATION (A-10)
UNITED STATES	6,649	4,850	978,615	29,943,448	5,104	1,207	1,249	1,238	152	387	5,690	6,004
Alabama	138	91	17,714	564,443	110	15	20	19	2	4	117	125
Alaska	27	23	1,677	57,154	17	1	0	0	0	0	19	24
Arizona	91	68	11,047	395,981	80	12	15	15	0	6	80	75
Arkansas	96	72	11,071	343,605	63	10	13	13	2	3	89	92
California	548	295	68,201	2,466,879	488	154	103	105	1	27	449	489
Colorado	86	74	11,477	360,111	67	17	18	16	0	3	76	79
Connecticut	63	53	13,697	373,962	53	23	30	29	5	14	52	51
Delaware	13	12	2,445	90,232	11	5	5	5	1	1	9	10
District of Columbia	17	16	7,840	197,482	16	7	13	14	0	6	16	14
Florida	288	199	47,959	1,510,296	254	44	33	35	1	10	206	258
Georgia	203	136	26,632	879,875	141	26	25	25	1	8	177	180
Hawaii	26	23	3,703	109,133	18	8	10	10	0	1	20	23
Idaho	50	39	3,197	98,322	18	8	3	3	0	0	45	45
Illinois	247	205	49,768	1,497,532	226	96	66	65	7	20	208	228
Indiana	135	112	22,009	677,775	108	21	21	20	2	4	83	125
Iowa	134	100	14,043	378,048	76	11	18	17	5	3	128	128
Kansas	160	114	12,211	309,287	72	13	14	13	1	1	154	146
Kentucky	123	93	15,867	516,049	96	11	17	16	0	4	117	118
Louisiana	173	127	19,871	564,189	131	13	27	26	3	7	149	162
Maine	44	37	4,606	142,205	40	11	6	5	0	1	42	40
Maryland	82	65	17,171	610,731	75	12	28	27	3	10	56	65
Massachusetts	157	128	28,941	820,102	140	51	52	54	8	18	133	139
Michigan	205	163	31,990	951,912	181	33	45	46	3	18	180	188
Minnesota	167	124	18,565	507,014	101	13	18	20	0	5	157	160
Mississippi	115	56	12,399	331,586	61	11	7	7	0	2	103	105
Missouri	160	95	21,902	668,797	112	29	29	27	8	11	135	149
Montana	62	47	4,255	107,991	20	1	0	0	0	0	55	59
Nebraska	102	63	8,226	194,379	43	13	14	14	1	2	93	97
Nevada	31	21	2,930	94,998	19	3	5	5	0	0	24	28
New Hampshire	40	32	4,086	131,530	34	12	3	3	0	1	37	31
New Jersey	119	103	33,400	1,127,227	105	44	46	43	17	13	104	105
New Mexico	60	48	4,865	177,928	44	6	8	8	0	2	46	51
New York	305	259	95,274	2,221,302	280	72	120	120	9	53	243	266
North Carolina	155	117	23,744	810,751	126	11	19	22	4	6	145	140
North Dakota	57	52	5,050	105,661	25	9	9	10	0	0	51	52
Ohio	224	186	45,975	1,491,466	194	70	55	52	16	25	215	209
Oklahoma	137	107	13,026	395,518	79	18	16	18	0	3	112	129
Oregon	77	55	7,774	280,828	56	22	10	10	0	2	66	69
Pennsylvania	302	226	54,433	1,730,928	253	65	86	86	34	33	256	270
Rhode Island	19	17	4,187	134,749	17	4	8	8	1	5	14	17
South Carolina	89	71	12,240	435,611	65	12	14	13	0	3	73	74
South Dakota	66	48	4,577	107,945	26	6	3	3	1	0	58	61
Tennessee	156	107	23,134	728,133	138	19	26	26	4	8	131	147
Texas	537	332	59,118	1,838,640	382	48	68	64	2	18	473	473
Utah	52	41	4,660	183,044	34	9	8	8	0	1	42	46
Vermont	18	17	2,140	62,337	16	4	4	4	0	2	15	17
Virginia	135	106	25,921	740,646	122	31	26	26	8	7	112	116
Washington	110	84	13,115	517,541	73	35	19	19	0	4	94	97
West Virginia	68	56	8,679	271,797	53	9	13	13	1	3	61	62
Wisconsin	148	110	19,468	579,708	124	27	30	28	1	9	139	141
Wyoming	32	25	2,335	50,088	21	2	3	3	0	0	31	29
U.S. ASSOCIATED AREAS	62	46	8,607	337,447	31	6	15	17	0	2	37	47
American Samoa	1	0	0	0	0	0	0	0	0	0	0	1
Canal Zone	0	0	0	0	0	0	0	0	0	0	0	0
Guam	2	1	55	3,344	1	0	0	0	0	0	0	1
Marshall Islands	1	0	0	0	0	0	0	0	0	0	0	0
Puerto Rico	56	44	8,465	330,773	30	6	15	17	0	2	37	44
Virgin Islands	2	1	87	3,330	0	0	0	0	0	0	0	1

Table

11

Revenue in Community Hospitals

AREA	ALL COMMUNITY HOSPITALS: HOSP-ITALS	Percent of Total (gross inpatient revenue)	Percent of Total (gross outpatient revenue)	Net Patient Revenue (in thousands)	Net Total Revenue (in thousands)	NONGOVERNMENT NOT-FOR-PROFIT: HOSPI-TALS	Percent of Total (gross inpatient revenue)	Percent of Total (gross outpatient revenue)	Net Patient Revenue (in thousands)	Net Total Revenue (in thousands)
UNITED STATES	5,384	77.4	22.6	$195,539,641	$211,842,938	3,191	77.6	22.4	$146,754,476	$156,852,531
6-24 beds	226	55.6	44.4	402,960	471,011	75	53.5	46.5	155,888	177,610
25-49	935	64.7	35.3	3,735,152	4,065,551	408	62.8	37.2	1,963,130	2,103,273
50-99	1,263	69.3	30.7	12,212,289	12,898,600	634	67.7	32.3	6,495,181	6,836,922
100-199	1,306	73.1	26.9	32,722,196	34,664,978	778	72.3	27.7	20,801,343	22,056,445
200-299	739	76.4	23.6	37,980,386	40,304,966	562	75.8	24.2	29,467,583	31,194,467
300-399	408	79.0	21.0	32,224,062	34,705,463	331	78.8	21.2	26,404,934	28,218,002
400-499	222	79.8	20.2	24,417,827	26,336,462	179	79.8	20.2	19,340,759	20,510,995
500 or more	285	81.5	18.5	51,844,769	58,395,906	224	81.8	18.2	42,125,658	45,754,817
CENSUS DIVISION 1, NEW ENGLAND	229	73.7	26.3	11,648,552	12,651,526	209	73.8	26.2	10,853,866	11,810,622
Connecticut	35	75.9	24.1	2,845,381	2,999,476	34	76.1	23.9	2,764,218	2,908,754
Maine	39	74.1	25.9	888,126	936,108	35	74.5	25.5	827,872	872,159
Massachusetts	101	73.0	27.0	5,966,997	6,637,560	89	72.9	27.1	5,398,699	6,037,161
New Hampshire	27	71.6	28.4	811,256	857,178	24	72.0	28.0	726,284	771,344
Rhode Island	12	73.1	26.9	785,524	853,546	12	73.1	26.9	785,524	853,546
Vermont	15	71.5	28.5	351,268	367,658	15	71.5	28.5	351,268	367,658
CENSUS DIVISION 2, MIDDLE ATLANTIC	568	78.3	21.7	35,229,104	38,672,808	510	78.2	21.8	31,568,382	34,022,346
New Jersey	95	80.0	20.0	6,368,764	6,764,768	91	80.1	19.9	6,123,771	6,454,742
New York	235	78.3	21.7	16,992,847	19,190,742	194	78.1	21.9	13,711,533	15,004,718
Pennsylvania	238	77.7	22.3	11,867,493	12,717,298	225	77.7	22.3	11,733,079	12,562,887
CENSUS DIVISION 3, SOUTH ATLANTIC	803	78.8	21.2	33,196,706	35,381,913	416	78.8	21.2	20,896,675	21,982,075
Delaware	8	76.1	23.9	556,925	585,734	8	76.1	23.9	556,925	585,734
District of Columbia	11	83.5	16.5	1,320,856	1,454,735	10	84.0	16.0	1,272,775	1,351,355
Florida	224	79.9	20.1	10,841,866	11,475,697	98	79.2	20.8	5,767,984	6,084,655
Georgia	163	78.4	21.6	4,938,159	5,322,299	39	82.1	17.9	2,101,226	2,219,858
Maryland	52	78.5	21.5	3,241,615	3,409,146	50	78.4	21.6	3,131,989	3,293,290
North Carolina	120	77.6	22.4	4,502,948	4,819,990	72	78.0	22.0	2,816,351	2,952,622
South Carolina	69	77.9	22.1	2,284,872	2,459,821	29	77.1	22.9	1,228,243	1,288,298
Virginia	97	77.8	22.2	4,035,411	4,318,625	77	76.4	23.6	2,854,019	2,986,261
West Virginia	59	74.7	25.3	1,474,054	1,535,865	33	75.3	24.7	1,167,164	1,220,001
CENSUS DIVISION 4, EAST NORTH CENTRAL	818	75.2	24.8	34,984,164	37,738,272	643	75.5	24.5	31,110,738	33,211,894
Illinois	210	78.7	21.3	9,659,891	10,799,051	163	78.9	21.1	8,981,663	9,822,718
Indiana	113	74.6	25.4	4,347,498	4,660,499	56	76.3	23.7	3,139,858	3,353,109
Michigan	176	71.3	28.7	7,978,295	8,432,485	137	71.6	28.4	7,315,117	7,693,813
Ohio	190	75.6	24.4	9,593,495	10,245,232	165	75.5	24.5	8,601,225	9,105,183
Wisconsin	129	73.7	26.3	3,404,984	3,601,006	122	73.5	26.5	3,072,875	3,237,071
CENSUS DIVISION 5, EAST SOUTH CENTRAL	464	79.4	20.6	11,875,477	12,653,626	195	80.3	19.7	6,569,733	6,990,483
Alabama	120	80.6	19.4	3,135,666	3,405,746	39	80.7	19.3	1,280,102	1,368,320
Kentucky	107	77.7	22.3	2,734,338	2,879,167	68	77.2	22.8	1,824,441	1,931,730
Mississippi	103	78.4	21.6	1,593,371	1,690,365	32	80.6	19.4	679,795	714,932
Tennessee	134	79.9	20.1	4,412,101	4,678,349	56	82.0	18.0	2,785,394	2,975,501
CENSUS DIVISION 6, WEST NORTH CENTRAL	742	76.6	23.4	14,054,934	15,227,385	429	77.3	22.7	10,961,095	11,803,454
Iowa	124	75.1	24.9	2,085,236	2,297,293	57	76.2	23.8	1,496,991	1,586,480
Kansas	138	76.1	23.9	1,710,994	1,809,355	62	76.6	23.4	1,130,188	1,194,690
Minnesota	152	76.5	23.5	3,284,886	3,540,244	86	77.8	22.2	2,515,910	2,684,088
Missouri	135	76.8	23.2	4,736,257	5,174,650	84	77.2	22.8	3,987,512	4,364,485
Nebraska	90	77.3	22.7	1,192,366	1,280,181	46	76.3	23.7	813,642	877,928
North Dakota	50	78.3	21.7	563,747	601,810	49	78.6	21.4	552,696	590,068
South Dakota	53	80.2	19.8	481,448	523,851	45	80.4	19.6	464,155	505,715
CENSUS DIVISION 7, WEST SOUTH CENTRAL	765	78.4	21.6	18,407,509	20,417,478	247	80.3	19.7	10,196,749	10,816,420
Arkansas	86	78.8	21.2	1,690,629	1,798,680	42	79.4	20.6	1,168,237	1,240,060
Louisiana	140	78.0	22.0	3,404,758	3,819,625	34	80.2	19.8	1,705,479	1,792,853
Oklahoma	111	80.3	19.7	2,028,697	2,171,190	39	82.5	17.5	1,250,730	1,325,152
Texas	428	78.2	21.8	11,283,424	12,627,982	132	80.1	19.9	6,072,303	6,458,355
CENSUS DIVISION 8, MOUNTAIN	355	76.4	23.6	8,774,343	9,377,691	196	77.0	23.0	6,013,795	6,379,328
Arizona	61	78.6	21.4	2,409,927	2,593,103	46	79.5	20.5	2,020,977	2,142,872
Colorado	69	76.1	23.9	2,262,115	2,435,691	35	75.9	24.1	1,633,218	1,751,986
Idaho	43	70.9	29.1	520,570	552,030	11	70.0	30.0	274,829	290,003
Montana	55	77.6	22.4	544,212	585,022	42	77.8	22.2	520,866	553,831
Nevada	21	82.4	17.6	822,096	857,282	6	81.9	18.1	286,164	298,514
New Mexico	37	70.3	29.7	885,288	957,194	23	74.9	25.1	452,061	481,669
Utah	42	73.7	26.3	1,082,901	1,126,857	24	73.0	27.0	730,012	760,060
Wyoming	27	72.4	27.6	247,233	270,511	9	74.8	25.2	95,668	100,391
CENSUS DIVISION 9, PACIFIC	640	77.9	22.1	27,368,853	29,722,239	346	78.7	21.3	18,583,445	19,835,910
Alaska	16	75.6	24.4	303,576	324,459	7	74.3	25.7	205,547	220,116
California	445	78.8	21.2	21,520,402	23,416,308	237	79.8	20.2	14,070,813	15,050,039
Hawaii	18	78.1	21.9	623,802	749,480	10	78.6	21.4	542,843	588,082
Oregon	70	71.4	28.6	1,880,152	1,993,787	43	71.6	28.4	1,519,673	1,608,956
Washington	91	73.7	26.3	3,040,920	3,238,205	49	74.8	25.2	2,244,569	2,368,718

Tables 12-13

Notes

In the 1980 edition of *AHA Hospital Statistics,* tables 13A and 13B included hospitals, units, and beds, by inpatient service area, for the first time. In previous editions, inpatient units and beds were included in tables 12A and 12B.

Table 14 contains U.S. nonregistered hospital data, which, previous to 1980, were listed in table 13.

Table

12

Facilities and Services

The facilities and services presented in tables 12A and 12B are listed below in alphabetical order by major heading, referencing the page numbers on which they appear.

Table 12A Page	12B Page	
		Acquired immune-deficiency syndrome (AIDS) services
208	218	General inpatient care for AIDS/ARC
208	218	AIDS/ARC unit
208	218	Specialized outpatient program for AIDS/ARC
208	218	Alcohol/drug abuse or dependency outpatient services
208	218	Arthritis treatment center
208	218	Birthing room/LDRP Room
		Cardiac services
208	218	Angioplasty
209	219	Cardiac catheterization laboratory
209	219	Cardiac rehabilitation program
209	219	Non-invasive cardiac assessment
209	219	Open heart surgery
209	219	Chronic obstructive pulmonary disease services
		Emergency services
209	219	Emergency department
209	219	Trauma center (certified)
210	220	Extracorporeal shock wave lithotripter (ESWL)
210	220	Fitness center
210	220	Genetic counseling/screening
		Geriatric services
210	220	Adult day care program
210	220	Alzheimer's diagnostic/assessment services
210	220	Comprehensive geriatric assessment
210	220	Emergency response (geriatric)
211	221	Geriatric acute care unit
211	221	Geriatric clinics
211	221	Respite care
211	221	Senior membership program
		Health promotion services
211	221	Patient education
211	221	Community health promotion
211	221	Worksite health promotion
212	222	Health sciences library
212	222	Hemodialysis
212	222	Home health services
212	222	Hospice
		Laboratory services
212	222	Histopathology laboratory
212	222	Blood bank
212	222	Occupational health services

Table 12 Continued

Table

12A

Facilities and Services in the United States

For definitions of facilities and services, see Definitions of Terms, page xxiii. These data include only hospital-based facilities and services as reported by responding hospitals in Section C of the 1990 AHA Annual Survey, beginning on page 242. No estimates have been made for nonresponding hospitals.

CLASSIFICATION	HOSPITALS REPORTING	ACQUIRED IMMUNE-DEFICIENCY SYNDROME (AIDS) SERVICES: GENERAL INPATIENT CARE FOR AIDS/ARC		AIDS/ARC UNIT		SPECIALIZED OUTPATIENT PROGRAM FOR AIDS/ARC		ALCOHOL/DRUG ABUSE OR DEPENDENCY OUTPATIENT SERVICES		ARTHRITIS TREATMENT CENTER		BIRTHING ROOM/ LDRP ROOM		CARDIAC SERVICES: ANGIOPLASTY	
		Number	Percent	Number	Percent	Number	Percent	Number	Percent	Number	Percent	Number	Percent	Number	Percent
UNITED STATES	**6,105**	**3,745**	**61.3**	**146**	**2.4**	**389**	**6.4**	**1,508**	**24.7**	**418**	**6.8**	**3,394**	**55.6**	**1,101**	**18.0**
6-24 beds	254	69	27.2	1	0.4	4	1.6	23	9.1	2	0.8	113	44.5	1	0.4
25-49	974	359	36.9	2	0.2	6	0.6	101	10.4	14	1.4	473	48.6	5	0.5
50-99	1,451	649	44.7	6	0.4	15	1.0	247	17.0	49	3.4	697	48.0	29	2.0
100-199	1,439	950	66.0	21	1.5	54	3.8	366	25.4	70	4.9	841	58.4	148	10.3
200-299	804	686	85.3	19	2.4	62	7.7	244	30.3	76	9.5	514	63.9	259	32.2
300-399	485	417	86.0	20	4.1	56	11.5	183	37.7	57	11.8	329	67.8	238	49.1
400-499	265	233	87.9	15	5.7	60	22.6	115	43.4	44	16.6	185	69.8	157	59.2
500 or more	433	382	88.2	62	14.3	132	30.5	229	52.9	106	24.5	242	55.9	264	61.0
Federal	**301**	**210**	**69.8**	**23**	**7.6**	**90**	**29.9**	**215**	**71.4**	**42**	**14.0**	**98**	**32.6**	**59**	**19.6**
Psychiatric	17	14	82.4	0	0.0	1	5.9	16	94.1	2	11.8	0	0.0	0	0.0
General and other special	284	196	69.0	23	8.1	89	31.3	199	70.1	40	14.1	98	34.5	59	20.8
Nonfederal	**5,804**	**3,535**	**60.9**	**123**	**2.1**	**299**	**5.2**	**1,293**	**22.3**	**376**	**6.5**	**3,296**	**56.8**	**1,042**	**18.0**
Psychiatric	609	78	12.8	3	0.5	3	0.5	249	40.9	0	0.0	1	0.2	1	0.2
Nongovernment not-for-profit	106	5	4.7	0	0.0	0	0.0	68	64.2	0	0.0	1	0.9	0	0.0
Investor-owned (for-profit)	272	9	3.3	0	0.0	0	0.0	153	56.3	0	0.0	0	0.0	0	0.0
State and local government	231	64	27.7	3	1.3	3	1.3	28	12.1	0	0.0	0	0.0	1	0.4
TB and other respiratory diseases	3	2	66.7	0	0.0	0	0.0	0	0.0	0	0.0	0	0.0	0	0.0
Nongovernment not-for-profit	1	0	0.0	0	0.0	0	0.0	0	0.0	0	0.0	0	0.0	0	0.0
Investor-owned (for-profit)	0	0	0.0	0	0.0	0	0.0	0	0.0	0	0.0	0	0.0	0	0.0
State and local government	2	2	100.0	0	0.0	0	0.0	0	0.0	0	0.0	0	0.0	0	0.0
Long-term general and other special	119	37	31.1	7	5.9	2	1.7	6	5.0	14	11.8	3	2.5	1	0.8
Nongovernment not-for-profit	54	17	31.5	0	0.0	0	0.0	2	3.7	8	14.8	1	1.9	1	1.9
Investor-owned (for-profit)	16	0	0.0	0	0.0	0	0.0	1	6.3	1	6.3	0	0.0	0	0.0
State and local government	49	20	40.8	7	14.3	2	4.1	3	6.1	5	10.2	2	4.1	0	0.0
Short-term general and other special	5,073	3,418	67.4	113	2.2	294	5.8	1,038	20.5	362	7.1	3,292	64.9	1,040	20.5
6-24 beds	209	60	28.7	1	0.5	1	0.5	8	3.8	1	0.5	97	46.4	1	0.5
25-49	868	339	39.1	2	0.2	4	0.5	56	6.5	12	1.4	443	51.0	5	0.6
50-99	1,157	624	53.9	5	0.4	12	1.0	113	9.8	45	3.9	676	58.4	29	2.5
100-199	1,225	887	72.4	18	1.5	42	3.4	257	21.0	55	4.5	820	66.9	146	11.9
200-299	719	653	90.8	18	2.5	49	6.8	204	28.4	70	9.7	509	70.8	252	35.0
300-399	400	377	94.3	14	3.5	43	10.8	149	37.3	51	12.8	325	81.3	221	55.3
400-499	215	207	96.3	11	5.1	50	23.3	96	44.7	38	17.7	181	84.2	150	69.8
500 or more	280	271	96.8	44	15.7	93	33.2	155	55.4	90	32.1	241	86.1	236	84.3
Nongovernment not-for-profit	3,079	2,260	73.4	70	2.3	200	6.5	787	25.6	268	8.7	2,141	69.5	778	25.3
6-24 beds	71	24	33.8	0	0.0	1	1.4	5	7.0	1	1.4	39	54.9	0	0.0
25-49	383	159	41.5	0	0.0	1	0.3	33	8.6	8	2.1	210	54.8	2	0.5
50-99	601	331	55.1	2	0.3	7	1.2	67	11.1	25	4.2	366	60.9	15	2.5
100-199	748	542	72.5	9	1.2	29	3.9	175	23.4	37	4.9	515	68.9	83	11.1
200-299	552	510	92.4	13	2.4	38	6.9	172	31.2	59	10.7	399	72.3	184	33.3
300-399	326	309	94.8	8	2.5	28	8.6	128	39.3	38	11.7	268	82.2	179	54.9
400-499	175	168	96.0	9	5.1	35	20.0	82	46.9	28	16.0	150	85.7	120	68.6
500 or more	223	217	97.3	29	13.0	61	27.4	125	56.1	72	32.3	194	87.0	195	87.4
Investor-owned (for-profit)	636	399	62.7	11	1.7	12	1.9	99	15.6	43	6.8	320	50.3	127	20.0
6-24 beds	14	1	7.1	0	0.0	0	0.0	0	0.0	0	0.0	1	7.1	1	7.1
25-49	62	19	30.6	0	0.0	1	1.6	6	9.7	1	1.6	19	30.6	1	1.6
50-99	178	84	47.2	2	1.1	3	1.7	17	9.6	15	8.4	78	43.8	8	4.5
100-199	248	180	72.6	5	2.0	5	2.0	51	20.6	15	6.0	142	57.3	46	18.5
200-299	90	76	84.4	2	2.2	2	2.2	15	16.7	8	8.9	48	53.3	41	45.6
300-399	29	25	[illegible]	2	6.9	1	3.4	7	24.1	2	6.9	21	72.4	17	58.6
400-499	12	11	91.7	0	0.0	0	0.0	2	16.7	1	8.3	8	66.7	10	83.3
500 or more	3	3	100.0	0	0.0	0	0.0	1	33.3	1	33.3	3	100.0	3	100.0
State and local government	1,358	759	55.9	32	2.4	82	6.0	152	11.2	51	3.8	831	61.2	135	9.9
6-24 beds	124	35	28.2	1	0.8	0	0.0	3	2.4	0	0.0	57	46.0	0	0.0
25-49	423	161	38.1	2	0.5	2	0.5	17	4.0	3	0.7	214	50.6	2	0.5
50-99	378	209	55.3	1	0.3	2	0.5	29	7.7	5	1.3	232	61.4	6	1.6
100-199	229	165	72.1	4	1.7	8	3.5	31	13.5	3	1.3	163	71.2	17	7.4
200-299	77	67	87.0	3	3.9	9	11.7	17	22.1	3	3.9	62	80.5	27	35.1
300-399	45	43	95.6	4	8.9	14	31.1	14	31.1	11	24.4	36	80.0	25	55.6
400-499	28	28	100.0	2	7.1	15	53.6	12	42.9	9	32.1	23	82.1	20	71.4
500 or more	54	51	94.4	15	27.8	32	59.3	29	53.7	17	31.5	44	81.5	38	70.4
Hospital units of institutions	17	5	29.4	4	23.5	4	23.5	3	17.6	1	5.9	0	0.0	0	0.0
Community hospitals	5,056	3,413	67.5	109	2.2	290	5.7	1,035	20.5	361	7.1	3,292	65.1	1,040	20.6

CLASSIFICATION	HOSPITALS REPORTING	CARDIAC SERVICES, continued: CARDIAC CATHETERIZATION LABORATORY		CARDIAC REHABILITATION PROGRAM		NON-INVASIVE CARDIAC ASSESSMENT SERVICES		OPEN HEART SURGERY		CHRONIC OBSTRUCTIVE PULMONARY DISEASE SERVICES		EMERGENCY SERVICES: EMERGENCY DEPARTMENT		TRAUMA CENTER (CERTIFIED)	
		Number	Percent	Number	Percent	Number	Percent	Number	Percent	Number	Percent	Number	Percent	Number	Percent
UNITED STATES	6,105	1,470	24.1	2,148	35.2	2,949	48.3	898	14.7	3,647	59.7	5,024	82.3	664	10.9
6-24 beds	254	1	0.4	18	7.1	41	16.1	0	0.0	84	33.1	217	85.4	3	1.2
25-49	974	4	0.4	131	13.4	229	23.5	1	0.1	374	38.4	837	85.9	22	2.3
50-99	1,451	29	2.0	286	19.7	458	31.6	6	0.4	647	44.6	1,074	74.0	47	3.2
100-199	1,439	235	16.3	500	34.7	747	51.9	77	5.4	918	63.8	1,199	83.3	130	9.0
200-299	804	391	48.6	456	56.7	574	71.4	187	23.3	661	82.2	718	89.3	135	16.8
300-399	485	316	65.2	317	65.4	381	78.6	216	44.5	396	81.6	419	86.4	98	20.2
400-499	265	198	74.7	178	67.2	204	77.0	152	57.4	224	84.5	228	86.0	73	27.5
500 or more	433	296	68.4	262	60.5	315	72.7	259	59.8	343	79.2	332	76.7	156	36.0
Federal	301	79	26.2	108	35.9	177	58.8	51	16.9	202	67.1	250	83.1	11	3.7
Psychiatric	17	0	0.0	6	35.3	9	52.9	0	0.0	16	94.1	5	29.4	0	0.0
General and other special	284	79	27.8	102	35.9	168	59.2	51	18.0	186	65.5	245	86.3	11	3.9
Nonfederal	5,804	1,391	24.0	2,040	35.1	2,772	47.8	847	14.6	3,445	59.4	4,774	82.3	653	11.3
Psychiatric	609	0	0.0	2	0.3	12	2.0	0	0.0	17	2.8	24	3.9	2	0.3
Nongovernment not-for-profit	106	0	0.0	0	0.0	2	1.9	0	0.0	2	1.9	5	4.7	0	0.0
Investor-owned (for-profit)	272	0	0.0	0	0.0	3	1.1	0	0.0	0	0.0	6	2.2	1	0.4
State and local government	231	0	0.0	2	0.9	7	3.0	0	0.0	15	6.5	13	5.6	1	0.4
TB and other respiratory diseases	3	0	0.0	0	0.0	0	0.0	0	0.0	3	100.0	0	0.0	0	0.0
Nongovernment not-for-profit	1	0	0.0	0	0.0	0	0.0	0	0.0	1	100.0	0	0.0	0	0.0
Investor-owned (for-profit)	0	0	0.0	0	0.0	0	0.0	0	0.0	0	0.0	0	0.0	0	0.0
State and local government	2	0	0.0	0	0.0	0	0.0	0	0.0	2	100.0	0	0.0	0	0.0
Long-term general and other special	119	1	0.8	13	10.9	9	7.6	0	0.0	51	42.9	13	10.9	0	0.0
Nongovernment not-for-profit	54	1	1.9	8	14.8	4	7.4	0	0.0	18	33.3	4	7.4	0	0.0
Investor-owned (for-profit)	16	0	0.0	1	6.3	0	0.0	0	0.0	6	37.5	2	12.5	0	0.0
State and local government	49	0	0.0	4	8.2	5	10.2	0	0.0	27	55.1	7	14.3	0	0.0
Short-term general and other special	5,073	1,390	27.4	2,025	39.9	2,751	54.2	847	16.7	3,374	66.5	4,737	93.4	651	12.8
6-24 beds	209	1	0.5	17	8.1	34	16.3	0	0.0	77	36.8	184	88.0	3	1.4
25-49	868	4	0.5	131	15.1	221	25.5	1	0.1	364	41.9	792	91.2	22	2.5
50-99	1,157	29	2.5	276	23.9	445	38.5	6	0.5	620	53.6	1,037	89.6	47	4.1
100-199	1,225	232	18.9	482	39.3	712	58.1	77	6.3	858	70.0	1,148	93.7	127	10.4
200-299	719	382	53.1	439	61.1	548	76.2	184	25.6	628	87.3	695	96.7	132	18.4
300-399	400	296	74.0	296	74.0	352	88.0	202	50.5	362	90.5	393	98.3	97	24.3
400-499	215	188	87.4	169	78.6	186	86.5	145	67.4	204	94.9	214	99.5	72	33.5
500 or more	280	258	92.1	215	76.8	253	90.4	232	82.9	261	93.2	274	97.9	151	53.9
Nongovernment not-for-profit	3,079	1,024	33.3	1,502	48.8	1,901	61.7	651	21.1	2,201	71.5	2,894	94.0	476	15.5
6-24 beds	71	0	0.0	7	9.9	10	14.1	0	0.0	22	31.0	60	84.5	1	1.4
25-49	383	2	0.5	69	18.0	108	28.2	0	0.0	163	42.6	342	89.3	8	2.1
50-99	601	15	2.5	163	27.1	239	39.8	3	0.5	329	54.7	535	89.0	24	4.0
100-199	748	125	16.7	334	44.7	459	61.4	42	5.6	533	71.3	706	94.4	87	11.6
200-299	552	283	51.3	353	63.9	436	79.0	138	25.0	482	87.3	534	96.7	110	19.9
300-399	326	238	73.0	253	77.6	292	89.6	161	49.4	296	90.8	322	98.8	78	23.9
400-499	175	152	86.9	141	80.6	152	86.9	117	66.9	167	95.4	175	100.0	53	30.3
500 or more	223	209	93.7	182	81.6	205	91.9	190	85.2	209	93.7	220	98.7	115	51.6
Investor-owned (for-profit)	636	176	27.7	170	26.7	320	50.3	89	14.0	421	66.2	551	86.6	47	7.4
6-24 beds	14	0	0.0	1	7.1	1	7.1	0	0.0	4	28.6	8	57.1	0	0.0
25-49	62	0	0.0	3	4.8	16	25.8	1	1.6	25	40.3	48	77.4	2	3.2
50-99	178	9	5.1	28	15.7	65	36.5	3	1.7	100	56.2	143	80.3	7	3.9
100-199	248	76	30.6	69	27.8	141	56.9	28	11.3	172	69.4	223	89.9	21	8.5
200-299	90	53	58.9	39	43.3	59	65.6	29	32.2	80	88.9	85	94.4	10	11.1
300-399	29	23	79.3	18	62.1	25	86.2	15	51.7	26	89.7	29	100.0	2	6.9
400-499	12	12	100.0	9	75.0	10	83.3	10	83.3	11	91.7	12	100.0	2	16.7
500 or more	3	3	100.0	3	100.0	3	100.0	3	100.0	3	100.0	3	100.0	3	100.0
State and local government	1,358	190	14.0	353	26.0	530	39.0	107	7.9	752	55.4	1,292	95.1	128	9.4
6-24 beds	124	1	0.8	9	7.3	23	18.5	0	0.0	51	41.1	116	93.5	2	1.6
25-49	423	2	0.5	59	13.9	97	22.9	0	0.0	176	41.6	402	95.0	12	2.8
50-99	378	5	1.3	85	22.5	141	37.3	0	0.0	191	50.5	359	95.0	16	4.2
100-199	229	31	13.5	79	34.5	112	48.9	7	3.1	153	66.8	219	95.6	19	8.3
200-299	77	46	59.7	47	61.0	53	68.8	17	22.1	66	85.7	76	98.7	12	15.6
300-399	45	35	77.8	25	55.6	35	77.8	26	57.8	40	88.9	42	93.3	17	37.8
400-499	28	24	85.7	19	67.9	24	85.7	18	64.3	26	92.9	27	96.4	17	60.7
500 or more	54	46	85.2	30	55.6	45	83.3	39	72.2	49	90.7	51	94.4	33	61.1
Hospital units of institutions	17	0	0.0	1	5.9	3	17.6	0	0.0	3	17.6	9	52.9	0	0.0
Community hospitals	5,056	1,390	27.5	2,024	40.0	2,748	54.4	847	16.8	3,371	66.7	4,728	93.5	651	12.9

(continued on next page)

Table

12A (Continued)

Facilities and Services in the United States

For definitions of facilities and services, see Definitions of Terms, page xxiii. These data include only hospital-based facilities and services as reported by responding hospitals in Section C of the 1990 AHA Annual Survey, beginning on page 242. No estimates have been made for nonresponding hospitals.

CLASSIFICATION	HOSPITALS REPORTING	EXTRACORPOREAL SHOCK WAVE LITHOTRIPTER (ESWL)		FITNESS CENTER		GENETIC COUNSELING/ SCREENING		GERIATRIC SERVICES: ADULT DAY CARE PROGRAM		GERIATRIC SERVICES: ALZHEIMER'S DIAGNOSTIC/ ASSESSMENT SERVICES		GERIATRIC SERVICES: COMPREHENSIVE GERIATRIC ASSESSMENT		GERIATRIC SERVICES: EMERGENCY RESPONSE (GERIATRIC)	
		Number	Percent	Number	Percent	Number	Percent	Number	Percent	Number	Percent	Number	Percent	Number	Percent
UNITED STATES	6,105	327	5.4	850	13.9	553	9.1	427	7.0	570	9.3	1,202	19.7	1,853	30.4
6-24 beds	254	0	0.0	17	6.7	3	1.2	9	3.5	2	0.8	15	5.9	50	19.7
25-49	974	2	0.2	58	6.0	12	1.2	36	3.7	8	0.8	70	7.2	256	26.3
50-99	1,451	17	1.2	118	8.1	27	1.9	84	5.8	48	3.3	174	12.0	381	26.3
100-199	1,439	40	2.8	176	12.2	75	5.2	61	4.2	85	5.9	222	15.4	433	30.1
200-299	804	70	8.7	155	19.3	96	11.9	60	7.5	87	10.8	195	24.3	305	37.9
300-399	485	57	11.8	127	26.2	93	19.2	60	12.4	91	18.8	150	30.9	191	39.4
400-499	265	35	13.2	73	27.5	82	30.9	29	10.9	62	23.4	121	45.7	97	36.6
500 or more	433	106	24.5	126	29.1	165	38.1	88	20.3	187	43.2	255	58.9	140	32.3
Federal	301	7	2.3	59	19.6	45	15.0	39	13.0	81	26.9	128	42.5	41	13.6
Psychiatric	17	0	0.0	5	29.4	2	11.8	7	41.2	9	52.9	14	82.4	4	23.5
General and other special	284	7	2.5	54	19.0	43	15.1	32	11.3	72	25.4	114	40.1	37	13.0
Nonfederal	5,804	320	5.5	791	13.6	508	8.8	388	6.7	489	8.4	1,074	18.5	1,812	31.2
Psychiatric	609	1	0.2	44	7.2	5	0.8	48	7.9	77	12.6	120	19.7	28	4.6
Nongovernment not-for-profit	106	0	0.0	11	10.4	2	1.9	12	11.3	15	14.2	17	16.0	1	0.9
Investor-owned (for-profit)	272	0	0.0	20	7.4	2	0.7	16	5.9	20	7.4	22	8.1	5	1.8
State and local government	231	1	0.4	13	5.6	1	0.4	20	8.7	42	18.2	81	35.1	22	9.5
TB and other respiratory diseases	3	0	0.0	0	0.0	0	0.0	0	0.0	0	0.0	0	0.0	0	0.0
Nongovernment not-for-profit	1	0	0.0	0	0.0	0	0.0	0	0.0	0	0.0	0	0.0	0	0.0
Investor-owned (for-profit)	0	0	0.0	0	0.0	0	0.0	0	0.0	0	0.0	0	0.0	0	0.0
State and local government	2	0	0.0	0	0.0	0	0.0	0	0.0	0	0.0	0	0.0	0	0.0
Long-term general and other special	119	0	0.0	9	7.6	5	4.2	18	15.1	16	13.4	34	28.6	6	5.0
Nongovernment not-for-profit	54	0	0.0	6	11.1	3	5.6	5	9.3	6	11.1	15	27.8	3	5.6
Investor-owned (for-profit)	16	0	0.0	2	12.5	0	0.0	1	6.3	0	0.0	1	6.3	0	0.0
State and local government	49	0	0.0	1	2.0	2	4.1	12	24.5	10	20.4	18	36.7	3	6.1
Short-term general and other special	5,073	319	6.3	738	14.5	498	9.8	322	6.3	396	7.8	920	18.1	1,778	35.0
6-24 beds	209	0	0.0	10	4.8	1	0.5	7	3.3	2	1.0	13	6.2	47	22.5
25-49	868	2	0.2	47	5.4	9	1.0	35	4.0	7	0.8	66	7.6	250	28.8
50-99	1,157	16	1.4	95	8.2	20	1.7	62	5.4	25	2.2	143	12.4	372	32.2
100-199	1,225	40	3.3	160	13.1	65	5.3	49	4.0	63	5.1	188	15.3	428	34.9
200-299	719	69	9.6	149	20.7	90	12.5	53	7.4	71	9.9	160	22.3	300	41.7
300-399	400	56	14.0	112	28.0	87	21.8	45	11.3	64	16.0	105	26.3	178	44.5
400-499	215	34	15.8	62	28.8	75	34.9	25	11.6	47	21.9	96	44.7	90	41.9
500 or more	280	102	36.4	103	36.8	151	53.9	46	16.4	117	41.8	149	53.2	113	40.4
Nongovernment not-for-profit	3,079	219	7.1	533	17.3	384	12.5	241	7.8	314	10.2	661	21.5	1,243	40.4
6-24 beds	71	0	0.0	4	5.6	1	1.4	4	5.6	2	2.8	5	7.0	21	29.6
25-49	383	2	0.5	23	6.0	7	1.8	12	3.1	4	1.0	31	8.1	120	31.3
50-99	601	7	1.2	48	8.0	11	1.8	32	5.3	15	2.5	84	14.0	208	34.6
100-199	748	20	2.7	96	12.8	49	6.6	37	4.9	44	5.9	118	15.8	301	40.2
200-299	552	45	8.2	123	22.3	79	14.3	51	9.2	64	11.6	133	24.1	255	46.2
300-399	326	41	12.6	96	29.4	65	19.9	42	12.9	52	16.0	88	27.0	157	48.2
400-499	175	23	13.1	53	30.3	59	33.7	24	13.7	37	21.1	79	45.1	79	45.1
500 or more	223	81	36.3	90	40.4	113	50.7	39	17.5	96	43.0	123	55.2	102	45.7
Investor-owned (for-profit)	636	45	7.1	75	11.8	22	3.5	6	0.9	23	3.6	68	10.7	91	14.3
6-24 beds	14	0	0.0	0	0.0	0	0.0	0	0.0	0	0.0	0	0.0	0	0.0
25-49	62	0	0.0	2	3.2	0	0.0	1	1.6	1	1.6	5	8.1	6	9.7
50-99	178	6	3.4	7	3.9	3	1.7	1	0.6	4	2.2	12	6.7	22	12.4
100-199	248	14	5.6	39	15.7	10	4.0	2	0.8	10	4.0	33	13.3	45	18.1
200-299	90	16	17.8	17	18.9	4	4.4	1	1.1	3	3.3	6	6.7	13	14.4
300-399	29	3	10.3	5	17.2	3	10.3	1	3.4	3	10.3	6	20.7	4	13.8
400-499	12	3	25.0	4	33.3	1	8.3	0	0.0	1	8.3	4	33.3	1	8.3
500 or more	3	3	100.0	1	33.3	1	33.3	0	0.0	1	33.3	2	66.7	0	0.0
State and local government	1,358	55	4.1	130	9.6	92	6.8	75	5.5	59	4.3	191	14.1	444	32.7
6-24 beds	124	0	0.0	6	4.8	0	0.0	3	2.4	0	0.0	8	6.5	26	21.0
25-49	423	0	0.0	22	5.2	2	0.5	22	5.2	2	0.5	30	7.1	124	29.3
50-99	378	3	0.8	40	10.6	6	1.6	29	7.7	6	1.6	47	12.4	142	37.6
100-199	229	6	2.6	25	10.9	6	2.6	10	4.4	9	3.9	37	16.2	82	35.8
200-299	77	8	10.4	9	11.7	7	9.1	1	1.3	4	5.2	21	27.3	32	41.6
300-399	45	12	26.7	11	24.4	19	42.2	2	4.4	9	20.0	11	24.4	17	37.8
400-499	28	8	28.6	5	17.9	15	53.6	1	3.6	9	32.1	13	46.4	10	35.7
500 or more	54	18	33.3	12	22.2	37	68.5	7	13.0	20	37.0	24	44.4	11	20.4
Hospital units of institutions	17	0	0.0	1	5.9	3	17.6	1	5.9	1	5.9	2	11.8	2	11.8
Community hospitals	5,056	319	6.3	737	14.6	495	9.8	321	6.3	395	7.8	918	18.2	1,776	35.1

Table 12A (Continued)

CLASSIFICATION	HOSPITALS REPORTING	GERIATRIC SERVICES, continued								HEALTH PROMOTION SERVICES					
		GERIATRIC ACUTE CARE UNIT		GERIATRIC CLINICS		RESPITE CARE		SENIOR MEMBERSHIP PROGRAM		PATIENT EDUCATION		COMMUNITY HEALTH PROMOTION		WORKSITE HEALTH PROMOTION	
		Number	Percent	Number	Percent	Number	Percent	Number	Percent	Number	Percent	Number	Percent	Number	Percent
UNITED STATES	6,105	666	10.9	461	7.6	1,005	16.5	1,159	19.0	5,125	83.9	4,366	71.5	3,233	53.0
6-24 beds	254	21	8.3	5	2.0	55	21.7	8	3.1	159	62.6	122	48.0	85	33.5
25-49	974	72	7.4	25	2.6	212	21.8	59	6.1	677	69.5	559	57.4	310	31.8
50-99	1,451	108	7.4	26	1.8	224	15.4	128	8.8	1,134	78.2	956	65.9	651	44.9
100-199	1,439	125	8.7	55	3.8	187	13.0	275	19.1	1,284	89.2	1,134	78.8	841	58.4
200-299	804	84	10.4	68	8.5	106	13.2	287	35.7	758	94.3	679	84.5	513	63.8
300-399	485	68	14.0	67	13.8	70	14.4	186	38.4	457	94.2	394	81.2	344	70.9
400-499	265	56	21.1	63	23.8	39	14.7	99	37.4	254	95.8	217	81.9	193	72.8
500 or more	433	132	30.5	152	35.1	112	25.9	117	27.0	402	92.8	305	70.4	296	68.4
Federal	301	76	25.2	98	32.6	127	42.2	7	2.3	291	96.7	197	65.4	222	73.8
Psychiatric	17	9	52.9	8	47.1	15	88.2	1	5.9	17	100.0	5	29.4	13	76.5
General and other special	284	67	23.6	90	31.7	112	39.4	6	2.1	274	96.5	192	67.6	209	73.6
Nonfederal	5,804	590	10.2	363	6.3	878	15.1	1,152	19.8	4,834	83.3	4,169	71.8	3,011	51.9
Psychiatric	609	67	11.0	27	4.4	14	2.3	3	0.5	378	62.1	218	35.8	230	37.8
Nongovernment not-for-profit	106	11	10.4	3	2.8	1	0.9	0	0.0	63	59.4	42	39.6	35	33.0
Investor-owned (for-profit)	272	12	4.4	1	0.4	1	0.4	0	0.0	166	61.0	142	52.2	103	37.9
State and local government	231	44	19.0	23	10.0	12	5.2	3	1.3	149	64.5	34	14.7	92	39.8
TB and other respiratory diseases	3	0	0.0	0	0.0	0	0.0	0	0.0	2	66.7	1	33.3	2	66.7
Nongovernment not-for-profit	1	0	0.0	0	0.0	0	0.0	0	0.0	0	0.0	0	0.0	0	0.0
Investor-owned (for-profit)	0	0	0.0	0	0.0	0	0.0	0	0.0	0	0.0	0	0.0	0	0.0
State and local government	2	0	0.0	0	0.0	0	0.0	0	0.0	2	100.0	1	50.0	2	100.0
Long-term general and other special	119	14	11.8	4	11.8	21	17.6	7	5.9	72	60.5	41	34.5	44	37.0
Nongovernment not-for-profit	54	3	5.6	6	11.1	7	13.0	5	9.3	33	61.1	19	35.2	21	38.9
Investor-owned (for-profit)	16	0	0.0	0	0.0	0	0.0	0	0.0	8	50.0	6	37.5	4	25.0
State and local government	49	11	22.4	8	16.3	14	28.6	2	4.1	31	63.3	16	32.7	19	38.8
Short-term general and other special	5,073	509	10.0	322	6.3	843	16.6	1,142	22.5	4,382	86.4	3,909	77.1	2,735	53.9
6-24 beds	209	18	8.6	4	1.9	55	26.3	7	3.3	121	57.9	89	42.6	53	25.4
25-49	868	70	8.1	24	2.8	207	23.8	59	6.8	602	69.4	498	57.4	262	30.2
50-99	1,157	97	8.4	21	1.8	217	18.8	125	10.8	953	82.4	820	70.9	537	46.4
100-199	1,225	105	8.6	40	3.3	159	13.0	272	22.2	1,135	92.7	1,026	83.8	742	60.6
200-299	719	69	9.6	52	7.2	86	12.0	286	39.8	695	96.7	651	90.5	473	65.8
300-399	400	44	11.0	40	10.0	46	11.5	183	45.8	390	97.5	367	91.8	290	72.5
400-499	215	43	20.0	51	23.7	27	12.6	97	45.1	212	98.6	204	94.9	163	75.8
500 or more	280	63	22.5	90	32.1	46	16.4	113	40.4	274	97.9	254	90.7	215	76.8
Nongovernment not-for-profit	3,079	332	10.8	244	7.9	516	16.8	850	27.6	2,835	92.1	2,595	84.3	1,878	61.0
6-24 beds	71	9	12.7	2	2.8	21	29.6	5	7.0	52	73.2	37	52.1	22	31.0
25-49	383	30	7.8	11	2.9	85	22.2	30	7.8	302	78.9	249	65.0	132	34.5
50-99	601	58	9.7	12	2.0	117	19.5	71	11.8	522	86.9	459	76.4	308	51.2
100-199	748	57	7.6	29	3.9	108	14.4	167	22.3	708	94.7	655	87.6	485	64.8
200-299	552	57	10.3	49	8.9	78	14.1	228	41.3	539	97.6	514	93.1	373	67.6
300-399	326	37	11.3	30	9.2	41	12.6	158	48.5	317	97.2	305	93.6	243	74.5
400-499	175	33	18.9	42	24.0	25	14.3	86	49.1	173	98.9	168	96.0	134	76.6
500 or more	223	51	22.9	69	30.9	41	18.4	105	47.1	222	99.6	208	93.3	181	81.2
Investor-owned (for-profit)	636	40	6.3	8	1.3	23	3.6	171	26.9	523	82.2	453	71.2	325	51.1
6-24 beds	14	1	7.1	0	0.0	1	7.1	1	7.1	5	35.7	0	0.0	2	14.3
25-49	62	4	6.5	2	3.2	5	8.1	4	6.5	33	53.2	35	56.5	20	32.3
50-99	178	7	3.9	1	0.6	5	2.8	28	15.7	133	74.7	107	60.1	75	42.1
100-199	248	18	7.3	4	1.6	11	4.4	76	30.6	223	89.9	194	78.2	140	56.5
200-299	90	5	5.6	0	0.0	0	0.0	39	43.3	85	94.4	78	86.7	53	58.9
300-399	29	2	6.9	1	3.4	1	3.4	15	51.7	29	100.0	25	86.2	23	79.3
400-499	12	3	25.0	0	0.0	0	0.0	6	50.0	12	100.0	11	91.7	10	83.3
500 or more	3	0	0.0	0	0.0	0	0.0	2	66.7	3	100.0	3	100.0	2	66.7
State and local government	1,358	137	10.1	70	5.2	304	22.4	121	8.9	1,024	75.4	861	63.4	532	39.2
6-24 beds	124	8	6.5	2	1.6	33	26.6	1	0.8	64	51.6	52	41.9	29	23.4
25-49	423	36	8.5	11	2.6	117	27.7	25	5.9	267	63.1	214	50.6	110	26.0
50-99	378	32	8.5	8	2.1	95	25.1	26	6.9	298	78.8	254	67.2	154	40.7
100-199	229	30	13.1	7	3.1	40	17.5	29	12.7	204	89.1	177	77.3	117	51.1
200-299	77	7	9.1	3	3.9	8	10.4	19	24.7	71	92.2	59	76.6	47	61.0
300-399	45	5	11.1	9	20.0	4	8.9	10	22.2	44	97.8	37	82.2	24	53.3
400-499	28	7	25.0	9	32.1	2	7.1	5	17.9	27	96.4	25	89.3	19	67.9
500 or more	54	12	22.2	21	38.9	5	9.3	6	11.1	49	90.7	43	79.6	32	59.3
Hospital units of institutions	17	1	5.9	2	11.8	2	11.8	0	0.0	14	82.4	7	41.2	8	47.1
Community hospitals	5,056	508	10.0	320	6.3	841	16.6	1,142	22.6	4,368	86.4	3,902	77.2	2,727	53.9

(continued on next page)

Table

12A (Continued)

Facilities and Services in the United States

For definitions of facilities and services, see Definitions of Terms, page xxiii. These data include only hospital-based facilities and services as reported by responding hospitals in Section C of the 1990 AHA Annual Survey, beginning on page 242. No estimates have been made for nonresponding hospitals.

CLASSIFICATION	HOSPITALS REPORTING	HEALTH SCIENCES LIBRARY		HEMODIALYSIS		HOME HEALTH SERVICES		HOSPICE		LABORATORY SERVICES: HISTOPATHOLOGY		LABORATORY SERVICES: BLOOD BANK		OCCUPATIONAL HEALTH SERVICES	
		Number	Percent	Number	Percent	Number	Percent	Number	Percent	Number	Percent	Number	Percent	Number	Percent
UNITED STATES	6,105	2,544	41.7	1,451	23.8	1,921	31.5	868	14.2	3,571	58.5	3,757	61.5	2,377	38.9
6-24 beds	254	30	11.8	2	0.8	58	22.8	20	7.9	40	15.7	105	41.3	31	12.2
25-49	974	115	11.8	12	1.2	271	27.8	66	6.8	225	23.1	463	47.5	125	12.8
50-99	1,451	326	22.5	64	4.4	361	24.9	128	8.8	571	39.4	725	50.0	345	23.8
100-199	1,439	615	42.7	259	18.0	422	29.3	202	14.0	1,032	71.7	968	67.3	584	40.6
200-299	804	537	66.8	368	45.8	292	36.3	145	18.0	698	86.8	613	76.2	469	58.3
300-399	485	370	76.3	284	58.6	208	42.9	119	24.5	415	85.6	357	73.6	325	67.0
400-499	265	214	80.8	172	64.9	114	43.0	78	29.4	233	87.9	209	78.9	188	70.9
500 or more	433	337	77.8	290	67.0	195	45.0	110	25.4	357	82.4	317	73.2	310	71.6
Federal	301	220	73.1	98	32.6	101	33.6	36	12.0	224	74.4	231	76.7	198	65.8
Psychiatric	17	14	82.4	2	11.8	3	17.6	1	5.9	12	70.6	9	52.9	12	70.6
General and other special	284	206	72.5	96	33.8	98	34.5	35	12.3	212	74.6	222	78.2	186	65.5
Nonfederal	5,804	2,324	40.0	1,353	23.3	1,820	31.4	832	14.3	3,347	57.7	3,526	60.8	2,179	37.5
Psychiatric	609	131	21.5	1	0.2	7	1.1	2	0.3	43	7.1	13	2.1	126	20.7
Nongovernment not-for-profit	106	26	24.5	0	0.0	3	2.8	0	0.0	4	3.8	3	2.8	14	13.2
Investor-owned (for-profit)	272	27	9.9	0	0.0	0	0.0	1	0.4	7	2.6	4	1.5	41	15.1
State and local government	231	78	33.8	1	0.4	4	1.7	1	0.4	32	13.9	6	2.6	71	30.7
TB and other respiratory diseases	3	2	66.7	0	0.0	0	0.0	0	0.0	2	66.7	1	33.3	1	33.3
Nongovernment not-for-profit	1	0	0.0	0	0.0	0	0.0	0	0.0	0	0.0	0	0.0	1	100.0
Investor-owned (for-profit)	0	0	0.0	0	0.0	0	0.0	0	0.0	0	0.0	0	0.0	0	0.0
State and local government	2	2	100.0	0	0.0	0	0.0	0	0.0	2	100.0	1	50.0	0	0.0
Long-term general and other special	119	38	31.9	4	3.4	12	10.1	13	10.9	28	23.5	18	15.1	47	39.5
Nongovernment not-for-profit	54	18	33.3	2	3.7	9	16.7	6	11.1	5	9.3	4	7.4	23	42.6
Investor-owned (for-profit)	16	2	12.5	0	0.0	0	0.0	0	0.0	3	18.8	1	6.3	7	43.8
State and local government	49	18	36.7	2	4.1	3	6.1	7	14.3	20	40.8	13	26.5	17	34.7
Short-term general and other special	5,073	2,153	42.4	1,348	26.6	1,801	35.5	817	16.1	3,274	64.5	3,494	68.9	2,005	39.5
6-24 beds	209	16	7.7	2	1.0	53	25.4	20	9.6	33	15.8	86	41.1	18	8.6
25-49	868	93	10.7	12	1.4	261	30.1	65	7.5	203	23.4	434	50.0	98	11.3
50-99	1,157	271	23.4	64	5.5	357	30.9	123	10.6	543	46.9	694	60.0	280	24.2
100-199	1,225	537	43.8	250	20.4	410	33.5	196	16.0	970	79.2	918	74.9	515	42.0
200-299	719	493	68.6	351	48.8	273	38.0	140	19.5	664	92.4	587	81.6	434	60.4
300-399	400	322	80.5	262	65.5	193	48.3	112	28.0	381	95.3	333	83.3	280	70.0
400-499	215	184	85.6	160	74.4	105	48.8	72	33.5	207	96.3	192	89.3	159	74.0
500 or more	280	237	84.6	247	88.2	149	53.2	89	31.8	273	97.5	250	89.3	221	78.9
Nongovernment not-for-profit	3,079	1,663	54.0	1,036	33.6	1,252	40.7	618	20.1	2,238	72.7	2,242	72.8	1,488	48.3
6-24 beds	71	4	5.6	2	2.8	24	33.8	8	11.3	8	11.3	31	43.7	8	11.3
25-49	383	53	13.8	7	1.8	113	29.5	32	8.4	108	28.2	198	51.7	58	15.1
50-99	601	175	29.1	34	5.7	196	32.6	68	11.3	301	50.1	365	60.7	161	26.8
100-199	748	394	52.7	172	23.0	292	39.0	144	19.3	618	82.6	567	75.8	360	48.1
200-299	552	412	74.6	275	49.8	235	42.6	126	22.8	508	92.0	450	81.5	359	65.0
300-399	326	276	84.7	217	66.6	171	52.5	99	30.4	310	95.1	271	83.1	234	71.8
400-499	175	155	88.6	129	73.7	92	52.6	65	37.1	167	95.4	159	90.9	128	73.1
500 or more	223	194	87.0	200	89.7	129	57.8	76	34.1	218	97.8	201	90.1	180	80.7
Investor-owned (for-profit)	636	152	23.9	135	21.2	106	16.7	35	5.5	426	67.0	432	67.9	213	33.5
6-24 beds	14	2	14.3	0	0.0	2	14.3	0	0.0	2	14.3	3	21.4	1	7.1
25-49	62	5	8.1	0	0.0	13	21.0	3	4.8	19	30.6	28	45.2	10	16.1
50-99	178	32	18.0	14	7.9	30	16.9	5	2.8	82	46.1	106	59.6	47	26.4
100-199	248	59	23.8	53	21.4	39	15.7	20	8.1	194	78.2	184	74.2	89	35.9
200-299	90	29	32.2	44	48.9	14	15.6	5	5.6	85	94.4	77	85.6	38	42.2
300-399	29	15	51.7	14	48.3	7	24.1	2	6.9	29	100.0	24	82.8	17	58.6
400-499	12	7	58.3	8	66.7	1	8.3	0	0.0	12	100.0	8	66.7	8	66.7
500 or more	3	3	100.0	2	66.7	0	0.0	0	0.0	3	100.0	2	66.7	3	100.0
State and local government	1,358	338	24.9	177	13.0	443	32.6	164	12.1	610	44.9	820	60.4	304	22.4
6-24 beds	124	10	8.1	0	0.0	27	21.8	12	9.7	23	18.5	52	41.9	9	7.3
25-49	423	35	8.3	5	1.2	135	31.9	30	7.1	76	18.0	208	49.2	30	7.1
50-99	378	64	16.9	16	4.2	131	34.7	50	13.2	160	42.3	223	59.0	72	19.0
100-199	229	84	36.7	25	10.9	79	34.5	32	14.0	158	69.0	167	72.9	66	28.8
200-299	77	52	67.5	32	41.6	24	31.2	9	11.7	71	92.2	60	77.9	37	48.1
300-399	45	31	68.9	31	68.9	15	33.3	11	24.4	42	93.3	38	84.4	29	64.4
400-499	28	22	78.6	23	82.1	12	42.9	7	25.0	28	100.0	25	89.3	23	82.1
500 or more	54	40	74.1	45	83.3	20	37.0	13	24.1	52	96.3	47	87.0	38	70.4
Hospital units of institutions	17	3	17.6	1	5.9	0	0.0	0	0.0	2	11.8	1	5.9	3	17.6
Community hospitals	5,056	2,150	42.5	1,347	26.6	1,801	35.6	817	16.2	3,272	64.7	3,493	69.1	2,002	39.6

Table 12A (Continued)

CLASSIFICATION	HOSPITALS REPORTING	ORGANIZED OUTPATIENT SERVICES		PSYCHIATRIC SERVICES: CHILD/ADOLESCENT		CONSULTATION-LIAISON		EDUCATION		EMERGENCY		GERIATRIC		OUTPATIENT	
		Number	Percent	Number	Percent	Number	Percent	Number	Percent	Number	Percent	Number	Percent	Number	Percent
UNITED STATES	6,105	4,866	79.7	1,424	23.3	2,223	36.4	1,733	28.4	2,311	37.9	1,652	27.1	1,600	26.2
6-24 beds	254	179	70.5	16	6.3	27	10.6	23	9.1	33	13.0	2	0.8	33	13.0
25-49	974	745	76.5	61	6.3	109	11.2	73	7.5	124	12.7	41	4.2	91	9.3
50-99	1,451	1,056	72.8	257	17.7	329	22.7	259	17.8	350	24.1	214	14.7	238	16.4
100-199	1,439	1,175	81.7	315	21.9	512	35.6	370	25.7	540	37.5	341	23.7	337	23.4
200-299	804	712	88.6	256	31.8	421	52.4	324	40.3	445	55.3	322	40.0	263	32.7
300-399	485	410	84.5	185	38.1	297	61.2	238	49.1	313	64.5	248	51.1	216	44.5
400-499	265	232	87.5	120	45.3	183	69.1	166	62.6	183	69.1	159	60.0	130	49.1
500 or more	433	357	82.4	214	49.4	345	79.7	280	64.7	323	74.6	325	75.1	292	67.4
Federal	301	293	97.3	53	17.6	232	77.1	154	51.2	210	69.8	137	45.5	269	89.4
Psychiatric	17	16	94.1	0	0.0	16	94.1	7	41.2	14	82.4	16	94.1	17	100.0
General and other special	284	277	97.5	53	18.7	216	76.1	147	51.8	196	69.0	121	42.6	252	88.7
Nonfederal	5,804	4,573	78.8	1,371	23.6	1,991	34.3	1,579	27.2	2,101	36.2	1,515	26.1	1,331	22.9
Psychiatric	609	178	29.2	427	70.1	408	67.0	444	72.9	382	62.7	398	65.4	312	51.2
Nongovernment not-for-profit	106	45	42.5	82	77.4	73	68.9	85	80.2	62	58.5	60	56.6	71	67.0
Investor-owned (for-profit)	272	95	34.9	228	83.8	214	78.7	219	80.5	184	67.6	167	61.4	161	59.2
State and local government	231	38	16.5	117	50.6	121	52.4	140	60.6	136	58.9	171	74.0	80	34.6
TB and other respiratory diseases	3	2	66.7	0	0.0	1	33.3	0	0.0	0	0.0	0	0.0	0	0.0
Nongovernment not-for-profit	1	1	100.0	0	0.0	0	0.0	0	0.0	0	0.0	0	0.0	0	0.0
Investor-owned (for-profit)	0	0	0.0	0	0.0	0	0.0	0	0.0	0	0.0	0	0.0	0	0.0
State and local government	2	1	50.0	0	0.0	1	50.0	0	0.0	0	0.0	0	0.0	0	0.0
Long-term general and other special	119	71	59.7	14	11.8	38	31.9	16	13.4	9	7.6	22	18.5	19	16.0
Nongovernment not-for-profit	54	38	70.4	9	16.7	19	35.2	7	13.0	3	5.6	8	14.8	11	20.4
Investor-owned (for-profit)	16	9	56.3	0	0.0	2	12.5	2	12.5	0	0.0	1	6.3	3	18.8
State and local government	49	24	49.0	5	10.2	17	34.7	7	14.3	6	12.2	13	26.5	5	10.2
Short-term general and other special	5,073	4,322	85.2	930	18.3	1,544	30.4	1,119	22.1	1,710	33.7	1,095	21.6	1,000	19.7
6-24 beds	209	141	67.5	5	2.4	10	4.8	9	4.3	20	9.6	2	1.0	9	4.3
25-49	868	677	78.0	19	2.2	44	5.1	21	2.4	71	8.2	14	1.6	35	4.0
50-99	1,157	931	80.5	60	5.2	142	12.3	69	6.0	186	16.1	81	7.0	75	6.5
100-199	1,225	1,060	86.5	193	15.8	358	29.2	231	18.9	405	33.1	228	18.6	202	16.5
200-299	719	663	92.2	221	30.7	363	50.5	276	38.4	398	55.4	266	37.0	209	29.1
300-399	400	370	92.5	155	38.8	245	61.3	191	47.8	257	64.3	187	46.8	171	42.8
400-499	215	209	97.2	105	48.8	151	70.2	133	61.9	153	71.2	120	55.8	107	49.8
500 or more	280	271	96.8	172	61.4	231	82.5	189	67.5	220	78.6	197	70.4	192	68.6
Nongovernment not-for-profit	3,079	2,709	88.0	725	23.5	1,178	38.3	876	28.5	1,274	41.4	842	27.3	769	25.0
6-24 beds	71	50	70.4	4	5.6	6	8.5	7	9.9	14	19.7	2	2.8	7	9.9
25-49	383	314	82.0	10	2.6	28	7.3	10	2.6	36	9.4	9	2.3	17	4.4
50-99	601	485	80.7	33	5.5	84	14.0	42	7.0	112	18.6	48	8.0	38	6.3
100-199	748	658	88.0	152	20.3	254	34.0	158	21.1	280	37.4	151	20.2	142	19.0
200-299	552	510	92.4	177	32.1	296	53.6	230	41.7	323	58.5	214	38.8	176	31.9
300-399	326	306	93.9	129	39.6	204	62.6	163	50.0	214	65.6	159	48.8	145	44.5
400-499	175	170	97.1	87	49.7	124	70.9	112	64.0	122	69.7	100	57.1	89	50.9
500 or more	223	216	96.9	133	59.6	182	81.6	154	69.1	173	77.6	159	71.3	155	69.5
Investor-owned (for-profit)	636	543	85.4	58	9.1	129	20.3	81	12.7	128	20.1	83	13.1	67	10.5
6-24 beds	14	10	71.4	0	0.0	1	7.1	1	7.1	1	7.1	0	0.0	0	0.0
25-49	62	45	72.6	3	4.8	6	9.7	2	3.2	4	6.5	0	0.0	3	4.8
50-99	178	147	82.6	9	5.1	21	11.8	11	6.2	15	8.4	11	6.2	15	8.4
100-199	248	217	87.5	17	6.9	59	23.8	35	14.1	57	23.0	38	15.3	30	12.1
200-299	90	84	93.3	18	20.0	26	28.9	20	22.2	29	32.2	21	23.3	11	12.2
300-399	29	25	86.2	6	20.7	8	27.6	7	24.1	12	41.4	9	31.0	5	17.2
400-499	12	12	100.0	3	25.0	6	50.0	4	33.3	8	66.7	3	25.0	2	16.7
500 or more	3	3	100.0	2	66.7	2	66.7	1	33.3	2	66.7	1	33.3	1	33.3
State and local government	1,358	1,070	78.8	147	10.8	237	17.5	162	11.9	308	22.7	170	12.5	164	12.1
6-24 beds	124	81	65.3	1	0.8	3	2.4	1	0.8	5	4.0	0	0.0	2	1.6
25-49	423	318	75.2	6	1.4	10	2.4	9	2.1	31	7.3	5	1.2	15	3.5
50-99	378	299	79.1	18	4.8	37	9.8	16	4.2	59	15.6	22	5.8	22	5.8
100-199	229	185	80.8	24	10.5	45	19.7	38	16.6	68	29.7	39	17.0	30	13.1
200-299	77	69	89.6	26	33.8	41	53.2	26	33.8	46	59.7	31	40.3	22	28.6
300-399	45	39	86.7	20	44.4	33	73.3	21	46.7	31	68.9	19	42.2	21	46.7
400-499	28	27	96.4	15	53.6	21	75.0	17	60.7	23	82.1	17	60.7	16	57.1
500 or more	54	52	96.3	37	68.5	47	87.0	34	63.0	45	83.3	37	68.5	36	66.7
Hospital units of institutions	17	13	76.5	5	29.4	10	58.8	8	47.1	11	64.7	3	17.6	11	64.7
Community hospitals	5,056	4,309	85.2	925	18.3	1,534	30.3	1,111	22.0	1,699	33.6	1,092	21.6	989	19.6

(continued on next page)

Table

12A

(Continued)

Facilities and Services in the United States

For definitions of facilities and services, see Definitions of Terms, page xxiii. These data include only hospital-based facilities and services as reported by responding hospitals in Section C of the 1990 AHA Annual Survey, beginning on page 242. No estimates have been made for nonresponding hospitals.

CLASSIFICATION	HOSPITALS REPORTING	PSYCHIATRIC PARTIAL HOSPITALIZATION PROGRAM		RADIATION THERAPY: MEGAVOLTAGE RADIATION THERAPY		RADIATION THERAPY: RADIOACTIVE IMPLANTS		RADIATION THERAPY: THERAPEUTIC RADIOISOTOPE FACILITY		RADIATION THERAPY: X-RAY RADIATION THERAPY		RADIOLOGY (DIAGNOSTIC): CT SCANNER		RADIOLOGY (DIAGNOSTIC): DIAGNOSTIC RADIOISOTOPE FACILITY	
		Number	Percent	Number	Percent	Number	Percent	Number	Percent	Number	Percent	Number	Percent	Number	Percent
UNITED STATES	6,105	1,078	17.7	1,038	17.0	1,305	21.4	1,345	22.0	1,027	16.8	3,728	61.1	3,367	55.2
6-24 beds	254	12	4.7	0	0.0	0	0.0	0	0.0	1	0.4	20	7.9	17	6.7
25-49	974	43	4.4	3	0.3	4	0.4	7	0.7	7	0.7	275	28.2	194	19.9
50-99	1,451	197	13.6	19	1.3	35	2.4	45	3.1	26	1.8	711	49.0	580	40.0
100-199	1,439	228	15.8	141	9.8	209	14.5	227	15.8	146	10.1	1,060	73.7	964	67.0
200-299	804	186	23.1	226	28.1	318	39.6	325	40.4	211	26.2	692	86.1	660	82.1
300-399	485	135	27.8	240	49.5	292	60.2	290	59.8	231	47.6	414	85.4	398	82.1
400-499	265	91	34.3	154	58.1	177	66.8	176	66.4	154	58.1	225	84.9	222	83.8
500 or more	433	186	43.0	255	58.9	270	62.4	275	63.5	251	58.0	331	76.4	332	76.7
Federal	301	107	35.5	41	13.6	41	13.6	62	20.6	38	12.6	172	57.1	160	53.2
Psychiatric	17	8	47.1	0	0.0	0	0.0	0	0.0	0	0.0	2	11.8	5	29.4
General and other special	284	99	34.9	41	14.4	41	14.4	62	21.8	38	13.4	170	59.9	155	54.6
Nonfederal	5,804	971	16.7	997	17.2	1,264	21.8	1,283	22.1	989	17.0	3,556	61.3	3,207	55.3
Psychiatric	609	283	46.5	0	0.0	0	0.0	2	0.3	3	0.5	4	0.7	17	2.8
Nongovernment not-for-profit	106	70	66.0	0	0.0	0	0.0	0	0.0	0	0.0	1	0.9	2	1.9
Investor-owned (for-profit)	272	164	60.3	0	0.0	0	0.0	0	0.0	1	0.4	1	0.4	2	0.7
State and local government	231	49	21.2	0	0.0	0	0.0	2	0.9	2	0.9	2	0.9	13	5.6
TB and other respiratory diseases	3	0	0.0	0	0.0	0	0.0	0	0.0	0	0.0	0	0.0	1	33.3
Nongovernment not-for-profit	1	0	0.0	0	0.0	0	0.0	0	0.0	0	0.0	0	0.0	0	0.0
Investor-owned (for-profit)	0	0	0.0	0	0.0	0	0.0	0	0.0	0	0.0	0	0.0	0	0.0
State and local government	2	0	0.0	0	0.0	0	0.0	0	0.0	0	0.0	0	0.0	1	50.0
Long-term general and other special	119	4	3.4	3	2.5	2	1.7	2	1.7	2	1.7	7	5.9	15	12.6
Nongovernment not-for-profit	54	2	3.7	1	1.9	1	1.9	1	1.9	0	0.0	2	3.7	4	7.4
Investor-owned (for-profit)	16	1	6.3	0	0.0	0	0.0	0	0.0	0	0.0	0	0.0	1	6.3
State and local government	49	1	2.0	2	4.1	1	2.0	1	2.0	2	4.1	5	10.2	10	20.4
Short-term general and other special	5,073	684	13.5	994	19.6	1,262	24.9	1,279	25.2	984	19.4	3,545	69.9	3,174	62.6
6-24 beds	209	5	2.4	0	0.0	0	0.0	0	0.0	1	0.5	17	8.1	17	8.1
25-49	868	16	1.8	2	0.2	4	0.5	7	0.8	5	0.6	274	31.6	189	21.8
50-99	1,157	55	4.8	19	1.6	35	3.0	44	3.8	25	2.2	699	60.4	566	48.9
100-199	1,225	136	11.1	140	11.4	207	16.9	219	17.9	144	11.8	1,018	83.1	927	75.7
200-299	719	158	22.0	222	30.9	313	43.5	316	43.9	209	29.1	668	92.9	632	87.9
300-399	400	113	28.3	230	57.5	281	70.3	274	68.5	222	55.5	388	97.0	374	93.5
400-499	215	76	35.3	148	68.8	170	79.1	170	79.1	149	69.3	209	97.2	201	93.5
500 or more	280	125	44.6	233	83.2	252	90.0	249	88.9	229	81.8	272	97.1	268	95.7
Nongovernment not-for-profit	3,079	512	16.6	801	26.0	981	31.9	1,004	32.6	776	25.2	2,372	77.0	2,190	71.1
6-24 beds	71	4	5.6	0	0.0	0	0.0	0	0.0	0	0.0	5	7.0	9	12.7
25-49	383	5	1.3	2	0.5	4	1.0	6	1.6	3	0.8	140	36.6	91	23.8
50-99	601	25	4.2	8	1.3	22	3.7	28	4.7	12	2.0	367	61.1	309	51.4
100-199	748	93	12.4	103	13.8	135	18.0	146	19.5	104	13.9	633	84.6	601	80.3
200-299	552	130	23.6	174	31.5	244	44.2	255	46.2	161	29.2	520	94.2	493	89.3
300-399	326	95	29.1	196	60.1	229	70.2	226	69.3	185	56.7	317	97.2	307	94.2
400-499	175	61	34.9	126	72.0	141	80.6	140	80.0	125	71.4	171	97.7	166	94.9
500 or more	223	99	44.4	192	86.1	206	92.4	203	91.0	186	83.4	219	98.2	214	96.0
Investor-owned (for-profit)	636	53	8.3	49	7.7	113	17.8	100	15.7	61	9.6	477	75.0	396	62.3
6-24 beds	14	0	0.0	0	0.0	0	0.0	0	0.0	0	0.0	1	7.1	3	21.4
25-49	62	3	4.8	0	0.0	0	0.0	0	0.0	0	0.0	16	25.8	11	17.7
50-99	178	12	6.7	1	0.6	7	3.9	4	2.2	2	1.1	122	68.5	88	49.4
100-199	248	21	8.5	16	6.5	43	17.3	44	17.7	23	9.3	216	87.1	181	73.0
200-299	90	9	10.0	13	14.4	32	35.6	24	26.7	14	15.6	80	88.9	74	82.2
300-399	29	5	17.2	11	37.9	19	65.5	16	55.2	13	44.8	28	96.6	26	89.7
400-499	12	2	16.7	5	41.7	9	75.0	9	75.0	6	50.0	11	91.7	10	83.3
500 or more	3	1	33.3	3	100.0	3	100.0	3	100.0	3	100.0	3	100.0	3	100.0
State and local government	1,358	119	8.8	144	10.6	168	12.4	175	12.9	147	10.8	696	51.3	588	43.3
6-24 beds	124	1	0.8	0	0.0	0	0.0	0	0.0	1	0.8	11	8.9	5	4.0
25-49	423	8	1.9	0	0.0	0	0.0	1	0.2	2	0.5	118	27.9	87	20.6
50-99	378	18	4.8	10	2.6	6	1.6	12	3.2	11	2.9	210	55.6	169	44.7
100-199	229	22	9.6	21	9.2	29	12.7	29	12.7	17	7.4	169	73.8	145	63.3
200-299	77	19	24.7	35	45.5	37	48.1	37	48.1	34	44.2	68	88.3	65	84.4
300-399	45	13	28.9	23	51.1	33	73.3	32	71.1	24	53.3	43	95.6	41	91.1
400-499	28	13	46.4	17	60.7	20	71.4	21	75.0	18	64.3	27	96.4	25	89.3
500 or more	54	25	46.3	38	70.4	43	79.6	43	79.6	40	74.1	50	92.6	51	94.4
Hospital units of institutions	17	6	35.3	0	0.0	0	0.0	0	0.0	1	5.9	1	5.9	1	5.9
Community hospitals	5,056	678	13.4	994	19.7	1,262	25.0	1,279	25.3	983	19.4	3,544	70.1	3,173	62.8

Table 12A (Continued)

CLASSIFICATION	HOSPITALS REPORTING	RADIOLOGY (DIAGNOSTIC) continued: MAGNETIC RESONANCE IMAGING (MRI)		SINGLE PHOTON EMISSION COMPUTERIZED TOMOGRAPHY (SPECT)		ULTRASOUND		REHABILITATION OUTPATIENT SERVICES		REPRODUCTIVE HEALTH		SOCIAL WORK SERVICES: ORGANIZED		OUTPATIENT	
		Number	Percent	Number	Percent	Number	Percent	Number	Percent	Number	Percent	Number	Percent	Number	Percent
UNITED STATES	6,105	955	15.6	988	16.2	4,563	74.7	2,924	47.9	2,269	37.2	4,864	79.7	2,785	45.6
6-24 beds	254	0	0.0	0	0.0	115	45.3	38	15.0	73	28.7	79	31.1	47	18.5
25-49	974	12	1.2	19	2.0	593	60.9	229	23.5	287	29.5	464	47.6	237	24.3
50-99	1,451	62	4.3	66	4.5	959	66.1	513	35.4	420	28.9	1,112	76.6	521	35.9
100-199	1,439	169	11.7	204	14.2	1,177	81.8	708	49.2	517	35.9	1,281	89.0	657	45.7
200-299	804	223	27.7	233	29.0	722	89.8	562	69.9	378	47.0	768	95.5	494	61.4
300-399	485	167	34.4	186	38.4	418	86.2	337	69.5	223	46.0	473	97.5	315	64.9
400-499	265	113	42.6	96	36.2	232	87.5	196	74.0	147	55.5	262	98.9	189	71.3
500 or more	433	209	48.3	184	42.5	347	80.1	341	78.8	224	51.7	425	98.2	325	75.1
Federal	301	32	10.6	51	16.9	273	90.7	191	63.5	125	41.5	281	93.4	274	91.0
Psychiatric	17	0	0.0	0	0.0	12	70.6	17	100.0	0	0.0	15	88.2	15	88.2
General and other special	284	32	11.3	51	18.0	261	91.9	174	61.3	125	44.0	266	93.7	259	91.2
Nonfederal	5,804	923	15.9	937	16.1	4,290	73.9	2,733	47.1	2,144	36.9	4,583	79.0	2,511	43.3
Psychiatric	609	3	0.5	2	0.3	8	1.3	45	7.4	4	0.7	512	84.1	214	35.1
Nongovernment not-for-profit	106	1	0.9	1	0.9	1	0.9	15	14.2	1	0.9	86	81.1	54	50.9
Investor-owned (for-profit)	272	0	0.0	0	0.0	0	0.0	6	2.2	0	0.0	219	80.5	89	32.7
State and local government	231	2	0.9	1	0.4	7	3.0	24	10.4	3	1.3	207	89.6	71	30.7
TB and other respiratory diseases	3	0	0.0	0	0.0	1	33.3	1	33.3	0	0.0	3	100.0	1	33.3
Nongovernment not-for-profit	1	0	0.0	0	0.0	0	0.0	1	100.0	0	0.0	1	100.0	1	100.0
Investor-owned (for-profit)	0	0	0.0	0	0.0	0	0.0	0	0.0	0	0.0	0	0.0	0	0.0
State and local government	2	0	0.0	0	0.0	1	50.0	0	0.0	0	0.0	2	100.0	0	0.0
Long-term general and other special	119	1	0.8	1	0.8	17	14.3	77	64.7	8	6.7	108	90.8	63	52.9
Nongovernment not-for-profit	54	0	0.0	1	1.9	7	13.0	42	77.8	6	11.1	50	92.6	38	70.4
Investor-owned (for-profit)	16	0	0.0	0	0.0	1	6.3	13	81.3	0	0.0	15	93.8	10	62.5
State and local government	49	1	2.0	0	0.0	9	18.4	22	44.9	2	4.1	43	87.8	15	30.6
Short-term general and other special	5,073	919	18.1	934	18.4	4,264	84.1	2,610	51.4	2,132	42.0	3,960	78.1	2,233	44.0
6-24 beds	209	0	0.0	0	0.0	90	43.1	30	14.4	49	23.4	46	22.0	22	10.5
25-49	868	11	1.3	18	2.1	557	64.2	210	24.2	256	29.5	377	43.4	173	19.9
50-99	1,157	62	5.4	64	5.5	930	80.4	462	39.9	391	33.8	867	74.9	383	33.1
100-199	1,225	166	13.6	194	15.8	1,122	91.6	647	52.8	487	39.8	1,094	89.3	551	45.0
200-299	719	220	30.6	226	31.4	691	96.1	526	73.2	371	51.6	691	96.1	445	61.9
300-399	400	160	40.0	175	43.8	389	97.3	303	75.8	218	54.5	393	98.3	267	66.8
400-499	215	107	49.8	91	42.3	212	98.6	177	82.3	143	66.5	213	99.1	161	74.9
500 or more	280	193	68.9	166	59.3	273	97.5	255	91.1	217	77.5	279	99.6	231	82.5
Nongovernment not-for-profit	3,079	670	21.8	721	23.4	2,713	88.1	1,864	60.5	1,352	43.9	2,645	85.9	1,659	53.9
6-24 beds	71	0	0.0	0	0.0	24	33.8	13	18.3	18	25.4	21	29.6	13	18.3
25-49	383	6	1.6	11	2.9	263	68.7	112	29.2	109	28.5	200	52.2	98	25.6
50-99	601	31	5.2	40	6.7	483	80.4	276	45.9	200	33.3	475	79.0	242	40.3
100-199	748	97	13.0	130	17.4	700	93.6	432	57.8	292	39.0	693	92.6	387	51.7
200-299	552	168	30.4	183	33.2	529	95.8	427	77.4	281	50.9	537	97.3	372	67.4
300-399	326	123	37.7	147	45.1	320	98.2	251	77.0	171	52.5	324	99.4	230	70.6
400-499	175	85	48.6	78	44.6	174	99.4	147	84.0	112	64.0	173	98.9	136	77.7
500 or more	223	160	71.7	132	59.2	220	98.7	206	92.4	169	75.8	222	99.6	181	81.2
Investor-owned (for-profit)	636	114	17.9	84	13.2	547	86.0	268	42.1	241	37.9	475	74.7	173	27.2
6-24 beds	14	0	0.0	0	0.0	7	50.0	0	0.0	0	0.0	3	21.4	0	0.0
25-49	62	3	4.8	1	1.6	45	72.6	13	21.0	20	32.3	28	45.2	11	17.7
50-99	178	20	11.2	8	4.5	139	78.1	60	33.7	54	30.3	124	69.7	45	25.3
100-199	248	46	18.5	38	15.3	225	90.7	118	47.6	98	39.5	201	81.0	71	28.6
200-299	90	26	28.9	21	23.3	89	98.9	52	57.8	46	51.1	80	88.9	30	33.3
300-399	29	11	37.9	10	34.5	27	93.1	16	55.2	14	48.3	24	82.8	9	31.0
400-499	12	5	41.7	3	25.0	12	100.0	6	50.0	7	58.3	12	100.0	5	41.7
500 or more	3	3	100.0	3	100.0	3	100.0	3	100.0	2	66.7	3	100.0	2	66.7
State and local government	1,358	135	9.9	129	9.5	1,004	73.9	478	35.2	539	39.7	840	61.9	401	29.5
6-24 beds	124	0	0.0	0	0.0	59	47.6	17	13.7	31	25.0	22	17.7	9	7.3
25-49	423	2	0.5	6	1.4	249	58.9	85	20.1	127	30.0	149	35.2	64	15.1
50-99	378	11	2.9	16	4.2	308	81.5	126	33.3	137	36.2	268	70.9	96	25.4
100-199	229	23	10.0	26	11.4	197	86.0	97	42.4	97	42.4	200	87.3	93	40.6
200-299	77	26	33.8	22	28.6	73	94.8	47	61.0	44	57.1	74	96.1	43	55.8
300-399	45	26	57.8	18	40.0	42	93.3	36	80.0	33	73.3	45	100.0	28	62.2
400-499	28	17	60.7	10	35.7	26	92.9	24	85.7	24	85.7	28	100.0	20	71.4
500 or more	54	30	55.6	31	57.4	50	92.6	46	85.2	46	85.2	54	100.0	48	88.9
Hospital units of institutions	17	0	0.0	0	0.0	2	11.8	4	23.5	3	17.6	7	41.2	7	41.2
Community hospitals	5,056	919	18.2	934	18.5	4,262	84.3	2,606	51.5	2,129	42.1	3,953	78.2	2,226	44.0

(continued on next page)

Table

12A (Continued)

Facilities and Services in the United States

For definitions of facilities and services, see Definitions of Terms, page xxiii. These data include only hospital-based facilities and services as reported by responding hospitals in Section C of the 1990 AHA Annual Survey, beginning on page 242. No estimates have been made for nonresponding hospitals.

CLASSIFICATION	HOSPITALS REPORTING	SOCIAL WORK SERVICES continued: EMERGENCY DEPARTMENT		SPORTS MEDICINE CLINIC/SERVICES		SUPPLEMENTARY PATIENT ASSISTANCE: HOSPITAL AUXILIARY		PATIENT REPRESENTATIVE SERVICES		VOLUNTEER SERVICES DEPARTMENT		SURGERY SERVICES: OUTPATIENT		ORGAN/TISSUE TRANSPLANT	
		Number	Percent	Number	Percent	Number	Percent	Number	Percent	Number	Percent	Number	Percent	Number	Percent
UNITED STATES	6,105	2,440	40.0	1,060	17.4	4,405	72.2	3,210	52.6	4,027	66.0	5,070	83.0	558	9.1
6-24 beds	254	27	10.6	19	7.5	138	54.3	56	22.0	67	26.4	191	75.2	2	0.8
25-49	974	142	14.6	69	7.1	662	68.0	259	26.6	339	34.8	813	83.5	18	1.8
50-99	1,451	347	23.9	172	11.9	964	66.4	535	36.9	724	49.9	1,105	76.2	28	1.9
100-199	1,439	598	41.6	258	17.9	1,063	73.9	822	57.1	1,055	73.3	1,237	86.0	82	5.7
200-299	804	491	61.1	200	24.9	656	81.6	564	70.1	721	89.7	734	91.3	93	11.6
300-399	485	333	68.7	139	28.7	398	82.1	378	77.9	447	92.2	422	87.0	89	18.4
400-499	265	196	74.0	77	29.1	212	80.0	224	84.5	254	95.8	231	87.2	72	27.2
500 or more	433	306	70.7	126	29.1	312	72.1	372	85.9	420	97.0	337	77.8	174	40.2
Federal	301	185	61.5	34	11.3	102	33.9	254	84.4	256	85.0	249	82.7	30	10.0
Psychiatric	17	7	41.2	1	5.9	5	29.4	15	88.2	15	88.2	5	29.4	0	0.0
General and other special	284	178	62.7	33	11.6	97	34.2	239	84.2	241	84.9	244	85.9	30	10.6
Nonfederal	5,804	2,255	38.9	1,026	17.7	4,303	74.1	2,956	50.9	3,771	65.0	4,821	83.1	528	9.1
Psychiatric	609	80	13.1	1	0.2	91	14.9	216	35.5	251	41.2	9	1.5	1	0.2
Nongovernment not-for-profit	106	16	15.1	1	0.9	30	28.3	33	31.1	48	45.3	2	1.9	0	0.0
Investor-owned (for-profit)	272	33	12.1	0	0.0	6	2.2	56	20.6	22	8.1	3	1.1	0	0.0
State and local government	231	31	13.4	0	0.0	55	23.8	127	55.0	181	78.4	4	1.7	1	0.4
TB and other respiratory diseases	3	0	0.0	0	0.0	1	33.3	1	33.3	2	66.7	1	33.3	0	0.0
Nongovernment not-for-profit	1	0	0.0	0	0.0	0	0.0	0	0.0	0	0.0	0	0.0	0	0.0
Investor-owned (for-profit)	0	0	0.0	0	0.0	0	0.0	0	0.0	0	0.0	0	0.0	0	0.0
State and local government	2	0	0.0	0	0.0	1	50.0	1	50.0	2	100.0	1	50.0	0	0.0
Long-term general and other special	119	9	7.6	11	9.2	58	48.7	50	42.0	88	73.9	17	14.3	1	0.8
Nongovernment not-for-profit	54	3	5.6	5	9.3	34	63.0	24	44.4	45	83.3	6	11.1	1	1.9
Investor-owned (for-profit)	16	1	6.3	4	25.0	2	12.5	4	25.0	7	43.8	1	6.3	0	0.0
State and local government	49	5	10.2	2	4.1	22	44.9	22	44.9	36	73.5	10	20.4	0	0.0
Short-term general and other special	5,073	2,166	42.7	1,014	20.0	4,153	81.9	2,689	53.0	3,430	67.6	4,794	94.5	526	10.4
6-24 beds	209	12	5.7	14	6.7	123	58.9	34	16.3	44	21.1	169	80.9	2	1.0
25-49	868	109	12.6	58	6.7	644	74.2	218	25.1	293	33.8	780	89.9	18	2.1
50-99	1,157	298	25.8	164	14.2	917	79.3	450	38.9	635	54.9	1,069	92.4	28	2.4
100-199	1,225	550	44.9	251	20.5	1,017	83.0	721	58.9	945	77.1	1,182	96.5	78	6.4
200-299	719	467	65.0	198	27.5	629	87.5	516	71.8	653	90.8	707	98.3	89	12.4
300-399	400	305	76.3	135	33.8	368	92.0	314	78.5	378	94.5	396	99.0	81	20.3
400-499	215	178	82.8	73	34.0	196	91.2	185	86.0	206	95.8	214	99.5	70	32.6
500 or more	280	247	88.2	121	43.2	259	92.5	251	89.6	276	98.6	277	98.9	160	57.1
Nongovernment not-for-profit	3,079	1,667	54.1	737	23.9	2,715	88.2	1,852	60.1	2,394	77.8	2,948	95.7	402	13.1
6-24 beds	71	8	11.3	8	11.3	47	66.2	17	23.9	20	28.2	55	77.5	0	0.0
25-49	383	65	17.0	29	7.6	298	77.8	107	27.9	158	41.3	345	90.1	15	3.9
50-99	601	196	32.6	100	16.6	511	85.0	253	42.1	382	63.6	555	92.3	21	3.5
100-199	748	397	53.1	169	22.6	674	90.1	464	62.0	618	82.6	727	97.2	57	7.6
200-299	552	396	71.7	165	29.9	502	90.9	408	73.9	513	92.9	544	98.6	71	12.9
300-399	326	260	79.8	108	33.1	310	95.1	257	78.8	314	96.3	326	100.0	59	18.1
400-499	175	148	84.6	58	33.1	166	94.9	147	84.0	170	97.1	175	100.0	54	30.9
500 or more	223	197	88.3	100	44.8	207	92.8	199	89.2	219	98.2	221	99.1	125	56.1
Investor-owned (for-profit)	636	148	23.3	101	15.9	344	54.1	322	50.6	421	66.2	581	91.4	47	7.4
6-24 beds	14	0	0.0	0	0.0	5	35.7	1	7.1	1	7.1	12	85.7	1	7.1
25-49	62	4	6.5	4	6.5	23	37.1	13	21.0	18	29.0	51	82.3	2	3.2
50-99	178	26	14.6	20	11.2	87	48.9	70	39.3	99	55.6	154	86.5	4	2.2
100-199	248	68	27.4	50	20.2	148	59.7	148	59.7	191	77.0	234	94.4	14	5.6
200-299	90	28	31.1	16	17.8	54	60.0	55	61.1	73	81.1	88	97.8	11	12.2
300-399	29	12	41.4	7	24.1	17	58.6	22	75.9	25	86.2	28	96.6	9	31.0
400-499	12	7	58.3	3	25.0	7	58.3	11	91.7	11	91.7	11	91.7	4	33.3
500 or more	3	3	100.0	1	33.3	3	100.0	2	66.7	3	100.0	3	100.0	2	66.7
State and local government	1,358	351	25.8	176	13.0	1,094	80.6	515	37.9	615	45.3	1,265	93.2	77	5.7
6-24 beds	124	4	3.2	6	4.8	71	57.3	16	12.9	23	18.5	102	82.3	1	0.8
25-49	423	40	9.5	25	5.9	323	76.4	98	23.2	117	27.7	384	90.8	1	0.2
50-99	378	76	20.1	44	11.6	319	84.4	127	33.6	154	40.7	360	95.2	3	0.8
100-199	229	85	37.1	32	14.0	195	85.2	109	47.6	136	59.4	221	96.5	7	3.1
200-299	77	43	55.8	17	22.1	73	94.8	53	68.8	67	87.0	75	97.4	7	9.1
300-399	45	33	73.3	20	44.4	41	91.1	35	77.8	39	86.7	42	93.3	13	28.9
400-499	28	23	82.1	12	42.9	23	82.1	27	96.4	25	89.3	28	100.0	12	42.9
500 or more	54	47	87.0	20	37.0	49	90.7	50	92.6	54	100.0	53	98.1	33	61.1
Hospital units of institutions	17	4	23.5	6	35.3	1	5.9	1	5.9	3	17.6	6	35.3	0	0.0
Community hospitals	5,056	2,162	42.8	1,008	19.9	4,152	82.1	2,688	53.2	3,427	67.8	4,788	94.7	526	10.4

Table 12A (Continued)

CLASSIFICATION	HOSPITALS REPORTING	SURGERY SERVICES continued: ORTHOPEDIC Number	SURGERY SERVICES continued: ORTHOPEDIC Percent	THERAPY SERVICES: OCCUPATIONAL Number	OCCUPATIONAL Percent	PHYSICAL Number	PHYSICAL Percent	RECREATIONAL Number	RECREATIONAL Percent	RESPIRATORY Number	RESPIRATORY Percent	SPEECH Number	SPEECH Percent	WOMEN'S HEALTH CENTER/SERVICES Number	WOMEN'S HEALTH CENTER/SERVICES Percent
UNITED STATES	6,105	3,980	65.2	3,206	52.5	4,822	79.0	2,475	40.5	4,944	81.0	2,746	45.0	1,170	19.2
6-24 beds	254	45	17.7	24	9.4	122	48.0	23	9.1	135	53.1	26	10.2	10	3.9
25-49	974	371	38.1	181	18.6	617	63.3	140	14.4	714	73.3	182	18.7	55	5.6
50-99	1,451	796	54.9	523	36.0	1,056	72.8	439	30.3	1,063	73.3	431	29.7	112	7.7
100-199	1,439	1,093	76.0	773	53.7	1,179	81.9	534	37.1	1,240	86.2	631	43.8	265	18.4
200-299	804	707	87.9	619	77.0	733	91.2	420	52.2	749	93.2	514	63.9	244	30.3
300-399	485	415	85.6	421	86.8	452	93.2	335	69.1	434	89.5	356	73.4	182	37.5
400-499	265	227	85.7	247	93.2	253	95.5	194	73.2	234	88.3	215	81.1	109	41.1
500 or more	433	326	75.3	418	96.5	410	94.7	390	90.1	375	86.6	391	90.3	193	44.6
Federal	301	184	61.1	184	61.1	277	92.0	162	53.8	239	79.4	165	54.8	93	30.9
Psychiatric	17	0	0.0	16	94.1	17	100.0	17	100.0	17	100.0	15	88.2	6	35.3
General and other special	284	184	64.8	168	59.2	260	91.5	145	51.1	222	78.2	150	52.8	87	30.6
Nonfederal	5,804	3,796	65.4	3,022	52.1	4,545	78.3	2,313	39.9	4,705	81.1	2,581	44.5	1,077	18.6
Psychiatric	609	6	1.0	406	66.7	153	25.1	546	89.7	38	6.2	162	26.6	25	4.1
Nongovernment not-for-profit	106	1	0.9	58	54.7	15	14.2	86	81.1	5	4.7	14	13.2	4	3.8
Investor-owned (for-profit)	272	2	0.7	162	59.6	23	8.5	242	89.0	6	2.2	44	16.2	17	6.3
State and local government	231	3	1.3	186	80.5	115	49.8	218	94.4	27	11.7	104	45.0	4	1.7
TB and other respiratory diseases	3	0	0.0	1	33.3	2	66.7	1	33.3	3	100.0	1	33.3	0	0.0
Nongovernment not-for-profit	1	0	0.0	1	100.0	1	100.0	0	0.0	1	100.0	1	100.0	0	0.0
Investor-owned (for-profit)	0	0	0.0	0	0.0	0	0.0	0	0.0	0	0.0	0	0.0	0	0.0
State and local government	2	0	0.0	0	0.0	1	50.0	1	50.0	2	100.0	0	0.0	0	0.0
Long-term general and other special	119	10	8.4	101	84.9	108	90.8	103	86.6	80	67.2	93	78.2	2	1.7
Nongovernment not-for-profit	54	2	3.7	49	90.7	51	94.4	48	88.9	33	61.1	45	83.3	0	0.0
Investor-owned (for-profit)	16	0	0.0	15	93.8	15	93.8	14	87.5	12	75.0	15	93.8	1	6.3
State and local government	49	8	16.3	37	75.5	42	85.7	41	83.7	35	71.4	33	67.3	1	2.0
Short-term general and other special	5,073	3,780	74.5	2,514	49.6	4,282	84.4	1,663	32.8	4,584	90.4	2,325	45.8	1,050	20.7
6-24 beds	209	43	20.6	22	10.5	99	47.4	19	9.1	130	62.2	25	12.0	8	3.8
25-49	868	353	40.7	145	16.7	571	65.8	90	10.4	688	79.3	163	18.8	43	5.0
50-99	1,157	774	66.9	355	30.7	970	83.8	212	18.3	1,009	87.2	358	30.9	99	8.6
100-199	1,225	1,048	85.6	617	50.4	1,086	88.7	356	29.1	1,163	94.9	557	45.5	235	19.2
200-299	719	683	95.0	552	76.8	677	94.2	344	47.8	708	98.5	475	66.1	232	32.3
300-399	400	391	97.8	348	87.0	389	97.3	254	63.5	395	98.8	302	75.5	174	43.5
400-499	215	213	99.1	202	94.0	211	98.1	148	68.8	213	99.1	179	83.3	97	45.1
500 or more	280	275	98.2	273	97.5	279	99.6	240	85.7	278	99.3	266	95.0	162	57.9
Nongovernment not-for-profit	3,079	2,538	82.4	1,393	61.5	2,778	90.2	1,258	40.9	2,848	92.5	1,737	56.4	756	24.6
6-24 beds	71	18	25.4	8	11.3	39	54.9	11	15.5	41	57.7	11	15.5	6	8.5
25-49	383	185	48.3	90	23.5	277	72.3	53	13.8	299	78.1	91	23.8	28	7.3
50-99	601	430	71.5	228	37.9	527	87.7	141	23.5	525	87.4	227	37.8	55	9.2
100-199	748	663	88.6	444	59.4	692	92.5	245	32.8	717	95.9	399	53.3	134	17.9
200-299	552	529	95.8	448	81.2	528	95.7	279	50.5	547	99.1	393	71.2	186	33.7
300-399	326	320	98.2	293	89.9	321	98.5	214	65.6	324	99.4	255	78.2	136	41.7
400-499	175	174	99.4	165	94.3	172	98.3	125	71.4	174	99.4	149	85.1	76	43.4
500 or more	223	219	98.2	217	97.3	222	99.6	190	85.2	221	99.1	212	95.1	135	60.5
Investor-owned (for-profit)	636	484	76.1	228	35.8	503	79.1	155	24.4	589	92.6	196	30.8	145	22.8
6-24 beds	14	4	28.6	0	0.0	2	14.3	1	7.1	5	35.7	2	14.3	0	0.0
25-49	62	26	41.9	14	22.6	40	64.5	9	14.5	52	83.9	11	17.7	4	6.5
50-99	178	116	65.2	43	24.2	138	77.5	36	20.2	166	93.3	49	27.5	22	12.4
100-199	248	212	85.5	93	37.5	209	84.3	57	23.0	239	96.4	74	29.8	66	26.6
200-299	90	84	93.3	48	53.3	74	82.2	31	34.4	85	94.4	38	42.2	29	32.2
300-399	29	28	96.6	17	58.6	26	89.7	13	44.8	28	96.6	14	48.3	15	51.7
400-499	12	11	91.7	10	83.3	11	91.7	5	41.7	11	91.7	5	41.7	6	50.0
500 or more	3	3	100.0	3	100.0	3	100.0	3	100.0	3	100.0	3	100.0	3	100.0
State and local government	1,358	758	55.8	393	28.9	1,001	73.7	250	18.4	1,147	84.5	392	28.9	149	11.0
6-24 beds	124	21	16.9	14	11.3	58	46.8	7	5.6	84	67.7	12	9.7	2	1.6
25-49	423	142	33.6	41	9.7	254	60.0	28	6.6	337	79.7	61	14.4	11	2.6
50-99	378	228	60.3	84	22.2	305	80.7	35	9.3	318	84.1	82	21.7	22	5.8
100-199	229	173	75.5	80	34.9	185	80.8	54	23.6	207	90.4	84	36.7	35	15.3
200-299	77	70	90.9	56	72.7	75	97.4	34	44.2	76	98.7	44	57.1	17	22.1
300-399	45	43	95.6	38	84.4	42	93.3	27	60.0	43	95.6	33	73.3	23	51.1
400-499	28	28	100.0	27	96.4	28	100.0	18	64.3	28	100.0	25	89.3	15	53.6
500 or more	54	53	98.1	53	98.1	54	100.0	47	87.0	54	100.0	51	94.4	24	44.4
Hospital units of institutions	17	3	17.6	4	23.5	11	64.7	7	41.2	5	29.4	2	11.8	5	29.4
Community hospitals	5,056	3,777	74.7	2,510	49.6	4,271	84.5	1,656	32.8	4,579	90.6	2,323	45.9	1,045	20.7

Table
12B

Facilities and Services in U.S. Census Divisions and States

For definitions of facilities and services, see Definitions of Terms, page xxiii. These data include only hospital-based facilities and services as reported by responding hospitals in Section C of the 1990 AHA Annual Survey, beginning on page 242. No estimates have been made for nonresponding hospitals.

CLASSIFICATION	HOSPITALS REPORTING	ACQUIRED IMMUNE-DEFICIENCY SYNDROME (AIDS) SERVICES						ALCOHOL/DRUG ABUSE OR DEPENDENCY OUTPATIENT SERVICES		ARTHRITIS TREATMENT CENTER		BIRTHING ROOM/ LDRP ROOM		CARDIAC SERVICES	
		GENERAL INPATIENT CARE FOR AIDS/ARC		AIDS/ARC UNIT		SPECIALIZED OUTPATIENT PROGRAM FOR AIDS/ARC								ANGIOPLASTY	
		Number	Percent	Number	Percent	Number	Percent	Number	Percent	Number	Percent	Number	Percent	Number	Percent
UNITED STATES	6,105	3,745	61.3	146	2.4	389	6.4	1,508	24.7	418	6.8	3,394	55.6	1,101	18.0
CENSUS DIVISION 1, NEW ENGLAND	315	213	67.6	8	2.5	34	10.8	107	34.0	34	10.8	157	49.8	35	11.1
Connecticut	60	38	63.3	1	1.7	8	13.3	27	45.0	6	10.0	26	43.3	9	15.0
Maine	42	28	66.7	0	0.0	1	2.4	19	45.2	2	4.8	33	78.6	2	4.8
Massachusetts	140	94	67.1	6	4.3	20	14.3	41	29.3	19	13.6	53	37.9	15	10.7
New Hampshire	36	25	69.4	0	0.0	1	2.8	10	27.8	4	11.1	24	66.7	5	13.9
Rhode Island	19	16	84.2	1	5.3	3	15.8	6	31.6	2	10.5	8	42.1	2	10.5
Vermont	18	12	66.7	0	0.0	1	5.6	4	22.2	1	5.6	13	72.2	2	11.1
CENSUS DIVISION 2, MIDDLE ATLANTIC	681	485	71.2	38	5.6	91	13.4	197	28.9	71	10.4	359	52.7	123	18.1
New Jersey	114	92	80.7	6	5.3	23	20.2	49	43.0	10	8.8	57	50.0	19	16.7
New York	288	204	70.8	28	9.7	53	18.4	91	31.6	29	10.1	158	54.9	51	17.7
Pennsylvania	279	189	67.7	4	1.4	15	5.4	57	20.4	32	11.5	144	51.6	53	19.0
CENSUS DIVISION 3, SOUTH ATLANTIC	963	600	62.3	25	2.6	54	5.6	199	20.7	42	4.4	470	48.8	168	17.4
Delaware	13	9	69.2	0	0.0	2	15.4	2	15.4	1	7.7	6	46.2	2	15.4
District of Columbia	16	13	81.3	2	12.5	6	37.5	7	43.8	6	37.5	7	43.8	7	43.8
Florida	260	178	68.5	10	3.8	12	4.6	49	18.8	15	5.8	98	37.7	70	26.9
Georgia	188	101	53.7	2	1.1	6	3.2	35	18.6	6	3.2	99	52.7	20	10.6
Maryland	78	56	71.8	5	6.4	5	6.4	31	39.7	4	5.1	34	43.6	11	14.1
North Carolina	135	84	62.2	3	2.2	10	7.4	20	14.8	2	1.5	85	63.0	22	16.3
South Carolina	84	50	59.5	2	2.4	2	2.4	10	11.9	0	0.0	43	51.2	8	9.5
Virginia	124	76	61.3	1	0.8	7	5.6	34	27.4	7	5.6	66	53.2	22	17.7
West Virginia	65	33	50.8	0	0.0	4	6.2	11	16.9	1	1.5	32	49.2	6	9.2
CENSUS DIVISION 4, EAST NORTH CENTRAL	918	608	66.2	16	1.7	51	5.6	294	32.0	87	9.5	569	62.0	192	20.9
Illinois	231	158	68.4	7	3.0	13	5.6	79	34.2	25	10.8	148	64.1	59	25.5
Indiana	131	87	66.4	1	0.8	3	2.3	40	30.5	4	3.1	84	64.1	27	20.6
Michigan	201	123	61.2	2	1.0	8	4.0	62	30.8	12	6.0	108	53.7	33	16.4
Ohio	214	144	67.3	6	2.8	16	7.5	68	31.8	15	7.0	125	58.4	50	23.4
Wisconsin	141	96	68.1	0	0.0	11	7.8	45	31.9	31	22.0	104	73.8	23	16.3
CENSUS DIVISION 5, EAST SOUTH CENTRAL	492	275	55.9	4	0.8	16	3.3	79	16.1	18	3.7	220	44.7	69	14.0
Alabama	119	62	52.1	3	2.5	6	5.0	22	18.5	7	5.9	47	39.5	23	19.3
Kentucky	117	61	52.1	0	0.0	3	2.6	17	14.5	4	3.4	61	52.1	14	12.0
Mississippi	110	61	55.5	1	0.9	3	2.7	13	11.8	0	0.0	27	24.5	1	0.9
Tennessee	146	91	62.3	0	0.0	4	2.7	27	18.5	7	4.8	85	58.2	31	21.2
CENSUS DIVISION 6, WEST NORTH CENTRAL	810	409	50.5	7	0.9	24	3.0	190	23.5	54	6.7	506	62.5	108	13.3
Iowa	134	58	43.3	0	0.0	2	1.5	33	24.6	9	6.7	103	76.9	21	15.7
Kansas	147	65	44.2	0	0.0	2	1.4	24	16.3	5	3.4	88	59.9	14	9.5
Minnesota	158	94	59.5	4	2.5	8	5.1	50	31.6	5	3.2	116	73.4	15	9.5
Missouri	159	99	62.3	2	1.3	10	6.3	43	27.0	24	15.1	48	30.2	40	25.2
Nebraska	91	43	47.3	1	1.1	1	1.1	19	20.9	3	3.3	63	69.2	9	9.9
North Dakota	55	25	45.5	0	0.0	1	1.8	11	20.0	5	9.1	44	80.0	6	10.9
South Dakota	66	25	37.9	0	0.0	0	0.0	10	15.2	3	4.5	44	66.7	3	4.5
CENSUS DIVISION 7, WEST SOUTH CENTRAL	862	453	52.6	11	1.3	31	3.6	177	20.5	49	5.7	437	50.7	162	18.8
Arkansas	91	50	54.9	0	0.0	2	2.2	8	8.8	5	5.5	52	57.1	17	18.7
Louisiana	146	70	47.9	3	2.1	8	5.5	39	26.7	12	8.2	66	45.2	35	24.0
Oklahoma	112	44	39.3	0	0.0	2	1.8	23	20.5	3	2.7	68	60.7	15	13.4
Texas	513	289	56.3	8	1.6	19	3.7	107	20.9	29	5.7	251	48.9	95	18.5
CENSUS DIVISION 8, MOUNTAIN	422	241	57.1	4	0.9	16	3.8	100	23.7	21	5.0	283	67.1	77	18.2
Arizona	80	51	63.8	0	0.0	4	5.0	22	27.5	4	5.0	50	62.5	18	22.5
Colorado	82	54	65.9	1	1.2	5	6.1	22	26.8	6	7.3	59	72.0	22	26.8
Idaho	45	22	48.9	0	0.0	0	0.0	6	13.3	1	2.2	34	75.6	4	8.9
Montana	58	35	60.3	0	0.0	1	1.7	7	12.1	0	0.0	38	65.5	6	10.3
Nevada	23	14	60.9	1	4.3	1	4.3	7	30.4	0	0.0	14	60.9	7	30.4
New Mexico	55	23	41.8	1	1.8	2	3.6	16	29.1	4	7.3	29	52.7	6	10.9
Utah	49	25	51.0	1	2.0	3	6.1	13	26.5	6	12.2	37	75.5	12	24.5
Wyoming	30	17	56.7	0	0.0	0	0.0	7	23.3	0	0.0	22	73.3	2	6.7
CENSUS DIVISION 9, PACIFIC	642	461	71.8	33	5.1	72	11.2	165	25.7	42	6.5	393	61.2	167	26.0
Alaska	21	11	52.4	0	0.0	1	4.8	8	38.1	1	4.8	18	85.7	2	9.5
California	436	314	72.0	28	6.4	53	12.2	111	25.5	30	6.9	239	54.8	124	28.4
Hawaii	20	15	75.0	1	5.0	4	20.0	4	20.0	0	0.0	14	70.0	4	20.0
Oregon	68	47	69.1	0	0.0	3	4.4	16	23.5	3	4.4	54	79.4	14	20.6
Washington	97	74	76.3	4	4.1	11	11.3	26	26.8	8	8.2	68	70.1	23	23.7

Table 12B (Continued)

CLASSIFICATION	HOSPITALS REPORTING	CARDIAC SERVICES, continued: CARDIAC CATHETERIZATION LABORATORY		CARDIAC REHABILITATION PROGRAM		NON-INVASIVE CARDIAC ASSESSMENT SERVICES		OPEN HEART SURGERY		CHRONIC OBSTRUCTIVE PULMONARY DISEASE SERVICES		EMERGENCY SERVICES: EMERGENCY DEPARTMENT		TRAUMA CENTER (CERTIFIED)	
		Number	Percent	Number	Percent	Number	Percent	Number	Percent	Number	Percent	Number	Percent	Number	Percent
UNITED STATES	6,105	1,470	24.1	2,148	35.2	2,949	48.3	898	14.7	3,647	59.7	5,024	82.3	664	10.9
CENSUS DIVISION 1, NEW ENGLAND	315	59	18.7	150	47.6	166	52.7	28	8.9	198	62.9	226	71.7	45	14.3
Connecticut	60	19	31.7	25	41.7	24	40.0	7	11.7	31	51.7	38	63.3	8	13.3
Maine	42	5	11.9	23	54.8	27	64.3	2	4.8	26	61.9	40	95.2	6	14.3
Massachusetts	140	21	15.0	67	47.9	78	55.7	14	10.0	96	68.6	93	66.4	21	15.0
New Hampshire	36	9	25.0	18	50.0	19	52.8	2	5.6	24	66.7	26	72.2	8	22.2
Rhode Island	19	4	21.1	7	36.8	9	47.4	2	10.5	11	57.9	13	68.4	1	5.3
Vermont	18	1	5.6	10	55.6	9	50.0	1	5.6	10	55.6	16	88.9	1	5.6
CENSUS DIVISION 2, MIDDLE ATLANTIC	681	135	19.8	261	38.3	365	53.6	81	11.9	450	66.1	524	76.9	60	8.8
New Jersey	114	26	22.8	42	36.8	67	58.8	14	12.3	81	71.1	87	76.3	6	5.3
New York	288	59	20.5	88	30.6	141	49.0	29	10.1	178	61.8	226	78.5	33	11.5
Pennsylvania	279	50	17.9	131	47.0	157	56.3	38	13.6	191	68.5	211	75.6	21	7.5
CENSUS DIVISION 3, SOUTH ATLANTIC	963	288	29.9	303	31.5	462	48.0	132	13.7	584	60.6	758	78.7	103	10.7
Delaware	13	2	15.4	7	53.8	8	61.5	1	7.7	9	69.2	10	76.9	1	7.7
District of Columbia	16	9	56.3	6	37.5	11	68.8	7	43.8	10	62.5	11	68.8	5	31.3
Florida	260	100	38.5	87	33.5	140	53.8	55	21.2	160	61.5	201	77.3	23	8.8
Georgia	188	40	21.3	34	18.1	65	34.6	17	9.0	112	59.6	151	80.3	22	11.7
Maryland	78	31	39.7	29	37.2	38	48.7	7	9.0	50	64.1	52	66.7	12	15.4
North Carolina	135	37	27.4	46	34.1	64	47.4	18	13.3	78	57.8	116	85.9	16	11.9
South Carolina	84	19	22.6	28	33.3	37	44.0	8	9.5	46	54.8	68	81.0	2	2.4
Virginia	124	37	29.8	47	37.9	67	54.0	15	12.1	79	63.7	95	76.6	15	12.1
West Virginia	65	13	20.0	19	29.2	32	49.2	4	6.2	40	61.5	54	83.1	7	10.8
CENSUS DIVISION 4, EAST NORTH CENTRAL	918	279	30.4	464	50.5	563	61.3	151	16.4	612	66.7	787	85.7	138	15.0
Illinois	231	82	35.5	110	47.6	139	60.2	44	19.0	144	62.3	201	87.0	76	32.9
Indiana	131	41	31.3	72	55.0	85	64.9	24	18.3	91	69.5	112	85.5	10	7.6
Michigan	201	51	25.4	84	41.8	112	55.7	27	13.4	124	61.7	166	82.6	23	11.4
Ohio	214	75	35.0	110	51.4	140	65.4	38	17.8	152	71.0	184	86.0	29	13.6
Wisconsin	141	30	21.3	88	62.4	87	61.7	18	12.8	101	71.6	124	87.9	0	0.0
CENSUS DIVISION 5, EAST SOUTH CENTRAL	492	108	22.0	101	20.5	163	33.1	65	13.2	274	55.7	418	85.0	30	6.1
Alabama	119	28	23.5	24	20.2	43	36.1	18	15.1	58	48.7	103	86.6	11	9.2
Kentucky	117	31	26.5	36	30.8	49	41.9	13	11.1	62	53.0	99	84.6	6	5.1
Mississippi	110	12	10.9	1	0.9	3	2.7	9	8.2	62	56.4	93	84.5	0	0.0
Tennessee	146	37	25.3	40	27.4	68	46.6	25	17.1	92	63.0	123	84.2	13	8.9
CENSUS DIVISION 6, WEST NORTH CENTRAL	810	119	14.7	317	39.1	326	40.2	87	10.7	426	52.6	722	89.1	89	11.0
Iowa	134	21	15.7	72	53.7	60	44.8	12	9.0	70	52.2	125	93.3	11	8.2
Kansas	147	14	9.5	37	25.2	42	28.6	11	7.5	65	44.2	131	89.1	5	3.4
Minnesota	158	15	9.5	63	39.9	55	34.8	16	10.1	69	43.7	137	86.7	14	8.9
Missouri	159	45	28.3	77	48.4	97	61.0	31	19.5	125	78.6	138	86.8	48	30.2
Nebraska	91	14	15.4	37	40.7	39	42.9	8	8.8	40	44.0	82	90.1	6	6.6
North Dakota	55	7	12.7	13	23.6	12	21.8	6	10.9	26	47.3	50	90.9	3	5.5
South Dakota	66	3	4.5	18	27.3	21	31.8	3	4.5	31	47.0	59	89.4	2	3.0
CENSUS DIVISION 7, WEST SOUTH CENTRAL	862	194	22.5	207	24.0	378	43.9	147	17.1	443	51.4	694	80.5	50	5.8
Arkansas	91	25	27.5	22	24.2	39	42.9	13	14.3	53	58.2	82	90.1	2	2.2
Louisiana	146	40	27.4	38	26.0	68	46.6	31	21.2	69	47.3	109	74.7	5	3.4
Oklahoma	112	19	17.0	19	17.0	41	36.6	14	12.5	54	48.2	100	89.3	11	9.8
Texas	513	110	21.4	128	25.0	230	44.8	89	17.3	267	52.0	403	78.6	32	6.2
CENSUS DIVISION 8, MOUNTAIN	422	80	19.0	128	30.3	192	45.5	66	15.6	240	56.9	354	83.9	52	12.3
Arizona	80	19	23.8	27	33.8	41	51.3	21	26.3	53	66.3	66	82.5	17	21.3
Colorado	82	21	25.6	35	42.7	38	46.3	19	23.2	51	62.2	71	86.6	9	11.0
Idaho	45	4	8.9	11	24.4	18	40.0	2	4.4	27	60.0	39	86.7	7	15.6
Montana	58	8	13.8	15	25.9	33	56.9	4	6.9	30	51.7	54	93.1	2	3.4
Nevada	23	7	30.4	7	30.4	11	47.8	6	26.1	16	69.6	18	78.3	4	17.4
New Mexico	55	6	10.9	11	20.0	16	29.1	4	7.3	23	41.8	40	72.7	5	9.1
Utah	49	12	24.5	16	32.7	20	40.8	8	16.3	22	44.9	40	81.6	8	16.3
Wyoming	30	3	10.0	6	20.0	15	50.0	2	6.7	18	60.0	26	86.7	0	0.0
CENSUS DIVISION 9, PACIFIC	642	208	32.4	217	33.8	334	52.0	141	22.0	420	65.4	541	84.3	97	15.1
Alaska	21	2	9.5	3	14.3	7	33.3	1	4.8	7	33.3	19	90.5	0	0.0
California	436	152	34.9	158	36.2	232	53.2	113	25.9	301	69.0	354	81.2	50	11.5
Hawaii	20	5	25.0	7	35.0	10	50.0	4	20.0	11	55.0	16	80.0	3	15.0
Oregon	68	20	29.4	16	23.5	37	54.4	10	14.7	43	63.2	65	95.6	35	51.5
Washington	97	29	29.9	33	34.0	48	49.5	13	13.4	58	59.8	87	89.7	9	9.3

(continued on next page)

Table

12B (Continued) Facilities and Services in U.S. Census Divisions and States

For definitions of facilities and services, see Definitions of Terms, page xxiii. These data include only hospital-based facilities and services as reported by responding hospitals in Section C of the 1990 AHA Annual Survey, beginning on page 242. No estimates have been made for nonresponding hospitals.

CLASSIFICATION	HOSPITALS REPORTING	EXTRACORPOREAL SHOCK WAVE LITHOTRIPTER (ESWL)		FITNESS CENTER		GENETIC COUNSELING/ SCREENING		GERIATRIC SERVICES: ADULT DAY CARE PROGRAM		GERIATRIC SERVICES: ALZHEIMER'S DIAGNOSTIC/ ASSESSMENT SERVICES		GERIATRIC SERVICES: COMPREHENSIVE GERIATRIC ASSESSMENT		GERIATRIC SERVICES: EMERGENCY RESPONSE (GERIATRIC)	
		Number	Percent	Number	Percent	Number	Percent	Number	Percent	Number	Percent	Number	Percent	Number	Percent
UNITED STATES	6,105	327	5.4	850	13.9	553	9.1	427	7.0	570	9.3	1,202	19.7	1,853	30.4
CENSUS DIVISION 1, NEW ENGLAND	315	23	7.3	31	9.8	47	14.9	28	8.9	50	15.9	92	29.2	116	36.8
Connecticut	60	4	6.7	9	15.0	10	16.7	4	6.7	16	26.7	24	40.0	17	28.3
Maine	42	0	0.0	5	11.9	4	9.5	4	9.5	3	7.1	7	16.7	19	45.2
Massachusetts	140	13	9.3	8	5.7	26	18.6	14	10.0	24	17.1	45	32.1	56	40.0
New Hampshire	36	6	16.7	5	13.9	2	5.6	4	11.1	4	11.1	8	22.2	12	33.3
Rhode Island	19	0	0.0	2	10.5	4	21.1	2	10.5	3	15.8	5	26.3	5	26.3
Vermont	18	0	0.0	2	11.1	1	5.6	0	0.0	0	0.0	3	16.7	7	38.9
CENSUS DIVISION 2, MIDDLE ATLANTIC	681	31	4.6	66	9.7	114	16.7	71	10.4	100	14.7	218	32.0	188	27.6
New Jersey	114	0	0.0	10	8.8	27	23.7	19	16.7	22	19.3	43	37.7	47	41.2
New York	288	16	5.6	20	6.9	55	19.1	36	12.5	41	14.2	104	36.1	66	22.9
Pennsylvania	279	15	5.4	36	12.9	32	11.5	16	5.7	37	13.3	71	25.4	75	26.9
CENSUS DIVISION 3, SOUTH ATLANTIC	963	71	7.4	135	14.0	75	7.8	34	3.5	71	7.4	145	15.1	255	26.5
Delaware	13	0	0.0	3	23.1	2	15.4	1	7.7	0	0.0	2	15.4	1	7.7
District of Columbia	16	2	12.5	1	6.3	6	37.5	1	6.3	2	12.5	4	25.0	3	18.8
Florida	260	19	7.3	52	20.0	14	5.4	10	3.8	25	9.6	42	16.2	58	22.3
Georgia	188	15	8.0	23	12.2	10	5.3	2	1.1	5	2.7	13	6.9	43	22.9
Maryland	78	2	2.6	10	12.8	12	15.4	8	10.3	12	15.4	18	23.1	21	26.9
North Carolina	135	13	9.6	16	11.9	13	9.6	4	3.0	11	8.1	28	20.7	48	35.6
South Carolina	84	7	8.3	11	13.1	4	4.8	4	4.8	1	1.2	10	11.9	36	42.9
Virginia	124	9	7.3	11	8.9	12	9.7	3	2.4	10	8.1	19	15.3	32	25.8
West Virginia	65	4	6.2	8	12.3	2	3.1	1	1.5	5	7.7	9	13.8	13	20.0
CENSUS DIVISION 4, EAST NORTH CENTRAL	918	44	4.8	164	17.9	99	10.8	79	8.6	128	13.9	217	23.6	377	41.1
Illinois	231	10	4.3	36	15.6	29	12.6	32	13.9	37	16.0	56	24.2	100	43.3
Indiana	131	8	6.1	28	21.4	8	6.1	7	5.3	12	9.2	29	22.1	68	51.9
Michigan	201	8	4.0	40	19.9	18	9.0	9	4.5	22	10.9	48	23.9	48	23.9
Ohio	214	4	1.9	39	18.2	28	13.1	16	7.5	26	12.1	47	22.0	80	37.4
Wisconsin	141	14	9.9	21	14.9	16	11.3	15	10.6	31	22.0	37	26.2	81	57.4
CENSUS DIVISION 5, EAST SOUTH CENTRAL	492	20	4.1	57	11.6	17	3.5	8	1.6	23	4.7	48	9.8	88	17.9
Alabama	119	1	0.8	9	7.6	3	2.5	1	0.8	4	3.4	9	7.6	27	22.7
Kentucky	117	2	1.7	13	11.1	3	2.6	3	2.6	7	6.0	16	13.7	22	18.8
Mississippi	110	5	4.5	15	13.6	6	5.5	0	0.0	3	2.7	7	6.4	1	0.9
Tennessee	146	12	8.2	20	13.7	5	3.4	4	2.7	9	6.2	16	11.0	38	26.0
CENSUS DIVISION 6, WEST NORTH CENTRAL	810	30	3.7	135	16.7	44	5.4	89	11.0	65	8.0	172	21.2	347	42.8
Iowa	134	5	3.7	34	25.4	3	2.2	20	14.9	10	7.5	27	20.1	90	67.2
Kansas	147	5	3.4	24	16.3	5	3.4	15	10.2	8	5.4	19	12.9	60	40.8
Minnesota	158	4	2.5	22	13.9	10	6.3	33	20.9	15	9.5	34	21.5	67	42.4
Missouri	159	9	5.7	29	18.2	21	13.2	2	1.3	24	15.1	56	35.2	53	33.3
Nebraska	91	5	5.5	13	14.3	4	4.4	8	8.8	5	5.5	11	12.1	33	36.3
North Dakota	55	1	1.8	5	9.1	0	0.0	7	12.7	3	5.5	12	21.8	23	41.8
South Dakota	66	1	1.5	8	12.1	1	1.5	4	6.1	0	0.0	13	19.7	21	31.8
CENSUS DIVISION 7, WEST SOUTH CENTRAL	862	43	5.0	114	13.2	48	5.6	33	3.8	39	4.5	100	11.6	166	19.3
Arkansas	91	5	5.5	7	7.7	3	3.3	2	2.2	3	3.3	15	16.5	25	27.5
Louisiana	146	5	3.4	23	15.8	8	5.5	10	6.8	9	6.2	14	9.6	25	17.1
Oklahoma	112	5	4.5	14	12.5	4	3.6	3	2.7	5	4.5	15	13.4	29	25.9
Texas	513	28	5.5	70	13.6	33	6.4	18	3.5	22	4.3	56	10.9	87	17.0
CENSUS DIVISION 8, MOUNTAIN	422	15	3.6	69	16.4	36	8.5	32	7.6	38	9.0	92	21.8	130	30.8
Arizona	80	6	7.5	8	10.0	7	8.8	10	12.5	6	7.5	17	21.3	10	12.5
Colorado	82	3	3.7	21	25.6	13	15.9	6	7.3	11	13.4	25	30.5	29	35.4
Idaho	45	1	2.2	7	15.6	0	0.0	7	15.6	2	4.4	9	20.0	11	24.4
Montana	58	0	0.0	12	20.7	2	3.4	6	10.3	6	10.3	15	25.9	18	31.0
Nevada	23	2	8.7	3	13.0	3	13.0	1	4.3	2	8.7	5	21.7	8	34.8
New Mexico	55	2	3.6	7	12.7	7	12.7	1	1.8	2	3.6	8	14.5	16	29.1
Utah	49	1	2.0	9	18.4	4	8.2	0	0.0	7	14.3	7	14.3	23	46.9
Wyoming	30	0	0.0	2	6.7	0	0.0	1	3.3	2	6.7	6	20.0	15	50.0
CENSUS DIVISION 9, PACIFIC	642	50	7.8	79	12.3	73	11.4	53	8.3	56	8.7	118	18.4	186	29.0
Alaska	21	0	0.0	2	9.5	4	19.0	1	4.8	2	9.5	2	9.5	8	38.1
California	436	33	7.6	48	11.0	48	11.0	37	8.5	36	8.3	75	17.2	110	25.2
Hawaii	20	1	5.0	1	5.0	2	10.0	3	15.0	1	5.0	6	30.0	4	20.0
Oregon	68	7	10.3	10	14.7	2	2.9	5	7.4	6	8.8	17	25.0	22	32.4
Washington	97	9	9.3	18	18.6	17	17.5	7	7.2	11	11.3	18	18.6	42	43.3

Table 12B (Continued)

CLASSIFICATION	HOSPITALS REPORTING	GERIATRIC SERVICES, continued								HEALTH PROMOTION SERVICES					
		GERIATRIC ACUTE CARE UNIT		GERIATRIC CLINICS		RESPITE CARE		SENIOR MEMBERSHIP PROGRAM		PATIENT EDUCATION		COMMUNITY HEALTH PROMOTION		WORKSITE HEALTH PROMOTION	
		Number	Percent	Number	Percent	Number	Percent	Number	Percent	Number	Percent	Number	Percent	Number	Percent
UNITED STATES	6,105	666	10.9	461	7.6	1,005	16.5	1,159	19.0	5,125	83.9	4,366	71.5	3,233	53.0
CENSUS DIVISION 1, NEW ENGLAND	315	47	14.9	43	13.7	45	14.3	35	11.1	275	87.3	237	75.2	204	64.8
Connecticut	60	9	15.0	11	18.3	7	11.7	7	11.7	51	85.0	41	68.3	43	71.7
Maine	42	3	7.1	2	4.8	2	4.8	10	23.8	38	90.5	36	85.7	21	50.0
Massachusetts	140	27	19.3	22	15.7	20	14.3	12	8.6	123	87.9	104	74.3	91	65.0
New Hampshire	36	3	8.3	3	8.3	7	19.4	4	11.1	34	94.4	28	77.8	25	69.4
Rhode Island	19	3	15.8	4	21.1	6	31.6	2	10.5	14	73.7	13	68.4	10	52.6
Vermont	18	2	11.1	1	5.6	3	16.7	0	0.0	15	83.3	15	83.3	14	77.8
CENSUS DIVISION 2, MIDDLE ATLANTIC	681	82	12.0	103	15.1	83	12.2	128	18.8	618	90.7	538	79.0	408	59.9
New Jersey	114	15	13.2	22	19.3	20	17.5	25	21.9	107	93.9	97	85.1	75	65.8
New York	288	50	17.4	52	18.1	24	8.3	40	13.9	254	88.2	219	76.0	151	52.4
Pennsylvania	279	17	6.1	29	10.4	39	14.0	63	22.6	257	92.1	222	79.6	182	65.2
CENSUS DIVISION 3, SOUTH ATLANTIC	963	80	8.3	49	5.1	140	14.5	144	15.0	816	84.7	668	69.4	496	51.5
Delaware	13	2	15.4	1	7.7	3	23.1	0	0.0	10	76.9	9	69.2	7	53.8
District of Columbia	16	3	18.8	1	6.3	2	12.5	2	12.5	13	81.3	13	81.3	10	62.5
Florida	260	19	7.3	13	5.0	20	7.7	55	21.2	223	85.8	190	73.1	129	49.6
Georgia	188	9	4.8	2	1.1	19	10.1	21	11.2	150	79.8	123	65.4	86	45.7
Maryland	78	9	11.5	12	15.4	8	10.3	13	16.7	70	89.7	50	64.1	38	48.7
North Carolina	135	17	12.6	9	6.7	39	28.9	9	6.7	115	85.2	90	66.7	75	55.6
South Carolina	84	6	7.1	1	1.2	23	27.4	13	15.5	74	88.1	68	81.0	55	65.5
Virginia	124	10	8.1	6	4.8	10	8.1	23	18.5	111	89.5	88	71.0	71	57.3
West Virginia	65	5	7.7	4	6.2	16	24.6	8	12.3	50	76.9	37	56.9	25	38.5
CENSUS DIVISION 4, EAST NORTH CENTRAL	918	138	15.0	95	10.3	195	21.2	269	29.3	832	90.6	724	78.9	580	63.2
Illinois	231	28	12.1	26	11.3	49	21.2	85	36.8	210	90.9	184	79.7	137	59.3
Indiana	131	17	13.0	6	4.6	24	18.3	36	27.5	116	88.5	103	78.6	87	66.4
Michigan	201	19	9.5	26	12.9	36	17.9	39	19.4	183	91.0	153	76.1	126	62.7
Ohio	214	22	10.3	19	8.9	27	12.6	70	32.7	196	91.6	170	79.4	140	65.4
Wisconsin	141	52	36.9	18	12.8	59	41.8	39	27.7	127	90.1	114	80.9	90	63.8
CENSUS DIVISION 5, EAST SOUTH CENTRAL	492	34	6.9	13	2.6	57	11.6	68	13.8	373	75.8	306	62.2	223	45.3
Alabama	119	5	4.2	3	2.5	12	10.1	25	21.0	82	68.9	67	56.3	39	32.8
Kentucky	117	6	5.1	5	4.3	10	8.5	18	15.4	95	81.2	74	63.2	53	45.3
Mississippi	110	9	8.2	0	0.0	27	24.5	1	0.9	77	70.0	62	56.4	42	38.2
Tennessee	146	14	9.6	5	3.4	8	5.5	24	16.4	119	81.5	103	70.5	89	61.0
CENSUS DIVISION 6, WEST NORTH CENTRAL	810	112	13.8	50	6.2	257	31.7	108	13.3	681	84.1	581	71.7	422	52.1
Iowa	134	14	10.4	9	6.7	60	44.8	31	23.1	124	92.5	108	80.6	92	68.7
Kansas	147	14	9.5	8	5.4	49	33.3	14	9.5	105	71.4	92	62.6	53	36.1
Minnesota	158	21	13.3	7	4.4	79	50.0	17	10.8	138	87.3	117	74.1	86	54.4
Missouri	159	36	22.6	17	10.7	18	11.3	29	18.2	143	89.9	129	81.1	110	69.2
Nebraska	91	7	7.7	3	3.3	17	18.7	9	9.9	75	82.4	57	62.6	31	34.1
North Dakota	55	10	18.2	2	3.6	21	38.2	4	7.3	45	81.8	36	65.5	18	32.7
South Dakota	66	10	15.2	4	6.1	13	19.7	4	6.1	51	77.3	42	63.6	32	48.5
CENSUS DIVISION 7, WEST SOUTH CENTRAL	862	65	7.5	26	3.0	98	11.4	157	18.2	663	76.9	550	63.8	368	42.7
Arkansas	91	9	9.9	8	8.8	8	8.8	10	11.0	77	84.6	70	76.9	40	44.0
Louisiana	146	9	6.2	0	0.0	13	8.9	37	25.3	117	80.1	93	63.7	65	44.5
Oklahoma	112	9	8.0	7	6.3	20	17.9	13	11.6	90	80.4	74	66.1	47	42.0
Texas	513	38	7.4	11	2.1	57	11.1	97	18.9	379	73.9	313	61.0	216	42.1
CENSUS DIVISION 8, MOUNTAIN	422	42	10.0	36	8.5	64	15.2	86	20.4	343	81.3	304	72.0	218	51.7
Arizona	80	7	8.8	8	10.0	13	16.3	17	21.3	68	85.0	63	78.8	46	57.5
Colorado	82	7	8.5	14	17.1	15	18.3	15	18.3	72	87.8	61	74.4	47	57.3
Idaho	45	5	11.1	2	4.4	10	22.2	6	13.3	35	77.8	32	71.1	26	57.8
Montana	58	10	17.2	2	3.4	9	15.5	12	20.7	42	72.4	38	65.5	26	44.8
Nevada	23	2	8.7	2	8.7	3	13.0	7	30.4	17	73.9	14	60.9	10	43.5
New Mexico	55	3	5.5	5	9.1	4	7.3	6	10.9	43	78.2	37	67.3	28	50.9
Utah	49	4	8.2	3	6.1	3	6.1	18	36.7	40	81.6	38	77.6	23	46.9
Wyoming	30	4	13.3	0	0.0	7	23.3	5	16.7	26	86.7	21	70.0	12	40.0
CENSUS DIVISION 9, PACIFIC	642	66	10.3	46	7.2	66	10.3	164	25.5	524	81.6	458	71.3	314	48.9
Alaska	21	0	0.0	0	0.0	3	14.3	3	14.3	17	81.0	16	76.2	9	42.9
California	436	43	9.9	27	6.2	30	6.9	114	26.1	356	81.7	307	70.4	205	47.0
Hawaii	20	3	15.0	2	10.0	2	10.0	2	10.0	14	70.0	11	55.0	12	60.0
Oregon	68	6	8.8	7	10.3	14	20.6	16	23.5	53	77.9	49	72.1	36	52.9
Washington	97	14	14.4	10	10.3	17	17.5	29	29.9	84	86.6	75	77.3	52	53.6

(continued on next page)

Table

12B (Continued)

Facilities and Services in U.S. Census Divisions and States

For definitions of facilities and services, see Definitions of Terms, page xxiii. These data include only hospital-based facilities and services as reported by responding hospitals in Section C of the 1990 AHA Annual Survey, beginning on page 242. No estimates have been made for nonresponding hospitals.

CLASSIFICATION	HOSPITALS REPORTING	HEALTH SCIENCES LIBRARY		HEMODIALYSIS		HOME HEALTH SERVICES		HOSPICE		LABORATORY SERVICES: HISTOPATHOLOGY		LABORATORY SERVICES: BLOOD BANK		OCCUPATIONAL HEALTH SERVICES	
		Number	Percent	Number	Percent	Number	Percent	Number	Percent	Number	Percent	Number	Percent	Number	Percent
UNITED STATES	6,105	2,544	41.7	1,451	23.8	1,921	31.5	868	14.2	3,571	58.5	3,757	61.5	2,377	38.9
CENSUS DIVISION 1, NEW ENGLAND	315	215	68.3	82	26.0	50	15.9	40	12.7	208	66.0	217	68.9	175	55.6
Connecticut	60	41	68.3	20	33.3	13	21.7	9	15.0	36	60.0	36	60.0	31	51.7
Maine	42	27	64.3	7	16.7	5	11.9	4	9.5	24	57.1	32	76.2	19	45.2
Massachusetts	140	98	70.0	38	27.1	21	15.0	19	13.6	101	72.1	97	69.3	82	58.6
New Hampshire	36	23	63.9	8	22.2	5	13.9	5	13.9	21	58.3	23	63.9	24	66.7
Rhode Island	19	17	89.5	8	42.1	4	21.1	0	0.0	16	84.2	14	73.7	10	52.6
Vermont	18	9	50.0	1	5.6	2	11.1	3	16.7	10	55.6	15	83.3	9	50.0
CENSUS DIVISION 2, MIDDLE ATLANTIC	681	426	62.6	236	34.7	194	28.5	118	17.3	526	77.2	499	73.3	325	47.7
New Jersey	114	84	73.7	36	31.6	31	27.2	30	26.3	95	83.3	90	78.9	57	50.0
New York	288	172	59.7	117	40.6	71	24.7	34	11.8	219	76.0	214	74.3	121	42.0
Pennsylvania	279	170	60.9	83	29.7	92	33.0	54	19.4	212	76.0	195	69.9	147	52.7
CENSUS DIVISION 3, SOUTH ATLANTIC	963	341	35.4	267	27.7	227	23.6	115	11.9	607	63.0	648	67.3	364	37.8
Delaware	13	8	61.5	5	38.5	5	38.5	1	7.7	10	76.9	9	69.2	6	46.2
District of Columbia	16	12	75.0	8	50.0	4	25.0	2	12.5	13	81.3	11	68.8	12	75.0
Florida	260	92	35.4	91	35.0	54	20.8	18	6.9	176	67.7	145	55.8	108	41.5
Georgia	188	43	22.9	42	22.3	19	10.1	20	10.6	100	53.2	135	71.8	56	29.8
Maryland	78	45	57.7	31	39.7	22	28.2	18	23.1	49	62.8	48	61.5	33	42.3
North Carolina	135	59	43.7	27	20.0	27	20.0	18	13.3	85	63.0	99	73.3	53	39.3
South Carolina	84	2	2.4	15	17.9	14	16.7	9	10.7	47	56.0	65	77.4	22	26.2
Virginia	124	58	46.8	35	28.2	60	48.4	21	16.9	86	69.4	87	70.2	54	43.5
West Virginia	65	22	33.8	13	20.0	22	33.8	8	12.3	41	63.1	49	75.4	20	30.8
CENSUS DIVISION 4, EAST NORTH CENTRAL	918	495	53.9	232	25.3	306	33.3	146	15.9	625	68.1	530	57.7	461	50.2
Illinois	231	124	53.7	63	27.3	97	42.0	55	23.8	169	73.2	155	67.1	117	50.6
Indiana	131	55	42.0	28	21.4	60	45.8	24	18.3	90	68.7	75	57.3	57	43.5
Michigan	201	97	48.3	42	20.9	39	19.4	20	10.0	130	64.7	143	71.1	93	46.3
Ohio	214	121	56.5	69	32.2	73	34.1	31	14.5	158	73.8	157	73.4	113	52.8
Wisconsin	141	98	69.5	30	21.3	37	26.2	16	11.3	78	55.3	0	0.0	81	57.4
CENSUS DIVISION 5, EAST SOUTH CENTRAL	492	194	39.4	92	18.7	123	25.0	43	8.7	238	48.4	346	70.3	109	22.2
Alabama	119	26	21.8	19	16.0	9	7.6	9	7.6	57	47.9	84	70.6	23	19.3
Kentucky	117	35	29.9	20	17.1	39	33.3	9	7.7	68	58.1	87	74.4	27	23.1
Mississippi	110	85	77.3	17	15.5	23	20.9	4	3.6	36	32.7	72	65.5	15	13.6
Tennessee	146	48	32.9	36	24.7	52	35.6	21	14.4	77	52.7	103	70.5	44	30.1
CENSUS DIVISION 6, WEST NORTH CENTRAL	810	226	27.9	130	16.0	336	41.5	167	20.6	327	40.4	460	56.8	284	35.1
Iowa	134	36	26.9	18	13.4	52	38.8	27	20.1	63	47.0	67	50.0	44	32.8
Kansas	147	32	21.8	10	6.8	54	36.7	15	10.2	51	34.7	72	49.0	40	27.2
Minnesota	158	41	25.9	25	15.8	59	37.3	51	32.3	62	39.2	100	63.3	56	35.4
Missouri	159	67	42.1	48	30.2	92	57.9	41	25.8	96	60.4	118	74.2	91	57.2
Nebraska	91	21	23.1	11	12.1	36	39.6	16	17.6	25	27.5	39	42.9	20	22.0
North Dakota	55	14	25.5	9	16.4	21	38.2	8	14.5	13	23.6	25	45.5	18	32.7
South Dakota	66	15	22.7	9	13.6	22	33.3	9	13.6	17	25.8	39	59.1	15	22.7
CENSUS DIVISION 7, WEST SOUTH CENTRAL	862	188	21.8	159	18.4	291	33.8	62	7.2	415	48.1	409	47.4	208	24.1
Arkansas	91	20	22.0	18	19.8	48	52.7	9	9.9	42	46.2	49	53.8	15	16.5
Louisiana	146	36	24.7	25	17.1	59	40.4	19	13.0	85	58.2	80	54.8	38	26.0
Oklahoma	112	32	28.6	16	14.3	42	37.5	6	5.4	41	36.6	55	49.1	27	24.1
Texas	513	100	19.5	100	19.5	142	27.7	28	5.5	247	48.1	225	43.9	128	25.0
CENSUS DIVISION 8, MOUNTAIN	422	157	37.2	82	19.4	156	37.0	60	14.2	210	49.8	263	62.3	148	35.1
Arizona	80	39	48.8	25	31.3	24	30.0	11	13.8	48	60.0	56	70.0	35	43.8
Colorado	82	36	43.9	19	23.2	37	45.1	16	19.5	49	59.8	48	58.5	43	52.4
Idaho	45	16	35.6	6	13.3	15	33.3	8	17.8	19	42.2	29	64.4	13	28.9
Montana	58	13	22.4	6	10.3	31	53.4	8	13.8	25	43.1	39	67.2	10	17.2
Nevada	23	9	39.1	3	13.0	3	13.0	3	13.0	15	65.2	19	82.6	6	26.1
New Mexico	55	13	23.6	10	18.2	16	29.1	8	14.5	21	38.2	28	50.9	20	36.4
Utah	49	17	34.7	10	20.4	21	42.9	5	10.2	22	44.9	27	55.1	16	32.7
Wyoming	30	14	46.7	3	10.0	9	30.0	1	3.3	11	36.7	17	56.7	5	16.7
CENSUS DIVISION 9, PACIFIC	642	302	47.0	171	26.6	238	37.1	117	18.2	415	64.6	385	60.0	303	47.2
Alaska	21	3	14.3	2	9.5	7	33.3	0	0.0	8	38.1	14	66.7	9	42.9
California	436	218	50.0	133	30.5	153	35.1	74	17.0	300	68.8	266	61.0	203	46.6
Hawaii	20	8	40.0	4	20.0	6	30.0	2	10.0	13	65.0	13	65.0	14	70.0
Oregon	68	31	45.6	14	20.6	44	64.7	24	35.3	41	60.3	51	75.0	31	45.6
Washington	97	42	43.3	18	18.6	28	28.9	17	17.5	53	54.6	41	42.3	46	47.4

Table 12B (Continued)

CLASSIFICATION	HOSPITALS REPORTING	ORGANIZED OUTPATIENT SERVICES		PSYCHIATRIC SERVICES: CHILD/ADOLESCENT		CONSULTATION-LIAISON		EDUCATION		EMERGENCY		GERIATRIC		OUTPATIENT	
		Number	Percent	Number	Percent	Number	Percent	Number	Percent	Number	Percent	Number	Percent	Number	Percent
UNITED STATES	6,105	4,866	79.7	1,424	23.3	2,223	36.4	1,733	28.4	2,311	37.9	1,652	27.1	1,600	26.2
CENSUS DIVISION 1, NEW ENGLAND	315	245	77.8	101	32.1	191	60.6	139	44.1	155	49.2	121	38.4	129	41.0
Connecticut	60	44	73.3	28	46.7	44	73.3	40	66.7	40	66.7	30	50.0	42	70.0
Maine	42	39	92.9	10	23.8	18	42.9	10	23.8	13	31.0	11	26.2	9	21.4
Massachusetts	140	109	77.9	40	28.6	88	62.9	63	45.0	70	50.0	56	40.0	59	42.1
New Hampshire	36	25	69.4	12	33.3	19	52.8	12	33.3	16	44.4	12	33.3	7	19.4
Rhode Island	19	14	73.7	6	31.6	13	68.4	10	52.6	9	47.4	6	31.6	8	42.1
Vermont	18	14	77.8	5	27.8	9	50.0	4	22.2	7	38.9	6	33.3	4	22.2
CENSUS DIVISION 2, MIDDLE ATLANTIC	681	549	80.6	198	29.1	359	52.7	255	37.4	333	48.9	269	39.5	245	36.0
New Jersey	114	96	84.2	39	34.2	73	64.0	49	43.0	64	56.1	49	43.0	51	44.7
New York	288	231	80.2	87	30.2	160	55.6	113	39.2	152	52.8	116	40.3	116	40.3
Pennsylvania	279	222	79.6	72	25.8	126	45.2	93	33.3	117	41.9	104	37.3	78	28.0
CENSUS DIVISION 3, SOUTH ATLANTIC	963	750	77.9	240	24.9	347	36.0	266	27.6	374	38.8	277	28.8	216	22.4
Delaware	13	9	69.2	6	46.2	7	53.8	6	46.2	7	53.8	3	23.1	5	38.5
District of Columbia	16	13	81.3	7	43.8	11	68.8	10	62.5	11	68.8	9	56.3	9	56.3
Florida	260	214	82.3	55	21.2	94	36.2	69	26.5	95	36.5	70	26.9	54	20.8
Georgia	188	143	76.1	42	22.3	57	30.3	41	21.8	60	31.9	43	22.9	40	21.3
Maryland	78	56	71.8	34	43.6	47	60.3	40	51.3	50	64.1	41	52.6	27	34.6
North Carolina	135	109	80.7	36	26.7	42	31.1	27	20.0	57	42.2	41	30.4	25	18.5
South Carolina	84	52	61.9	15	17.9	23	27.4	20	23.8	27	32.1	23	27.4	16	19.0
Virginia	124	99	79.8	35	28.2	45	36.3	38	30.6	48	38.7	32	25.8	29	23.4
West Virginia	65	55	84.6	10	15.4	21	32.3	15	23.1	19	29.2	15	23.1	11	16.9
CENSUS DIVISION 4, EAST NORTH CENTRAL	918	770	83.9	251	27.3	404	44.0	318	34.6	413	45.0	307	33.4	274	29.8
Illinois	231	189	81.8	76	32.9	103	44.6	89	38.5	106	45.9	88	38.1	74	32.0
Indiana	131	107	81.7	34	26.0	51	38.9	41	31.3	52	39.7	37	28.2	39	29.8
Michigan	201	157	78.1	39	19.4	93	46.3	66	32.8	89	44.3	63	31.3	53	26.4
Ohio	214	181	84.6	59	27.6	102	47.7	78	36.4	101	47.2	72	33.6	63	29.4
Wisconsin	141	136	96.5	43	30.5	55	39.0	44	31.2	65	46.1	47	33.3	45	31.9
CENSUS DIVISION 5, EAST SOUTH CENTRAL	492	346	70.3	81	16.5	124	25.2	103	20.9	145	29.5	82	16.7	76	15.4
Alabama	119	86	72.3	22	18.5	28	23.5	26	21.8	32	26.9	25	21.0	22	18.5
Kentucky	117	88	75.2	20	17.1	28	23.9	27	23.1	39	33.3	23	19.7	19	16.2
Mississippi	110	57	51.8	12	10.9	19	17.3	15	13.6	15	13.6	0	0.0	12	10.9
Tennessee	146	115	78.8	27	18.5	49	33.6	35	24.0	59	40.4	34	23.3	23	15.8
CENSUS DIVISION 6, WEST NORTH CENTRAL	810	654	80.7	150	18.5	215	26.5	182	22.5	250	30.9	185	22.8	192	23.7
Iowa	134	122	91.0	29	21.6	37	27.6	34	25.4	51	38.1	36	26.9	35	26.1
Kansas	147	96	65.3	23	15.6	27	18.4	27	18.4	32	21.8	23	15.6	22	15.0
Minnesota	158	129	81.6	30	19.0	41	25.9	34	21.5	51	32.3	36	22.8	44	27.8
Missouri	159	145	91.2	43	27.0	76	47.8	58	36.5	69	43.4	60	37.7	57	35.8
Nebraska	91	70	76.9	11	12.1	15	16.5	12	13.2	20	22.0	14	15.4	14	15.4
North Dakota	55	37	67.3	9	16.4	11	20.0	11	20.0	16	29.1	10	18.2	12	21.8
South Dakota	66	55	83.3	5	7.6	8	12.1	6	9.1	11	16.7	6	9.1	8	12.1
CENSUS DIVISION 7, WEST SOUTH CENTRAL	862	689	79.9	172	20.0	217	25.2	187	21.7	239	27.7	168	19.5	172	20.0
Arkansas	91	82	90.1	12	13.2	18	19.8	14	15.4	22	24.2	13	14.3	14	15.4
Louisiana	146	118	80.8	28	19.2	35	24.0	28	19.2	39	26.7	28	19.2	29	19.9
Oklahoma	112	87	77.7	20	17.9	30	26.8	21	18.8	31	27.7	18	16.1	25	22.3
Texas	513	402	78.4	112	21.8	134	26.1	124	24.2	147	28.7	109	21.2	104	20.3
CENSUS DIVISION 8, MOUNTAIN	422	349	82.7	100	23.7	141	33.4	117	27.7	163	38.6	89	21.1	116	27.5
Arizona	80	69	86.3	21	26.3	32	40.0	25	31.3	35	43.8	18	22.5	27	33.8
Colorado	82	73	89.0	26	31.7	30	36.6	28	34.1	36	43.9	25	30.5	26	31.7
Idaho	45	33	73.3	4	8.9	7	15.6	7	15.6	12	26.7	4	8.9	6	13.3
Montana	58	51	87.9	7	12.1	12	20.7	8	13.8	16	27.6	6	10.3	6	10.3
Nevada	23	19	82.6	5	21.7	7	30.4	6	26.1	7	30.4	6	26.1	7	30.4
New Mexico	55	43	78.2	15	27.3	24	43.6	15	27.3	22	40.0	12	21.8	18	32.7
Utah	49	38	77.6	16	32.7	22	44.9	22	44.9	25	51.0	12	24.5	20	40.8
Wyoming	30	23	76.7	6	20.0	7	23.3	6	20.0	10	33.3	6	20.0	6	20.0
CENSUS DIVISION 9, PACIFIC	642	514	80.1	131	20.4	225	35.0	166	25.9	239	37.2	154	24.0	180	28.0
Alaska	21	15	71.4	6	28.6	8	38.1	6	28.6	14	66.7	5	23.8	7	33.3
California	436	351	80.5	91	20.9	164	37.6	121	27.8	148	33.9	104	23.9	127	29.1
Hawaii	20	12	60.0	5	25.0	8	40.0	6	30.0	9	45.0	6	30.0	6	30.0
Oregon	68	58	85.3	11	16.2	15	22.1	11	16.2	28	41.2	17	25.0	14	20.6
Washington	97	78	80.4	18	18.6	30	30.9	22	22.7	40	41.2	22	22.7	26	26.8

(continued on next page)

Table

12B (Continued)

Facilities and Services in U.S. Census Divisions and States

For definitions of facilities and services, see Definitions of Terms, page xxiii. These data include only hospital-based facilities and services as reported by responding hospitals in Section C of the 1990 AHA Annual Survey, beginning on page 242. No estimates have been made for nonresponding hospitals.

CLASSIFICATION	HOSPITALS REPORTING	PSYCHIATRIC PARTIAL HOSPITALIZATION PROGRAM		RADIATION THERAPY: MEGAVOLTAGE RADIATION THERAPY		RADIATION THERAPY: RADIOACTIVE IMPLANTS		RADIATION THERAPY: THERAPEUTIC RADIOISOTOPE FACILITY		RADIATION THERAPY: X-RAY RADIATION THERAPY		RADIOLOGY (DIAGNOSTIC): CT SCANNER		RADIOLOGY (DIAGNOSTIC): DIAGNOSTIC RADIOISOTOPE FACILITY	
		Number	Percent	Number	Percent	Number	Percent	Number	Percent	Number	Percent	Number	Percent	Number	Percent
UNITED STATES	6,105	1,078	17.7	1,038	17.0	1,305	21.4	1,345	22.0	1,027	16.8	3,728	61.1	3,367	55.2
CENSUS DIVISION 1, NEW ENGLAND	315	84	26.7	59	18.7	53	16.8	64	20.3	58	18.4	192	61.0	189	60.0
Connecticut	60	37	61.7	19	31.7	17	28.3	17	28.3	19	31.7	34	56.7	33	55.0
Maine	42	6	14.3	6	14.3	4	9.5	9	21.4	7	16.7	23	54.8	27	64.3
Massachusetts	140	31	22.1	26	18.6	25	17.9	29	20.7	26	18.6	88	62.9	86	61.4
New Hampshire	36	6	16.7	4	11.1	4	11.1	6	16.7	4	11.1	23	63.9	20	55.6
Rhode Island	19	4	21.1	2	10.5	2	10.5	2	10.5	1	5.3	12	63.2	11	57.9
Vermont	18	0	0.0	2	11.1	1	5.6	1	5.6	1	5.6	12	66.7	12	66.7
CENSUS DIVISION 2, MIDDLE ATLANTIC	681	146	21.4	175	25.7	200	29.4	223	32.7	169	24.8	465	68.3	469	68.9
New Jersey	114	25	21.9	37	32.5	47	41.2	50	43.9	36	31.6	86	75.4	81	71.1
New York	288	79	27.4	75	26.0	79	27.4	92	31.9	75	26.0	181	62.8	200	69.4
Pennsylvania	279	42	15.1	63	22.6	74	26.5	81	29.0	58	20.8	198	71.0	188	67.4
CENSUS DIVISION 3, SOUTH ATLANTIC	963	143	14.8	162	16.8	198	20.6	209	21.7	160	16.6	639	66.4	557	57.8
Delaware	13	3	23.1	1	7.7	1	7.7	3	23.1	2	15.4	9	69.2	9	69.2
District of Columbia	16	7	43.8	7	43.8	6	37.5	9	56.3	7	43.8	11	68.8	12	75.0
Florida	260	37	14.2	49	18.8	79	30.4	63	24.2	52	20.0	186	71.5	153	58.8
Georgia	188	23	12.2	22	11.7	31	16.5	32	17.0	21	11.2	108	57.4	99	52.7
Maryland	78	19	24.4	16	20.5	14	17.9	17	21.8	15	19.2	49	62.8	48	61.5
North Carolina	135	10	7.4	23	17.0	21	15.6	23	17.0	20	14.8	105	77.8	80	59.3
South Carolina	84	12	14.3	10	11.9	10	11.9	14	16.7	12	14.3	51	60.7	46	54.8
Virginia	124	25	20.2	24	19.4	25	20.2	33	26.6	22	17.7	80	64.5	69	55.6
West Virginia	65	7	10.8	10	15.4	11	16.9	15	23.1	9	13.8	40	61.5	41	63.1
CENSUS DIVISION 4, EAST NORTH CENTRAL	918	194	21.1	204	22.2	235	25.6	261	28.4	195	21.2	645	70.3	600	65.4
Illinois	231	48	20.8	58	25.1	72	31.2	75	32.5	57	24.7	173	74.9	159	68.8
Indiana	131	28	21.4	30	22.9	34	26.0	36	27.5	30	22.9	94	71.8	80	61.1
Michigan	201	47	23.4	35	17.4	38	18.9	45	22.4	34	16.9	113	56.2	120	59.7
Ohio	214	43	20.1	58	27.1	68	31.8	74	34.6	52	24.3	174	81.3	164	76.6
Wisconsin	141	28	19.9	23	16.3	23	16.3	31	22.0	22	15.6	91	64.5	77	54.6
CENSUS DIVISION 5, EAST SOUTH CENTRAL	492	53	10.8	73	14.8	90	18.3	100	20.3	62	12.6	314	63.8	256	52.0
Alabama	119	13	10.9	19	16.0	26	21.8	25	21.0	17	14.3	72	60.5	65	54.6
Kentucky	117	15	12.8	13	11.1	21	17.9	24	20.5	13	11.1	85	72.6	54	46.2
Mississippi	110	5	4.5	10	9.1	8	7.3	18	16.4	1	0.9	52	47.3	55	50.0
Tennessee	146	20	13.7	31	21.2	35	24.0	33	22.6	31	21.2	105	71.9	82	56.2
CENSUS DIVISION 6, WEST NORTH CENTRAL	810	118	14.6	90	11.1	112	13.8	121	14.9	95	11.7	358	44.2	310	38.3
Iowa	134	22	16.4	14	10.4	18	13.4	22	16.4	15	11.2	55	41.0	40	29.9
Kansas	147	10	6.8	16	10.9	17	11.6	20	13.6	16	10.9	60	40.8	56	38.1
Minnesota	158	24	15.2	13	8.2	18	11.4	22	13.9	17	10.8	56	35.4	48	30.4
Missouri	159	39	24.5	30	18.9	36	22.6	38	23.9	32	20.1	123	77.4	107	67.3
Nebraska	91	10	11.0	12	13.2	13	14.3	11	12.1	10	11.0	27	29.7	26	28.6
North Dakota	55	10	18.2	4	7.3	6	10.9	6	10.9	4	7.3	18	32.7	16	29.1
South Dakota	66	3	4.5	1	1.5	4	6.1	2	3.0	1	1.5	19	28.8	17	25.8
CENSUS DIVISION 7, WEST SOUTH CENTRAL	862	133	15.4	93	10.8	147	17.1	131	15.2	96	11.1	466	54.1	405	47.0
Arkansas	91	5	5.5	8	8.8	13	14.3	15	16.5	5	5.5	60	65.9	53	58.2
Louisiana	146	20	13.7	21	14.4	29	19.9	27	18.5	20	13.7	80	54.8	73	50.0
Oklahoma	112	13	11.6	19	17.0	16	14.3	18	16.1	20	17.9	55	49.1	48	42.9
Texas	513	95	18.5	45	8.8	89	17.3	71	13.8	51	9.9	271	52.8	231	45.0
CENSUS DIVISION 8, MOUNTAIN	422	75	17.8	46	10.9	71	16.8	66	15.6	50	11.8	215	50.9	189	44.8
Arizona	80	18	22.5	9	11.3	23	28.8	20	25.0	11	13.8	49	61.3	43	53.8
Colorado	82	21	25.6	14	17.1	19	23.2	17	20.7	15	18.3	50	61.0	47	57.3
Idaho	45	2	4.4	5	11.1	5	11.1	6	13.3	4	8.9	19	42.2	16	35.6
Montana	58	4	6.9	3	5.2	6	10.3	5	8.6	4	6.9	22	37.9	18	31.0
Nevada	23	4	17.4	2	8.7	3	13.0	4	17.4	2	8.7	12	52.2	10	43.5
New Mexico	55	9	16.4	5	9.1	7	12.7	6	10.9	7	12.7	22	40.0	21	38.2
Utah	49	16	32.7	5	10.2	6	12.2	5	10.2	5	10.2	25	51.0	19	38.8
Wyoming	30	1	3.3	3	10.0	2	6.7	3	10.0	2	6.7	16	53.3	15	50.0
CENSUS DIVISION 9, PACIFIC	642	132	20.6	136	21.2	199	31.0	170	26.5	142	22.1	434	67.6	392	61.1
Alaska	21	4	19.0	1	4.8	2	9.5	2	9.5	0	0.0	9	42.9	6	28.6
California	436	94	21.6	99	22.7	154	35.3	126	28.9	107	24.5	310	71.1	278	63.8
Hawaii	20	5	25.0	4	20.0	5	25.0	5	25.0	4	20.0	12	60.0	11	55.0
Oregon	68	11	16.2	12	17.6	16	23.5	14	20.6	10	14.7	43	63.2	43	63.2
Washington	97	18	18.6	20	20.6	22	22.7	23	23.7	21	21.6	60	61.9	54	55.7

CLASSIFICATION	HOSPITALS REPORTING	RADIOLOGY (DIAGNOSTIC) continued: MAGNETIC RESONANCE IMAGING (MRI)		SINGLE PHOTON EMISSION COMPUTERIZED TOMOGRAPHY (SPECT)		ULTRASOUND		REHABILITATION OUTPATIENT SERVICES		REPRODUCTIVE HEALTH		SOCIAL WORK SERVICES: ORGANIZED		OUTPATIENT	
		Number	Percent	Number	Percent	Number	Percent	Number	Percent	Number	Percent	Number	Percent	Number	Percent
UNITED STATES	6,105	955	15.6	988	16.2	4,563	74.7	2,924	47.9	2,269	37.2	4,864	79.7	2,785	45.6[r]
CENSUS DIVISION 1, NEW ENGLAND	315	48	15.2	45	14.3	224	71.1	203	64.4	114	36.2	294	93.3	196	62.2[r]
Connecticut	60	11	18.3	8	13.3	37	61.7	35	58.3	20	33.3	57	95.0	43	71.7
Maine	42	2	4.8	4	9.5	35	83.3	25	59.5	16	38.1	37	88.1	22	52.4
Massachusetts	140	24	17.1	22	15.7	97	69.3	100	71.4	49	35.0	136	97.1	92	65.7
New Hampshire	36	7	19.4	8	22.2	26	72.2	23	63.9	16	44.4	28	77.8	20	55.6
Rhode Island	19	3	15.8	3	15.8	14	73.7	10	52.6	6	31.6	19	100.0	12	63.2
Vermont	18	1	5.6	0	0.0	15	83.3	10	55.6	7	38.9	17	94.4	7	38.9[r]
CENSUS DIVISION 2, MIDDLE ATLANTIC	681	87	12.8	137	20.1	538	79.0	414	60.8	285	41.9	646	94.9	426	62.6[r]
New Jersey	114	12	10.5	32	28.1	93	81.6	73	64.0	58	50.9	110	96.5	85	74.6
New York	288	37	12.8	51	17.7	230	79.9	176	61.1	122	42.4	270	93.8	180	62.5
Pennsylvania	279	38	13.6	54	19.4	215	77.1	165	59.1	105	37.6	266	95.3	161	57.7[r]
CENSUS DIVISION 3, SOUTH ATLANTIC	963	170	17.7	170	17.7	736	76.4	432	44.9	353	36.7	813	84.4	396	41.1[r]
Delaware	13	2	15.4	1	7.7	10	76.9	7	53.8	4	30.8	11	84.6	3	23.1
District of Columbia	16	5	31.3	5	31.3	13	81.3	11	68.8	10	62.5	15	93.8	13	81.3
Florida	260	55	21.2	56	21.5	204	78.5	134	51.5	82	31.5	224	86.2	106	40.8
Georgia	188	28	14.9	14	7.4	130	69.1	65	34.6	68	36.2	131	69.7	64	34.0
Maryland	78	18	23.1	23	29.5	54	69.2	42	53.8	33	42.3	74	94.9	37	47.4
North Carolina	135	26	19.3	25	18.5	113	83.7	54	40.0	50	37.0	118	87.4	51	37.8
South Carolina	84	8	9.5	16	19.0	65	77.4	28	33.3	32	38.1	71	84.5	37	44.0
Virginia	124	22	17.7	17	13.7	94	75.8	64	51.6	50	40.3	113	91.1	52	41.9
West Virginia	65	6	9.2	13	20.0	53	81.5	27	41.5	24	36.9	56	86.2	33	50.8[r]
CENSUS DIVISION 4, EAST NORTH CENTRAL	918	164	17.9	214	23.3	739	80.5	542	59.0	356	38.8	807	87.9	531	57.8[r]
Illinois	231	42	18.2	62	26.8	185	80.1	130	56.3	87	37.7	205	88.7	134	58.0
Indiana	131	22	16.8	31	23.7	107	81.7	73	55.7	42	32.1	114	87.0	69	52.7
Michigan	201	28	13.9	37	18.4	158	78.6	119	59.2	74	36.8	169	84.1	108	53.7
Ohio	214	39	18.2	46	21.5	185	86.4	126	58.9	80	37.4	191	89.3	123	57.5
Wisconsin	141	33	23.4	38	27.0	104	73.8	94	66.7	73	51.8	128	90.8	97	68.8[r]
CENSUS DIVISION 5, EAST SOUTH CENTRAL	492	75	15.2	41	8.3	374	76.0	165	33.5	152	30.9	379	77.0	140	28.5[r]
Alabama	119	19	16.0	11	9.2	97	81.5	34	28.6	28	23.5	87	73.1	36	30.3
Kentucky	117	13	11.1	14	12.0	99	84.6	43	36.8	33	28.2	83	70.9	41	35.0
Mississippi	110	10	9.1	0	0.0	64	58.2	28	25.5	35	31.8	86	78.2	3	2.7
Tennessee	146	33	22.6	16	11.0	114	78.1	60	41.1	56	38.4	123	84.2	60	41.1[r]
CENSUS DIVISION 6, WEST NORTH CENTRAL	810	98	12.1	96	11.9	515	63.6	364	44.9	318	39.3	537	66.3	310	38.3[r]
Iowa	134	18	13.4	10	7.5	91	67.9	51	38.1	62	46.3	91	67.9	53	39.6
Kansas	147	10	6.8	13	8.8	82	55.8	55	37.4	39	26.5	82	55.8	37	25.2
Minnesota	158	20	12.7	14	8.9	88	55.7	72	45.6	57	36.1	104	65.8	47	29.7
Missouri	159	36	22.6	41	25.8	132	83.0	113	71.1	88	55.3	142	89.3	102	64.2
Nebraska	91	7	7.7	9	9.9	52	57.1	32	35.2	29	31.9	53	58.2	30	33.0
North Dakota	55	5	9.1	7	12.7	29	52.7	18	32.7	18	32.7	34	61.8	20	36.4
South Dakota	66	2	3.0	2	3.0	41	62.1	23	34.8	25	37.9	31	47.0	21	31.8[r]
CENSUS DIVISION 7, WEST SOUTH CENTRAL	862	122	14.2	103	11.9	605	70.2	284	32.9	253	29.4	585	67.9	311	36.1[r]
Arkansas	91	12	13.2	11	12.1	76	83.5	33	36.3	27	29.7	63	69.2	34	37.4
Louisiana	146	22	15.1	18	12.3	104	71.2	40	27.4	37	25.3	104	71.2	58	39.7
Oklahoma	112	12	10.7	11	9.8	77	68.8	34	30.4	32	28.6	68	60.7	38	33.9
Texas	513	76	14.8	63	12.3	348	67.8	177	34.5	157	30.6	350	68.2	181	35.3[r]
CENSUS DIVISION 8, MOUNTAIN	422	77	18.2	60	14.2	307	72.7	191	45.3	171	40.5	297	70.4	175	41.5[r]
Arizona	80	16	20.0	18	22.5	65	81.3	44	55.0	39	48.8	66	82.5	40	50.0
Colorado	82	22	26.8	16	19.5	60	73.2	58	70.7	35	42.7	58	70.7	38	46.3
Idaho	45	8	17.8	6	13.3	27	60.0	17	37.8	14	31.1	22	48.9	11	24.4
Montana	58	5	8.6	4	6.9	38	65.5	18	31.0	20	34.5	31	53.4	18	31.0
Nevada	23	3	13.0	3	13.0	19	82.6	7	30.4	10	43.5	18	78.3	10	43.5
New Mexico	55	8	14.5	6	10.9	36	65.5	21	38.2	24	43.6	44	80.0	25	45.5
Utah	49	12	24.5	4	8.2	35	71.4	16	32.7	17	34.7	38	77.6	25	51.0
Wyoming	30	3	10.0	3	10.0	27	90.0	10	33.3	12	40.0	20	66.7	8	26.7[r]
CENSUS DIVISION 9, PACIFIC	642	114	17.8	122	19.0	525	81.8	329	51.2	267	41.6	506	78.8	300	46.7[r]
Alaska	21	3	14.3	2	9.5	18	85.7	5	23.8	11	52.4	15	71.4	9	42.9
California	436	90	20.6	93	21.3	359	82.3	225	51.6	183	42.0	351	80.5	196	45.0
Hawaii	20	1	5.0	5	25.0	12	60.0	11	55.0	6	30.0	16	80.0	10	50.0
Oregon	68	9	13.2	9	13.2	59	86.8	34	50.0	28	41.2	49	72.1	29	42.6
Washington	97	11	11.3	13	13.4	77	79.4	54	55.7	39	40.2	75	77.3	56	57.7

(continued on next page)

Table

12B (Continued)

Facilities and Services in U.S. Census Divisions and States

For definitions of facilities and services, see Definitions of Terms, page xxiii. These data include only hospital-based facilities and services as reported by responding hospitals in Section C of the 1990 AHA Annual Survey, beginning on page 242. No estimates have been made for nonresponding hospitals.

CLASSIFICATION	HOSPITALS REPORTING	SOCIAL WORK SERVICES continued: EMERGENCY DEPARTMENT		SPORTS MEDICINE CLINIC/SERVICES		SUPPLEMENTARY PATIENT ASSISTANCE: HOSPITAL AUXILIARY		PATIENT REPRESENTATIVE SERVICES		VOLUNTEER SERVICES DEPARTMENT		SURGERY SERVICES: OUTPATIENT		ORGAN/TISSUE TRANSPLANT	
		Number	Percent	Number	Percent	Number	Percent	Number	Percent	Number	Percent	Number	Percent	Number	Percent
UNITED STATES	6,105	2,440	40.0	1,060	17.4	4,405	72.2	3,210	52.6	4,027	66.0	5,070	83.0	558	9.1
CENSUS DIVISION 1, NEW ENGLAND	315	171	54.3	65	20.6	237	75.2	182	57.8	261	82.9	235	74.6	25	7.9
Connecticut	60	32	53.3	11	18.3	46	76.7	38	63.3	50	83.3	38	63.3	5	8.3
Maine	42	28	66.7	7	16.7	37	88.1	21	50.0	31	73.8	40	95.2	1	2.4
Massachusetts	140	75	53.6	31	22.1	102	72.9	84	60.0	119	85.0	100	71.4	17	12.1
New Hampshire	36	16	44.4	10	27.8	26	72.2	17	47.2	28	77.8	27	75.0	1	2.8
Rhode Island	19	11	57.9	2	10.5	13	68.4	10	52.6	17	89.5	14	73.7	0	0.0
Vermont	18	9	50.0	4	22.2	13	72.2	12	66.7	16	88.9	16	88.9	1	5.6
CENSUS DIVISION 2, MIDDLE ATLANTIC	681	385	56.5	131	19.2	532	78.1	463	68.0	598	87.8	545	80.0	75	11.0
New Jersey	114	63	55.3	20	17.5	98	86.0	92	80.7	109	95.6	90	78.9	11	9.6
New York	288	177	61.5	43	14.9	222	77.1	205	71.2	254	88.2	237	82.3	27	9.4
Pennsylvania	279	145	52.0	68	24.4	212	76.0	166	59.5	235	84.2	218	78.1	37	13.3
CENSUS DIVISION 3, SOUTH ATLANTIC	963	355	36.9	143	14.8	640	66.5	525	54.5	639	66.4	776	80.6	83	8.6
Delaware	13	6	46.2	4	30.8	8	61.5	7	53.8	11	84.6	10	76.9	1	7.7
District of Columbia	16	11	68.8	2	12.5	10	62.5	12	75.0	15	93.8	12	75.0	6	37.5
Florida	260	96	36.9	46	17.7	170	65.4	138	53.1	156	60.0	201	77.3	24	9.2
Georgia	188	49	26.1	26	13.8	117	62.2	90	47.9	90	47.9	150	79.8	12	6.4
Maryland	78	36	46.2	8	10.3	58	74.4	57	73.1	63	80.8	57	73.1	8	10.3
North Carolina	135	48	35.6	14	10.4	96	71.1	72	53.3	103	76.3	117	86.7	8	5.9
South Carolina	84	35	41.7	10	11.9	57	67.9	45	53.6	67	79.8	70	83.3	7	8.3
Virginia	124	45	36.3	23	18.5	85	68.5	84	67.7	92	74.2	101	81.5	12	9.7
West Virginia	65	29	44.6	10	15.4	39	60.0	20	30.8	42	64.6	58	89.2	5	7.7
CENSUS DIVISION 4, EAST NORTH CENTRAL	918	492	53.6	245	26.7	744	81.0	526	57.3	710	77.3	801	87.3	116	12.6
Illinois	231	133	57.6	48	20.8	183	79.2	130	56.3	175	75.8	203	87.9	28	12.1
Indiana	131	56	42.7	28	21.4	103	78.6	74	56.5	95	72.5	113	86.3	10	7.6
Michigan	201	93	46.3	55	27.4	159	79.1	112	55.7	147	73.1	172	85.6	14	7.0
Ohio	214	120	56.1	72	33.6	175	81.8	137	64.0	187	87.4	187	87.4	22	10.3
Wisconsin	141	90	63.8	42	29.8	124	87.9	73	51.8	106	75.2	126	89.4	42	29.8
CENSUS DIVISION 5, EAST SOUTH CENTRAL	492	129	26.2	59	12.0	285	57.9	245	49.8	278	56.5	404	82.1	32	6.5
Alabama	119	35	29.4	12	10.1	66	55.5	54	45.4	63	52.9	95	79.8	3	2.5
Kentucky	117	40	34.2	14	12.0	74	63.2	59	50.4	67	57.3	97	82.9	6	5.1
Mississippi	110	2	1.8	10	9.1	72	65.5	56	50.9	54	49.1	83	75.5	1	0.9
Tennessee	146	52	35.6	23	15.8	73	50.0	76	52.1	94	64.4	129	88.4	22	15.1
CENSUS DIVISION 6, WEST NORTH CENTRAL	810	252	31.1	158	19.5	672	83.0	329	40.6	437	54.0	718	88.6	55	6.8
Iowa	134	42	31.3	25	18.7	122	91.0	47	35.1	64	47.8	125	93.3	6	4.5
Kansas	147	30	20.4	10	6.8	106	72.1	42	28.6	59	40.1	133	90.5	5	3.4
Minnesota	158	35	22.2	36	22.8	134	84.8	67	42.4	86	54.4	139	88.0	8	5.1
Missouri	159	95	59.7	45	28.3	136	85.5	114	71.7	135	84.9	134	84.3	25	15.7
Nebraska	91	23	25.3	17	18.7	75	82.4	24	26.4	39	42.9	87	95.6	7	7.7
North Dakota	55	13	23.6	13	23.6	47	85.5	18	32.7	31	56.4	47	85.5	3	5.5
South Dakota	66	14	21.2	12	18.2	52	78.8	17	25.8	23	34.8	53	80.3	1	1.5
CENSUS DIVISION 7, WEST SOUTH CENTRAL	862	228	26.5	95	11.0	564	65.4	378	43.9	430	49.9	693	80.4	71	8.2
Arkansas	91	28	30.8	9	9.9	78	85.7	35	38.5	43	47.3	81	89.0	8	8.8
Louisiana	146	43	29.5	14	9.6	87	59.6	77	52.7	82	56.2	113	77.4	10	6.8
Oklahoma	112	23	20.5	11	9.8	83	74.1	39	34.8	56	50.0	96	85.7	8	7.1
Texas	513	134	26.1	61	11.9	316	61.6	227	44.2	249	48.5	403	78.6	45	8.8
CENSUS DIVISION 8, MOUNTAIN	422	153	36.3	71	16.8	288	68.2	221	52.4	240	56.9	342	81.0	36	8.5
Arizona	80	41	51.3	9	11.3	46	57.5	44	55.0	54	67.5	63	78.8	13	16.3
Colorado	82	30	36.6	26	31.7	61	74.4	61	74.4	51	62.2	68	82.9	8	9.8
Idaho	45	8	17.8	7	15.6	36	80.0	17	37.8	23	51.1	38	84.4	2	4.4
Montana	58	16	27.6	6	10.3	46	79.3	20	34.5	24	41.4	48	82.8	2	3.4
Nevada	23	10	43.5	2	8.7	15	65.2	12	52.2	14	60.9	19	82.6	4	17.4
New Mexico	55	18	32.7	7	12.7	32	58.2	28	50.9	25	45.5	39	70.9	4	7.3
Utah	49	25	51.0	11	22.4	33	67.3	23	46.9	32	65.3	41	83.7	3	6.1
Wyoming	30	5	16.7	3	10.0	19	63.3	16	53.3	17	56.7	26	86.7	0	0.0
CENSUS DIVISION 9, PACIFIC	642	275	42.8	93	14.5	443	69.0	341	53.1	434	67.6	556	86.6	65	10.1
Alaska	21	10	47.6	1	4.8	9	42.9	8	38.1	9	42.9	15	71.4	0	0.0
California	436	182	41.7	56	12.8	296	67.9	242	55.5	298	68.3	378	86.7	47	10.8
Hawaii	20	7	35.0	1	5.0	12	60.0	10	50.0	15	75.0	13	65.0	2	10.0
Oregon	68	29	42.6	11	16.2	54	79.4	25	36.8	42	61.8	62	91.2	6	8.8
Washington	97	47	48.5	24	24.7	72	74.2	56	57.7	70	72.2	88	90.7	10	10.3

Table 12B (Continued)

CLASSIFICATION	HOSPITALS REPORTING	SURGERY SERVICES continued		THERAPY SERVICES										WOMEN'S HEALTH CENTER/SERVICES	
		ORTHOPEDIC		OCCUPATIONAL		PHYSICAL		RECREATIONAL		RESPIRATORY		SPEECH			
		Number	Percent	Number	Percent	Number	Percent	Number	Percent	Number	Percent	Number	Percent	Number	Percent
UNITED STATES	6,105	3,980	65.2	3,206	52.5	4,822	79.0	2,475	40.5	4,944	81.0	2,746	45.0	1,170	19.2
CENSUS DIVISION 1, NEW ENGLAND	315	214	67.9	245	77.8	271	86.0	159	50.5	251	79.7	184	58.4	80	25.4
Connecticut	60	34	56.7	42	70.0	48	80.0	37	61.7	41	68.3	33	55.0	15	25.0
Maine	42	33	78.6	27	64.3	40	95.2	10	23.8	38	90.5	14	33.3	7	16.7
Massachusetts	140	95	67.9	119	85.0	122	87.1	73	52.1	116	82.9	94	67.1	38	27.1
New Hampshire	36	25	69.4	29	80.6	30	83.3	19	52.8	26	72.2	19	52.8	13	36.1
Rhode Island	19	13	68.4	13	68.4	15	78.9	9	47.4	15	78.9	12	63.2	4	21.1
Vermont	18	14	77.8	15	83.3	16	88.9	11	61.1	15	83.3	12	66.7	3	16.7
CENSUS DIVISION 2, MIDDLE ATLANTIC	681	494	72.5	471	69.2	605	88.8	399	58.6	568	83.4	427	62.7	137	20.1
New Jersey	114	89	78.1	80	70.2	106	93.0	63	55.3	97	85.1	76	66.7	28	24.6
New York	288	200	69.4	205	71.2	254	88.2	188	65.3	243	84.4	177	61.5	53	18.4
Pennsylvania	279	205	73.5	186	66.7	245	87.8	148	53.0	228	81.7	174	62.4	56	20.1
CENSUS DIVISION 3, SOUTH ATLANTIC	963	629	65.3	482	50.1	739	76.7	405	42.1	766	79.5	411	42.7	200	20.8
Delaware	13	9	69.2	7	53.8	11	84.6	9	69.2	9	69.2	6	46.2	1	7.7
District of Columbia	16	11	68.8	13	81.3	14	87.5	11	68.8	15	93.8	13	81.3	6	37.5
Florida	260	180	69.2	144	55.4	197	75.8	106	40.8	206	79.2	116	44.6	64	24.6
Georgia	188	102	54.3	69	36.7	125	66.5	68	36.2	137	72.9	62	33.0	31	16.5
Maryland	78	54	69.2	56	71.8	61	78.2	51	65.4	62	79.5	40	51.3	14	17.9
North Carolina	135	98	72.6	54	40.0	117	86.7	48	35.6	117	86.7	61	45.2	22	16.3
South Carolina	84	52	61.9	38	45.2	60	71.4	27	32.1	66	78.6	21	25.0	17	20.2
Virginia	124	85	68.5	77	62.1	102	82.3	64	51.6	97	78.2	65	52.4	34	27.4
West Virginia	65	38	58.5	24	36.9	52	80.0	21	32.3	57	87.7	27	41.5	11	16.9
CENSUS DIVISION 4, EAST NORTH CENTRAL	918	713	77.7	585	63.7	789	85.9	432	47.1	792	86.3	563	61.3	223	24.3
Illinois	231	170	73.6	136	58.9	191	82.7	113	48.9	200	86.6	140	60.6	56	24.2
Indiana	131	103	78.6	66	50.4	109	83.2	55	42.0	107	81.7	77	58.8	27	20.6
Michigan	201	146	72.6	130	64.7	171	85.1	94	46.8	169	84.1	118	58.7	46	22.9
Ohio	214	175	81.8	145	67.8	193	90.2	104	48.6	191	89.3	145	67.8	53	24.8
Wisconsin	141	119	84.4	108	76.6	125	88.7	66	46.8	125	88.7	83	58.9	41	29.1
CENSUS DIVISION 5, EAST SOUTH CENTRAL	492	251	51.0	140	28.5	370	75.2	119	24.2	411	83.5	123	25.0	76	15.4
Alabama	119	62	52.1	35	29.4	88	73.9	30	25.2	97	81.5	25	21.0	17	14.3
Kentucky	117	67	57.3	34	29.1	94	80.3	28	23.9	102	87.2	35	29.9	23	19.7
Mississippi	110	40	36.4	16	14.5	65	59.1	15	13.6	83	75.5	15	13.6	10	9.1
Tennessee	146	82	56.2	55	37.7	123	84.2	46	31.5	129	88.4	48	32.9	26	17.8
CENSUS DIVISION 6, WEST NORTH CENTRAL	810	440	54.3	373	46.0	646	79.8	287	35.4	611	75.4	335	41.4	97	12.0
Iowa	134	86	64.2	52	38.8	110	82.1	53	39.6	114	85.1	48	35.8	17	12.7
Kansas	147	59	40.1	61	41.5	112	76.2	37	25.2	117	79.6	45	30.6	12	8.2
Minnesota	158	94	59.5	81	51.3	129	81.6	56	35.4	105	66.5	63	39.9	14	8.9
Missouri	159	118	74.2	122	76.7	146	91.8	91	57.2	137	86.2	122	76.7	35	22.0
Nebraska	91	44	48.4	26	28.6	69	75.8	17	18.7	65	71.4	27	29.7	7	7.7
North Dakota	55	17	30.9	15	27.3	36	65.5	19	34.5	29	52.7	12	21.8	5	9.1
South Dakota	66	22	33.3	16	24.2	44	66.7	14	21.2	44	66.7	18	27.3	7	10.6
CENSUS DIVISION 7, WEST SOUTH CENTRAL	862	501	58.1	314	36.4	564	65.4	257	29.8	681	79.0	233	27.0	138	16.0
Arkansas	91	59	64.8	31	34.1	66	72.5	13	14.3	80	87.9	27	29.7	13	14.3
Louisiana	146	84	57.5	56	38.4	84	57.5	48	32.9	110	75.3	39	26.7	26	17.8
Oklahoma	112	57	50.9	36	32.1	85	75.9	31	27.7	88	78.6	31	27.7	11	9.8
Texas	513	301	58.7	191	37.2	329	64.1	165	32.2	403	78.6	136	26.5	88	17.2
CENSUS DIVISION 8, MOUNTAIN	422	253	60.0	191	45.3	314	74.4	159	37.7	315	74.6	159	37.7	84	19.9
Arizona	80	54	67.5	47	58.8	63	78.8	28	35.0	57	71.3	39	48.8	15	18.8
Colorado	82	51	62.2	53	64.6	70	85.4	37	45.1	72	87.8	43	52.4	20	24.4
Idaho	45	25	55.6	19	42.2	34	75.6	14	31.1	35	77.8	15	33.3	9	20.0
Montana	58	29	50.0	15	25.9	36	62.1	13	22.4	35	60.3	12	20.7	9	15.5
Nevada	23	15	65.2	11	47.8	14	60.9	8	34.8	19	82.6	8	34.8	3	13.0
New Mexico	55	24	43.6	22	40.0	39	70.9	19	34.5	34	61.8	16	29.1	11	20.0
Utah	49	31	63.3	16	32.7	35	71.4	32	65.3	38	77.6	15	30.6	17	34.7
Wyoming	30	24	80.0	8	26.7	23	76.7	8	26.7	25	83.3	11	36.7	0	0.0
CENSUS DIVISION 9, PACIFIC	642	485	75.5	405	63.1	524	81.6	258	40.2	549	85.5	311	48.4	135	21.0
Alaska	21	10	47.6	10	47.6	16	76.2	6	28.6	16	76.2	5	23.8	3	14.3
California	436	334	76.6	288	66.1	354	81.2	187	42.9	370	84.9	229	52.5	91	20.9
Hawaii	20	13	65.0	15	75.0	16	80.0	14	70.0	12	60.0	8	40.0	3	15.0
Oregon	68	56	82.4	36	52.9	59	86.8	19	27.9	64	94.1	25	36.8	15	22.1
Washington	97	72	74.2	56	57.7	79	81.4	32	33.0	87	89.7	44	45.4	23	23.7

Table

13

Hospitals, Units, and Beds, by Inpatient Service Areas

The facilities and services presented in tables 13A and 13B are listed below in alphabetical order by major heading, referencing the page numbers on which they appear.

Table

13A

Hospitals, Units, and Beds, by Inpatient Service Area in the United States

These data include hospitals, units, and beds as reported by hospitals responding to Section D, Beds and Utilization by Inpatient Service, of the 1990 AHA Annual Survey, beginning on page 242. A difference may exist between the total number of hospitals reporting for a particular classification and the sum of the specific hospital service components of that classification because the number of total reporting hospitals includes specialty service hospitals, which do not fall into any of the specific hospital service components.

		GENERAL MEDICAL AND SURGICAL											
		ADULT				PEDIATRIC				OBSTETRICS			
		HOSPITALS		UNITS		HOSPITALS		UNITS		HOSPITALS		UNITS	
CLASSIFICATION	HOSPITALS REPORTING	Number	Beds	Number	Beds	Number	Beds	Number	Beds	Number	Beds	Number	Beds
UNITED STATES	**6,105**	**5,129**	**557,705**	**142**	**8,621**	**42**	**5,096**	**2,387**	**39,859**	**12**	**818**	**3,438**	**60,549**
6-24 beds	254	228	3,817	10	157	0	0	29	108	0	0	76	273
25-49	974	872	25,842	11	286	0	0	183	857	0	0	452	2,173
50-99	1,451	1,116	51,145	22	1,059	4	211	361	2,570	2	71	708	5,776
100-199	1,439	1,205	101,324	29	2,280	21	2,026	629	7,272	8	522	850	11,692
200-299	804	728	107,608	9	667	14	2,124	466	7,899	1	96	546	11,617
300-399	485	420	85,927	10	415	3	735	311	6,822	1	129	347	9,511
400-499	265	231	60,716	7	587	0	0	170	4,490	0	0	201	6,992
500 or more	433	329	121,326	44	3,170	0	0	238	9,841	0	0	258	12,515
Federal	**301**	**278**	**32,973**	**22**	**1,908**	**0**	**0**	**84**	**977**	**0**	**0**	**106**	**1,688**
Psychiatric	17	0	0	17	869	0	0	0	0	0	0	0	0
General and other special	284	278	32,973	5	1,039	0	0	84	977	0	0	106	1,688
Nonfederal	**5,804**	**4,851**	**524,732**	**120**	**6,713**	**42**	**5,096**	**2,303**	**38,882**	**12**	**818**	**3,332**	**58,861**
Psychiatric	609	0	0	39	1,196	0	0	3	23	0	0	1	5
Nongovernment not-for-profit	106	0	0	3	81	0	0	2	10	0	0	1	5
Investor-owned (for-profit)	272	0	0	5	109	0	0	1	13	0	0	0	0
State and local government	231	0	0	31	1,006	0	0	0	0	0	0	0	0
TB and other respiratory diseases	3	0	0	1	85	0	0	0	0	0	0	0	0
Nongovernment not-for-profit	1	0	0	0	0	0	0	0	0	0	0	0	0
Investor-owned (for-profit)	0	0	0	0	0	0	0	0	0	0	0	0	0
State and local government	2	0	0	1	85	0	0	0	0	0	0	0	0
Long-term general and other special	119	15	786	12	606	1	70	5	90	0	0	2	29
Nongovernment not-for-profit	54	7	359	1	10	1	70	1	19	0	0	1	27
Investor-owned (for-profit)	16	1	52	1	7	0	0	1	3	0	0	0	0
State and local government	49	7	375	10	589	0	0	3	68	0	0	1	2
Short-term general and other special	5,073	4,836	523,946	68	4,826	41	5,026	2,295	38,769	12	818	3,329	58,827
6-24 beds	209	193	3,374	10	157	0	0	20	71	0	0	61	179
25-49	868	827	24,764	10	279	0	0	158	707	0	0	420	1,882
50-99	1,157	1,083	49,843	14	871	3	141	342	2,395	2	71	685	5,407
100-199	1,225	1,154	97,448	24	1,908	21	2,026	608	6,979	8	522	828	11,248
200-299	719	697	103,581	5	577	14	2,124	458	7,765	1	96	539	11,444
300-399	400	392	80,982	2	90	3	735	307	6,733	1	129	343	9,392
400-499	215	215	57,418	0	0	0	0	166	4,344	0	0	197	6,811
500 or more	280	275	106,536	3	944	0	0	236	9,775	0	0	256	12,464
Nongovernment not-for-profit	3,079	2,919	377,402	35	2,776	41	5,026	1,654	28,814	5	440	2,182	42,194
6-24 beds	71	60	1,046	6	93	0	0	10	54	0	0	21	79
25-49	383	358	10,659	3	91	0	0	83	515	0	0	199	941
50-99	601	554	24,978	8	563	3	141	214	1,531	0	0	375	2,993
100-199	748	698	60,099	13	1,027	21	2,026	412	4,717	4	311	516	6,959
200-299	552	533	79,069	3	433	14	2,124	363	6,021	0	0	422	8,844
300-399	326	320	66,406	1	72	3	735	253	5,418	1	129	282	7,720
400-499	175	175	47,179	0	0	0	0	131	3,304	0	0	162	5,407
500 or more	223	221	87,966	1	497	0	0	188	7,254	0	0	205	9,251
Investor-owned (for-profit)	636	584	57,198	15	711	0	0	178	2,563	7	378	309	4,905
6-24 beds	14	12	214	1	11	0	0	0	0	0	0	0	0
25-49	62	53	1,732	3	79	0	0	4	6	0	0	16	78
50-99	178	155	8,583	2	100	0	0	28	286	2	71	72	678
100-199	248	231	21,556	8	440	0	0	88	1,116	4	211	139	2,096
200-299	90	89	14,082	1	81	0	0	32	550	1	96	49	1,113
300-399	29	29	6,365	0	0	0	0	15	288	0	0	22	547
400-499	12	12	3,646	0	0	0	0	9	210	0	0	8	305
500 or more	3	3	1,020	0	0	0	0	2	107	0	0	3	88
State and local government	1,358	1,333	89,346	18	1,339	0	0	463	7,392	0	0	838	11,728
6-24 beds	124	121	2,114	3	53	0	0	10	17	0	0	40	100
25-49	423	416	12,373	4	109	0	0	71	186	0	0	205	863
50-99	378	374	16,282	4	208	0	0	100	578	0	0	238	1,736
100-199	229	225	15,793	3	441	0	0	108	1,146	0	0	173	2,193
200-299	77	75	10,430	1	63	0	0	63	1,194	0	0	68	1,487
300-399	45	43	8,211	1	18	0	0	39	1,027	0	0	39	1,125
400-499	28	28	6,593	0	0	0	0	26	830	0	0	27	1,099
500 or more	54	51	17,550	2	447	0	0	46	2,414	0	0	48	3,125
Hospital units of institutions	17	0	0	16	607	0	0	0	0	0	0	1	19
Community hospitals	5,056	4,836	523,946	52	4,219	41	5,026	2,295	38,769	12	818	3,328	58,808

CLASSIFICATION	HOSPITALS REPORTING	BURN CARE		NEONATAL INTERMEDIATE CARE		INTENSIVE CARE: NEONATAL		INTENSIVE CARE: PEDIATRIC		INTENSIVE CARE: CARDIAC		INTENSIVE CARE: MIXED OR OTHER	
		Units	Beds	Units	Beds	Units	Beds	Units	Beds	Units	Beds	Units	Beds
UNITED STATES	6,105	137	1,500	404	4,537	737	12,364	335	2,881	1,182	11,850	4,226	63,298
CENSUS DIVISION 1, NEW ENGLAND	315	5	61	10	109	27	491	12	109	53	451	219	2,820
Connecticut	60	1	9	0	0	10	166	4	23	14	148	36	659
Maine	42	1	2	2	20	1	25	0	0	6	50	39	311
Massachusetts	140	3	50	8	89	9	177	6	74	28	217	91	1,324
New Hampshire	36	0	0	0	0	5	43	1	4	1	8	26	235
Rhode Island	19	0	0	0	0	1	60	1	8	4	28	12	157
Vermont	18	0	0	0	0	1	20	0	0	0	0	15	134
CENSUS DIVISION 2, MIDDLE ATLANTIC	681	22	195	55	527	106	1,796	41	309	195	2,006	521	8,390
New Jersey	114	2	23	14	124	20	291	7	44	35	402	92	1,429
New York	288	12	100	12	161	46	924	24	167	88	843	221	3,376
Pennsylvania	279	8	72	29	242	40	581	10	98	72	761	208	3,585
CENSUS DIVISION 3, SOUTH ATLANTIC	963	17	220	85	974	119	1,970	59	556	240	2,511	692	12,355
Delaware	13	0	0	2	26	1	24	2	27	3	18	8	235
District of Columbia	16	2	29	5	90	9	171	2	30	5	70	12	347
Florida	260	4	51	23	274	38	606	20	203	72	888	195	4,130
Georgia	188	3	55	23	244	25	289	7	72	37	306	118	1,748
Maryland	78	1	10	2	22	11	248	3	37	22	195	57	1,160
North Carolina	135	3	43	12	113	13	253	10	73	34	381	107	1,921
South Carolina	84	0	0	8	80	8	136	3	18	20	212	58	925
Virginia	124	3	28	8	106	11	189	9	74	30	314	92	1,336
West Virginia	65	1	4	2	19	3	54	3	22	17	127	45	553
CENSUS DIVISION 4, EAST NORTH CENTRAL	918	28	302	60	623	111	2,412	55	432	200	2,139	697	10,598
Illinois	231	6	71	28	264	30	579	20	127	47	524	181	2,475
Indiana	131	3	26	10	115	21	357	7	63	26	299	103	1,697
Michigan	201	8	78	5	69	21	499	11	99	46	428	136	1,869
Ohio	214	9	111	11	135	25	684	11	98	67	772	173	2,941
Wisconsin	141	2	16	6	40	14	293	6	45	14	116	104	1,616
CENSUS DIVISION 5, EAST SOUTH CENTRAL	492	9	69	26	300	44	693	21	149	99	941	316	5,044
Alabama	119	3	25	3	28	9	182	5	41	30	301	83	1,265
Kentucky	117	2	8	8	59	11	164	4	29	21	203	80	1,059
Mississippi	110	1	16	5	64	11	130	4	16	27	171	53	741
Tennessee	146	3	20	10	149	13	217	8	63	21	266	100	1,979
CENSUS DIVISION 6, WEST NORTH CENTRAL	810	14	127	40	394	59	852	32	278	92	790	475	5,507
Iowa	134	3	28	4	46	11	108	5	32	17	126	95	926
Kansas	147	2	20	5	45	8	119	4	27	8	99	65	544
Minnesota	158	3	40	12	115	10	161	7	81	19	163	93	1,052
Missouri	159	5	37	13	141	14	277	8	85	22	256	118	2,091
Nebraska	91	0	0	1	9	7	113	3	23	13	76	44	457
North Dakota	55	0	0	4	32	6	49	2	12	5	34	31	258
South Dakota	66	1	2	1	6	3	25	3	18	8	36	29	179
CENSUS DIVISION 7, WEST SOUTH CENTRAL	862	16	247	63	836	107	1,645	46	405	115	1,102	528	7,100
Arkansas	91	1	14	4	74	7	128	2	20	10	90	64	1,016
Louisiana	146	3	38	8	71	29	372	11	86	13	123	92	1,018
Oklahoma	112	3	46	4	38	12	175	3	23	20	169	65	694
Texas	513	9	149	47	653	59	970	30	276	72	720	307	4,372
CENSUS DIVISION 8, MOUNTAIN	422	9	93	21	233	38	720	22	199	48	497	272	3,079
Arizona	80	2	29	3	42	5	163	5	54	14	185	54	862
Colorado	82	4	29	7	86	13	206	4	36	12	105	61	712
Idaho	45	0	0	0	0	4	54	3	11	7	40	29	227
Montana	58	0	0	2	23	4	47	1	4	2	11	36	279
Nevada	23	1	12	1	3	4	109	4	40	5	81	16	249
New Mexico	55	1	10	3	26	2	30	2	14	3	29	27	314
Utah	49	1	13	3	41	6	111	2	35	4	42	25	298
Wyoming	30	0	0	2	12	0	0	1	5	1	4	24	138
CENSUS DIVISION 9, PACIFIC	642	17	186	44	541	126	1,785	47	444	140	1,413	506	8,405
Alaska	21	1	7	4	30	2	44	2	13	4	25	13	81
California	436	13	135	26	374	106	1,413	37	363	112	1,132	342	6,286
Hawaii	20	0	0	2	36	3	47	1	6	3	23	13	212
Oregon	68	1	12	4	33	5	106	3	20	8	90	62	729
Washington	97	2	32	8	68	10	175	4	42	13	143	76	1,097

(continued on next page)

Table

13B (Continued)

Hospitals, Units, and Beds, by Inpatient Service Area in U.S. Census Divisions and States

These data include hospitals, units, and beds as reported by hospitals responding to Section D, Beds and Utilization by Inpatient Service, of the 1990 AHA Annual Survey, beginning on page 242. A difference may exist between the total number of hospitals reporting for a particular classification and the sum of the specific hospital service components of that classification because the number of total reporting hospitals includes specialty service hospitals, which do not fall into any of the specific hospital service components.

CLASSIFICATION	HOSPITALS REPORTING	LONG-TERM CARE				PSYCHIATRIC				MENTAL RETARDATION			
		SKILLED NURSING		OTHER		HOSPITALS		UNITS		HOSPITALS		UNITS	
		Units	Beds	Units	Beds	Number	Beds	Number	Beds	Number	Beds	Number	Beds
UNITED STATES	6,105	1,251	70,985	629	40,236	557	105,020	1,602	61,704	12	6,042	37	3,404
CENSUS DIVISION 1, NEW ENGLAND	315	32	1,863	30	2,220	42	6,197	108	2,939	0	0	1	86
Connecticut	60	4	507	5	501	15	2,208	25	698	0	0	0	0
Maine	42	10	227	7	330	2	374	11	302	0	0	0	0
Massachusetts	140	8	769	7	684	16	2,766	50	1,518	0	0	1	86
New Hampshire	36	6	212	6	433	4	376	11	206	0	0	0	0
Rhode Island	19	0	0	1	34	3	353	5	120	0	0	0	0
Vermont	18	4	148	4	238	2	120	6	95	0	0	0	0
CENSUS DIVISION 2, MIDDLE ATLANTIC	681	151	14,318	68	6,700	73	25,169	243	11,584	1	138	1	24
New Jersey	114	17	2,695	7	514	10	3,651	51	2,391	0	0	0	0
New York	288	73	7,917	30	3,315	34	13,582	95	6,169	0	0	1	24
Pennsylvania	279	61	3,706	31	2,871	29	7,936	97	3,024	1	138	0	0
CENSUS DIVISION 3, SOUTH ATLANTIC	963	155	10,135	90	5,281	107	21,019	263	9,992	2	2,192	4	777
Delaware	13	1	60	3	134	3	446	5	105	0	0	0	0
District of Columbia	16	1	120	2	50	2	1,512	8	336	0	0	0	0
Florida	260	20	1,841	14	706	32	5,684	62	2,903	0	0	0	0
Georgia	188	31	3,494	9	820	21	2,458	36	1,417	0	0	3	699
Maryland	78	11	776	7	280	13	2,978	35	1,248	0	0	0	0
North Carolina	135	35	1,367	18	838	10	3,316	47	1,543	1	906	1	78
South Carolina	84	16	788	3	144	6	1,176	19	555	0	0	0	0
Virginia	124	26	1,097	25	1,924	17	3,045	39	1,535	1	1,286	0	0
West Virginia	65	14	592	9	385	3	404	12	350	0	0	0	0
CENSUS DIVISION 4, EAST NORTH CENTRAL	918	195	11,961	85	5,323	80	16,077	309	12,134	1	76	17	1,376
Illinois	231	74	3,704	23	1,361	18	4,115	87	4,109	0	0	6	618
Indiana	131	24	751	17	592	14	2,541	38	1,459	0	0	5	358
Michigan	201	32	2,432	20	1,044	19	4,029	67	2,679	0	0	2	329
Ohio	214	30	2,164	11	1,345	19	3,828	78	2,871	1	76	4	71
Wisconsin	141	35	2,910	14	981	10	1,564	39	1,016	0	0	0	0
CENSUS DIVISION 5, EAST SOUTH CENTRAL	492	81	4,039	56	3,778	33	6,171	117	4,155	0	0	2	92
Alabama	119	15	1,317	12	961	7	1,949	31	1,200	0	0	1	44
Kentucky	117	24	607	13	302	9	1,427	28	804	0	0	1	48
Mississippi	110	24	1,267	10	684	6	686	13	650	0	0	0	0
Tennessee	146	18	848	21	1,831	11	2,109	45	1,501	0	0	0	0
CENSUS DIVISION 6, WEST NORTH CENTRAL	810	219	10,172	128	5,972	43	7,288	163	6,753	5	2,301	5	813
Iowa	134	29	820	33	1,538	6	794	30	1,085	2	974	0	0
Kansas	147	30	642	29	1,306	7	1,445	22	918	2	799	0	0
Minnesota	158	67	4,657	13	528	10	2,031	27	1,257	1	528	5	813
Missouri	159	49	1,513	18	815	15	2,151	57	2,592	0	0	0	0
Nebraska	91	19	1,091	14	673	3	565	12	381	0	0	0	0
North Dakota	55	13	869	5	338	1	242	8	221	0	0	0	0
South Dakota	66	12	580	16	774	1	60	7	299	0	0	0	0
CENSUS DIVISION 7, WEST SOUTH CENTRAL	862	151	4,226	70	3,544	95	10,558	151	5,592	0	0	4	173
Arkansas	91	21	924	5	216	4	243	13	501	0	0	0	0
Louisiana	146	37	885	13	395	19	1,838	26	817	0	0	0	0
Oklahoma	112	15	242	7	202	9	1,009	20	779	0	0	0	0
Texas	513	78	2,175	45	2,731	63	7,468	92	3,495	0	0	4	173
CENSUS DIVISION 8, MOUNTAIN	422	111	4,438	44	2,510	41	4,540	75	2,079	2	547	0	0
Arizona	80	16	720	5	341	12	1,198	12	388	0	0	0	0
Colorado	82	21	1,016	12	887	8	1,407	19	626	0	0	0	0
Idaho	45	16	623	2	18	2	159	5	126	1	202	0	0
Montana	58	31	1,290	3	136	1	22	6	146	0	0	0	0
Nevada	23	6	157	4	71	2	156	4	79	0	0	0	0
New Mexico	55	6	136	6	602	8	677	9	225	1	345	0	0
Utah	49	5	87	6	150	6	614	15	415	0	0	0	0
Wyoming	30	10	409	6	305	2	307	5	74	0	0	0	0
CENSUS DIVISION 9, PACIFIC	642	156	9,833	58	4,908	43	8,001	173	6,476	1	788	3	63
Alaska	21	2	45	5	76	2	194	5	54	0	0	0	0
California	436	115	8,185	29	3,562	36	5,653	117	4,876	1	788	2	55
Hawaii	20	12	362	7	499	1	205	7	226	0	0	1	8
Oregon	68	11	598	9	552	2	676	18	491	0	0	0	0
Washington	97	16	643	8	219	2	1,273	26	829	0	0	0	0

CLASSIFICATION	HOSPITALS REPORTING	ALCOHOLISM/ CHEMICAL DEPENDENCY				OTHER				REHABILITATION			
		HOSPITALS		UNITS		HOSPITALS		UNITS		HOSPITALS		UNITS	
		Number	Beds	Number	Beds	Number	Beds	Number	Beds	Number	Beds	Number	Beds
UNITED STATES	6,105	55	3,770	1,169	30,309	28	5,250	620	20,089	128	9,861	781	19,079
CENSUS DIVISION 1, NEW ENGLAND	315	2	226	45	1,147	15	3,210	42	2,096	11	1,312	41	847
Connecticut	60	0	0	10	235	2	318	14	501	1	101	14	240
Maine	42	0	0	7	209	0	0	1	21	0	0	5	82
Massachusetts	140	0	0	17	479	12	2,618	24	1,291	9	1,109	10	288
New Hampshire	36	2	226	7	129	0	0	0	0	1	102	3	64
Rhode Island	19	0	0	2	46	1	274	2	273	0	0	6	111
Vermont	18	0	0	2	49	0	0	1	10	0	0	3	62
CENSUS DIVISION 2, MIDDLE ATLANTIC	681	11	1,100	122	3,206	3	476	83	3,661	27	2,500	120	3,216
New Jersey	114	0	0	15	413	0	0	11	334	6	592	11	251
New York	288	5	497	59	1,864	3	476	51	2,894	4	401	59	1,860
Pennsylvania	279	6	603	48	929	0	0	21	433	17	1,507	50	1,105
CENSUS DIVISION 3, SOUTH ATLANTIC	963	14	870	173	4,139	4	380	96	2,871	23	1,497	87	2,339
Delaware	13	0	0	1	12	0	0	0	0	0	0	3	68
District of Columbia	16	0	0	5	156	1	80	2	84	1	160	2	28
Florida	260	5	309	47	1,017	0	0	35	1,091	8	511	23	674
Georgia	188	2	106	36	1,020	0	0	12	352	3	203	15	320
Maryland	78	1	88	22	416	2	241	17	720	1	135	10	304
North Carolina	135	2	174	15	375	0	0	8	183	3	224	11	426
South Carolina	84	3	123	7	212	0	0	5	69	2	64	4	80
Virginia	124	1	70	30	684	1	59	12	313	2	80	16	375
West Virginia	65	0	0	10	247	0	0	5	59	3	120	3	64
CENSUS DIVISION 4, EAST NORTH CENTRAL	918	12	747	238	6,253	2	711	132	3,672	15	1,185	162	3,777
Illinois	231	2	126	62	1,639	1	679	38	1,133	3	353	41	1,030
Indiana	131	2	152	37	1,060	1	32	19	348	1	60	23	572
Michigan	201	2	116	46	1,253	0	0	17	457	6	362	33	705
Ohio	214	2	208	59	1,561	0	0	27	719	4	314	39	951
Wisconsin	141	4	145	34	740	0	0	31	1,015	1	96	26	519
CENSUS DIVISION 5, EAST SOUTH CENTRAL	492	2	144	96	2,253	1	41	40	2,402	8	614	39	1,172
Alabama	119	2	144	27	518	0	0	13	411	3	220	9	262
Kentucky	117	0	0	14	353	0	0	6	472	2	165	6	118
Mississippi	110	0	0	15	448	0	0	12	1,257	1	104	5	110
Tennessee	146	0	0	40	934	1	41	9	262	2	125	19	682
CENSUS DIVISION 6, WEST NORTH CENTRAL	810	1	38	141	4,174	0	0	48	1,076	9	490	75	1,636
Iowa	134	0	0	29	793	0	0	8	294	0	0	8	241
Kansas	147	0	0	23	572	0	0	4	29	2	126	12	196
Minnesota	158	0	0	32	1,228	0	0	13	258	0	0	11	308
Missouri	159	0	0	37	1,000	0	0	15	404	3	124	33	665
Nebraska	91	0	0	12	302	0	0	3	14	1	51	2	80
North Dakota	55	1	38	5	206	0	0	1	50	1	42	5	77
South Dakota	66	0	0	3	73	0	0	4	27	2	147	4	69
CENSUS DIVISION 7, WEST SOUTH CENTRAL	862	5	231	173	4,535	2	390	53	999	25	1,672	94	2,239
Arkansas	91	0	0	10	327	0	0	7	60	4	241	5	102
Louisiana	146	1	28	34	821	1	366	11	136	3	301	17	403
Oklahoma	112	0	0	21	480	0	0	3	116	1	26	14	360
Texas	513	4	203	108	2,907	1	24	32	687	17	1,104	58	1,374
CENSUS DIVISION 8, MOUNTAIN	422	3	90	52	1,229	0	0	31	619	7	463	52	1,062
Arizona	80	0	0	9	215	0	0	7	114	0	0	12	267
Colorado	82	0	0	13	297	0	0	13	166	3	258	14	242
Idaho	45	1	22	3	61	0	0	2	13	1	50	5	80
Montana	58	0	0	6	124	0	0	2	4	0	0	5	98
Nevada	23	1	50	5	110	0	0	2	243	0	0	5	124
New Mexico	55	1	18	4	113	0	0	2	23	2	75	2	36
Utah	49	0	0	8	184	0	0	3	56	1	80	7	189
Wyoming	30	0	0	4	125	0	0	0	0	0	0	2	26
CENSUS DIVISION 9, PACIFIC	642	5	324	129	3,373	1	42	95	2,693	3	128	111	2,791
Alaska	21	0	0	4	53	0	0	2	4	0	0	1	16
California	436	3	178	91	2,417	1	42	68	1,997	3	128	77	2,089
Hawaii	20	0	0	1	20	0	0	3	51	0	0	0	0
Oregon	68	0	0	12	259	0	0	5	137	0	0	11	260
Washington	97	2	146	21	624	0	0	17	504	0	0	22	426

Table

14

Table		Page
14	**Utilization, Personnel, and Finances in U.S. AHA Nonregistered Hospitals**	240

Notes

Data in table 14 represent U.S. hospitals that did not have AHA registration status but were open and operating as of October 1, 1990. Hospitals within this group fall into three major classifications: nonregistered osteopathic hospitals, provisional AHA members, and nonregistered, nonmember hospitals. These hospitals have been identified primarily through American Hospital Association files, the files of the National Center for Health Statistics, and various directories of the hospital industry. Data for these hospitals are not included in tables 1 through 13.

Table
14

Utilization, Personnel, and Finances in U.S. Nonregistered Hospitals

The data for nonregistered hospitals are not included in any other table in this publication.

CLASSIFICATION	HOSPITALS	BEDS	ADMISSIONS	INPATIENT DAYS	ADJUSTED PATIENT DAYS	OCCUPANCY, percent	AVERAGE DAILY CENSUS	ADJUSTED AVERAGE DAILY CENSUS	AVERAGE STAY, days	SURGICAL OPERATIONS	OUTPATIENT VISITS			NEWBORNS	
											Emergency	Other	Total	Bassinets	Births
U.S. NONREGISTERED	157	11,742	148,116	2,834,791		66.3	7,790			54,099	313,556	953,053	1,266,609	154	4,954
6-24 beds	27	490	11,718	86,211		48.8	239			5,455	49,584	217,467	267,051	21	811
25-49	45	1,584	24,463	295,209		51.1	809			5,080	79,282	262,525	341,807	22	422
50-99	55	3,988	41,377	912,063		63.2	2,520			10,426	62,382	192,048	254,430	39	1,517
100-199	21	2,829	41,604	713,777		69.1	1,956			16,548	86,804	213,706	300,510	56	1,687
200-299	6	1,486	26,233	389,791		71.7	1,066			16,539	35,285	66,499	101,784	16	517
300-399	1	338	190	106,061		86.1	291			51	219	808	1,027	0	0
400-499	1	496	1,010	150,597		83.3	413			0	0	0	0	0	0
500 or more	1	531	1,521	181,082		93.4	496			0	0	0	0	0	0
Psychiatric	86	6,661	56,607	1,719,524		70.7	4,712			75	15,742	352,039	367,781	12	0
Hospitals	83	6,073	56,295	1,532,376		69.1	4,199			0	15,418	350,844	366,262	12	0
Institutions for mentally retarded	3	588	312	187,148		87.2	513			75	324	1,195	1,519	0	0
General	51	2,832	70,092	510,107		50.1	1,420			40,639	283,726	517,773	801,499	142	4,954
Hospitals	51	2,832	70,092	510,107		50.1	1,420			40,639	283,726	517,773	801,499	142	4,954
Hospital units of institutions	0	0	0	0		00.0	0			0	0	0	0	0	0
TB and other respiratory diseases	0	0	0	0		00.0	0			0	0	0	0	0	0
Obstetrics and gynecology	2	32	739	3,104		25.0	8			1,466	8,055	3,957	12,012	0	0
Eye, ear, nose, and throat	0	0	0	0		00.0	0			0	0	0	0	0	0
Rehabilitation	8	801	4,640	204,687		70.0	561			0	611	45,304	45,915	0	0
Orthopedic	1	88	466	25,412		79.5	70			52	1,701	9,171	10,872	0	0
Chronic disease	2	290	11,388	75,189		71.0	206			10,238	0	3,625	3,625	0	0
All other	7	1,038	4,184	296,768		78.3	813			1,629	3,721	21,184	24,905	0	0
Federal	2	258	12,927	64,967		69.0	178			11,594	21,351	99,591	120,942	6	561
Psychiatric	0	0	0	0		00.0	0			0	0	0	0	0	0
General and other special	2	258	12,927	64,967		69.0	178			11,594	21,351	99,591	120,942	6	561
Nonfederal	155	11,484	135,189	2,769,824		66.3	7,612			42,505	292,205	853,462	1,145,667	148	4,393
Psychiatric	86	6,661	56,607	1,719,524		70.7	4,712			75	15,742	352,039	367,781	12	0
Hospitals	83	6,073	56,295	1,532,376		69.1	4,199			0	15,418	350,844	366,262	12	0
Institutions for mentally retarded	3	588	312	187,148		87.2	513			75	324	1,195	1,519	0	0
TB and other respiratory diseases	0	0	0	0		00.0	0			0	0	0	0	0	0
Long-term general and other special	11	1,588	5,533	454,788		78.6	1,248			283	5,421	47,004	52,425	0	0
Short-term general and other special	58	3,235	73,049	595,512		51.1	1,652			42,147	271,042	454,419	725,461	136	4,393
Hospital units of institutions	0	0	0	0		00.0	0			0	0	0	0	0	0
Community hospitals*	58	3,235	73,049	595,512	845,153	51.1	1,652	2,347	8.2	42,147	271,042	454,419	725,461	136	4,393
6-24 beds	15	259	6,833	33,413	73,257	35.5	92	204	4.9	4,099	26,325	21,958	48,283	15	250
25-49	19	633	13,511	82,689	122,626	35.5	225	334	6.1	5,080	69,934	97,897	167,831	22	422
50-99	16	1,157	19,982	219,556	289,262	53.8	622	824	11.0	10,303	55,416	95,095	150,511	39	1,517
100-199	7	982	25,977	216,338	292,939	60.5	594	801	8.3	16,524	85,795	185,590	271,385	44	1,687
200-299	1	204	6,746	43,516	67,069	58.3	119	184	6.5	6,141	33,572	53,879	87,451	16	517
300-399	0	0	0	0	0	00.0	0	0	0.0	0	0	0	0	0	0
400-499	0	0	0	0	0	00.0	0	0	0.0	0	0	0	0	0	0
500 or more	0	0	0	0	0	00.0	0	0	0.0	0	0	0	0	0	0
Nongovernment not-for-profit	20	1,628	37,868	317,766	457,277	54.9	893	1,284	8.4	24,760	144,649	301,561	446,210	49	2,193
Investor-owned (for-profit)	22	888	21,214	146,905	208,744	45.3	402	573	6.9	12,449	77,951	89,131	167,082	44	1,393
State and local government	16	719	13,967	130,841	179,132	49.7	357	490	9.4	4,938	48,442	63,727	112,169	43	807

Table 14 (Continued)

CLASSIFICATION	FULL-TIME EQUIVALENT PERSONNEL: Physicians and Dentists	Registered Nurses	Licensed Practical Nurses	Other Salaried Personnel	Total Personnel	FULL-TIME EQUIVALENT TRAINEES: Medical and Dental Residents	Other Trainees	Total Trainees	EXPENSES — LABOR: Payroll (in thousands)	Employee Benefits (in thousands)	Total (in thousands)	Percent of Total	EXPENSES — TOTAL: Amount (in thousands)	Adjusted, per Admission	Adjusted, per Inpatient Day
U.S. NONREGISTERED	412	3,681	1,375	19,786	25,254	184	32	216	$ 635,799	$ 119,337	$ 755,136	59.3	$ 1,274,292		
6-24 beds	35	189	97	1,176	1,497	0	0	0	30,476	6,190	36,667	57.1	64,165		
25-49	43	437	223	2,598	3,301	40	0	40	71,235	14,516	85,751	55.9	153,497		
50-99	74	1,261	392	5,968	7,695	13	5	18	192,407	39,979	232,386	54.3	427,736		
100-199	58	1,116	289	4,353	5,816	7	8	15	155,389	34,856	190,246	57.7	330,001		
200-299	171	551	219	3,036	3,977	124	1	125	118,845	19,958	138,802	66.7	208,248		
300-399	6	27	27	679	739	0	18	18	15,922	3,831	19,753	80.7	24,483		
400-499	8	44	87	962	1,101	0	0	0	21,539	6	21,545	87.8	24,526		
500 or more	17	56	41	1,014	1,128	0	0	0	29,986	0	29,986	72.0	41,636		
Psychiatric	193	1,530	546	9,858	12,127	55	29	84	326,997	65,759	392,756	62.0	632,971		
Hospitals	183	1,457	482	8,680	10,802	55	3	58	300,755	59,083	359,838	60.8	592,319		
Institutions for mentally retarded	10	73	64	1,178	1,325	0	26	26	26,242	6,676	32,918	81.0	40,652		
General	63	1,511	494	5,271	7,339	68	2	70	162,549	33,215	195,764	50.8	385,687		
Hospitals	63	1,511	494	5,271	7,339	68	2	70	162,549	33,215	195,764	50.8	385,687		
Hospital units of institutions	0	0	0	0	0	0	0	0	0	0	0	0.0	0		
TB and other respiratory diseases	0	0	0	0	0	0	0	0	0	0	0	0.0	0		
Obstetrics and gynecology	0	11	7	46	64	0	0	0	1,490	278	1,768	52.0	3,398		
Eye, ear, nose, and throat	0	0	0	0	0	0	0	0	0	0	0	0.0	0		
Rehabilitation	18	234	95	1.450	1,797	6	0	6	38,716	8,206	46,923	60.1	78,064		
Orthopedic	3	30	13	221	267	0	0	0	7,467	1,620	9,087	63.6	14,298		
Chronic disease	114	199	75	1.065	1,453	53	1	54	46,802	3,302	50,104	63.9	78,425		
All other	21	166	145	1.875	2,207	2	0	2	51,779	6,956	58,735	72.1	81,448		
Federal	128	227	66	1 159	1,580	53	1	54	44,244	3,248	47,492	64.3	73,804		
Psychiatric	0	0	0	0	0	0	0	0	0	0	0	0.0	0		
General and other special	128	227	66	1 159	1,580	53	1	54	44,244	3,248	47,492	64.3	73,804		
Nonfederal	284	3,454	1,309	18 627	23,674	131	31	162	591,555	116,089	707,644	58.9	1,200,487		
Psychiatric	193	1,530	546	9 858	12,127	55	29	84	326,997	65,759	392,756	62.0	632,971		
Hospitals	183	1,457	482	8 680	10,802	55	3	58	300,755	59,083	359,838	60.8	592,319		
Institutions for mentally retarded	10	73	64	1 178	1,325	0	26	26	26,242	6,676	32,918	81.0	40,652		
TB and other respiratory diseases	0	0	0	0	0	0	0	0	0	0	0	0.0	0		
Long-term general and other special	32	334	223	2 926	3,515	2	0	2	83,628	14,845	98,473	69.2	142,383		
Short-term general and other special	59	1,590	540	5 843	8,032	74	2	76	180,931	35,484	216,415	50.9	425,134		
Hospital units of institutions	0	0	0	0	0	0	0	0	0	0	0	0.0	0		
Community hospitals*	59	1,590	540	5 843	8,032	74	2	76	180,931	35,484	216,415	50.9	425,134	$3,864.26	$503.03
6-24 beds	9	88	63	397	557	0	0	0	11,914	2,031	13,945	50.6	27,575	1,767.60	376.41
25-49	4	194	151	979	1,328	0	0	0	22,104	4,053	26,158	49.5	52,889	2,581.44	431.30
50-99	13	479	141	1 927	2,560	6	2	8	53,714	10,159	63,873	47.2	135,304	4,837.64	467.76
100-199	15	647	125	1 864	2,651	3	0	3	66,442	13,922	80,364	52.9	152,044	4,275.33	519.03
200-299	18	182	60	676	936	65	0	65	26,757	5,319	32,076	56.0	57,323	5,513.45	854.69
300-399	0	0	0	0	0	0	0	0	0	0	0	0.0	0	0.00	0.00
400-499	0	0	0	0	0	0	0	0	0	0	0	0.0	0	0.00	0.00
500 or more	0	0	0	0	0	0	0	0	0	0	0	0.0	0	0.00	0.00
Nongovernment not-for-profit	42	937	263	3 481	4,723	68	0	68	114,100	22,512	136,612	52.1	262,113	4,721.82	573.20
Investor-owned (for-profit)	5	371	139	1 383	1,898	6	0	6	43,680	8,800	52,481	46.5	112,853	3,273.19	540.63
State and local government	12	282	138	979	1,411	0	2	2	23,150	4,172	27,322	54.5	50,168	2,504.91	280.06

American
Hospital
Association

1990 Annual Survey of Hospital

Please return to:
American Hospital Association
840 North Lake Shore Drive
Chicago, Illinois 60611

Please return by:

ENERAL INSTRUCTIONS

vo copies of the Annual Survey questionnaire are enclosed. Please check and correct any label information as printed on e front of the survey. Return one completed copy in the enclosed return envelope to the American Hospital Association and tain the second completed copy in your files for reference. Also, please forward a photocopy of the completed iestionnaire to your state hospital association.

equested return date is listed on the cover page, but if additional time is necessary to complete the survey, please notify us calling 312/280-6463.

eport utilization and financial information for a full 12-month period, preferably the period ending September 30, 1990. **If u prefer, you may use your fiscal year as the reporting period.**

eport personnel figures according to the number of full-time, part-time, and trainees on payroll as of September 30, 1990, gardless of the reporting period used. For hospitals that operate a nursing home-type unit, the nursing home/unit staff embers should not be included in the personnel occupational categories. There is a separate question that requests the tal number of full-time and part-time nursing home/unit staff.

ake an entry for every item on the form. Enter "NA" only if data is not available. Enter "0" if zero is appropriate.

assistance is needed, please contact the American Hospital Association Annual Survey staff at 312/280-6463. You may so contact your state hospital association or other state agency if so directed by survey return instructions.

1990 Annual Survey of Hospitals

AMERICAN HOSPITAL ASSOCIATION
PLEASE REFER TO THE INSTRUCTIONS AND DEFINITIONS

A. REPORTING PERIOD

Report data for a full 12-month period, preferably 10/01/89 through 09/30/90 (365 days). (Use the same reporting period for data reported in sections D, E and F.)

1. Reporting Period used (beginning and ending date) .... ____/____/____ to ____/____/____
   Month Day Year Month Day Year

2 a. Were you in operation 12 full months at the end of your reporting period? ....YES ☐ NO ☐

b. Number of days open during reporting period .... ☐

3. Indicate the beginning of your current fiscal year .... ____/____/____
   Month Day Year

B. ORGANIZATIONAL STRUCTURE

1. CONTROL

Indicate the type of organization that is responsible for establishing policy for overall operation of your hospital. CHECK ONLY ONE.

Government, nonfederal
- ☐ 12 State
- ☐ 13 County
- ☐ 14 City
- ☐ 15 City–County
- ☐ 16 Hospital district or authority

Nongovernment, not-for-profit (NFP)
- ☐ 21 Church-operated
- ☐ 23 Other not-for-profit (including NFP Corporation)

Investor-owned, for-profit
- ☐ 31 Individual
- ☐ 32 Partnership
- ☐ 33 Corporation

Government, federal
- ☐ 41 Air Force
- ☐ 42 Army
- ☐ 43 Navy
- ☐ 44 Public Health Service
- ☐ 45 Veterans Administration
- ☐ 46 Federal other than 41–45 or 47–48
- ☐ 47 PHS Indian Service
- ☐ 48 Department of Justice

2. SERVICE

Indicate the ONE category that BEST describes your hospital or the type of service it provides to the MAJORITY of admissions:

- ☐ 10 General medical and surgical
- ☐ 11 Hospital unit of an institution (prison hospital, college infirmary)
- ☐ 12 Hospital unit within an institution for the mentally retarded
- ☐ 22 Psychiatric
- ☐ 33 Tuberculosis and other respiratory diseases
- ☐ 44 Obstetrics and gynecology
- ☐ 45 Eye, ear, nose, and throat
- ☐ 46 Rehabilitation
- ☐ 47 Orthopedic
- ☐ 48 Chronic disease
- ☐ 62 Institution for mentally retarded
- ☐ 82 Alcoholism and other chemical dependency
- ☐ 49 Other-specify treatment area: ____________________

3. OTHER

a. Does your hospital restrict admissions primarily to children? ....YES ☐ NO ☐

b. Is your hospital primarily osteopathic? ....YES ☐ NO ☐

c. Does your hospital have a formal written contract with:

(1) Health maintenance organization (HMO) that specifies the obligations of each party. ....YES ☐ NO ☐

(2) Preferred provider organization (PPO) that specifies the obligations of each party ....YES ☐ NO ☐

d. Is the hospital part of a health care system? If yes, please provide the name, city and state of the system headquarters: ......YES ☐ NO ☐

Name: ______________________________

City: ______________________ State: ________

e. Is the hospital a division or subsidiary of a holding company? ....YES ☐ NO ☐

f. Does the hospital itself operate subsidiary corporations? ....YES ☐ NO ☐

g. Is the hospital contract managed? If yes, please provide the name, city and state of the organization that manages the hospital: .....YES ☐ NO ☐

Name: ______________________________

City: ______________________ State: ________

h. Is the hospital a member of an alliance? If yes, please provide the name(s), city, and state of the alliance headquarters: ....YES ☐ NO ☐

Name: ______________________________ ______________________________

City: ______________________ State: ________ ______________________State: ________

AMERICAN HOSPITAL ASSOCIATION

INSTRUCTIONS AND DEFINITIONS FOR ANNUAL SURVEY OF HOSPITALS 1990

HOSPITAL. For purposes of this survey, a hospital is defined as the organization or corporate entity licensed or registered as a hospital by a state to provide diagnostic and therapeutic patient services for a variety of medical conditions, both surgical and nonsurgical.

SECTION A
REPORTING PERIOD
Instructions

Record the beginning and ending dates of the reporting period in a six-digit number: for example, January 1, 1990, should be shown as 01/01/90. Number of days should equal the time span between the two dates that the hospital was open. If you are reporting for less than 365 days, utilization and finances should be presented for days reported only.

SECTION B
ORGANIZATIONAL STRUCTURE
Instructions and Definitions

1. CONTROL

Check the box to the left of the type of organization that is responsible for establishing policy for overall operation of the hospital.

Government, nonfederal.

State. Controlled by an agency of state government.
County. Controlled by an agency of county government.
City. Controlled by an agency of municipal government.
City-County. Controlled jointly by agencies of municipal and county governments.
Hospital district or authority. Controlled by a political subdivision of a state, county or city created solely for the purpose of establishing and maintaining medical care or health-related care institutions.

Nongovernment, not-for-profit. Hospitals controlled by not-for-profit organizations, including religious organizations (Catholic hospitals, for example), community hospitals, cooperative hospitals, hospitals operated by fraternal societies, and so forth.

Investor-owned, for-profit. Hospitals controlled on a for-profit basis by an individual, partnership, or a profit-making corporation.

Government, federal. Hospitals controlled by an agency or department of the federal government.

2. SERVICE

Indicate the ONE category that best describes the type of service that your hospital provides to the majority of admissions.

General medical and surgical. Provides diagnostic and therapeutic services to patients for a variety of medical conditions, both surgical and nonsurgical.

Hospital unit of an institution. Provides diagnostic and therapeutic services to patients in an institution.

Hospital unit within an institution for the mentally retarded. Provides diagnostic and therapeutic services to patients in an institution for the mentally retarded.

Psychiatric. Provides diagnostic and therapeutic services to patients with mental or emotional disorders.

Tuberculosis and other respiratory diseases. Provides medical care and rehabilitative services to patients for whom the primary diagnosis is tuberculosis or other respiratory diseases.

Obstetrics and gynecology. Provides medical and surgical treatment to pregnant women and to mothers following delivery. Also provides diagnostic and therapeutic services to women with diseases or disorders of the reproductive organs.

Eye, ear, nose and throat. Provides diagnosis and treatment of diseases and injuries of the eyes, ears, nose, and throat.

Rehabilitation. Provides a comprehensive array of restoration services for the disabled and all support services necessary to help them attain their maximum functional capacity.

Orthopedic. Provides corrective treatment of deformities, diseases, and ailments of the locomotive apparatus, especially affecting the limbs, bones, muscles, and joints.

Chronic disease. Provides medical and skilled nursing services to patients with long-term illnesses who are not in an acute phase, but who require an intensity of services not available in nursing homes.

Institution for the mentally retarded. Provides health related care on a regular basis to patients with psychiatric or developmental impairment who cannot be treated in a skilled nursing unit.

Alcoholism and other chemical dependency. Provides diagnosis and therapeutic services to patients with alcoholism or other drug dependencies.

3. OTHER

b. **Osteopathic.** Osteopathic medicine is a medical practice based on a theory that diseases are due chiefly to a loss of structural integrity which can be restored by manipulation of the neuro-muscular and skeletal system, supplemented by therapeutic measures (as use of medicine or surgery).

c. (1) **Health maintenance organization (HMO).** An organization that has management responsibility for providing comprehensive health care services on a prepayment basis to voluntarily enrolled persons within a designated population.

(2) **Preferred provider organization (PPO).** A formal arrangement whereby the services of a select panel of health care providers are marketed on the basis of cost efficiency to purchasers, for which payment is on a prospectively negotiated, predominately fee-for-service basis, and in which subscribers have an economic incentive to use the select panel.

d. **Healthcare system.** A corporate body that may own and/or manage health provider facilities or health related subsidiaries as well as non-health related facilities including freestanding facilities and/or subsidiary corporations.

e. **Holding company.** Any company, incorporated or unincorporated, that is in a position to control or materially influence the management of one or more other companies by virtue of its ownership of securities and/or its right to appoint directors in the other company or companies.

f. **Subsidiary.** A company that is wholly controlled by another or one that is more than 50% owned by another organization.

g. **Contract managed.** General day to day management of an entire organization by another organization under a formal contract. Managing organization reports directly to the board of trustees or owners of the managed organization; managed organization retains total legal responsibility and ownership of the facility's assets and liabilities.

h. **Alliance.** A formal organization, usually owned by shareholder/members that works on behalf of its individual members in the provision of services and products and in the promotion of activities and ventures. Examples of alliances: Voluntary Hospitals of America, Consolidated Catholic Health Care and American HealthCare System.

C. FACILITIES AND SERVICES

For each service or facility listed below, please check all those provided by your hospital as of the last day of the reporting period. If a service is not maintained in the hospital but is available through a FORMAL CONTRACTUAL ARRANGEMENT with another hospital or provider (include joint ventures), please check column (2). **If neither column (1) nor (2) applies for a particular service, please leave it blank.** Facilities and services added to the survey since last year are underlined.

	(1) Provided by the Hospital	(2) Provided under Arrangement with Another Hospital or Provider
1. Acquired immune–deficiency syndrome (AIDS) services:		
a. General inpatient care for AIDS/ARC	☐	☐
b. AIDS/ARC unit	☐	☐
c. Specialized outpatient program for AIDS/ARC	☐	☐
d. HIV testing	☐	☐
2. Alcohol/drug abuse or dependency outpatient services	☐	☐
3. Arthritis treatment center	☐	☐
4. Birthing room/Labor, delivery, recovery, postpartum room (LDRP room)	☐	☐
5. Cardiac services:		
a. Cardiac catheterization laboratory	☐	☐
b. Non-invasive cardiac assessment services	☐	☐
c. Open heart surgery	☐	☐
d. Angioplasty	☐	☐
e. Cardiac rehabilitation	☐	☐
6. Chronic obstructive pulmonary disease services	☐	☐
7. Emergency services:		
a. Emergency department	☐	☐
b. Certified trauma center	☐	☐
(1) Level of unit # ________ Source of designation: ________________		
8. Extracorporeal shock wave lithotripter (ESWL) [check one: Fixed( ) or Mobile( )]	☐	☐
9. Fitness center	☐	☐
10. Genetic counseling/screening	☐	☐
11. Geriatric services:		
a. Adult day care program	☐	☐
b. Alzheimer's diagnostic/assessment services	☐	☐
c. Comprehensive geriatric assessment	☐	☐
d. Emergency response system	☐	☐
e. Geriatric acute care unit	☐	☐
f. Geriatric clinics	☐	☐
g. Respite care	☐	☐
h. Senior membership program	☐	☐

SECTION C
FACILITIES AND SERVICES
Definitions

C. FACILITIES AND SERVICES

1a. General inpatient care for AIDS/ARC. Inpatient diagnosis and treatment for AIDS/ARC patients, but dedicated unit is not available.

1b. AIDS/ARC unit. Special unit or team designated and equipped specifically for diagnosis, treatment, continuing care planning, and counseling services for AIDS/ARC patients and their families.

1c. Specialized oupatient program for AIDS/ARC. Special outpatient program providing diagnostic, treatment, continuing care planning, and counseling for AIDS/ARC patients and their families.

1d. HIV testing. Service providing blood and laboratory testing to detect the presence of the HIV virus.

2. Alcohol/drug abuse or dependency outpatient services. Organized hospital services that provide medical care and/or rehabilitative treatment services to outpatients for whom the primary diagnosis is alcoholism or other chemical dependency.

3. Arthritis treatment center. Specifically equipped and staffed center for the diagnosis and treatment of arthritis and other joint disorders.

4. Birthing room/Labor, delivery, recovery, postpartum room (LDRP room). Combination labor and delivery unit with home like setting for parents who have completed specified childbirth courses and wish to participate jointly in the birth of their child.

5a. Cardiac catheterization laboratory. Facilities offering special diagnostic procedures for cardiac patients. Available procedures must include, but need not be limited to, introduction of a catheter into the interior of the heart by way of a vein or artery or by direct needle puncture. Procedures must be performed in a laboratory or a special procedure room.

5b. Non-invasive cardiac assessment services. Includes cardiac studies, tests and evaluations not conducted in the cardiac catherization laboratory or operating room. Non-invasive cardiac assessment services include at a minimum: echocardiography and exercise stress testing (stress EKG); and may additionally include cardiac nuclear medicine studies.

5c. Open heart surgery. Heart surgery where the chest has been opened and the blood recirculated and oxygenated with the proper equipment and the necessary staff to perform the surgery.

5d. Angioplasty. The reconstruction or restructuring of a blood vessel by operative means or by nonsurgical techniques such as balloon dilation or laser.

5e. Cardiac rehabilitation. Restorative services whereby a patient is reconditioned from a state of cardiac injury, or high risk to resume daily activities of living at an optimum level. Programs often include counselling, education and exercise. Patient instruction in self monitoring of their cardiac condition, stress management and dietary counselling are often components of these programs. Cardiac rehab services are used after open heart surgery, angioplasty, acute myocardial infarction (heart attack), and for patients identified as being at high risk for adverse cardiovascular events.

6. Chronic obstructive pulmonary disease services. Services provided for the treatment of disorders such as asthma, chronic bronchitis, and emphysema which are marked by persistant obstruction of bronchial air flow.

7a. Emergency department. Hospital facilities for the provision of unscheduled outpatient services to patients whose conditions require immediate care. **Must be available 24 hours a day.**

7b. Certified trauma center. A facility certified to provide emergency and specialized intensive care to critically ill and injured patients. **Level 1** is a regional resource trauma center, which is capable of providing total care for every aspect of injury and plays a leadership role in trauma research and education. **Level 2** is a community trauma center, which is capable of providing trauma care to all but the most severely injured patients who require highly specialized care. **Level 3** is a rural trauma hospital, which is capable of providing care to a large number of injury victims and can resusitate and stabilize more severely injured patients so that they can be transported to level 1 or 2 facilities. Source of designation should be listed on the line provided, which may include: city/county, regional, American College of Surgeons (ACS), self, etc. Please provide explanation on page 34 if necessary.

8. Extracorporeal shock wave lithotripter (ESWL). A medical device used for treating stones in the kidney or ureter. The device disintegrates kidney stones noninvasively through the transmission of acoustic shock waves directed at the stones.

9. Fitness center. Provides exercise, testing or evaluation programs and fitness activities to the community and hospital employees.

10. Genetic counseling/screening. A service equipped with adequate laboratory facilities and directed by a qualified physician to advise parents and prospective parents on potential problems in cases of genetic defects. Service provides antenatal diagnosis including amniocentesis, chorionic villi sampling, fetal blood sampling and MRI imaging. Service shall have appropriate ultrasound evaluation capacity.

11a. Adult day care program. Program providing supervision, medical and psychological care, and social activities for older adults who live at home or in another family setting, but cannot be alone or prefer to be with others during the day. May include intake assessment, health monitoring, occupational therapy, personal care, noon meal, and transportation services.

11b. Alzheimer's diagnostic/assessment services. Specially organized program to diagnose and evaluate people suspected of having Alzheimer's disease. Includes the assessment of medical, social and behavioral conditions and development of a treatment plan addressing family preferences and financial options as well as medical concerns.

11c. Comprehensive geriatric assessment. Diagnostic and evaluation services that assist in determining elderly patients' short-term and long-term needs for health care and related services. Includes the assessment of medical conditions, functional abilities, and mental health and emotional needs, and incorporates these into a treatment plan that addresses family and financial concerns as well as medical needs.

11d. Emergency response system. A program for disabled and/or homebound elderly individuals whereby subscribers have an emergency response unit attached to their telephone, linking them to the hospital emergency department and allowing them to automatically call for help by pressing a button.

11e. Geriatric acute care unit. Provides acute care to older patients in a special unit in the hospital. Care is provided by a multi–disciplinary team trained in geriatrics. The unit may also offer architectural/design modifications to accommodate the special needs of older adults.

11f. Geriatric clinics. Special medical or surgical clinics providing services targeted to older adults such as arthritis, primary geriatric and podiatric clinics.

11g. Respite care. Facilities and services that provide for short–term placement of elderly or disabled individuals to help family care-givers handle emergencies or take planned absences from home (such as vacations or hospitalization), or to allow them to shop or do errands.

11h. Senior membership program. A senior enrollment program which offers older adults service benefits such as information, claims assistance, education and senior wellness programs, and discounts for other hospital services. May or may not charge an application fee.

C. FACILITIES AND SERVICES (continued)

	(1) Provided by the Hospital	(2) Provided under Arrangement with Another Hospital or Provider
12. Health promotion:		
a. Patient education	☐	☐
b. Community health promotion	☐	☐
c. Worksite health promotion	☐	☐
13. Hemodialysis	☐	☐
14. Home health services	☐	☐
15. Hospice	☐	☐
16. Laboratory services:		
a. Histopathology	☐	☐
b. Blood bank	☐	☐
17. Long–term care services:		
a. Medicare–certified distinct–part skilled nursing unit	☐	☐
b. Other skilled nursing care	☐	☐
18. Occupational health services	☐	☐
19. Outpatient services:		
a. Hospital based outpatient care center/services	☐	☐
b. Freestanding outpatient care center	☐	☐
20. Psychiatric services:		
a. Psychiatric child/adolescent services	☐	☐
b. Psychiatric consultation–liaison services	☐	☐
c. Psychiatric education services	☐	☐
d. Psychiatric emergency services	☐	☐
e. Psychiatric geriatric services	☐	☐
f. Psychiatric outpatient services	☐	☐
g. Psychiatric partial hospitalization program	☐	☐
21. Radiation therapy:		
a. Megavoltage radiation therapy	☐	☐
b. Radioactive implants	☐	☐
c. <u>Stereotactic radiosurgery</u>	☐	☐
d. Therapeutic radioisotope facility	☐	☐
e. X–ray radiation therapy	☐	☐

C. FACILITIES AND SERVICES

22a. CT scanner. Computed tomographic scanner for head or whole body scans.

22b. Diagnostic radioisotope facility. The use of radioactive isotopes (radiopharmaceuticals) as tracers or indicators to detect an abnormal condition or disease.

22c. Magnetic resonance imaging (MRI). The use of a uniform magnetic field and radio frequencies to study tissue and structure of the body. This procedure enables the visualization of biochemical activity of the cell in vivo without the use of ionizing radiation, radioisotopic substances, or high-frequency sound.

22d. PET. PET is a nuclear medicine imaging technology which uses radioactive (positron emitting) isotopes created in a cyclotron or generator and computers to produce composite pictures of the brain and heart at work. PET Scanning produces sectional images depicting metabolic activity or blood flow rather than anatomy.

22e. SPECT. SPECT is a nuclear medicine imaging technology which combines existing technology of gamma camera imaging with computed tomographic imaging technology to provide a more precise and clear image.

22f. Ultrasound. The use of acoustic waves above the range of 20,000 cycles per second to visualize internal body structures.

23. Rehabilitation outpatient services. Outpatient program providing medical, health-related, therapy, social and/or vocational services to help disabled persons attain or retain their maximum functional capacity.

24a. Fertility counseling. A service which counsels and educates on infertility problems and includes laboratory and surgical workup and management for individuals having problems conceiving children.

24b. In vitro fertilization. Program providing for the induction of fertilization of a surgically removed ovum by donated sperm in a culture medium followed by a short incubation period. The embryo is then reimplanted in the female womb.

24c. Sterilization. A service with capacity to perform total occlusion or ligation as appropriate for women and vasectomy for men.

25a. Organized social work services. Services that are properly directed and sufficiently staffed by qualified individuals who provide assistance and counseling to patients and their families in dealing with social, emotional, and environmental problems associated with illness or disability, often in the context of financial or discharge planning coordination.

25b. Outpatient social work services. Social work services provided in ambulatory care areas.

25c. Emergency department social work services. Social work services provided to emergency department patients by social workers dedicated to the emergency department or on call.

26. Sports medicine clinic/services. Provision of diagnostic screening and assessment, clinical and rehabilitation services for the prevention and treatment of sports related injuries.

27a. Hospital auxiliary. A volunteer community organization formed to assist the institution in carrying out its purpose and to serve as a link between the institution and the community.

27b. Patient representative services. Organized hospital services providing personnel through whom patients and staff can seek solutions to institutional problems affecting the delivery of high-quality care and services.

27c. Volunteer services department. An organized hospital department responsible for coordinating the services of volunteers working within the institution.

28a. Outpatient surgery. Scheduled surgical services provided to patients who do not remain in the hospital overnight. The surgery may be performed in operating suites also used for inpatient surgery, specially designated surgical suites for outpatient surgery, or procedure rooms within an outpatient care facility.

28b. Orthopedic surgery. Surgical treatment of the skeletal system, its articulations, and associated structures.

28c. Kidney transplant. Service offering specially trained and equipped staff to perform the surgical removal of a viable kidney from either a living donor or a deceased person immediately after death, and the surgical grafting of the kidney to a suitably evaluated and prepared patient.

28d. Organ transplant (other than kidney). Service offering specially trained and equipped staff to perform the surgical removal of viable human organs from either a living or deceased person immediately after death, and the surgical grafting of the organ into a suitably evaluated and prepared patient.

28e. Tissue transplant. Service offering specially trained and equipped staff to perform the surgical removal of viable human tissue from either a living or deceased person immediately after death, and the surgical grafting of the tissue into a suitably evaluated and prepared patient.

28f. Bone marrow transplant program. Bone marrow transplants are typically performed on select cancer patients as part of their rescue treatment following extensive chemotherapy and radiation therapy. A bone marrow program involves a significant dollar investment in special facilities and trained staff for bone marrow procurement, compatibility testing, frozen storage, transplantation; as well as appropriately trained physicians, critical care nurses and lab facilities for managing the severely immunocompromised patient following completion of bone marrow transplant procedures.

29a. Occupational therapy. Facilities for the provision of occupational therapy services prescribed by physicians and administered by, or under the direction of, a qualified occupational therapist.

29b. Physical therapy. Facilities for the provision of physical therapy services prescribed by physicians and administered by, or under the direction of, a qualified physical therapist.

29c. Recreational therapy. Facilities for the provision of recreational therapy services prescribed by physicians and administered by, or under the direction of, a qualified recreational therapist.

29d. Respiratory therapy. The equipment and staff necessary for the administration of oxygen and certain potent drugs through inhalation or positive pressure.

29e. Speech therapy. Service providing evaluation and treatment to inpatients or outpatients with speech and language disorders.

30. Women's health center/services. An area set aside for coordinated education and treatment services specifically for and promoted to women as provided by this special unit. Services may or may not include obstetrics but include a range of services other than OB.

31. Health sciences library. A facility that maintains an organized collection of printed and/or other library materials, has a staff trained to provide and interpret such materials as required to meet informational or educational needs, and keeps an established schedule in which services of the staff are available to clientele.

D. BEDS AND UTILIZATION BY INPATIENT SERVICE

Account for all adult and pediatric inpatient beds set up and staffed for use at the end of the reporting period. Do not include normal newborn bassinets. List beds for a particular service area only if a unit is specifically designated for the service area. Hospitals with skilled nursing and/or other institutional care (on lines 18-21) should complete the section on page 13 for separate nursing home type unit/facility data.

	(1) Beds Set Up & Staffed on last day of the Reporting Period	(2) Total Inpatient Days for the Reporting Period
1. General medical/surgical (adult, include gynecology)	_____	_____
2. General medical/surgical (pediatric)	_____	_____
3. Obstetrics (circle unit level: 1 2 or 3, see page 12 definitions)	_____	_____
4. Other acute (Specify type: __________)	_____	_____
5. Medical/surgical intensive care (include mixed ICU/CCU)	_____	_____
6. Cardiac intensive care	_____	_____
7. Neonatal intensive care (exclude normal newborns listed on page 13)	_____	_____
8. Neonatal intermediate care (exclude normal newborns listed on page 13)	_____	_____
9. Pediatric intensive care	_____	_____
10. Burn care	_____	_____
11. Other special care	_____	_____
12. Other intensive care (Specify type: __________)	_____	_____
13. Rehabilitation	_____	_____
14. Chronic disease	_____	_____
15. Hospice	_____	_____
16. Psychiatric care	_____	_____
17. Alcoholism/drug abuse or dependency care	_____	_____
18. Mental retardation	_____	_____
19. Skilled nursing care	_____	_____
20. Intermediate care	_____	_____
21. Residential care/elderly housing	_____	_____
22. Other subacute (Specify type: __________)	_____	_____
23. TOTAL FACILITY (excluding swing bed utilization. Add lines 1 to 22)	_____	_____

24. SWING-BEDS

a. Is your hospital certified by Medicare to provide swing bed services as defined on page 12? ..... YES ☐ NO ☐

b. If YES, please report the total number of acute care beds from the above that were utilized by the hospital as swing beds. (Please do not include beds for newborn or beds for intensive care units). _____

c. Please report the number of admissions and inpatient days for the reporting period that the swing-beds (Medicare certified) were used in the provision of long-term care swing services.

	(1) Admissions	(2) Inpatient Days
(1) Skilled nursing swing bed utilization	_____	_____
(2) Intermediate care swing bed utilization	_____	_____

25. TOTAL FACILITY INPATIENT DAY TOTAL (including swing bed utilization) (Add lines 23, 24c(1) and 24c(2); This number should equal that reported on 2e, page 13) ..... _____

SECTION D
BEDS AND UTILIZATION BY INPATIENT SERVICE
Instructions and Definitions

Account for all adult and pediatric inpatient beds set up and staffed for use at the end of the reporting period. List beds for a particular service area only if a unit is specifically designated for the service area. Do not include normal newborn bassinets.

TOTAL FACILITY beds set up and staffed (page 11, line 23, column 1) should equal beds (page 13 line 2c, column 1). Inpatient days (page 11, line 25) should equal inpatient days (page 13, line 2e, column 1). Do not count beds more than once. Please list data under the appropriate service area only if a specific ward, wing, floor, or other unit has been designated exclusively for that service. For example, if pediatric inpatients are lodged in the same units as adults, separate bed and utilization data should not be reported for pediatric patients. If obstetric, rehabilitation, or other patients are placed in general medical and surgical units, no separate data for these service areas should be reported. Similarly, if alcoholism/drug abuse or dependency patients are treated in psychiatric inpatient units, utilization data for these patients should be included as part of the psychiatric unit.

If ACTUAL UTILIZATION DATA by unit cannot be readily obtained, please provide ESTIMATES for service area utilization.

BEDS SET UP AND STAFFED. The number of beds at the **end of the reporting period** that are staffed and ready for use.

1. **Medical/Surgical, Acute.** Provides acute care to patients in medical and surgical units on the basis of physicians' orders and approved nursing care plans.
2. **Pediatric, Acute.** Provides acute care to pediatric patients on the basis of physicians' orders and approved nursing care plans.
3. **Obstetric Care Unit.** Levels should be designated: (1) unit provides services for uncomplicated maternity and newborn cases; (2) unit provides services for uncomplicated cases, the majority of complicated problems, and special neonatal services; and (3) unit provides services for all serious illnesses and abnormalities and is supervised by a full time maternal/fetal specialist.
5. **Medical/Surgical Intensive Care.** Provides patient care of a more intensive nature than the usual medical and surgical care, on the basis of physicians' orders and approved nursing care plans. These units are staffed with specially trained nursing personnel and contain monitoring and specialized support equipment for patients who, because of shock, trauma, or other life-threatening conditions, require intensified, comprehensive observation and care. Includes mixed intensive care units.
6. **Cardiac Intensive Care.** Provides patient care of a more specialized nature than the usual medical and surgical care, on the basis of physicians' orders and approved nursing care plans. The unit is staffed with specially trained nursing personnel and contains monitoring and specialized support or treatment equipment for patients who, because of heart seizure, open-heart surgery, or other life-threatening conditions, require intensified, comprehensive observation and care. May include myocardial infarction, pulmonary care, and heart transplant units.
7. **Neonatal Intensive Care.** A unit that must be separate from the newborn nursery providing intensive care to all sick infants including those with the very lowest birth weights (less than 1500 grams). NICU has potential for providing mechanical ventilation, neonatal surgery and special care for the sickest infants born in the hospital or transferred from another institution. A full-time neonatologist serves as director of the NICU.
8. **Neonatal Intermediate Care.** A unit that must be separate from the normal newborn nursery and that provides intermediate and/or recovery care and some specialized services, including immediate resuscitation, intravenous therapy, and capacity for prolonged oxygen therapy and monitoring.
9. **Pediatric Intensive Care.** Provides care to pediatric patients that is of a more intensive nature than that usually provided to pediatric patients. The unit is staffed with specially trained personnel and contains monitoring and specialized support equipment for treatment of patients who, because of shock, trauma, or other life-threatening conditions, require intensified, comprehensive observation and care.
10. **Burn Care.** Provides care to severely burned patients. Severely burned patients are those with any of the following: 1) second-degree burns of more than 25% total body surface area for adults or 20% total body surface area for children; 2) third-degree burns of more than 10% total body surface area; 3) any severe burns of the hands, face, eyes, ears, or feet; or 4) all inhalation injuries, electrical burns, complicated burn injuries involving fractures and other major traumas, and all other poor risk factors.
11. **Other Special Care.** Provides care to patients requiring care more intensive than that provided in the acute area, yet not sufficiently intensive to require admission to an intensive care unit. Patients admitted to this area are usually transferred here from an intensive care unit once their condition has improved. These units are sometimes referred to as definitive observation, step-down, or progressive care units.
13. **Rehabilitation.** Provides care encompassing a comprehensive array of restoration services for the disabled and all support services necessary to help patients attain their maximum functional capacity.
14. **Chronic Disease.** Provides medical and skilled nursing care to patients with long term illnesses who are not in the acute phase, but who require an intensity of services not available in nursing homes.
15. **Hospice.** Provides palliative care, chiefly medical relief of pain, and supportive services for terminally ill patients and their families.
16. **Psychiatric Care.** Provides acute or long term care to emotionally disturbed patients, including patients admitted for diagnosis and those admitted for treatment of psychiatric problems, on the basis of physicians' orders and approved nursing care plans. Long term care may include intensive supervision to the chronically mentally ill, mentally disordered, or other mentally incompetent persons.
17. **Alcoholism/Drug Abuse or Dependency Care.** Provides diagnosis and therapeutic services to patients with alcoholism or other drug dependencies. Includes care for inpatient/residential treatment for patients whose course of treatment involves more intensive care than provided in an outpatient setting or where patient requires supervised withdrawal.
18. **Mental Retardation.** Provides on a regular basis, health-related care and services to patients with psychiatric or developmental impairment who do not require the degree of care or treatment that a skilled nursing unit is designed to provide.
19. **Skilled Nursing Care.** Provides non-acute medical and nursing care services, therapy and social services under the supervision of a licensed registered nurse on a 24-hour basis.
20. **Intermediate Care.** Provides health-related services (nursing care and social services) to residents with a variety of physical conditions or functional disabilities. These residents do not require the care provided by a hospital or skilled nursing facility, but do need supervision and supportive services.
21. **Residential Care/Elderly Housing.** The provision of residential services for those who do not require daily medical or nursing services, but may require some assistance in the activities of daily living. Includes sheltered care facilities for developmentally disabled or long term psychiatric patients as well as elderly housing.
24. **Swing Beds.** A licensed acute care bed that has been designated by a hospital to provide either acute or long-term care services. The beds should meet the following conditions under section 1883,b1 of the Social Security Act.
    1) A hospital must be located in a "rural" area.
    2) A hospital must have less than 100 acute care beds.
    3) When applicable, a hospital must receive a certificate-of-need (CON) for the provision of long-term services from its state health planning and development agency.

E. TOTAL FACILITY BEDS AND UTILIZATION

Inpatient days and beds reported on this page should be consistant with these items as reported on page 11.

1. **BED CHANGES** (for all facility beds excluding newborn nursery bassinets)

   a. Was there a permanent or significant temporary change in the total number of beds set up and staffed for use during the reporting period? ....YES ☐ NO ☐

   b. If YES, please provide the following information on changes:

	(+ or −) Number of Beds	Date of Change Month/Day/Year
(1) 1st Change		/ /
(2) 2nd Change		/ /

(Please list additional changes on page 34)

2. **BEDS AND UTILIZATION** (exclude newborn nursery, include neonatal, intensive and intermediate care units):

   a. Does your hospital maintain a separate nursing home type of long–term care unit/facility? (Please refer to the instructions and definitions on page 14.) ....YES ☐ NO ☐

If NO, report total facility statistics only in column (1) below. **If YES, report data for all three columns**

***Because of unit transfers, column (1) may be less than the sum of columns (2) and (3)**

	(1) Total Facility	(2) Hospital	(3) Nursing Home-Type Unit/Facility
b. Licensed bed capacity. The maximum number of beds authorized by state licensing (certifying) agency. If state does not regulate number, please report "NONE"			
c. Beds set up and staffed for use at the end of the reporting period (include neonatal & swing beds) (should match bed total on page 11 line 23.)			
d. Admissions (exclude newborns, include neonatal & swing admissions)*			
e. Inpatient days (exclude newborns, include neonatal & swing days) (should match TOTAL FACILITY inpatient day total on page 11, line 25)			
f. Discharges (exclude newborns, include neonatal, swing discharges & deaths)*			
g. Discharge days (exclude newborns, include neonatal, swing days & deaths)			
h. Census (number of inpatients occupying beds on the last day of reporting period. Exclude newborn, include neonatal.)			

3. **MEDICARE/MEDICAID UTILIZATION** (excl. newborns, incl. neonatal & swing)

	(1)	(2)	(3)
a. Total Medicare (Title XVIII) inpatient discharges*			
b. Total Medicare (Title XVIII) inpatient days			
c. Total Medicaid (Title XIX) inpatient discharges*			
d. Total Medicaid (Title XIX) inpatient days			

4. **NEWBORN NURSERY**

   a. Number of bassinets set up and staffed for use at the end of the reporting period (exclude pediatric and neonatal beds listed on page 11) .... ______

   b. Total births (exclude fetal deaths) .... ______

   c. Newborn days (exclude neonatal listed on page 11) .... ______

5. **SURGICAL OPERATIONS** (whether major or minor.)

   a. Inpatient .... ______

   b. Outpatient .... ______

   c. Total .... ______

6. **OUTPATIENT VISITS** (Please report outpatient visits as defined on page 14 and not occasions of service.) **Visits**

   a. Emergency .... ______

   b. Other (all nonemergency visits including physician referrals and outpatient surgeries) .... ______

   c. Total .... ______

SECTION E
TOTAL FACILITY BEDS AND UTILIZATION
Instructions and Definitions

1. a. A significant temporary change occurs when beds are temporarily out of use and not included in the bed count; it is not considered a permanent change. Report in a six-digit number, the date(s) when bed change(s) occurred; for example, January 7, 1990, should be shown as 01/07/90. If there have been more than two changes during the reporting period, please report all additional changes as supplemental information on page 34.

2. a. Information pertaining to nursing home type units/facilities that provide non-acute medical and nursing services and are owned and operated by the hospital should be included if the following conditions are met:

(1) Hospital and nursing home-type unit/facility are governed by a common governing board.

(2) Only one legal entity may be vested with title to the physical property or operate under the authority of a duly executed lease of the physical property.

If above criteria are not met, no information related to a nursing home type unit/facility should appear on the questionnaire.

For purposes of this survey, nursing home-type unit is a unit/facility that offers primarily only the following type of services to the majority of all admissions:

Skilled Nursing, Intermediate Care, Residential Care/Elderly housing, or Mental Retardation. See page 12 for the definitions describing these care services.

b-h. All hospitals should fill out column 1, TOTAL FACILITY statistics. A combination facility that includes a hospital and nursing home-type unit/facility should give breakdowns for these units in columns 2 and 3. Include unit transfers in admission and discharge counts for a unit/facility; exclude unit/facility transfers in admissions and discharges reported for the total facility.

c. Report the number of beds regularly available (those set up and staffed for use) at the end of the reporting period. Report only operating beds, not constructed bed capacity. Include all bed facilities that are set up and staffed for use by inpatients who have no other bed facilities, such as pediatric bassinets, isolation units, quiet rooms, and reception and observation units assigned to or reserved for them. Exclude newborn bassinets and bed facilities for patients receiving special procedures for a portion of their stay and who have other bed facilities assigned to or reserved for them. Exclude, for example, labor room, postanesthesia, or postoperative recovery room beds, psychiatric holding beds, and beds that are used only as holding facilities for patients prior to their transfer to another hospital. Any difference between total beds reported in 1990 versus 1989 should be accounted for in E1b.

d. Include the number of adult and pediatric admissions only (exclude births). This figure should include all patients admitted during the reporting period. The sum of admissions for the units can be greater than the total reported for the entire facility because of unit transfers.

e. Report the number of adult and pediatric days of care rendered during the entire reporting period. Do not include days of care rendered for normal infants born in the hospital, but do include those for their mothers. Include days of care for infants born in the hospital and transferred into a neonatal care unit. Inpatient day of care (also commonly referred to as a **patient day** or a **census day,** or by some federal hospitals as an **occupied bed day)** is a period of service between the census-taking hours on two successive calendar days, the day of discharge being counted only when the patient was admitted the same day. For interward transfers between the hospital and nursing home unit/facility, report inpatient days only for the time spent in each unit/facility.

f. Report the number of adult and pediatric discharges only (exclude newborns). This figure should include all patients discharged during the reporting period. The sum of discharges for the units can be greater than the total reported for the entire facility because of unit transfers.

g. Report the total number of patient days of care rendered to patients discharged during the reporting period; include days of care rendered to those patients prior to the beginning of the reporting period. Do not report discharge days for patients transferred between the hospital and nursing home unit/facility, except for those patients discharged from the institution following transfer. In this case, report discharge days for both units according to the days of care rendered in each unit.

4. a. Record the number of normal newborn bassinets. DO NOT include neonatal intensive or intermediate care bassinets. These should be reported on page 11, D7 and D8 and on page 13, E2b and c.

c. Report the number of inpatient days for normal newborn nursery. DO NOT include neonatal intensive or intermediate care inpatient days as these should be reported on page 11, D7 and D8 and on page 13, E2e.

5. Count each patient undergoing surgery as one surgical operation regardless of the number of surgical procedures that were performed while the patient was in the operating or procedure room. For outpatient surgical operations, please record operations performed on patients who do not remain in the hospital overnight. Include all operations whether performed in the inpatient operating rooms or in procedure rooms located in an outpatient facility. Include an endoscopy only when used as an operative tool and not when used for diagnosis alone.

6. An outpatient visit is a visit to each emergency or nonemergency outpatient service area by a person who is not lodged in the hospital overnight while receiving medical, dental or other health related services. Include in the visit count each appearance of an outpatient in each emergency or nonemergency outpatient service area. (Report visits, not the number of diagnostic and/or therapeutic **treatments** the patient received in the ancillary departments.)

a. Emergency visits should reflect total number of patients seen in an emergency unit.

b. Other visits should reflect the number of scheduled or unscheduled visits to outpatient service areas other than the emergency room. Include physician referrals and outpatient surgeries. DO NOT INCLUDE OCCASIONS OF SERVICE (Note: an occasion of service is each test, examination, treatment, or procedure rendered to an outpatient in ancillary departments. For example: one other visit would be an outpatient receiving a blood test and an X-ray during a single appearance in the ancillary service area.

c. Compare the total outpatient visits with those that were reported last year and explain major differences (more than 50%). Use page 34 if explanation is lengthy.

F. FINANCIAL DATA

For reporting period only, as stated on page 3 of this survey. If final figures are not available, please estimate. Round to the nearest dollar.

1. STATEMENT OF REVENUES AND EXPENSES OF GENERAL FUNDS	All hospitals fill out column (1) (1) Total Facility	Only hospitals with separate units for nursing home type of long term care should fill out columns (2) & (3) (2) Hospital	(3) Nursing Home Type Unit/Facility
a. NET PATIENT SERVICE REVENUE**	.00	.00	.00
b. OTHER REVENUE**			
(1) Tax appropriations	.00	.00	
(2) Other (including operating gains)	.00	.00	
(3) TOTAL OTHER REVENUE [1b(1) + 1b(2)]	.00	.00	
c. TOTAL REVENUE** [1a + 1b(3)]	.00	.00	.00
d. PAYROLL EXPENSES			
(1) Medical & dental residents/interns and trainees	.00	.00	
(2) All other personnel	.00	.00	
(3) TOTAL PAYROLL EXPENSES [1d(1) + 1d(2)]	.00	.00	.00
e. NONPAYROLL EXPENSES			
(1) Employee benefits	.00	.00	
(2) Professional fees	.00	.00	
(3) Depreciation expense (for reporting period only)	.00	.00	
(4) Interest expense	.00	.00	
(5) Bad debt expense	.00	.00	
(6) All other operating expenses (including operating losses)	.00	.00	
(7) TOTAL NONPAYROLL EXPENSES (add 1e(1) thru 1e(6))	.00	.00	.00
f. TOTAL EXPENSES [1d(3) + 1e(7)]	.00	.00	.00
g. NONOPERATING GAINS**			
(1) Investment income	.00	.00	
(2) Other nonoperating gains (including extraordinary gains)	.00	.00	
(3) TOTAL NONOPERATING GAINS	.00	.00	.00
h. NONOPERATING LOSSES (including extraordinary losses)	.00	.00	.00
i. NET INCOME** (Revenue and gains in excess of expenses and losses) [(1c + 1g(3)) − (1f + 1h)]	.00	.00	.00

2. DETAIL OF PATIENT SERVICE REVENUE** (based on full established rates; include charity care in gross revenue)	(1)	(2)	(3)
a. GROSS REVENUE from service to INPATIENTS	.00	.00	
b. GROSS REVENUE from service to OUTPATIENTS	.00	.00	
c. TOTAL GROSS REVENUE from service to PATIENTS (2a + 2b)	.00	.00	.00
d. DEDUCTIONS FROM REVENUE			
(1) Medicare contractual adjustments	.00	.00	
(2) Medicaid contractual adjustments	.00	.00	
(3) Other governmental contractual adjustments	.00	.00	
(4) Self-pay adjustments	.00	.00	
(5) Third party payor contractual adjustments (include Blue Cross)	.00	.00	
(6) Other nongovernment contractual adjustments	.00	.00	
(7) Charity (revenue forgone at full established rates)	.00	.00	
(8) Total deductions [add 2d(1) thru 2d(7)]	.00	.00	.00
e. NET PATIENT SERVICE REVENUE [2c − 2d(8)] (should agree to line 1a.)	.00	.00	.00

This data will be treated as confidential and will not be released without written permission from the hospital.

SECTION F
FINANCIAL DATA
Instructions and Definitions

All financial data questions are based on the AICPA **Audits of Providers of Health Care Services** (July 1990). If final figures are not available, please estimate. Do not use "NA" to designate "not applicable"; enter "0" wherever appropriate.

All hospitals should fill out column 1. "Total Facility Statistics." A combination facility that includes a nursing home-type facility meeting the conditions outlined in the instructions for Section E.2.a. should give breakdowns for these units in columns (2) and (3).

1. STATEMENT OF REVENUES AND EXPENSES OF GENERAL FUNDS

General funds. Funds that are used to account for resources not restricted for identified purposes by donors and grantors. They account for all resources and obligations not recorded in donor restricted funds, including assets whose use is limited, agency funds, and property and equipment related to the general operations of the entity.

Activities associated with the provision of health care services constitute the ongoing major or central operations of providers of health care services. Revenue, expenses, gains and losses arising from those activities are classified as "operating." Gains and losses from transactions that are peripheral or incidental to the provision of health care services and from other events stemming from the environment that may be largely beyond the control of the entity and its management are classified as "nonoperating." The classification of items as revenue or gain and expense or loss depends on the individual health care provider. The same transaction may result in revenue to one hospital and gain to another.

Therefore, classify and report revenue, expenses, gains and losses on the appropriate survey line in a manner consistent with your hospital's financial statements prepared under the basis of generally accepted accounting principles. However, since no separate line items have been provided for operating gains and losses, include these in "other revenue" (1b(2)) and in "all other operating expenses" (1e(6)) respectively.

a. **Net patient service revenue.** Reported at the estimated net realizable amounts from patients, third party payors, and others for services rendered, including estimated retroactive adjustments under reimbursement agreements with third-party payors. Retroactive adjustments are accrued on an estimated basis in the period the related services are rendered and adjusted in future periods as final settlements are determined.

b. **Other revenue.** Revenue from services other than health care provided to patients, as well as sales and services to nonpatients. Revenue which arises from the normal day-to-day operations from services other than health care provided to patients. Includes sales and services to nonpatients, and revenue from miscellaneous sources (rental of hospital space, sale of cafeteria meals, gift shop sales) Also include operating gains in this category.

d(1) **Medical and dental residents/interns and trainees.** Salaries for professional personnel in training such as medical and dental residents/interns, and all technical trainees in medical technology, x-ray, therapy, laboratory, etc. Include persons who have not completed the necessary requirements for certification or met the qualifications required for full salary under the related title: Note; the salaries listed for residents/interns should correspond to personnel reported in Section G. (page 21, G1b(2) or b(4)) or total other trainees (page 23. G2).

e(1) **Employee benefits.** Includes social security, group insurance, retirement benefits, workman's compensation, unemployment insurance, etc.

e(2) **Professional fees.** Fees paid to physicians for patient care and supervisory activities and non-medical professional fees such as legal, auditing and consulting.

e(5) **Bad debt-expense.** The provision for actual or expected uncollectibles resulting from the extension of credit.

e(6) **All other operating expenses.** Include expenses for supplies, expenses for purchased services, utilities, income taxes, operating losses and any other expenses not included in the above categories.

2. DETAIL OF PATIENT SERVICE REVENUE

d. **Contractual adjustments.** Differences between revenue at established rates and amounts realized from third-party payors under contractual agreements.

d.(7) **Charity care.** Health services that were never expected to result in cash inflows. Charity care results from a provider's policy to provide health care services free of charge to individuals who met certain financial criteria. For purposes of this survey, charity care is measured on the basis of revenue forgone, at full established rates.

F. FINANCIAL DATA (Continued)

3. SOURCES OF PATIENT SERVICE REVENUE**	Total Facility Gross	Total Facility Net
a. GOVERNMENT		
(1) Medicare	.00	.00
(2) Medicaid	.00	.00
(3) Other (please specify: ______)	.00	.00
(4) Total government sources	.00	.00
b. NONGOVERNMENT		
(1) Self-pay	.00	.00
(2) Third party payors (include Blue Cross)	.00	.00
(3) Other (please specify: ______)	.00	.00
(4) Total nongovernment sources	.00	.00
c. TOTAL GROSS REVENUE from service to PATIENTS [3a(4) + 3b(4)] (total should agree with line 2c for gross & 2e for net on page 15)	.00	.00

4. BALANCE SHEET - GENERAL FUNDS**		
a. ASSETS		
(1) Current assets		
(a) Cash and cash equivalents	.00	
(b) Net patient accounts receivable	.00	
(c) Other accounts receivable	.00	
(d) Other current assets	.00	
(e) Total current assets (sum of above 4 lines)		.00
(2) Noncurrent assets whose use is limited		.00
(3) Property and equipment		
(a) Gross property and equipment	.00	
(b) Less: Accumulated depreciation	.00	
(c) Net property and equipment		.00
(4) Other assets		.00
(5) Total assets [4a(1)(e) + 4a(2) + 4a(3)(c) + 4a(4)]		.00
b. LIABILITIES AND FUND BALANCE		
(1) Current liabilities		.00
(2) Long-term debt		.00
(3) Other noncurrent liabilities		.00
(4) Fund balance		.00
(5) Total liabilities and fund balance [should agree to line 4a(5)]		.00

5. OTHER FUND BALANCES**	
a. DONOR RESTRICTED FUNDS (report fund balances only)	
(1) Specific purpose	.00
(2) Plant replacement and expansion	.00
(3) Endowment funds	.00
b. FOUNDATION (report total of general and restricted fund balances)	.00

6. CHANGES IN GENERAL FUND BALANCE**	
a. FUND BALANCE at beginning of year	.00
b. ADDITIONS	
(1) Net income (from line 1i on page 15 if positive, report 0 if value is negative)	.00
(2) Other (please specify: ______)	.00
(3) Total	.00
c. DEDUCTIONS (no negative amounts)	
(1) Net loss (absolute value of line 1i on page 15 if negative, report 0 if value is positive)	.00
(2) Other (please specify: ______)	.00
(3) Total	.00
d. FUND BALANCE at end of year [should agree to line 4b(4)]	.00

****This data will be treated as confidential and will not be released without written permission from the hospital.**

4. BALANCE SHEET - GENERAL FUNDS

The AICPA Guide allows both disaggregated (funds are layered) and aggregated (funds are combined) balance sheets. This survey utilizes the disaggregated, layered approach whereby several funds are reported in self-balancing layers. The two major divisions of the layered balance sheet are labeled "general" (or "unrestricted") and "restricted." Only the general funds should be reported in this section of the survey.

If your hospital prepares an aggregated balance sheet and combines all of its funds into a single non-layered balance sheet, the restricted funds must be separated (usually from assets whose use is limited) and reported in section 5 "Other Fund Balances" in order to conform to the format of this survey.

This section is most easily prepared by direct reference to your hospital's financial statements.

a.(1c) **Other accounts receivable.** Include estimated third party payor settlements, due from other funds, related party receivables, employee receivables, etc.

a.(1d) **Other current assets.** May include the current portion (i.e., required for current liabilities) of assets whose use is limited, prepaid expenses, supplies inventory, short-term investments.

a.(1e) **Total current assets.** This amount should agree to total current assets per your financial statements.

a.(2) **Noncurrent assets whose use is limited.** The noncurrent portion of general fund assets 1) set aside by the governing board for identified purposes (also referred to as board-designated assets) 2) proceeds of debt issues and funds of the health care entity deposited with a trustee and limited to use in accordance with the requirements of an indenture or a similar agreement and 3) other assets limited to use for identified purposes through an agreement between the health care entity and outside party other than a donor or grantor (includes assets set aside under a self-insurance funding arrangement and assets set aside under agreements with third-party payors to meet depreciation funding requirements.)

a.(3a) **Gross property and equipment.** Include land, buildings, and equipment. Include actual or estimated value of property/equipment that is leased.

a.(3b) **Accumulated depreciation.** Depreciation accumulated over the years including the depreciation applicable to the current year.

a.(3c) **Net property and equipment.** Gross property and equipment less accumulated depreciation.

a.(4) **Other assets.** May include deferred financing costs/unamortized bond issue costs, investment in affiliated company/partnership, deferred third party reimbursement, deferred pension expense, deferred pension asset, long-term receivables.

b.(1) **Current liabilities.** May include accounts payable, accrued expenses, current portion of long-term debt, borrowings under line of credit, estimated third-party settlements, advances from third party payors due to donor-restricted funds, accrued interest payable, unexpended grants/gifts/income, accrued payroll and related liabilities. This amount should agree to "total current liabilities" per your financial statements.

b.(2) **Long-term debt.** May include revenue and other bonds, mortgages payable, notes payable loans/contracts payable.

b.(3) **Other noncurrent liabilities.** May include estimated malpractice/self insurance costs, deferred compensation payable, deferred third-party reimbursement, accrued pension/deferred pension liability.

b.(4) **Fund balance.** The excess of assets over liabilities (net equity). An excess of liabilities is reflected as a deficit.

5. OTHER FUND BALANCES

Report fund balances only.

a. **Donor-restricted funds.** Funds restricted for specific purposes by donors and grantors--for example, endowment funds or funds restricted to plant replacement and expansion.

a.(1) **Specific purpose funds.** Funds restricted for a specific purpose or project. Board-designated funds do not constitute specific purpose funds.

a.(3) **Endowment funds.** Funds for which a donor has stipulated, as a condition of a gift, that the principal of the fund is to be maintained inviolate and in perpetuity and that only income may be expended.

b. **Foundation.** An organization that is 1) under the control of (or common control with) the hospital (but not consolidated or combined with the hospital) and 2) solicits funds solely for the benefit of the hospital.

F. FINANCIAL DATA (Continued)

7. CAPITAL ACCOUNTS**

Include capitalized leases in the appropriate category, for example, a building under capital lease should be included in "Buildings and improvements". Record lines (1) to (5) as historical costs.

Long-term debt which has been refinanced should be shown as both an addition and a retirement. Include capital lease obligations in long-term debt.

	(1) Balance at Beginning of Year	(2) Additions and Transfers-in	(3) Retirements, Disposals and Transfers-out	(1) + (2) − (3) Balance at End of Year
a. ACCOUNTS				
(1) Land	.00	.00	.00	.00
(2) Buildings and improvements	.00	.00	.00	.00
(3) Equipment	.00	.00	.00	.00
(4) Construction in progress	.00	.00	.00	.00
(5) Total cost [balance at end of year should agree to line 4a(3)(a) on page 17]	.00			.00
b. Less: Accumulated Depreciation [balance at end of year should agree to line 4a(3)(b) on page 17]	.00			.00
c. NET BOOK VALUE [balance at end of year should agree to line 4a(3)(c) on page 17]	.00			.00

	(1) Balance at Beginning of Year	(2) Additions	(3) Payments and Retirements	(1) + (2) − (3) Balance at End of Year
d. LONG-TERM DEBT [balance at end of year should agree to line 4b(2) on page 17]	.00	.00	.00	.00

This data will be treated as confidential and will not be released without written permission from the hospital.

7. CAPITAL ACCOUNTS

This section captures some of the detail and activity of the property and equipment and long-term debt sections of the general fund balance sheet.

a. (1) **Land.** Include all land and nondepreciable improvements.

(2) **Buildings and improvements.** Include land improvements, if depreciable.

(3) **Equipment.** Includes all fixed and movable equipment.

(4) **Construction in progress.** Include costs incurred for uncompleted buildings and equipment (i.e., depreciation has not commenced). Amounts for completed construction projects should be transfered-out of the construction in progress account to the appropriate asset account.

G. PERSONNEL ON PAYROLL AS OF SEPTEMBER 30, 1990

1. HOSPITAL PERSONNEL BY OCCUPATIONAL CATEGORY

Report full-time and part-time personnel including trainees who were on the payroll as of SEPTEMBER 30, 1990 and whose payroll expenses are reported in F1d. If full-time and part-time are not available, please report full-time equivalent (FTE) personnel in column (1) and zero in column (2). For those hospitals that operate a nursing home-type unit/facility as reported in E2a, DO NOT INCLUDE NURSING HOME STAFF HERE. If there are staff positions that are shared between the hospital and nursing home-type unit/facility, please record these staff as part-time employees in each area. This means that one full-time employee would be counted as a part-time employee under the appropriate hospital occupational category and also as one part-time employee in total nursing home personnel. Include members of religious orders for whom dollar equivalents were reported.

	(1) Full-Time (35 hr/wk or more) On Payroll	(2) Part-Time (less than 33 hr/wk) On Payroll
a. Administration:		
(1) Administrator and assistant administrators	______	______
b. Physician and dental services:		
(1) Physicians	______	______
(2) Medical residents/interns	______	______
(3) Dentists	______	______
(4) Dental residents/interns	______	______
c. Nursing services:		
(1) Registered nurses	______	______
(2) Licensed practical (vocational) nurses	______	______
(3) Ancillary nursing personnel	______	______
d. Physician's assistants	______	______
e. Nurse practitioners	______	______
f. Medical record services:		
(1) Medical record administrators	______	______
(2) Medical record technicians	______	______
g. Pharmacy:		
(1) Pharmacists, licensed	______	______
(2) Pharmacy technicians	______	______
h. Clinical laboratory services:		
(1) Medical technologists	______	______
(2) Other laboratory personnel	______	______
i. Dietary services:		
(1) Dietitians	______	______
(2) Dietetic technicians	______	______
j. Radiological services:		
(1) Radiographers (radiologic technologists)	______	______
(2) Radiation therapy technologists	______	______
(3) Nuclear medicine technologists	______	______
(4) Other radiologic personnel	______	______

SECTION G
PERSONNEL ON PAYROLL AS OF SEPTEMBER 30, 1990
Instructions and Definitions

Report the number of full-time and part-time personnel in the categories specified and as defined below who were on the hospital payroll as of September 30, 1990, EVEN IF YOUR REPORTING PERIOD ENDED ON A DIFFERENT DATE. Exclude private-duty nurses, volunteers, and all personnel whose salary is financed entirely by outside research grants. Personnel who work in more than one area should be included only in the category of their primary responsibility and should be counted only once. Include trainees if on the hospital payroll as of September 30, 1990. Include members of religious orders for whom dollar equivalents were reported.

Full-time personnel. Persons whose regularly scheduled work-week is 35 hours or more.

Part-time personnel. Persons whose regularly scheduled work-week is less than 35 hours.

1 b. Include only those physicians and dentists engaged in clinical practice and on the payroll. Those who hold administrative positions should be reported under "Administration" (G1a). Exclude physicians and dentists who are paid on a fee basis.

OCCUPATIONAL DEFINITIONS - HOSPITAL PERSONNEL BY OCCUPATIONAL CATEGORY

1 a.(1) **Administrator and assistant administrators.** The top level position in the facility, the person in charge of policy development, activity coordination, procedural development, and planning of the institution. Also includes persons who work under the supervision of the facility administrator as department administration assistants for the areas of finance, organization, personnel, purchasing, accounting, and voluntary services.

c.(1) **Registered nurses.** Nurses who have graduated from approved schools of nursing and who are currently registered by a state. They are responsible for the nature and quality of all nursing care that patients receive. Do not include any registered nurses more appropriately reported in other occupational categories, such as facility administrators.

c.(2) **Licensed practical or vocational nurses.** Nurses who have graduated from an approved school of practical (vocational) nursing who work under the supervision of registered nurses and/or physicians.

c.(3) **Ancillary personnel.** Persons who assist the nursing staff by performing routine duties in caring for patients under the direct supervision of a nurse, including nursing aides, orderlies, attendants, operating room technicians, and so forth.

d. **Physician's assistants.** Persons who provide health care services customarily performed by a physician under responsible supervision of that qualified licensed physician and who have successfully completed an accredited education program for physician's assistants that is approved by the Committee on Allied Health Education and Accreditation or other recognized accrediting agencies or who have been certified, licensed, or registered by recognized agencies or commissions.

e. **Nurse practitioners.** Registered nurses who have successfully completed a formal program of study designed to prepare registered nurses to provide primary health care through diagnosis, clinical judgment, and management abilities to restore, maintain, and improve the health status of patients.

f.(1) **Medical record administrators (medical record librarians).** Persons who plan, design, develop, and manage systems of patient information, administrative and clinical statistical data, and patient medical records.

f.(2) **Medical record technicians.** Persons who assist the medical record administrator and perform the technical tasks associated with the maintenance and use of medical records.

g.(1) **Pharmacists, licensed.** Persons licensed within the state who are concerned with the preparation and distribution of medicinal products.

g.(2) **Pharmacy technicians.** Persons who assist the pharmacist with selected activities, including medication profile reviews for drug incompatibilities, typing labels and prescription packaging, handling of purchase records, and inventory control.

h.(1) **Medical technologists (biochemistry technologist, blood technologist, microbiology technologist).** Persons who perform a wide range of complex and specialized procedures in all general areas of the clinical laboratory, making independent and correlated judgments and working in conjunction with pathologists, physicians, and qualified scientists. They may supervise and/or teach laboratory personnel.

h.(2) **Other clinical laboratory personnel.** Other laboratory personnel performing specified tasks requiring special training or experience. This includes medical laboratory scientists, cytotechnologists, histologic technicians, medical laboratory technicians, certified laboratory assistants, and other laboratory personnel performing specified tasks requiring special training or experience.

i.(1) **Dietitians.** Persons who apply the principles of nutrition and management in administering institutional food service programs, planning special diets at the physician's request, and instructing individuals and groups in the application of nutrition principles to the selection of food.

i.(2) **Dietetic technicians.** Persons who function as service personnel in the nutritional care of patients in health care facilities, assist with the planning, implementation, and evaluation of food programs, and work with both the food service supervisor and the dietitian.

j.(1) **Radiographers (radiologic technologists).** Persons who accurately demonstrate anatomical structures on a radiograph by applying knowledge of anatomy, positioning, and radiographic technique. They may maintain equipment, process film, keep patient records, and perform various office tasks. Radiographers must be graduates of at least a two-year educational program.

j.(2) **Radiation therapy technologists.** Persons who assist the radiologist in all aspects of radiation therapy treatment. They may expose specific areas of patient's body to prescribed doses of ionizing radiation and operate a variety of laboratory equipment, including high energy linear accelerators, radioactive isotopes, and particle generators. They must be graduates of a 12-month or 2-year program in radiation therapy.

j.(3) **Nuclear medicine technologists.** Persons who work under the supervision of a physician in administering and measuring radioactive nucleotides in diagnostic and therapeutic applications. They must be graduates of a 12-month or longer educational program in nuclear medicine technology.

j.(4) **Other radiologic personnel.** Persons with the following titles: ultrasound technologists/technicians, radiation monitors, health physics technicians, personnel monitors, radiation protectors, radiologic assistants, and x-ray assistants. Also included under this category are radiologic technicians, radiation therapy technicians, and nuclear medicine technicians. A technician is one who has not completed the educational requirements specified above for the technologist level of the respective occupational area.

G. PERSONNEL ON PAYROLL AS OF SEPTEMBER 30, 1990 (Continued)

	(1) Full-Time (35 hr/wk or more) On Payroll	(2) Part-Time (less than 35 hr/wk) On Payroll
k. Therapeutic services:		
(1) Occupational therapists	______	______
(2) Occupational therapy assistants and aides	______	______
(3) Physical therapists	______	______
(4) Physical therapy assistants and aides	______	______
(5) Recreational therapists	______	______
l. Speech and hearing services:		
(1) Speech pathologists	______	______
(2) Audiologists	______	______
m. Respiratory therapy services:		
(1) Respiratory therapists	______	______
(2) Respiratory therapy technicians	______	______
n. Psychologists	______	______
o. Social workers	______	______
p. All other health professional and technical personnel	______	______
q. All other personnel	______	______
r. Total hospital personnel (add 1a through 1q)	______	______

2. TRAINEES ON PAYROLL
Report full-time and part-time trainees who were on payroll and included in TOTAL HOSPITAL PERSONNEL (line G1r) or NURSING HOME PERSONNEL (line G3). Please do not include medical and dental residents and interns, who are listed on line G1b. Note that corresponding payroll expense for trainees should be listed on page 15.(line F1d.(1))

	Full-Time (35 hr/wk or more)	Part-Time (less than 35 hr/wk)
TOTAL OTHER TRAINEES (exclude medical and dental residents)	______	______

3. NURSING HOME PERSONNEL ON PAYROLL
Complete only if hospital has a separate nursing home-type unit/facility as reported on Page 13. (E.2a) Report full-time and part-time nursing home personnel who were on the payroll as of September 30, 1990. If personnel is shared with the hospital, report personnel as part-time employees here and on lines a-r.

	Full-Time (35 hr/wk or more)	Part-Time (less than 35 hr/wk)
a. Registered Nurses	______	______
b. Licensed practical (vocational) nurses	______	______
c. All other personnel	______	______
d. Total nursing home personnel (3a + 3b + 3c)	______	______

4. TOTAL FACILITY PERSONNEL ON PAYROLL
Report full-time and part-time hospital plus nursing home personnel who were on the payroll as of September 30, 1990. If no nursing home-type unit/facility is present, please zero fill nursing home personnel and carry down the total hospital personnel figures to these lines.

	Full-Time (35 hr/wk or more)	Part-Time (less than 35 hr/wk)
TOTAL FACILITY PERSONNEL (Hospital plus Nursing Home Unit/Facility)	______	______

5. 1990 TOTAL PAID MAN HOURS
Please report TOTAL PAID MAN-HOURS for all personnel who were on payroll during the current reporting year. Refer to top of page 3 for your hospitals reporting period. See definitions on page 24.

a. Medical and dental residents/interns and trainees Paid Man-hours (year's total hours).. ______

b. Total Personnel Paid Man-Hours (year's total hours)........... ______

G. PERSONNEL ON PAYROLL AS OF SEPTEMBER 30, 1990 (Continued)

1\. k.(1) **Occupational therapists.** Persons who evaluate the self-care, work, or leisure time and task performance skills of well and disabled patients of all age ranges. They plan and implement programs and social and interpersonal activities designed to restore, develop, and/or maintain the patient's ability to satisfactorily accomplish those daily living tasks required to his specific age and necessary to his particular occupational role adjustment.

k.(2) **Occupational therapy assistants.** Persons who work under the supervision of an occupational therapist in evaluating patients and planning and implementing programs and who are prepared to function independently when working with patients.

k.(2) **Occupational therapy aides (or attendants).** Persons who assist occupational therapists in administering medically oriented occupational programs to assist in rehabilitating patients in hospitals and similar institutions.

k.(3) **Physical therapists.** Therapists who use physical agents, biomechanical and neurophysiological principles, and assistive devices in relieving pain, restoring maximum function, and preventing disability following disease, injury, or loss of bodily part.

k.(4) **Physical therapy assistants and aides.** Persons who assist the physical therapist by assembling equipment, carrying out specified treatment programs, and helping with complex treatment procedures. Other duties include responsibility for the personal care of patients, safety precautions, and routine clerical and maintenance work.

k.(5) **Recreational therapists.** Persons who plan, organize, and direct medically approved recreation programs such as sports, trips, dramatics, and arts and crafts, either to help patients in recovery from illness or in coping with a temporary or permanent disability. In pediatric settings, may be classified as child-life workers.

l.(1) **Speech pathologists.** Persons who diagnose and evaluate speech and language abilities and plan, direct, and conduct rehabilitative treatment programs to restore or develop communication skills.

l.(2) **Audiologists.** Persons who assess type and degree of hearing impairment and participate in aural rehabilitation programs that meet the needs of the individual patient.

m.(1) **Respiratory therapists.** Persons who specialize in the application of scientific knowledge and theory to practical, clinical problems of respiratory care. Knowledge and skills for performing these functions are usually achieved through two or more years of academic and clinical responsibility for all respiratory care modalities, including responsibilities involved in supervision of respiratory technician functions.

m.(2) **Respiratory therapy technicians.** Persons who specialize in the technical details of general respiratory therapeutics. The knowledge and skills of the technician are usually acquired through formal education programs of at least one year in length. They may assume clinical responsibility for specified respiratory care modalities involving the application of well-defined therapeutic techniques under the direct or indirect supervision of a therapist or physician.

n. **Psychologists.** Persons with a doctoral degree in psychology from an American Psychological Association approved program in clinical psychology or a masters level psychologist who has obtained recognition of competency through the American Board of Examiners for professional psychology, state certification or licensing, or through endorsement by his or her state psychological association.

o. **Social workers.** Persons who have completed a formal program of study providing preparation to identify and understand the social and emotional factors underlying a patient's illness and to communicate these factors to the health team. They assist patients and their families in understanding and accepting the treatment necessary to maximize medical benefits and in their adjustments to permanent and temporary effects of illness. They utilize resources, such as family and community agencies, in assisting patients to recovery.

p. **All other health professional and technical personnel.** Persons not previously included who work in health occupations requiring special education and training to allow them to function in a health setting.

q. **All other personnel.** Persons not previously counted. These include accounting, data processing, secretarial, and clerical; kitchen, laundry, housekeeping, and maintenance personnel; and so forth.

2\. Report the total number of trainees who were on the payroll as of September 30, 1990, and who were included in TOTAL HOSPITAL PERSONNEL, line G1r. A trainee is a person who has not completed the necessary requirements for certification or met the qualifications required for full salary under the related title. Exclude medical and dental residents and interns, as they are reported separately in lines G1b(2) and G1b(4).

5\. Report total paid man-hours for the entire reporting period as indicated on top of survey page 3. Paid man-hours consist of worked man-hours and nonworked man-hours. Worked man-hours include regular hours worked, overtime hours worked, hours worked when on call or on standby, hours spent in in-service education, and so forth. Nonworked man-hours should include paid vacations, holidays, sick days, military leave, educational leave, bereavement or funeral leave, jury duty and so forth.

H. MEDICAL STAFF

Indicate number of practitioners on ACTIVE and ASSOCIATE (do not include courtesy, consulting, honorary, provisional, or other) medical staff in the following specialty groups as of September 30, 1990. Do not report full-time equivalents. For physicians certified by more than one board, please include only the primary certification. If exact numbers are unavailable, give your best estimates.

	Active and Associate Medical Staff	
	(1) Total (Include Board Certified)	(2) Board Certified
1. MEDICAL SPECIALTIES		
a. General & family practice	______	______
b. Internal medicine	______	______
c. Pediatrics	______	______
d. Cardiovascular disease	______	______
e. Gastroenterology	______	______
f. Oncology	______	______
g. Neurology	______	______
h. Other medical specialties	______	______
2. SURGICAL SPECIALTIES		
a. Obstetrics & gynecology	______	______
b. Ophthalmology	______	______
c. Orthopedic surgery	______	______
d. Plastic surgery	______	______
e. General surgery	______	______
f. Thoracic surgery	______	______
g. Other surgical specialties	______	______
3. OTHER		
a. Anesthesiology	______	______
b. Emergency medicine	______	______
c. Nuclear medicine	______	______
d. Pathology	______	______
e. Psychiatry	______	______
f. Physical medicine & rehabilitation	______	______
g. Radiology	______	______
h. Other specialties	______	______
4. TOTAL	______	______

5. Does your hospital have a contractual arrangement with a physician who serves in a paid capacity (i.e., medical director or vice president for medical affairs) as liaison between hospital management and the medical staff? . . . . . YES ☐ NO ☐

I. MEDICARE PROVIDER NUMBERS

The following information should pertain only to units within this facility that have received certification by the Health Care Financing Administration (HCFA). Please refer to your most recent Medicare cost report.

1. Please provide the Medicare provider number for your facility ______

2. If applicable, please indicate the Medicare subprovider number for each of the following designated distinct part unit service areas:

	Subprovider Number
a. Rehabilitation	______
b. Psychiatric	______
c. Hospice	______
d. Home care	______
e. Alcoholism and other chemical dependency	______
f. Swing bed SNF	______
g. Hospital-based SNF	______
h. Other (Specify service: ______)	______

SECTION H
MEDICAL STAFF
Definitions

Active and associate. JCAHO categories of medical staff. Exclude those physicians in the following medical staff categories: courtesy, consulting, honorary, provisional, or other. Include all active and associate staff who are board certified.

Board certified. Physicians who have passed an examination given by a medical specialty board and have been certified by that board as specialists. Do not include board-eligible physicians. For physicians certified by more than one board, please include only the primary certification board.

1. **Medical specialties**

   Pediatrics. Includes pediatrics, pediatric allergy, and pediatric cardiology.

   Other medical specialties. Includes pulmonary diseases, nephrology, allergy, and dermatology.

2. **Surgical specialties**

   Other surgical specialties. Includes neurological surgery, otolaryngology, colon and rectal surgery, urology, head and neck surgery, traumatic surgery and pediatric surgery.

3. **Other**

   Pathology. Includes anatomical and clinical pathology and forensic pathology.
   Psychiatry. Includes child psychiatry.
   Radiology. Includes diagnostic radiology and radiation oncology.
   Other specialties. Includes aerospace medicine, occupational medicine, general preventive medicine and public health.

SUPPLEMENTAL INFORMATION

Use this space or an additional sheet if more space is required, to elaborate on any of the information supplied on this survey. Refer to the response by page, section, and item name.

I understand that certain parts of the financial data provided may be released only under the terms and conditions described in Section F, which includes release to the respective state hospital association upon request. The state hospital association may not release this data without written permission from the hospital.

Date of Completion

Signature of Administrator

_____/_____/_____

____

Thank you for your cooperation in completing this survey. If there are any questions about your responses to this survey, who should be contacted?

Name (please print)	Title	(Area Code) Telephone Number
Name (please print)	Title	(Area Code) Telephone Number

(   )
Hospital's Main Fax Number

NOTE: PLEASE COPY THE INFORMATION FOR YOUR HOSPITAL FILE BEFORE RETURNING THE ORIGINAL FORM TO THE AMERICAN HOSPITAL ASSOCIATION. ALSO, PLEASE FORWARD A PHOTOCOPY OF THE COMPLETED QUESTIONNAIRE TO YOUR STATE HOSPITAL ASSOCIATION. THANK YOU.

Index

The index is designed to help readers locate specific data in the statistical tables. Both table numbers and page numbers are provided.

Table (Page)

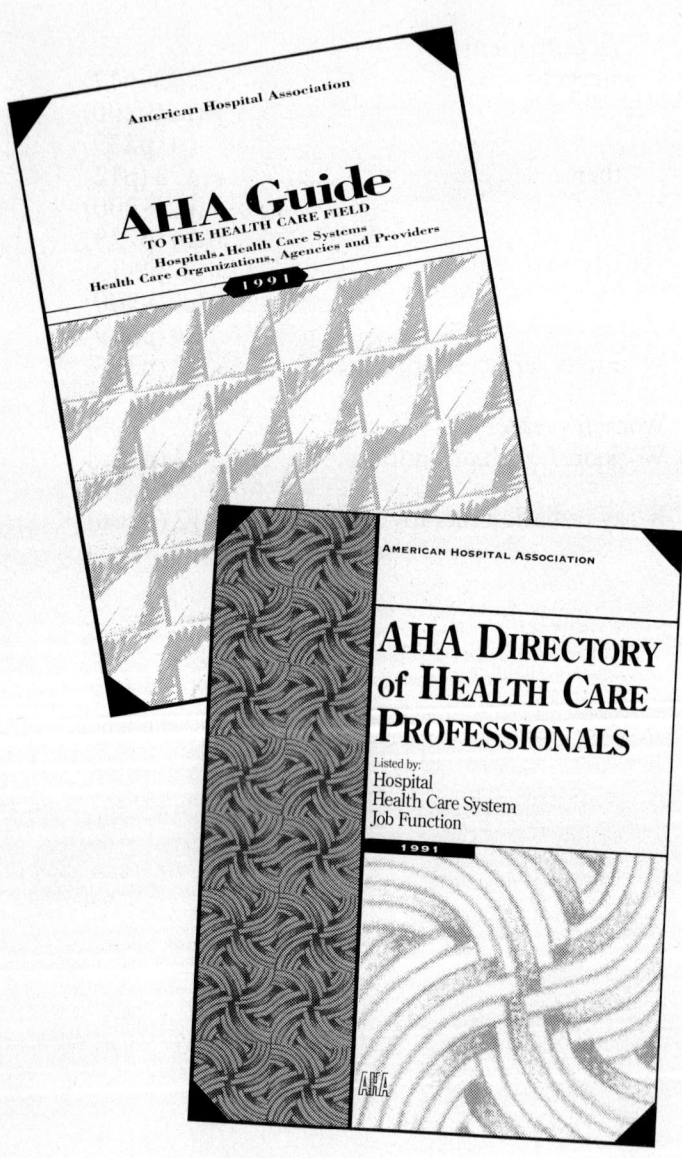

AHA Services, Inc.

Data Order Agreement

This order form can be used for obtaining AHA data products. Licensing terms and conditions on reverse.

Ordered by: Please print or type

Name Title

Organization

Address

City State Zip code

Telephone

The undersigned understands the conditions of the data agreements, as stated on the reverse side of this form, and agrees to abide by same. All orders must contain a signature that acknowledges acceptance of these conditions.

Signature of person placing order

Institution or associate member organization **Membership no.**

Ship to: Complete only if different from ordered by

Name Title

Organization

Address

City State Zip code

Please charge my ☐ **VISA** ☐ **MasterCard** ☐ **American Express**

Card no.

Cardholder's signature Expiration date

Purchase order no. **Date of order**

For billed order: Bill to attention of

Order Number	Title	Quantity	Institutional Member Price	Associate Member Price	Personal Member Price	Nonmember Price	Extended Price
G02-010091	1991 AHA Guide to the Health Care Field		$ 70	$ 70	$ 195	$ 195	
G02-011191	1991 AHA Guide to the Health Care Field Abridged Guide on Diskette (5¼" disks)		**	$1800	$2000	$2000	
G02-011291	1991 AHA Guide to the Health Care Field Abridged Guide on Diskette (3½" disks)		**	$1800	$2000	$2000	
G02-020091	1991 Directory of Health Care Professionals		$ 119	$ 119	$ 119	$ 289	
G02-082091	AHA Hospital Statistics 1991-92		$ 50	$ 50	$ 50	$ 125	
G02-084190	The National Hospital Panel Survey Report* (Printed version)		$ 150	$1350	$1500	$1500	
G02-084090	The National Hospital Panel Survey Report* (Diskette version with hardcopy reports)		**	$1620	$1800	$1800	

Telephone Orders
1-800-AHA-2626

FAX Orders:
312-280-6015

MasterCard, Visa, American Express or institutional/company purchase order number accepted. Telephone orders will usually be shipped within 48 hours.

Orders from individuals must be prepaid or charged to a credit card. Billed orders must be accompanied by a purchase order number.

Mail Orders

Mail all orders to:
AHA Services, Inc.
P.O. Box 92683
Chicago, IL 60675-2683

* **Note:** These data products are not returnable. Orders for these products cannot be processed prior to receipt of this signed Data Order Agreement.

** Please call for special discount price.

Foreign Orders
All foreign orders must be prepaid in U.S. funds only.

For surface mail: add 10% of merchandise price for shipping and handling. Delivery may take up to 8 weeks.

For airmail: add 20% of merchandise price for shipping and handling. Allow 4 weeks for delivery.

Sales tax:
Sales tax must be paid on orders shipped to CA, CO, GA, IL, MA, MO, NY, OH, and TX unless you provide us with a copy of your tax-exempt certificate.

Quantity discounts
Except where otherwise noted in the item description, quantity discounts are:

15%	11 to 50 copies
20%	51 to 100 copies
25%	101 to 1,000 copies

when shipped to one address.

Subtotal

Shipping and Handling

Sales Tax

Total
U.S. Funds Only

Shipping and handling charges apply to all domestic and Canadian orders

Up to $ 10.00	add $ 2.95
$10.01 to $ 20.00	add $ 4.95
$20.01 to $ 35.00	add $ 6.95
$35.01 to $ 50.00	add $ 7.95
$50.01 to $ 75.00	add $ 8.95
$75.01 to $100.00	add $10.95
$100.01 to $200.00	add $12.95
$200.01 to $300.00	add $14.95
$300.01 to $ 400.00	add $16.95
$400.01 to $ 500.00	add $18.95
$500.01 and above	add $27.50

American Hospital Association

AHA

Terms and Conditions

1. LICENSEE is granted a perpetual license to use the DATA at the site to which the DATA was shipped, in accordance with the Terms and Conditions of this Agreement.

2. LICENSEE acknowledges that the DATA is proprietary and confidential property of LICENSOR and constitutes valuable trade secret information and that LICENSEE acquires no right in the DATA except to use the DATA solely within its own organization and for its own business purposes, in accordance with this Agreement. Unless otherwise agreed upon in writing by AHA, LICENSEE agrees to hold the DATA in strict confidence and agrees not to provide, disclose, or otherwise make available any DATA to any third party, including but not limited to subsidiary and parent corporations, and that in no event shall LICENSEE release data which might reasonably be used to identify any particular institution without the prior express written permission of AHA and of such institution. Notwithstanding the foregoing, LICENSOR agrees that LICENSEE shall be permitted to disclose and extend use of such DATA to its employees, agents, and consultants whose assigned duties reasonably require such disclosure and use, and only to the extent necessary to enable such persons to reasonably perform their assigned duties. LICENSEE will take appropriate measures, by instruction, agreement or otherwise, to ensure compliance with this and the other provisions of this Agreement by LICENSEE, its employees, agents, and consultants. This provision shall survive the termination of this Agreement.

3. LICENSEE agrees not to use the DATA as a mailing source. LICENSEE agrees that if the DATA is supplied on magnetic tape, disk, or hard copy, no copies of the tape, disk, or hard copy report shall be made except that one copy may be made solely for back-up purposes.

4. LICENSOR acknowledges that LICENSEE may have contact with individual health care institutions which contribute to the DATA in the course of its normal business operation; however, LICENSEE agrees that it will not refer to the DATA during any such contact and will not contact such institutions regarding the DATA or information contained in the DATA. However, at LICENSEE's request and expense, LICENSOR will use its best efforts to clarify any questions LICENSEE may have with reference to the DATA.

5. LICENSEE recognizes that the DATA is collected by LICENSOR and while LICENSOR believes the DATA to be accurate, LICENSOR MAKES NO WARRANTIES OR REPRESENTATIONS, EXPRESS OR IMPLIED, INCLUDING, BUT NOT LIMITED TO, THE IMPLIED WARRANTY OF MERCHANTABILITY AND FITNESS FOR A PARTICULAR PURPOSE. In no event shall LICENSOR's liability for any damages, regardless of the form of action, exceed the fee paid by LICENSEE for use of the DATA. Under no circumstances shall LICENSOR be liable for incidental, consequential, special or exemplary damages of any kind or for lost profits.

6. Whenever LICENSOR has knowledge or reason to believe that LICENSEE has failed to observe the terms and conditions of this Agreement, LICENSOR will notify LICENSEE of the suspected breach. If, within 30 days of such notice, LICENSEE fails to make available for inspection by LICENSOR all records and documents of LICENSEE necessary to verify compliance, LICENSOR may terminate the license granted herein and prevent LICENSEE from obtaining future licenses from LICENSOR. Upon termination, LICENSEE shall immediately return all DATA to LICENSOR. This relief for breach shall in no way limit LICENSOR from pursuing whatever other relief it deems appropriate AND LICENSEE specifically agrees that in the event of a breach or threatened breach by LICENSEE, LICENSOR shall be entitled to an injunction restraining LICENSEE from further breaching action.

7. No waiver by LICENSOR of any breach on the part of LICENSEE or of any right or remedy incident thereto shall constitute a continuing waiver or a waiver of any breach or right or remedy incident thereto.

8. This agreement supercedes all prior agreements and understandings of any nature whatsoever, oral or written, and constitutes the entire understanding between the parties hereto.

9. Each paragraph and provision of this Agreement is severable from the entire Agreement, and if one provision shall be declared invalid, the other provisions shall remain in full force and effect without regard to the invalidity of said provision.

10. This Agreement may be modified only by a written instrument executed by both parties.

11. This Agreement shall be governed by the laws of the State of Illinois.